T0173102

'Any practitioner of Chinese medicine who wishes to expand their knowledge of paediatrics need not reach for other texts; Rebecca Avern thoroughly and thoughtfully presents the subject in exquisite detail. Every paediatric issue, including history, background, diagnosis and treatment, is analysed. A smart and sensitive exploration of childhood ailments for the 21st century.'
– *Dr Melanie Katin, DAMC, LAc, Faculty, Pacific College of Oriental Medicine, California, USA*

'Rebecca has an engaging, warm teaching style, which is reflected throughout this beautifully written book. It is thorough, clear and fully informed by her own learning and extensive experience. In short, it is an invaluable resource for students, teachers and practitioners of acupuncture who are interested in the treatment of children and adolescents, and I can see that the day will very soon come when we will all wonder how we ever managed without it!'
– *Julie Ann Reynolds, Joint Principal of the Acupuncture Academy, Leamington Spa, UK*

'This book is a delight. It is a wonderful resource for acupuncturists who deal with children, or indeed the parents of children. As well as being packed with wise advice about the causation and treatment of childhood illness, its descriptions of childhood illnesses are systematic, thorough and beautifully presented, and enriched throughout with case vignettes.'
– *Dr Clare Stephenson, MA(Cantab), BM BCh (Oxon),*
MSc (Public Health Medicine), LicAc (Licentiate in Acupuncture)

'The best book available on treating children! Rebecca runs a busy children's practice and, crucially, has two children of her own. It is clearly written, easy to read and you can dip into it to find an abundance of illustrations, tips and other gems.'
– *Angela and John Hicks, Co-Founders, College of Integrated Chinese Medicine, Reading, UK*

'In *Acupuncture for Babies, Children and Teenagers*, Rebecca Avern provides us with a comprehensive exploration of childhood and the treatment of common childhood conditions. The book stands out for its exploration of the psycho-emotional realm, the interpersonal skills needed to work with children of differing ages, and the integration of both traditional Chinese medicine patterns with Five Phase dynamics. For practitioners working with children, this source will be a valuable reference for common conditions and patterns, including acupuncture and *tui na* protocols to initiate care, and considerations regarding the child's experience and how to optimise interpersonal connections.'
– *David W. Miller, MD, FAAP, LAc, Dipl OM*

Acupuncture for Babies, Children and Teenagers

of related interest

The Art and Practice of Diagnosis in Chinese Medicine
Nigel Ching
Foreword by Jeremy Halpin
ISBN 978 1 84819 314 7
eISBN 978 0 85701 267 8

Returning to the Source
Han Dynasty Medical Classics in Modern Clinical Practice
Z'ev Rosenberg
Foreword by Dr Sabine Wilms
ISBN 978 1 84819 348 2
eISBN 978 0 85701 306 4

The Acupuncturist's Guide to Conventional Medicine, Second Edition
Clare Stephenson
ISBN 978 1 84819 302 4
eISBN 978 0 85701 255 5

The Fundamentals of Acupuncture
Nigel Ching
Foreword by Charles Buck
ISBN 978 1 84819 313 0
eISBN 978 0 85701 266 1

Intuitive Acupuncture
John Hamwee
ISBN 978 1 84819 273 7
eISBN 978 0 85701 220 3

The Acupuncture Points Functions Colouring Book
Rainy Hutchinson
Forewords by Richard Blackwell, and Angela Hicks and John Hicks
ISBN 978 1 84819 266 9
eISBN 978 0 85701 214 2

ACUPUNCTURE for BABIES, CHILDREN and TEENAGERS

TREATING BOTH THE ILLNESS AND THE CHILD

REBECCA AVERN

Illustrated by Sarah Hoyle

Foreword by Julian Scott

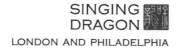

SINGING
DRAGON
LONDON AND PHILADELPHIA

First published in 2019
by Singing Dragon
an imprint of Jessica Kingsley Publishers
73 Collier Street
London N1 9BE, UK
and
400 Market Street, Suite 400
Philadelphia, PA 19106, USA

www.singingdragon.com

Library of Congress Cataloging in Publication Data
Names: Avern, Rebecca, author.
Title: Acupuncture for babies, children and teenagers : treating both the illness and the child / Rebecca Avern.
Description: London ; Philadelphia : Jessica Kingsley Publishers, 2018. | Includes bibliographical references and index.
Identifiers: LCCN 2017059752 (print) | LCCN 2017058215 (ebook) | ISBN 9780857012753 (ebook) | ISBN 9781848193222 (alk. paper)
Subjects: | MESH: Acupuncture Therapy | Medicine, Chinese Traditional | Child | Infant | Adolescent
Classification: LCC RJ53.A27 (print) | LCC RJ53.A27 (ebook) | NLM WB 369 | DDC 615.8/92083--dc23
LC record available at https://lccn.loc.gov/2017059752

British Library Cataloguing in Publication Data
A CIP catalogue record for this book is available from the British Library

ISBN 978 1 84819 322 2
eISBN 978 0 85701 275 3

Printed and bound by CPI Group (UK) Ltd, Croydon, CR0 4YY

For my daughters, Alathea and Leyla.

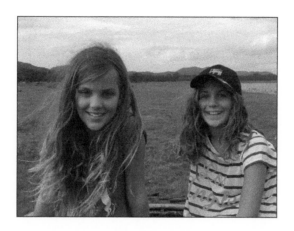

Contents

Foreword

Acupuncture for children continues to be a rapidly growing area of interest amongst both practitioners and parents. It is quicker and usually more effective than orthodox Western medicine, free from side effects and wholly suited to the treatment of so many conditions that plague children, such as earache and chronic cough. It is mainly ignorance of its capabilities that keeps people away. There is also, perhaps, a feeling that using needles is too invasive and will not be tolerated by many children. In this book there have been great strides in giving effective treatments in a gentle way, either with or without needles. Now there are easy-to-use press needles that can hardly be felt, there are hand-held laser 'pens' which are effective for more delicate children, and of course there is always moxa. Rebecca also includes comprehensive details of paediatric *tui na*, where appropriate, and shows how it may either be used on its own or combined with acupuncture treatment.

Another of the great advantages of acupuncture is that it is cheap to administer. There are no extra costs involved except a practitioner's time and some sterile needles. As the world becomes more unstable, with population migrations, and income differentials increasing, the great majority of people will not have access to, or will not be able to afford the expense of, Western drugs. It is my opinion that as crises become increasingly more common, acupuncture will be sorely needed. This book is therefore timely.

It is an exciting time for the acupuncture profession. When I started my practice, there were very few textbooks on acupuncture available in English; just a few point manuals, and sketchy translations from Chinese. Fortunately, that has now changed, and there are many excellent books and training courses to choose from, and many books covering specialist subjects.

This book is a wonderful contribution to the area of treating children, and it is very welcome. Welcome for many reasons, not least because it shows that acupuncture really can be learned by any good practitioner; welcome because it provides a different point of view, with a strong emphasis on the Five Element approach as taught by JR Worsley. There is also much new information, including causes of disease that were not so much seen in children only a few decades ago, differentiations of '21st-century conditions', such as chronic fatigue syndrome, details of 'red flag' signs that the practitioner should look out for and a focus on what goes on in the treatment room.

I have known Rebecca for many years and she brings to this book her compassionate approach to working with vulnerable teenagers. Here she shows how a combination of what is commonly known as TCM, together with a Five Element style, can be used to treat adolescents. It is of course difficult to take the first steps in treating children, but the chapters that Rebecca has devoted to teenage problems (including anorexia and self-harm) are a good place to start. Teenagers often have younger brothers and sisters, so gradually one can extend the age range towards the very young. Throughout the book Rebecca distinguishes the different approaches to treatment that are needed depending on the age of child being treated.

I can honestly say that treating children is one of the most rewarding areas of practice and I am delighted that more authors are joining the campaign to see acupuncture widely accepted for the treatment of babies and children.

Dr Julian Scott, MA, PhD, Cert.Ac. (China)
Fellow of BAcC

Acknowledgements

There may be one name on the cover of this book but the writing of it has been a team effort. While I am solely responsible for any mistakes and inadequacies, there would have been many more if it had not been for friends and colleagues.

I could not have even contemplated beginning without the full support of my husband, Peter Mole. He has given up countless hours of his time to read and comment upon chapters. He has taken on more than his fair share of domestic chores so that I have had more time to write. And he has believed in me when I have doubted myself. His love, support and generosity fundamentally underpin this book.

The following friends and colleagues all gave up their valuable time to read chapters and give me their insightful comments and suggestions: Helen Attwooll, Danny Blyth, Jess Buck, Emma Collins, Dr Michael Fitzpatrick, Marian Fixler, Sylvia Gulbenkian, Greg Lampert, Fiona Lyburn, Mary Kaspar, Stella King, Soreh Levy, Darrell Nightingale, Jane Roberts, Sandy Steele, Dr Clare Stephenson, Jenny Tune and Dr Hongchun Yin. They all graciously contributed, shared their knowledge and insights, and were prepared to debate knotty issues. Their collective contribution to the book is enormous.

I am truly grateful to Sarah Hoyle for putting into her wonderful illustrations exactly the ideas I wanted to convey. Nothing I asked of her (and I asked a lot) was ever too much trouble. Thank you also to Claire Wilson, my editor at Singing Dragon, who put her trust in me and patiently answered my many questions along the way. She and the rest of her team at Singing Dragon were professional, easy to communicate with and provided great expertise from beginning to end. My thanks also go to Tom Croft for skilfully taking the photograph for the front cover, and to Albie Davis-James for agreeing to be the model and entering into the spirit of it with such enthusiasm.

Many friends and family have also carried me along over the two years of writing, generously giving both emotional and practical support, namely Peter and Sue Avern, Anne Burns, Vicky, Christina and Bella Cuming, Tristan Hugh-Jones, Kanika Lang, Jo Payne, Adam Pearson, Letty Peppiatt and Clare Rule. Without them, and other friends and family members, it might have felt like a lonely road, but it never did.

I feel incredibly fortunate to have benefited from the wisdom of my Chinese medicine teachers (especially Angie and John Hicks, Giovanni Maciocia, Peter Mole and Julian Scott). All of the children who come to The Panda Clinic have also taught me something valuable and I continue to learn from them every day. Students at the College of Integrated Chinese Medicine have encouraged me to think more deeply with their searching questions, and their enthusiasm helps me to remain inspired.

This book is dedicated to my daughters, Alathea and Leyla. At times, my decision to write this book has been hard for them. Yet they have rarely complained. The experience of living with them and observing their truly amazing personalities warms my heart every day. Thank you both for being you.

Notes for the Reader

Prior knowledge

It is not the aim of this book to teach the basics of Chinese medicine. My aim is, rather, to teach suitably qualified practitioners how to practise paediatric acupuncture. I have therefore assumed a basic knowledge of the fundamental concepts of Chinese medicine. For those readers who may be unfamiliar with some of the concepts of Chinese medicine, I recommend two outstanding texts, namely *The Foundations of Chinese Medicine* and *The Practice of Chinese Medicine*, both by Giovanni Maciocia.

Neither is it my aim to teach the reader how to practise Five Element constitutional acupuncture, of which I am aware many may be unfamiliar. I practise an integrated style of what is commonly called TCM acupuncture, with the Five Element constitutional style. Therefore, although there is some explanation of and reference to this style throughout the book, the reader who is interested in practising it will need to explore further. I recommend the only thorough and comprehensive text on this style, which is *Five Element Constitutional Acupuncture* by Angela Hicks, John Hicks and Peter Mole.

In addition, I do not cover point location, except for a small number of points which are widely used in paediatric acupuncture and less so with adults. *A Manual of Acupuncture* by Peter Deadman, Mazin Al-Khafaji and Kevin Baker is, in my opinion, an unrivalled text on this aspect of practice.

My main sources

- My understanding of the full, empty and Phlegm-type child (as described in Chapter 13) is largely based on the teachings of Julian Scott and Teresa Barlow and their description laid out in their text *Acupuncture in the Treatment of Children* (1999).

- My understanding of the Five Element constitutional imbalance is based on the work of JR Worsley, which was taught to me at the College of Integrated Chinese Medicine, Reading, UK.

- I have included patterns that I see most often in paediatric clinical practice. Underpinning this is a knowledge of TCM patterns I gained from working with Giovanni Maciocia. My understanding of how some of the basic patterns manifest in children is also based on Julian Scott's teachings.

- The description of tendencies towards pathological movements of *qi* (as described in Chapter 13) is based on my own clinical experience.

- My use of paediatric *tui na* is based on what I learned from Dr Hongchun Yin, and is also influenced by Elisa Rossi and Fan Ya-li.

- My use of *shonishin* is based on what I learned from Stephen Birch.

Capital letters

When an organ is written with an initial capital letter, it describes one of the *zangfu*. When it is written with a small letter, it denotes an organ in the context of Western medicine. When a climatic factor such as cold is written with a small letter, it alludes to cold as used in common parlance. When it is written with an initial capital, it refers to the Chinese medicine concept of a Pathogenic Factor.

Gender pronouns

I have alternated between female and male gender pronouns throughout the book. I have attempted to do this in a balanced fashion and it is not my intention to favour either the male or the female.

Definition of constitutional imbalance

Throughout the book, the term 'constitutional imbalance' refers to each child's fundamental, possibly innate, constitutional imbalance in one of the Elements. This is what practitioners of the Worsley school refer to as the 'causative factor'. The constitutional imbalance is considered to be the root (*ben*), which may give rise to manifestations of dysfunction (*biao*) in any of the other Elements. For a full description, please see Chapter 14.

List of symbols
Age of child

These four symbols are used throughout the book to denote when a pattern or aetiology is particularly relevant for that age group. When used with patterns, it does not mean that the pattern can *only* be seen in that age group, but that it is more common.

 Baby

 Toddler

 School-age child

 Teenager

Movements of *qi*

These four symbols are used when a condition is typically characterised by *qi* flowing in a certain direction. For a fuller description, please see Chapter 13.

 Counterflow *qi*

 Qi dispersing outwards

 Qi descending

Qi retreating inwards

How to use this book

Parts 1, 2 and 3 provide the background and context for Parts 4 and 5. It is my hope that readers will take the time to read the first three parts, and then refer to Parts 4 and 5 when in the clinic or to research treatment of a particular illness. Parts 4 and 5 will be most useful when used in this way.

 Please go to www.rebeccaavern.com for videos of many of the techniques described in the text and to share paediatric case histories.

INTRODUCTION

There have always been challenges involved in being a child. The nature of these challenges largely depends on when and where a child is born. At times, just surviving childhood has been a feat that only the strongest and luckiest accomplish. Children born in the 21st century in the developed world are faced with unique challenges. Their survival is usually a given. Yet the ability to thrive, physically and psychologically, eludes many. These are the children who come to our clinics for acupuncture. This book is written for acupuncture practitioners who want to help them.

I have two main purposes in writing this book. The first is to encourage and enable more acupuncture practitioners to treat babies and young children. The second is to support and inspire those who are already doing so. I have attempted to align the approach to the treatment of children with the 21st century. My experience of treating children with acupuncture has all been gained in the developed world. It is my hope that any practitioner working in the developing world will find this book of some use too.

The key features that set this book apart from others in the English language on paediatric acupuncture are the following:

- Some of the causes of disease covered are recent phenomena or ones which have not previously been written about in the context of Chinese medicine, such as over-parenting, overstimulation and strain in the family.

- The book focuses on the conditions most seen in acupuncture clinics in the developed world in the 21st century. Most of these are chronic, such as digestive disturbances, headaches and eczema. Many are relatively new conditions that little or nothing has been written about in acupuncture literature, such as food allergies and intolerances. Some are conditions that are becoming more and more prevalent, such as early onset of puberty.

- The book also covers psychological, mental and emotional conditions, such as self-harm, anxiety, depression and eating disorders, about which little has been written for acupuncturists.

- I have highlighted the approaches to diagnosis and treatment that are needed when working with children of different ages, from zero to eighteen years. Little has been written before about the particular needs of teenagers and some of the conditions for which they seek treatment.

- There is an emphasis on using acupuncture to help children be free from symptoms, and also to help them thrive and become resilient adults.

- I also provide an overview of the key therapeutic techniques that can be used when treating children, such as *shonishin*, paediatric *tui na* and laser acupuncture. These have not previously been discussed in the same text.

- As well as differentiating diseases according to traditional Chinese medicine (TCM) patterns, the book also includes application of the Five Element constitutional style of acupuncture to the treatment of children.

- Little emphasis has been given to the treatment of infectious diseases, such as measles, because they are rarely seen in the clinic.

21st-century causes of disease in the developed world

Many of the causes of disease discussed in Part 1, such as over-parenting and overuse of social media, are primarily recent phenomena. External Pathogenic Factors (EPF) are not usually the threat that they used to be, in a time when children have warm clothing, centrally heated homes with instant hot water and are well nourished. Many modern causes of disease tend to be subtly pernicious and continue for a protracted period of time. Sometimes, they are almost imperceptible, such as a lack of laughter in the household or a teacher who induces a feeling of fear in the child each day. Very often, aspects of children's lives that are considered to be completely normal are the very things that are making them ill. Too many after-school activities, food that is laden with sugar or parents who do not like each other are examples of what make children ill today. As these causes of disease tend to be ongoing, they are most likely to cause chronic conditions. In particular, they are conducive to the development of psychological conditions and psychosomatic illnesses.

A decline in acute conditions and a different range of chronic conditions

Historically, children in the UK used to die during periodic epidemics of infectious diseases such as whooping cough, polio and influenza. If they did not die, they would often be left with significant morbidity, such as breathing problems or paralysis. Nowadays, in the developed world, improved living conditions and vaccinations mean that the incidence of these potentially fatal diseases has vastly reduced. Antibiotics and other modern medicines mean they can be treated before reaching a critical stage. Children nowadays may be left with residual problems as a result of other common childhood illnesses such as chickenpox or norovirus gastroenteritis. However, these tend to be much less severe, partly because the diseases are less severe and partly because a well-nourished child with good living conditions is more able to withstand them.

Yet children in the developed world in the 21st century are beleaguered by an altogether different array of chronic conditions. Respiratory and food allergies, asthma, stomach ache, headaches, chronic fatigue syndrome, sleep disturbances and behavioural problems, to name but a few, have become modern-day epidemics. These conditions are rarely fatal but can have a profound effect on a child's life. They detract from the carefree condition that should characterise childhood. These maladies may mean that the child rarely feels energetic or is dependent on medication, which brings with it unpleasant, and potentially serious, side effects. The children who come for acupuncture treatment today largely come with these chronic problems. We are rarely involved in their survival but we can play an important role in helping them to thrive.

A prevalence of psychological, emotional and psychosomatic conditions

There has been an enormous increase in the prevalence of psychological and emotional conditions in children and teenagers, such as eating disorders, anxiety, depression and self-harm. Being a child in the 21st century, it seems, is stressful in a previously unseen way. Children are especially prone to psychosomatic illnesses, where an emotion is expressed physically because, for a variety of reasons, it cannot be made conscious or expressed verbally. The Monday morning stomach ache is a classic example of this, as are pre-exam migraines or, also, asthma attacks just before a parent leaves for work. Psychosomatic conditions are just as real, and just as important to treat, as purely physical illnesses. Unfortunately, society often deems them to be less worthy of attention, and the people who suffer from them to be less in need of support.

Babies, children and teenagers

Paediatric acupuncture texts have generally focused on children up to the age of seven or eight, after which the diagnosis and treatment is said to be more similar to that of an adult. My experience is that the causes of disease, the diagnosis and the treatment of children all vary hugely according to their age. Treatments of a two-year-old, an eight-year-old and a fifteen-year-old each need to be approached in different ways. I have attempted to highlight these differences and guide practitioners in modifying their approach depending on the age of the child.

I have placed a particular emphasis on adolescence. Although paediatrics has been a speciality of Chinese medicine since at least the time of the Song dynasty (nearly one thousand years ago), information on adolescence remains elusive. This is largely because adolescence is a relatively recent construction of modern, 'developed' societies. An adolescent is neither a child nor fully an adult, inhabiting a kind of in-between existence where she is likely to feel pulled backwards and driven forwards at the same time. Many of the challenges faced during adolescence are unique to this time. In the developed world, there is an epidemic of teenage mental health problems. How well someone navigates adolescence is crucial to his future health. The benefits of acupuncture treatment during this transition can hardly be overstated.

What role does acupuncture have in the treatment of children?

The current model of primary care medical practice emerged from the historical experience of dealing with children with infectious diseases, which required quick diagnosis and treatment. In modern family doctor practices, the usual model is short and hurried consultations, maybe with a different physician each time. This means there is little opportunity for a child and family to develop a personal relationship with their doctor. By contrast, we acupuncturists are able to offer both longer consultations and continuity of personal care. This allows for deeper exploration of symptoms and family dynamics, as well as the chance of building up an ongoing therapeutic relationship. The contribution these factors may have for the current and future health of the child is enormous.

Many parents come to acupuncturists desperate to find some help for their child, who often has a condition that Western medicine may be ill-equipped to treat. They may have been sent away by doctors, or are unwilling to use long-term medication that brings about other problems. Acupuncture is especially well suited to the treatment of these children. Practitioners will know from treating adults with chronic conditions how effective acupuncture treatment can be. When treating children with the same conditions, the results are often spectacular. The chances of bringing about a complete 'cure' are much greater than they are when treating an adult, because a child's *qi* is more easily influenced and the disease usually not so deeply embedded.

The absence of illness is, in itself, a wonderful treatment outcome. Yet there are other benefits of treatment that are particularly pertinent to children. Having ill health as a child tends to shape a person's relationship to illness later in life. An adult who was chronically ill as a child is more likely to feel powerless or fearful in the face of illness. It can mean that a sense of confidence in one's physical body is never attained. Long-term poor health as a child also has a strong influence on emotional development. It may mean that certain key milestones are delayed or do not take place at all.

Acupuncture for children should not be purely about eradicating symptoms, however. Five Element constitutional acupuncture in particular helps to prevent illness. Chapter 1 of the *Su Wen* talks about treating a person after she has become ill as being as futile as beginning to dig a well after one has become weak with thirst. Preventive treatment enables a child to better withstand the pressures she may face, and to ride times of accelerated growth and development more smoothly. Ensuring that the movements of *qi* remain balanced and smooth also means that unhealthy emotional patterns, such as chronic worry or erratic expressions of anger, are less likely to set in and become etched in the child's personality forever. Furthermore, disharmonies of *qi* can prevent a child from fulfilling her potential. This is not about being a super achiever. On the contrary, it affects each child's ability to set out on the right path to eventually, as an adult, achieve her unique 'contract with heaven' (*ming*).

The delivery of acupuncture treatment to children in the 21st century

The biggest barrier to more children having acupuncture is their fear that it will hurt or the parent's fear that the child will not tolerate being needled. In order for acupuncture treatment to be successful, it must be an experience that is enjoyable for the child or, at the very least, devoid of stress. If the child grumbles between treatments that he hates going to see the person who sticks needles in him, the family are much less likely to persist with the course of treatment. The vast majority of children are accepting of acupuncture needles when the treatment is approached in the right way. Whilst some persuasion may be necessary for the child and his parent to accept the treatment, generally speaking the child's treatment needs to be something that he feels good about.

For the few children for whom we cannot find a way of them comfortably accepting needles, we are in the fortunate position to have many more treatment modalities available to us than we did as recently as a decade ago. Part 3 will discuss paediatric *tui na* and *shonishin*, which have only been described in English fairly recently. It will also discuss the use of modern techniques, such as laser acupuncture. I have only ever seen one child for whom I was unable to find any method of treatment that was acceptable to them. It is advisable for the paediatric acupuncturist to have a wide range of modalities with which to deliver the treatment at his disposal.

My background

In writing this book, to use Isaac Newton's phrase, I consider myself to be 'standing on the shoulders of giants'. I have been incredibly fortunate to have learned from and worked with some pioneering and insightful masters of Chinese medicine, both general and paediatric. I have also benefited enormously from those who have devoted years of their lives to learning Chinese and have subsequently translated key paediatric texts. In particular, Sabine Wilms's translations of Sun Simiao's writings on paediatrics have proved invaluable.

My initial training was in both traditional Chinese medicine (TCM) and the Five Element constitutional style developed by JR Worsley. I was privileged to learn Five Element constitutional acupuncture from Angie and John Hicks and Peter Mole, all of whom studied for many years with JR Worsley. I had the honour of working alongside Giovanni Maciocia for four years, which provided me with the most thorough grounding in TCM that I could imagine. My main paediatric training was a two-year course with Julian Scott, co-author of *Acupuncture in the Treatment of Children* (1999). The importance of his pioneering work in promoting the treatment of children can hardly be overstated. I would not have begun treating children, nor be here writing this book, without Julian's work having gone before me. I have also gained many valuable insights from Stephen Birch, Elisa Rossi, Dr Hongchun Yin and Peter Gigante. I continue to learn from every child that I treat at The Panda Clinic, an acupuncture clinic specifically for the treatment of children, which I set up in Oxford, UK.

The approach to the treatment of children laid out in this book is one which pulls together aspects from a variety of styles which derive from these teachers and others. It is an ever-evolving style which works for me in my clinic. Everyone reading this book will bring their own perspective. I strongly encourage practitioners to use this book as a starting point and a guide, but not to slavishly follow it. Whilst treatment must first and foremost be safe, based on sound theory and approached with intelligence and integrity, beyond this each practitioner needs to make it their own.

Sun Simiao described the art of 'nurturing the young' and it is as relevant today as it was when he wrote about it 1400 years ago. Twenty-first-century children need exactly the kind of help that we, as acupuncturists, can give. It is my greatest wish that more practitioners embrace the challenge of treating children. The benefits for the child, the family and indeed the practitioner can be nothing short of life-changing.

• Part 1 •

WHY DO CHILDREN BECOME ILL?

• Chapter 1 •

INTRODUCTION TO THE CAUSES OF DISEASE

The topics discussed in this chapter are:

- The importance of understanding the cause of illness
- Every child responds differently
- Causes of disease rarely occur in isolation
- How can something be both health-giving *and* a cause of disease?
- Lifestyle advice based on an understanding of the causes of disease
- Causes of disease are amplified in children

Introduction

One of my main reasons for writing this book is that the causes of disease in children in the developed world are very different from those seen when the classics of Chinese medicine were written. They are different, even, from a few decades ago when the first key English-language texts on acupuncture paediatrics were written. Flaws, in his book *A Handbook of TCM Paediatrics*, states very strongly that, although external, internal and miscellaneous causes of disease may all apply to children, diet is by far the most common cause of disease in children under the age of six. Scott and Barlow, in their book *Acupuncture in the Treatment of Children*, devote an equal part of their discussion on the causes of disease to External Pathogenic Factors and to diet, and briefly mention emotional and other miscellaneous factors. Diet and vulnerability to External Pathogenic Factors are still relevant in any discussion of why children become ill. However, there are many aspects of modern life that have become just as important. They warrant further discussion and understanding.

Life for children in the developed world in the 21st century is less physically precarious than it has ever been. However, there are new, insidious factors that cause children to become ill, or not to thrive. Childhood mortality rates have dropped dramatically. Yet many children live with some form of chronic disease that blights their enjoyment of life, diminishes their potential and makes them reliant on medication that may, in turn, cause other health problems.

The importance of understanding the cause of illness

Understanding why children become ill is just as important as it always has been. In Chinese medicine, the 'superior doctor' was one who understood both the condition and its cause. We may not be able to change the circumstances that are working against the child, but knowing what they are helps us to understand better and therefore treat her more effectively. A chronic illness or symptom nearly always arises within the context of the child's life, circumstances and individual nature. Treating the child without understanding this background is like taking a quote out of context. It often leads to misunderstanding. A chronic symptom or illness rarely, if ever, arises out of the blue. We may talk of being 'struck down' by illnesses that come 'out of nowhere', which is often the case in acute conditions. Chronic imbalances, however, are woven into the fabric of a child's individual story. The more we understand of this story (even though this may be difficult in some cases), the more effective our treatment and advice may be.

The practitioner may feel that whatever he does to help the child is a mere drop in the ocean beside the powerful forces at work in the child's life that are making her ill. How can treating a child who is bedwetting help when the cause of her symptom is the fear she feels due to her volatile father? Can treatment of a child with anxiety, due to pressure and expectation, enable her to feel calm when the pressure and expectation continues? At the very least, treatment may mean that the effect of the cause of disease is reduced. At best, what felt like pressure to a child with Spleen *qi* and Heart Blood deficiency, for example, may not feel like pressure once these patterns of imbalance are significantly lessened. But, more than this, miraculous things sometimes happen when treating children. A small shift in the *qi* of the child can cause a domino-like change in the *qi* of everybody in the family, so that the whole unit finds a new and healthier equilibrium.

Every child responds differently

It is important not to jump to conclusions about the impact that factors in a child's life are having upon her health. As Jung said, 'the shoe that fits one person pinches another'.[1] Every child has a different physical and emotional constitution (see Chapter 2), which means that there is a range of possible responses to the same aetiological factor. One child's poison is another child's cure. For example, one child may tolerate dairy food well, whilst in another it may cause appalling eczema. One child may be untroubled by her parents' rows, whilst another may become fearful and anxious. Some children thrive on lots of exercise, for others it is too depleting. We all come with our own biases as practitioners. Being aware of what these are helps us to remain open-minded as to what is the cause of the symptoms in each child that we see.

 In 2004, Professor Bruce Ellis of the University of Arizona developed the concept of 'dandelion and orchid' children. He proposed that some children (dandelions) can survive harsh environments without it having too strong an impact on them. Others (orchids) are more susceptible to their environment, in particular to their family circumstances. They may blossom if they have a largely nurturing experience, but the wrong circumstances will have a detrimental effect on them. He was, in essence, describing that some children have a more robust *shen* than others.

Causes of disease rarely occur in isolation

The causes of disease in the following chapters are divided into the categories first laid out in the *San Yin Fang* written in 1174, namely internal, external and miscellaneous. There is rarely only one causative agent in a child's illness. It is usually when several factors combine, against the background of a child's constitutional imbalance, that illness arises. The challenge for the practitioner is to consider all the causes of disease equally, and to be aware of her own bias in favouring one category over another. Any advice she gives should be related only to the causes that she considers are relevant for the individual child. A long list of 'shoulds' and 'should nots' is usually overwhelming and decreases the likelihood that any of them will be followed. Small pieces of pertinent advice tailored to the individual child are more likely to be taken up. Furthermore, most parents will resonate with suggestions that really are relevant to their child. The practitioner is sometimes only pointing out what the parent already knows, but it may take an outsider to remind him of it.

How can something be both health-giving *and* a cause of disease?

There is a fine line between a certain aspect of a child's life contributing to health or detracting from it. Exercise is a good example of this. The right amount of the right kind of exercise will contribute to a child's health. Either too much, too little or the wrong kind of exercise may make a child ill. The same applies to many causes of disease. A lack of nurture is likely to cause imbalance, whereas over-attentiveness may do the same. Finding a middle way that suits each individual can be difficult. Even more challenging may be incorporating it into the life of a family, the members of which may have needs that are at odds with one another.

> A brother and sister who came to the clinic for treatment could not have been more different in their needs. The older boy was a deficient child who became easily overstimulated and tired by being out and about and with other children. His younger sister, on the other hand, was an excess child who became restless and irritable if she spent too long at home or did not have a variety of activities each day.

Lifestyle advice based on an understanding of the causes of disease

Understanding why a child has become ill may enable the practitioner to offer appropriate advice to the child and parent. It can be invaluable to inform someone about the ways in which her lifestyle is creating stress on her particular areas of vulnerability. This is especially the case during childhood, when growth and development are at their most rapid. It may not only help her to become free of the problem with which she is presenting, but can prevent illnesses in the future.

As an acupuncture practitioner, it is relatively easy to advise a parent on how to change her child's diet or keep him covered up when he goes out in the cold. It is considerably more challenging to grapple with some of the causes of disease discussed here which are related to the family and parenting. Sometimes treatment of the child brings about a change without anything needing to be said. At other times, the simple presence of the practitioner acts as a mirror being held up to the child or parent who can then see that something needs to change. The practitioner will sometimes feel it is necessary to talk to the parent about a delicate, emotive and possibly painful issue he perceives is contributing to the child's illness. This may need to be done when the child is not present. It should always be done in a way which maintains rapport, and from a place of compassion. Parents are, most of the time, doing the best they can, sometimes in very difficult circumstances.

> I once asked a parent whose eight-year-old child suffered from painful digestive cramps to tell me the child's typical weekly schedule. As she began going through the various activities, she stopped and said, 'I feel exhausted just telling you about it.' In this moment, it became clear to her that her child had very little downtime at all in his weekly schedule.

Causes of disease are amplified in children

Children are far more vulnerable to their external environment because the fundamentals are not yet in place. The effect of every cause of disease is magnified. If an adult does not get sufficient sleep for a night or two, he probably will not feel at his most vital. The chances are, however, that when he manages to catch up on sleep, he will be back to his old self. In contrast, if a three-year-old fails to get enough sleep for a couple of nights, it is likely to affect many aspects of his being. He may not eat properly, may be either miserable or hyperactive, or alternate between the two. He may become overly emotional and even temporarily regress in key areas such as toilet training and speaking. Therefore, when speaking to parents, giving information about which aspects we perceive to be affecting the child's health is vital.

SUMMARY

» Understanding a child's story, and the background to her illness, often enables more effective treatment and lifestyle advice.

» Lifestyle advice should always be imparted sensitively and from a place of compassion.

» Long lists of 'dos and don'ts' should be avoided, and only advice pertinent to the individual child should be given.

» Children are more vulnerable to their external environment than adults.

• Chapter 2 •

THE NATURE OF CHILDREN

Gaining some knowledge of the unique nature of children is fundamental to understanding what makes them ill. The topics discussed in this chapter are:

- Children are delicate and incomplete

- Children are predominantly *yang*

- Children's *yin* is insubstantial

- A young child is not able to self-regulate

- A child's spirit is strongly influenced by what is going on around her

- The channel system (*jingmai*) and points are immature

Children are delicate and incomplete

In Volume 5 of the great work *Essential Prescriptions Worth a Thousand in Gold for Every Emergency* (*Bei Ji Qian Jin Yao Fang*), Sun Simiao stressed the great vulnerability of young children. He conveyed the idea that, because of their 'newness', young children need meticulous care and attention.

In the same vein, the later classics abound with phrases suggesting that children's bodies are fragile, tender and soft. *The Spiritual Pivot* (*Ling Shu*), for example, stated, 'Children's flesh is fragile, their blood is scanty, and their *qi* is weak.'[2] A baby does not come out of the womb fully formed. The *Treatise on the Origins of Paediatric Diseases and Their Treatments* (*Xiao Er Bing Yuan Fang Lun*) makes the same point:

> The skin and hair, muscles and flesh, sinews and bones, brain and marrow, the five viscera and six bowels, the constructive and defensive, and the *qi* and Blood of children as a whole are not hard and secure.[3]

If we plant a seedling outside, it is unlikely to flourish. It may struggle to defend itself from the elements and find enough food and water in the way that a mature plant can. That is why we nurture seedlings in greenhouses, providing them with protection and warmth. We need to apply the same level of care to children whilst all the aspects of their physical and psychological nature develop. As they mature and become more established in the world, they become less vulnerable to harm from external forces.

 The size of a baby's brain in relation to his body is bigger than that of all other mammals. Humans also have a relatively small pelvis in order that they can walk on two legs. As a result, babies are born at a much earlier stage of their development than nearly all other animals. This is why they need so much more care in the early months of life. They are incapable of meeting their own primary needs.

Interestingly, this idea of a child being very vulnerable at the start of life is reflected in modern psychology too. The psychologist and psychiatrist Robin Skynner writes, 'And inside the mother's body he was completely safe, protected, warm, dark, quiet – now he is suddenly vulnerable, unprotected, every single element in his environment is new and strange. And anything new and strange is frightening.'[4]

However, the delicacy of a baby or young child does not mean they should be wrapped in cotton wool. Some authors, for example Chen Wen Zhong in the 13th century,[5] actually stressed that it is only through being exposed to the elements that children grow strongly. Parents have the difficult task of discerning to what extent they must protect their child and how much they should expose him to the world outside. The nature of the child, the factors he is exposed to and the relationship between the two determine what may be too much or not enough.

One area that supports Chen Wen Zhong's point of view is that of allergies. In 1989, Professor David Strachan developed 'the hygiene hypothesis'.[6] He suggested that a lack of exposure to germs and infections during childhood was a possible cause of the rise in allergies. More recent research, which shows that children raised on farms have fewer allergies than those raised in cities, would appear to confirm this. Age-appropriate sensitive care and attention is vital; over- or under-exposure to the external environment may be detrimental.

Children are predominantly *yang*

Children are described as having a 'pure *yang*' constitution.[7] It is worth exploring what this actually means.

Yang qi enables a child to grow and develop. Whilst *yin* creates stability, *yang* enables change. We see in children an absolutely extraordinary ability to grow and change. Within the first year of life, most children will have learned how to make sounds, sit up, crawl, walk, point at things, hold things, chew… They have usually tripled their birth weight. Children have a form or a quality of *yang* that adults simply do not possess.

Young children are the very essence of *yang*. They have a great need to run around and be active in order for all their *yang qi* not to become stagnant. Most parents of a young child know that there will come a point in the day when they have to send their child outside to let off steam. The abundant enthusiasm and inquisitiveness that are characteristic of most young children is also an expression of their exuberant *yang*.

Despite the *yang* constitution of young children, they often suffer from conditions which are Cold and/or deficient in nature. This is because there are so many aspects of modern life, such as diet and some medications, which have a strongly cooling effect on the child's *qi*.

Twenty-first-century children often present with a complex picture. As well as being constitutionally '*yang*', many are also deficient and plagued by Cold and Damp. This may, in part, be due to the following factors:

» Twenty-first-century diets, often composed largely of energetically Cold- and Damp-forming foods.

» Children commonly being born to older mothers, who are themselves depleted.

» Widespread use of energetically Cold medicines, such as anaesthetics during childbirth, antibiotics and fever-suppressing medications.

» The nature of life (especially for city-dwellers) which is often over-scheduled and strongly depleting.

» Many children's activities are 'head-based', which constrains *yang qi* rather than allowing it to flow and expand.

Children's *yin* is insubstantial

Yin enables a child to be still, consistent and resilient. Whilst *yang* gives a child the ability to start things, *yin* enables her to stick with them. *Yang qi* may be abundant in children, but without a strong underpinning of *yin* to support it, children will quickly flag. A child may be running around quite happily in the playground enjoying himself, but then suddenly appear to have no capacity at all to walk home. His mood changes in an instant from exuberant to miserable.

When the classics of Chinese medicine wrote that children's *yin* is insubstantial, they were alluding to the fact that it is easy for them to come down with Hot diseases. A more relevant implication of a child having insubstantial *yin* today is that it causes a propensity for *yang* to rise to the head. This may lead to a wide variety of behavioural, emotional or sleep problems, which are commonly seen in the clinic.

Saying a child's *yin* is insubstantial is not to say that this is a pathological state. It is simply that *yin* (as with nearly everything else in a child's body) is still in the process of developing and therefore needs to be nurtured and protected.

 The combination of abundant *yang* and insubstantial *yin* is what makes children prone to fevers, and means that fevers may rise substantially and quickly.

A young child is not able to self-regulate

Every parent knows the alarming speed with which a child can become ill. A baby or toddler may be running around quite happily, then begin moaning and crying and be burning up with a high fever in minutes. Within an hour or so, if things go badly, the situation may even be life-threatening. Alternatively, the young child may be right as rain and enjoying a big breakfast by the following morning. These rapid changes may occur because the *qi* of a child moves rapidly and easily leaves its path.

There are other, subtle ways in which young children are not able to regulate their *qi*. A child may become upset by a relatively trivial event, such as not getting the first go on a swing. If an adult is not immediately at hand (and sometimes even if she is), within seconds the child may be screaming, crying, red in the face and almost inconsolable. This is another expression of the rapidity with which a child's *qi* leaves its path and becomes chaotic.

A three-year-old girl came to the clinic and dropped her biscuit as she walked in the door. In seconds, she turned from smiley and calm to distraught, throwing herself on the floor crying. She was unable to 'right herself' until she had sat on her mother's lap quietly for ten minutes. Her *qi* had been disrupted and she needed her mother's calm presence in order for it to refind an equilibrium.

A child's spirit is strongly influenced by what is going on around her

The Spleen is the root of post-natal *qi*. One of the functions of post-natal *qi* is to root the spirit. Spleen *qi* is inherently underdeveloped and weak in children, and therefore the spirit is not well rooted. This is why children can become so easily upset.

Sun Simiao also talked of young children having very little ability to protect themselves against their external environment. Anything loud or sudden or unfamiliar may upset a child's being, as his protective *qi* is weak and ineffective. Hence, Sun Simiao urges:

> Constantly beware of fright while rearing small children. Do not let them hear loud noises and, when holding them in your arms, be still and gentle. Do not let them be frightened or startled. Moreover, when there is thunder in the sky, plug the children's ears and at the same time make some other subtle noises in order to distract them.[8]

He also talked of the way in which unfamiliar people may be frightening or upsetting for a young child: 'In all sorts of situations where there are people coming in from the outside or strange things entering through the door, ensure that the child avoids them, and do not let them see the child.'[9]

Again, this is an idea which is mirrored in modern psychology. Skynner writes, 'The parents have to shield him almost completely from outside disturbance, keeping him warm and comfortable, seeing he doesn't get too hungry, protecting him from too much noise and upset.'[10]

> A mother reported that her one-year-old boy, who usually slept very well, had started waking regularly since he had moved to a different bedroom. He seemed disturbed by his new surroundings and it took him several weeks to settle into a good sleep pattern again.

The channel system (*jingmai*) and points are immature

Chapter 10 of *The Spiritual Pivot* (*Ling Shu*) says, '[After labour when the] *gu* [grains] come into the stomach, the vessel-meridian pathways are [all] connected, the blood and *qi* [begin to] move.'[11] This quote implies that *qi* and Blood only start flowing in the channels after the child is born. Birch speculates that the eight extraordinary meridians (*qijingbaomai*) are open and functioning in the foetus *in utero*.[12] After birth, they close up and the channel system (*jingmai*) begins to function. If this is the case, the channel system is immature at birth because it has not previously been functioning. It seems unlikely that a system as complex as the twelve channels would reach a state of maturity immediately, but that this would be a gradual process taking place over the first years of life.

There are two implications of this. First, anything that is not yet fully formed needs to be handled with great care and sensitivity. Too much intervention may cause disruption in a system that is in a state of flux. Second, an immature channel system would explain why techniques such as *shonishin* and paediatric *tui na* are so effective. Specifically defined points have not yet developed and so access to a child's *qi* can be made over wider areas.

 In the clinic, it is common to see an immediate change in a child simply from palpating an area on a channel near to an acupuncture point, rather than the point itself.

SUMMARY

» Children are 'a work in progress', and therefore the appropriate amount and the right kind of care and attention is vital.

» Being predominantly *yang*, children need opportunities to move and be active in order to 'discharge' some of their exuberance.

» Twenty-first-century children often have a mix of exuberant *yang* as well as having a Cold and Damp Lingering Pathogenic Factor.

» *Yang* has a propensity to flow upwards and to affect the head in children because their *yin* is insubstantial and unable to root the *yang*.

» Children may be easily and strongly upset by small events, and need help to find their equilibrium again.

» Children are strongly influenced by everything in their external environment.

» Too much treatment may aggravate the *qi* of a child because her channel system is still maturing and therefore somewhat volatile.

• Chapter 3 •

HOW CHILDREN GROW

The topics discussed in this chapter are:

- Children have intense phases of growth and development
- The first seven or eight years of life are concerned with gathering resources
- The ages from seven or eight to puberty are concerned with consolidating resources
- The changes between the seven- and eight-year cycles are times when imbalance may be thrown off or penetrate deeper
- Adolescence is driven by a surge in Kidney *yang*
- Liver *qi* is especially prone to stagnation during adolescence
- The Spleen is under strain during adolescence
- Different aspects of children grow and develop at varying speeds
- Twenty-first-century children in the developed world struggle more with development than with growth

Children have intense phases of growth and development

One of the ways in which babies grow and develop is through a process described by Sun Simiao as 'transformations and steamings' (*bian zheng*). These are phases that occur at various times during the first two years of life. 'Transformations' (*bian*) refers to an ascent of *qi*, whilst 'steamings' (*zheng*) refers to the presence of Heat.[13] In practice, this usually manifests as a mild fever. Teething can also be seen as a transformation and steaming. They may also manifest as a temporary increase in an outpouring of coloured mucus.

Transformations and steamings are considered to be normal physiological parts of a child's development. They can be seen as a process by which the infant burns off excess *yang*. Sun Simiao indeed says that, 'when the major and minor steamings are all finished, [the baby] has become a human being'.[14] Chinese medicine understands that children are born with Heat that arose in the womb, and that fevers are an opportunity for this Heat to be released.

This reflects the observation of many parents that an illness sometimes seems to allow a leap in development in some way.

> One parent reported that her three-year-old began sleeping well for the first time after recovering from a strong fever. Another said that she had been concerned that her nearly two-year-old boy had not begun speaking at all. Shortly after his second birthday, he was 'ill' for a week (hot, grumpy and lethargic). When he emerged from this illness, he began saying words for the first time.

There is a rather widespread trend in medicating infants to reduce even a mild fever. This arises partly out of a generalised fear of fevers which, in the past, were a major cause of death. Without extended family to call upon, it is sometimes the only way parents can send their infant to childcare and go to work. For these reasons, and perhaps also because most children are vaccinated against major febrile diseases, it often takes longer than the two years Sun Simiao spoke of for a child to complete all her necessary transformations and steamings. It may also be that some children never complete them. We can only speculate about what long-term effects this may have on a child. On a physical level, it may mean that a child develops various chronic symptoms of Heat which are a reflection of excess *yang* being trapped inside her. On a psychological and emotional level, it may even impinge upon a child's ability to become a fully fledged adult, who embraces being in the world.

The first seven or eight years of life are concerned with gathering resources

Chapter 1 of *The Simple Questions* (*Su Wen*) distinguishes between different phases of a person's life, each with different characteristics and tasks. The first phase lasts approximately until the age of seven in a girl, and eight in a boy. The rate at which a child develops physically and mentally during this time is quite extraordinary. Modern medicine tends to be focused on whether children are putting on weight at the expected rate, and meeting the key development milestones at the expected time. With the emphasis on these outward, discernible signs of growth and development, it is easy to forget that the main purpose of this time is much more hidden and subtle. The core building blocks of a person should be laid down during this phase. In order for this to happen, a young child must assemble and gather in all the necessary components that are needed. This is akin to assembling all the ingredients to make a dish. If some of the ingredients are missing, or if they are not of good quality, it will affect the quality of the final dish. In a child, these ingredients are primarily love, care and attention, good food and clean air.

The implications of this are twofold. First, it follows that if a small child is undertaking the enormous task of gathering in the resources he needs, too much activity and engagement with the world will draw his *qi* outwards and make this task harder. Second, a child will not have the ability to filter what he is drawing in. So, if there are harmful elements in his environment, he will take these in too and they will become a part of his foundations. Harmful elements may include, for example, exposure to intense or prolonged emotions, criticisms, poor quality food, air pollution, bacteria and viruses.

 Many pathologies that begin during the first seven or eight years of life are a result of too many of the child's resources being diverted outward rather than gathered inward. This is often due to him having a hectic schedule.

By the end of this phase, the bones should be strong and the flesh should be firm. The Brain should be filled with Marrow and the sense organs fully functioning. The *shen* should be firmly rooted in the Heart.

Interestingly there are some parallels in Western medicine to this idea that the core aspects of basic development are completed by around the age of seven. Dr Enders, in her book *Gut*, writes:

> By the age of seven, we have probably seen it all, or all that is important to our immune cells. By this time, our immune system has finished its schooling and can go to work for us for the rest of our lives.[15]

The ages from seven or eight to puberty are concerned with consolidating resources

By the age of seven or eight, with luck all the vital building blocks of *jing*, *qi* and *shen* will be in place but they have yet to be built upon and refined. This is the task of the next seven or eight years of a child's life.

Qi may now be directed to a secondary level of physical and mental growth. The second set of teeth will begin to come through. A child has more *qi* available to express her individuality and start exploring what really interests her in life. Everything will have become a bit more 'set' and so she will be less affected by her external environment. She should be better able to right herself after being upset, without needing a parent to help her. She may also be less prone to acute illnesses in this phase.

Another use that the Kidney *qi* (previously employed purely for the purposes of growing) will now be put to is preparing a child for the next transition into the third phase of development. Often from approximately the age of nine in a girl, and usually slightly later in a boy, there will be signs that the body is preparing for puberty. There may be physical signs such as the appearance of pubic hair, an increase in testicle size in boys and the appearance of breast buds in girls. There may be emotional and psychological signs such as the growth of self-consciousness and phases of showing less dependence on the family. These are the early stirrings of a process which will take the next four or so years to complete.

The changes between the seven- and eight-year cycles are times when imbalance may be thrown off or penetrate deeper

The times of transition between the seven- and eight-year cycles described in *Su Wen* Chapter 1 are especially important phases in a child's life. Times of intense change are also times of opening and opportunity. A child's *qi* is more easily influenced during these times. Therefore, if circumstances are conducive, the child may, for example, be able to throw off a Lingering Pathogenic Factor (LPF) (see Chapter 27). Or he may capitalise on the surge of *yang* that usually accompanies these times and become stronger and more robust. Alternatively, if the circumstances of his life are not favourable during these times, for example if he is overworked or his parents are going through a divorce, a pre-existing LPF may penetrate deeper. A deficiency of *qi* or Blood in any Organ may become more pronounced. With each changeover of cycle, it becomes harder to correct an imbalance. Therefore, just as during the transformations and steamings, extra care should be taken of a child during a transition phase to help ensure her future health.

> A three-year-old boy came for treatment for speech problems which were due to Phlegm in the channels of the face and head. The treatment was not successful and the Phlegm remained. He came back at the age of seven (as he was entering the transition phase to the next cycle) and responded to treatment quickly. After a few sessions, he had a big 'outpouring' of phlegm (snotty nose, chesty cough), and when that cleared his speech was immediately and significantly clearer.

Adolescence is driven by a surge in Kidney *yang*

The behind-the-scenes changes that began to appear in the latter stages of the previous cycle now burst forth. Subtle changes in the physical body become pronounced and overt. Many children in the preceding years will have played with the idea of being a little more independent. For example, they may have banned their parents from showing them any affection at the school gates and had phases of moodiness and stroppiness. During this transition phase, these changes will suddenly become more exaggerated and constant. What drives this enormous shift towards independence during the pubertal years is a huge surge of Kidney *yang*. During the previous phase, both Kidney *yin* and *yang* were rising. By the time of puberty, they have (in a healthy teenager) become abundant.

This surge of Kidney *yang* drives the enormous growth that happens during this time. Teenagers grow at a rate which is second only to that of babies. The expansion of the *ming men* also powers the sexual energy, which first appears during this phase. The increase in Kidney *yang* also, in part, explains why emotions may be expressed more vociferously than they have been before. Western psychiatry explains this by the chemical changes that are taking place in the body.

> But once he gets to puberty – the start of adolescence – it's as if the child can't keep those feelings under wraps any longer because they're getting multiplied and made much more intense by the chemical changes now going on. So out they burst.[16]

Liver *qi* is especially prone to stagnation during adolescence

However, a lack of smooth flow of Liver *qi* is the main reason for the moodiness, grumpiness, frustration, explosions of anger and tendency to become withdrawn which characterise so many teenagers. There are two key reasons why Liver *qi* stagnation is such a common pattern in the teenage years. First, the Kidneys pertain to the Water Element. On the *sheng* cycle, Water is the mother of Wood and therefore generates it. In practice, the surge in Kidney *yang* fuels Liver *qi* which becomes more powerful. This is necessary in order for an adolescent to make the leap of independence that rightly accompanies this stage. However, it also takes some time for a teenager to integrate this new *qi* and to be able to express it smoothly.

The second reason for the occurrence of Liver *qi* stagnation during adolescence is simply that there is commonly a mismatch between a teenager's desire for independence, and the amount of freedom he is allowed. Every time he feels thwarted, by not being able to stay out late, being banned from getting a tattoo or having to do the odd household chore, feelings of frustration are inevitable and Liver *qi* is likely to stagnate. This is a two-way process. Liver *qi* stagnation causes feelings of frustration, and the feelings of frustration cause Liver *qi* to stagnate.

> One parent said of her eleven-year-old daughter that she did not know 'who she was going to get' throughout the day as her daughter's moods had become so changeable. This is a classic sign of Liver *qi* stagnation.

The Spleen is under strain during adolescence

Any parent of a teenager will know that they will normally start eating more than they ever have before. This food is needed to help fuel the growth spurt that is taking place. It means, however, that the Spleen becomes more taxed, just as it did in the first year or two of life. Added to this, many teenagers are faced with an increase in academic work, which also depletes the Spleen.

It is common for teenagers who come to the clinic to have developed Spleen symptoms in the first years of puberty, at the time their appetite increased. One girl, previously known in her family as very laid back, had begun to worry a lot (usually a symptom of Spleen *qi* deficiency). Her Spleen was busy digesting and was no longer able to provide a residence for her *yi*.

Different aspects of children grow and develop at varying speeds

Chinese medicine has various perspectives on how children grow and develop. Most of them involve specific time scales. For example, Sun Simiao wrote that transformations and steamings (*bian zheng*) will have been completed within the first two years of life. The *Su Wen* describes distinct phases of a person's development that last seven years for a girl and eight years for a boy. The reality is far less black and white. A combination of the constitution of the child and the circumstances of her life means that certain aspects of development do not get completed. An eleven-year-old girl's physical development may be more typical of a fifteen-year-old but her emotional development may be more akin to that of a five-year-old. Therefore, with each child it is necessary to treat them in accordance with their level of development rather than simply according to their age.

A sixteen-year-old girl, who, due to a developmental disorder, had the emotional age of a six-year-old, responded to paediatric *tui na*, which is normally ineffective after the age of seven or eight.

Twenty-first-century children in the developed world struggle more with development than with growth

In previous eras, growth was a major problem (and currently is in certain parts of the world). There was often not enough food to go around, and a lack of medicine to treat childhood illnesses and infections. One of the reasons historically that women had so many children was the assumption that some of them would not survive into adulthood. Nowadays, in the so-called developed world, growth and survival are almost taken for granted. Development, on the other hand, has become much more challenging and troublesome.

In the UK, the infant mortality rate has been steadily declining since the 1960s.[17] Almost simultaneously, the number of developmental disorders, such as autistic spectrum disorders and attention deficit hyperactivity disorder (ADHD), has been increasing. The challenge with childhood today in the developed world is not how to survive it but how to emerge from it psychologically and emotionally fit and capable of living an independent, fulfilling and happy adult life.

SUMMARY

» Sun Simiao considered fevers an important and physiological part of childhood and one of the ways in which a child becomes more rooted in the world.

» Ideally, the focus of the first seven or eight years of life should be on supporting a child to gather in the resources he needs for strong growth and development.

» Between the ages of seven or eight and puberty, the task of children is to consolidate these resources.

» When a child is 'crossing' from one cycle to the next, he is particularly vulnerable to ill health but also has an opportunity to throw off illnesses.

» Adolescence is characterised by a surge in Kidney *yang*.

» The stereotypical moods and grumpiness of a teenager's years are often due to Liver *qi* stagnation.

» The Spleen comes under strain during adolescence as the child increases her food intake.

» If a certain aspect of development or growth was not completed at the expected time, the child has the opportunity to complete it during a different phase when circumstances may be more supportive.

» Children who visit acupuncture clinics in the developed world usually do so because of problems with development rather than growth.

• Chapter 4 •

INHERITED, PREGNANCY AND BIRTH FACTORS

The topics discussed in this chapter are:

* *Jing*
* Pregnancy factors
* Birth factors

Jing
Physical inheritance

Jing, usually translated as Essence, is the means by which imbalances in the *qi* are handed down from parent to child. One aspect of *jing*, which is termed 'pre-heavenly', comes about at the moment of conception from a blending of the *jing* of the mother and father. To some degree, the future health of the child is decided in this brief moment. Pre-heavenly *jing* also incorporates the nourishment that the growing foetus receives from the mother in the womb. For this reason, the health of the foetus is more influenced by the mother than the father.

There are some genetic conditions that are hereditary. They are straightforwardly passed down from parent to child via the *jing*. Other genetic conditions appear to arise from a spontaneous mutation in the genes, and yet others from an environmental trigger which affects a particular gene. In Chinese medicine terms, all these possibilities can be said to relate to pre-heavenly *jing*.

Jing, therefore, plays a large part in determining how strong a person's physical constitution is and what her particular susceptibilities to disease may be. *Jing* is stored in and governed by the Kidneys. However, its influence extends far beyond the Kidneys. Asthma, skin conditions, heart weaknesses and a multitude of other conditions affecting almost every part of the body may all be inherited, and therefore related to *jing*.

In particular, *jing* is said to follow cycles of approximately seven years in girls and eight years in boys. This goes some way to explaining the strong link between the age of onset of the menstrual cycle between a girl and her mother. The same applies for the age at which the menopause occurs; unless other significant health or environmental factors intervene, the age of menopause for mother and daughter is likely to be similar.

Emotional and psychological inheritance

What we inherit is certainly not confined to the physical body. The nature and health of a child's emotional and psychological world is in part handed down from her parents. The best term to describe this aspect of a child's being is *jingshen*, which means different things in different contexts. *The Spiritual Axis* (*Ling Shu*) says, 'The combination of blood and *qi*, the association of essences and spirits (*jingshen*), this is what makes life, perfectly fulfilling the natural destiny (*xing ming*) of each.'[18]

It is, of course, impossible to completely separate nature and nurture, but we see time and time again how children come into the world with similar emotional traits or propensities to one of their parents. We also see how very different each child's *shen* is. Whilst one sibling is naturally gregarious and bubbly, another may be quiet and contemplative. One child may sail through the challenges that life throws at her, whilst another may be floored by the smallest obstacle.

What constitutes a 'healthy' state of the parents?

If one or both of the parents is unhealthy at the time a baby is conceived, this imbalance in their *qi* may be passed on to the child. The term 'unhealthy' is a broad one. A parent may be healthy in the usual medical sense of the word, being free of disease. However, from the Chinese medicine perspective, they may be in a state of imbalance that becomes reflected in the foetus, baby and then child. If any of the following is present at the moment of conception, it may influence the child's constitution to some degree:

- A parent is particularly run down or exhausted.

- A parent is particularly stressed and anxious.

- A parent is under the influence of alcohol or recreational drugs.

- A parent is experiencing a particularly intense emotion, such as grief or anger.

On the other hand, a parent may be 'unhealthy' in the usual medical sense of the word but in a relative state of balance from the Chinese medical perspective. For example, the mother may suffer from Crohn's disease but be in a stable phase, eating a good diet and generally feeling well at the time of conception.

Pregnancy factors

When treating children, it is necessary to enquire about the mother's pregnancy so that we can better understand how the child has come to be ill. It may be possible to make suggestions for any future pregnancies. However, the past cannot be changed, and adding to a mother's already hefty dose of maternal guilt is entirely inappropriate and counter-productive.

The concept of *yang tai*, or 'nurturing the foetus', has been in existence in China since the early second century BCE. Its premise is that how a woman lives, eats, thinks and feels during her pregnancy will have an impact on the development, health and well-being of her baby. As Yousheng taught, 'From the beginning of pregnancy, the foetus grows by consuming the *qi* and Blood of the mother, and all the mother's joy or anger, cold or heat, activity or rest influence the child. The mother plants the seed, and the child bears the fruit.'[19]

Most mothers would say they feel intuitively that their state of mind and lifestyle during pregnancy will have an impact in some way on their baby. At the same time, knowledge of this may in itself feel like a pressure and adversely affect their state of mind. There was a time in the 20th century when mothers were blamed for everything that was 'wrong' with a child. It feels as if there has been a backlash to this and now women are given the message that, as long as they do not smoke, drink too much or eat certain foods, nothing else that they do or feel has much of an impact on their unborn baby.

Both of these views are somewhat missing the point. First, in Chinese culture, the state of the mother is not an isolated entity but dependent on the state of the whole 'unit', which would include the father, extended family and community. If the mother is not thriving, it is probably due to a malfunctioning in the family and wider community. Second, the view of Chinese medicine throughout the centuries is that the foetus and mother are one unit, so it is simply not plausible to suggest that everything that affects the mother will not also have an impact on the foetus. The 14th-century physician Zhu Danxi states:

While the child is in the uterus, it shares the same body with its mother. When there is heat, both become hot. When there is cold, both become cold. If there is disease, both are diseased. If healing occurs, both recuperate.[20]

The particular aspects of the pregnant woman's life that may affect the foetus are her:

- emotions
- physical activity
- rhythm and balance of life
- diet
- womb toxins
- womb diseases.

Emotions

Sun Simiao emphasised the importance of a good state of mind in pregnancy over and over again. Confirming this centuries-old knowledge, it is now known that the feeling states of the mother during pregnancy are transmitted to the foetus via shifts in hormonal and neuropeptide activity.[21] There is an ever-expanding body of research which shows that the foetus responds to maternal stress with his own stress response.[22] The emotional life of a pregnant woman is considered to be of the greatest importance during the first few months of pregnancy and less so in the latter stages.

Intense or prolonged emotions

Any emotion that is experienced over a long period of time during the mother's pregnancy, or even for a short time very intensely, will upset the *qi* of the mother in some way and have a similar impact on the baby. Sun Simiao said that during the third month of pregnancy the mother 'must avoid feelings of sorrow and grief, thought and preoccupation, fright and commotion'.[23]

Wang Fengyi* stressed that the most important thing for the mother was to achieve a peaceful, emotional state during her pregnancy. The stereotypical image comes to mind of a blissed-out pregnant woman, who floats around with a broad grin on her face, revelling in her state. As any woman who has been pregnant will know, the reality is often rather different. Pregnancies, particularly first ones, are often times of great change, stress and upheaval in a woman's life. The effort to achieve this 'peaceful state' can of its own accord take a woman further away from it. A balance needs to be found between holding an awareness of what the ideal may be and accepting that life is rarely, if ever, ideal.

Fear and fright

There is a particular emphasis in the classical texts on the need for a pregnant woman to avoid fear and fright. This includes one-off moments of alarm as well as more chronic states of agitation. In the *Nei Jing*, when asked why a baby may be ill from birth, Qi Bo answers, 'It is acquired in the abdomen. When the mother was extremely frightened, the *qi* rises and does not move down.'[24]

---

*   Wang Fengyi was a 19th-century healer and educator who introduced the Five Element style of 'virtue healing'.

The nourishment that a foetus receives in the womb comes primarily from the mother's Kidney *jing*. Fear is the emotion that resonates with the Kidneys, and this is perhaps why it was thought to be particularly detrimental during pregnancy. If fear makes the *qi* 'rise up' then the baby may not receive sufficient nourishment from the mother to develop and become constitutionally strong.

Any intense emotion, however, also affects the *shen* which resides in the Heart. There is a direct link between the Heart and the womb, via the *bao mai* extra channel. This may explain why any prolonged or intense emotion that affects the Heart of the mother may have a strong impact on the foetus. Babies who are born to women who have had a fright during pregnancy may be born with symptoms and signs of *shen* disturbance, such as poor sleep, jumpiness and an inability to settle.

> The mother of one boy who came for treatment for epileptic seizures told me that she had found out her mother had terminal cancer during the third month of her pregnancy. She had been profoundly shocked by this news and had always wondered if it had had an impact on her unborn child.

There are many childhood diseases which have historically been attributed to fright experienced by the mother whilst in the womb, or directly by the baby shortly after birth. For example, *The Secrets for Saving the Young* (*Hou You Xin Fa*), written by Nie Shang Heng during the Ming dynasty, talks of erysipelas in the baby being due to fright.[25] Sun Simiao's condition of Intrusive Upset (*ke wu*) is said to be due to a fright, caused by the baby being exposed suddenly to something unfamiliar. He also described a category of childhood seizures said to be caused by fright.

Anxiety

Sun Simiao stressed the importance of the mother having a calm state of mind during pregnancy. He wrote:

> *The most important thing for a pregnant woman's psyche is to always have a peaceful state of mind. If her heart and mind are not peaceful it brings harm to her body and is harmful for the foetus. The harm brought by anxiety is the greatest.*[26]

Wang Fengyi was more specific and said that anxiety in the mother would mean the baby would be born with a lack of courage. He also mentioned the very common anxiety of losing the child during pregnancy. Acupuncturists who work with women through fertility treatment, desperate and painful years of trying to conceive or through multiple miscarriages will know how pervasive this anxiety can be. It stems from the deep longing for a baby. However, many women in these scenarios are also particularly Kidney deficient, which makes them further prone to anxiety.

Maternal anxiety during pregnancy may lead to the baby being anxious, as she has imbibed the state of the mother throughout her nine months in the womb. A 2013 review in the *Journal of Child Psychology and Psychiatry* concluded that 'clinically significant links between maternal prenatal distress and child behavioral and cognitive outcomes have been reported'.[27] In particular links have been drawn between high levels of maternal anxiety and children with ADHD.

Physical activity

Sun Simiao wrote that in the seventh month, 'Have [the pregnant woman] tax her body and shake the limbs; do not allow her to be solid and motionless; make her engage in physical activities and bend and stretch, all in order to make the blood and *qi* flow.'[28] His words are reflected by modern attitudes. Women today with straightforward pregnancies are generally encouraged to exercise. There is an increasing swathe of evidence that points towards exercise during pregnancy having a vast range of benefits for both mother and baby. Pregnancy is a time of accumulation in the Lower Burner, which means that Liver *qi* tends to stagnate. Moderate movement and exercise help to prevent this natural stagnation becoming pathological.

However, we live in an exercise-conscious, one could argue exercise-obsessed, age. A moderate degree of exercise to keep the Blood and *qi* flowing is probably beneficial for most mothers and babies, but tough workouts in the gym and long runs, on the other hand, may be too depleting. If the mother's *qi* and Blood are diverted to meet the physical demands of exercise, the foetus may be less adequately nourished and the baby born deficient in *qi* and Blood. If exercise genuinely promotes the calm and well-being of the mother, it is probably a good thing for the foetus. If fitting the exercise into her busy schedule feels like an added pressure or she exercises to the point of exhaustion and does not balance it with enough rest, it is probably far from beneficial.

Rhythm and balance of life

A lifestyle that does not allow time for rest will deplete the Kidney *qi* of the mother, which will impact the *qi* and Blood of the foetus. It is hard work growing a baby, and ideally a woman will find a way to allow for this by adapting her lifestyle. Sadly, many women in the developed world are not supported during pregnancy in a way which makes this possible.

Finding a rhythm to life is also particularly important during pregnancy. Liu Yousheng* teaches that, 'During pregnancy, you must furthermore follow a consistent rhythm of work and rest, avoiding in particular to reverse day and night. To be active at night and to stay in bed during the day, this is harmful to the foetus health and growth.'[29]

A regular lifestyle, as opposed to a chaotic one, will become imprinted on the growing foetus who may then be more likely to settle into a balanced rhythm of feeding and sleeping after birth.

Diet

Sun Simiao's text includes very specific pieces of dietary advice for pregnant women, such as that a woman should eat the meat of birds of prey and wild beasts during the sixth month. The diet of most 21st-century women bears little resemblance to the women in Tang-dynasty China, so these specifics may make us raise an eyebrow but are of little clinical use.

The food that a pregnant woman eats is one of the key factors that determines the strength of her post-natal *qi*. The Spleen has a particularly important role in supporting the nourishment of the foetus. Therefore, the better her diet, the more post-natal *qi* there will be to nourish the growing foetus. It can appear miraculous that a baby born of a mother who vomited several times a day for the entire pregnancy is healthy and strong. In these circumstances, the mother's body cleverly prioritises the needs of the foetus. A woman who has suffered in this way throughout her pregnancy may be more depleted by the end of it because she has had to call upon her reserves of *qi* in order to nourish the foetus.

The way that a mother eats during pregnancy should be determined by her pre-existing tendencies and constitution. If she is prone to Damp, she should avoid too many Damp-forming foods. If she is Blood deficient, she should eat lots of Blood-nourishing foods. Any imbalance in the *qi* of the mother, which may be helped or hindered by her diet, will be passed on to the foetus.

However, there are some dietary habits in pregnancy which may negatively impact upon the *qi* of the growing foetus, regardless of the mother's pre-existing energetic state:

---

* Liu Yousheng is a living practitioner who follows the Confucian tradition of virtue healing promoted by Wang Fengyi.

- **A diet lacking in Blood-nourishing foods:** The foetus feeds off the *qi* and Blood of the mother in order to grow and develop. The tendency for women to become anaemic during pregnancy reflects the fact that Blood often becomes strained and depleted. Therefore, a diet which does not contain an abundance of Blood-nourishing foods, such as a poor vegetarian diet, may mean that both the mother and baby become *qi* and Blood deficient. It is striking that some women who have not eaten meat for years cannot resist eating steak when they are pregnant.

- **Too many heating foods:** Hot food, including alcohol, coffee, spicy food, shellfish and oranges, may create too much Heat in the foetus and agitate the nervous system. Some medications and recreational drugs will do the same. A woman who already has a Hot nature should be particularly careful with these.

- **Food additives:** Food additives generally create Heat in the system and may create an imbalance in the Liver of the foetus.

Womb toxins

Womb toxins may arise from foods or other substances which are not only unsuitable for the mother and foetus, but actually have the potential to cause harm. These toxins may include recreational drugs, such as heroin or cocaine, and pharmaceutical drugs, such as lithium, warfarin and ACE inhibitors, to name but a few. Various chemicals that may be present in some paints and glues, such as toluene, are also known to cause potential harm in the developing foetus when inhaled in large amounts.

Womb diseases

If the mother has an illness during pregnancy, this may be transmitted to the baby. Western medicine recognises that particular infections, such as rubella and toxoplasmosis, may have severe developmental consequences for the baby. However, from the Chinese medicine perspective, any illness in the mother may be transmitted to the foetus in the form of a Lingering Pathogenic Factor. It may not be that the baby has the same disease as the mother had, but one that has a similar energetic resonance.

> A mother brought her eleven-year-old daughter for treatment for behavioural problems. My diagnosis of the child was Heat in the Liver. The mother told me that she had developed acute fatty liver in the latter stages of her pregnancy, which in Chinese medicine is an exacerbation of Damp-Heat in the Liver. The child was born with a Liver imbalance, which probably came about in the womb. It had manifested as digestive symptoms in her early life and was now showing as behavioural problems.

A womb disease may be transmitted to the foetus as the maternal *qi* and Blood, which keep the foetus alive, are disturbed. It may also be passed on during birth via an infected birth canal, such as with the herpes simplex virus. Alternatively, it may be transmitted after birth during breastfeeding. The quality and quantity of breast milk is dependent on the state of *qi* and Blood of the mother.

Birth factors

Caesarean delivery

In some cases, caesarean deliveries save the lives of both mothers and babies. At the same time, they may have a negative impact on the *qi* of the baby. Some of the most common imbalances seen in babies born by caesarean section are the following:

- An elective caesarean birth, without any labour beforehand, means that the baby moves from the safety and warmth of the womb to the outside world within a few minutes without any warning or preparation. This may disturb the *shen* of the baby because it is a form of shock.

- The passage of the baby through the birth canal during a vaginal delivery is known to have several benefits. First, the baby picks up a layer of protective bacteria which is believed to strengthen the immune system and line the intestinal tract. Second, the muscles involved are thought to help the baby squeeze out amniotic fluid which may be in his lungs, thereby helping to avoid breathing difficulties after birth. It may be, therefore, that babies born by caesarean section are more prone to deficiency of *qi* in the Lungs and Large Intestine.

- A vaginal delivery requires hard work from both mother and baby. However, there is a benefit to this for the baby as long as the labour is not too long. To work his way down the birth passage means a baby needs to start exercising his muscles, which are governed by the Spleen. We can surmise, therefore, that a baby who is born by caesarean section has missed out on this opportunity and may have weaker Spleen *qi* as a result.

Forceps delivery

A baby's skull is made up of soft bony plates that are capable of compressing and overlapping in order to fit through the narrow birth canal. A baby also has one or two areas on his skull that are particularly soft, known as fontanelles; these are gaps in the bones of the skull which allow the brain to grow quickly in the first year of life. To clamp something which is relatively soft with a pair of hard, metal forceps can leave an energetic imprint in the *qi* of the head in the form of *qi* stagnation.

Difficult delivery

A difficult delivery may be due to many factors, such as poor birth management, umbilical cord compression, problems with the placenta, the position of the baby or the mother's emotional state. The importance of this transition from the safety of the womb to the harsh reality of the outside world can hardly be overstated. In many respects, it is the most vulnerable moment of a person's life. Sun Simiao devoted an entire chapter of the paediatric section of the *Bei Ji Qian Jin Yao Fang* to the moment of birth, discussing how best to manage it and some of the consequences of mismanagement.

A difficult delivery, especially one which involves birth asphyxia, may lead to lifelong developmental disorders, such as cerebral palsy and epilepsy. Symptoms may include mental retardation, spasticity, gait abnormality (ataxia) and involuntary movements (athetosis).

Long labour

Labour requires effort on the part of the baby as well as the mother. The baby needs to muster a lot of *qi* to work his way down the birth canal. A labour that lasts several days means the baby goes from having his every need met whilst in the womb to full-time work. This means that mother and baby, who are still so entwined after birth, both begin this new phase depleted, particularly in terms of Spleen *qi*.

Short labour

A very short labour, one which takes only a few minutes from start to finish, can have a similar impact on the *shen* of a baby to being born by caesarean section. The rapidity gives little time for the baby to prepare for its transition from womb to world and can leave the baby in a state of shock. Even an uncomplicated labour is stressful for a baby, evidenced by the fact that the baby produces large amounts of adrenaline and corticosteroids during labour. It is not hard to believe, therefore, that a very short labour may be even more stressful for the baby, leaving him prone to being born with a degree of *shen* disturbance.

> A mother brought her two-month-old baby to the clinic because he had barely slept and was not happy being put down. I diagnosed shock that I thought arose from the labour which had only been five minutes from beginning to end. I treated He 7 *shenmen* and taught the mother a paediatric *tui na* routine to calm the *shen* and within a week he was much calmer and sleeping.

Premature birth

The Lungs are the last Organ to fully form in a foetus. Just as with every aspect of the foetus, their formation relies solely on the mother's *qi*, Blood and *jing*. If a baby is born prematurely, he has to complete this work himself using his own supply of *qi*. Therefore, a premature baby may have poor respiratory function in the short or long term. It is widely recognised that babies born prematurely have a significantly higher incidence of lung problems such as wheezing and asthma when they are older (please see Chapter 53).

The digestive system is also not fully formed in a premature baby. The Spleen and Stomach of a newborn is under great strain as it has to immediately take over the work that was carried out by the umbilical cord and placenta. In a premature baby, this strain is greater and the chances of a digestive imbalance are increased.

Pain relief, anaesthetics and antibiotics during labour

Anaesthetics are energetically Cold. Mother and baby are one unit, and therefore anaesthetics given to the mother during labour will also have an impact on the *qi* of the baby. Many babies born to mothers who need anaesthetics or antibiotics during labour are born with a Cold and deficient digestive system. Even Entonox (nitrous oxide, often called 'gas and air'), which relieves pain in the mother, may disperse the *qi* of the child and cause it to be deficient.

However, the effects of birth may all be strongly mitigated by good-quality care and nurturing after birth.

Circumstances immediately after birth

As the British comedian John Cleese put it, 'Being born brings a distinct change in one's life-style, doesn't it?'[30]

In the womb, a baby has everything done for it. Breathing and digestion are all taken care of by the mother. The environment is warm, dark, safe and quiet. From the moment of birth, the change for the baby could hardly be starker (especially if he is born in a bright and noisy environment) or the learning curve steeper. Times of change are also times of great vulnerability, to the physical body and to emotional health. Therefore, anything that takes place during this precious time immediately after birth may have a profound impact on the child.

The following factors may all disturb the *shen* of a newborn baby:

- separation from the mother
- any medical interventions such as vitamin K injections, vaccinations or eye drops
- not being kept warm
- panic or anxiety in surrounding healthcare professionals or family members.

Of course, it is not always possible to create the perfect environment for a baby who has just emerged from the womb. Some babies, depending on their emotional constitution, will be able to cope better than others with a less than ideal post-birth environment. As practitioners, however, we need to be aware that *shen* disturbance in a child may be traced back to this time.

Conclusion

Inherited, pregnancy and birth factors stand out from other causes of disease in that, after the event, there is absolutely nothing we can do to change them. Furthermore, if a woman's pregnancy or the birth of her child did not go as she wished, she is sometimes full of guilt, sadness or anger, or a mix of emotions, for many years afterwards. Similarly, parents easily blame themselves if their child inherits ill health from them.

Therefore, whilst it is important to ask about these factors, it is paramount that we do so in a way which will not compound any conflicted feelings the mother has about them. On the contrary, we may be able to reassure the mother of a baby or young child that acupuncture treatment will help to correct any imbalance that may be present. This will usually help the mother to let go of any guilt she may be harbouring.

SUMMARY

» *Jing* determines, in part, the psychological and emotional traits of a child, as well as the physical ones.

» The mother's emotional world, lifestyle and diet all impact the developing foetus.

» Circumstances surrounding birth may leave an imprint on the *qi* of the baby.

» This may be compounded or mitigated by the circumstances immediately after birth.

• Chapter 5 •

EMOTIONS
· · · · · · · · · · · · · · · · · · · ·

The topics discussed in this chapter are:

- Nature versus nurture

- Emotions as a cause of disease

- How do emotions become a cause of imbalance in children?

- Emotions affect the child's spirit

- The seven emotions

Nature versus nurture

Children do not arrive in the world as blank slates. Every parent will know that the seeds of their child's personality are often present from the moment they are born. One child appears to have a contented and carefree demeanour, whilst another brings with her a large dose of existential angst. The nature versus nurture debate will no doubt continue to rage for many decades to come, and may never be fully resolved.

From the Chinese medicine perspective, the key point is that the interaction between a child's constitutional emotional nature and the circumstances and events of her life has the potential to create an internal imbalance in the *qi* of her Organs to some degree. Some life events, such as the misfortune of growing up without the basics of love and security, are likely to be a cause of imbalance whatever the child's constitutional emotional nature. Other events, such as the parents divorcing, may be a major trigger for imbalance for one child but not for another.

For example, a family are moving to a new town because the father has found a job. The parents decide to tell their five children whilst they are all eating supper. Each of the five children responds in a different way, as follows:

- One child responds with anger and shouts, 'But I don't *want* to leave. I had it all planned out that I was going to join the new football league here next season. I'm not going to go. You can't *make* me go.'

- The next child sounds worried and says, 'But how will we get to see Grandma so often if we move? And will I have to go to a different school? And how will you meet me from school, Dad, if you have a new job?'

- The next child looks sad and begins to cry. Later on at bedtime, she says, 'I will miss this house and my school so much.'

- Another child seems fearful of the new start and says, 'But we don't know anybody in this new town. I've heard it has a rough part to it. Everything will be so new and unknown.'

(And, just as the parents think they can't take any more...)

- The last child looks hurt and rejected and says, 'But if you loved me, you wouldn't make me move. You wouldn't make me leave all my friends.'

As practitioners, the focus should always be on careful observation of how a child has reacted to events in her life so far. Focusing on the event, rather than the child's response, betrays an underlying assumption that children all react to life in the same way. This is to miss the fundamental point that children are unique and that treating them should always be approached with this in mind.

Emotions as a cause of disease

Emotions are considered to be internal causes of disease. The *San Yin Fang* describes seven emotions. These are anger (*nu*), excess joy (*xi le*), sadness (*bei*), grief (*you*), overthinking or worry (*si*), fear (*kong*) and shock (*jing*). These translations should not be taken too narrowly, however. Anger, for example, also covers related feelings such as irritation, resentment, frustration and fury. Fear encompasses other related emotions such as anxiety and terror.

Feeling a wide range of emotions is a normal part of being human and life would be very one-dimensional if we did not. Chinese medicine does not consider emotions as a cause of disease in themselves. They only become detrimental to a child's well-being if they are felt particularly intensely, if they are experienced over a long period of time, or if they are repressed or unresolved. A chaotic emotional life, where a child experiences many different, intense emotions much of the time, may also create imbalances in many Organs and Elements.

Emotions can be both a cause and a manifestation of disease. Any emotion, whether experienced consciously or not, affects the flow of *qi* in a particular Organ and Element. Prolonged, intense, repressed or unresolved emotions have the potential to disrupt it. Once the flow of *qi* in a particular Organ is disrupted, the expression of the linked emotion may become distorted. There is a circle of interaction between the Organs and their related emotion (see Figure 5.1). For example, if a child experiences particularly intense or prolonged fear, her Kidney *qi* is likely to become weakened as a result. This in turn may mean that she finds herself prone to being fearful.

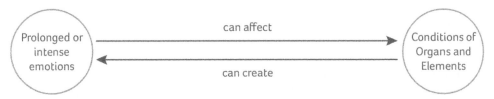

Figure 5.1 Interaction between emotions and their related Organs and Elements

How do emotions become a cause of imbalance in children?

> *Heaven lies about us in our infancy yet shades of the prison-house begin to close around the growing boy.*
>
> Wordsworth[31]

Chinese medical textbooks barely mention the emotions as a cause of disease in children. English-language books on TCM paediatrics generally only consider emotions as a cause of disease from the age of about seven or eight. This is because children are not generally believed to suppress their emotions until this time. Scott and Barlow, for example, say that young children 'usually do not restrain their emotions'.[32] They mention illnesses such as hay fever being rarely seen before the age of seven or eight because 'this is the age when the emotions develop and become controllable'.[33] However, there are other means by which emotions can have a profoundly deleterious effect and cause illness even in babies and toddlers.

Habitual or prolonged emotions

A particular emotion may become habitual in a child. Rather than having a reasonably balanced default emotional state, a child may have a strong tendency towards, for example, sadness or fear. Whatever happens in her life, she tends to respond to it with this emotion. This is largely determined by the child's emotional constitution. A child with a predisposition to feel hurt and rejected may feel this way when her best friend moves away, her mother starts working longer hours or she is dropped from the tennis team at school. Another child may respond to these same events with an entirely different emotion, such as anger or anxiety.

If a child has a tendency to respond to events in a certain way, then that emotion becomes habitual for her. Her *qi* becomes further disordered as a result. Worry, for example, knots *qi*. This may, over time, affect any of the functions of the Spleen and lead to a range of physical and/ or psychological symptoms. A vicious circle ensues as knotted *qi* will also perpetuate the child's tendency to worry.

Intense emotions

Depending on the nature of her emotional constitution, a child may be prone to expressing a particular emotion or several emotions with intensity. She may begin to get in trouble at school because when she gets angry, she has an explosion of physical rage. Or she becomes upset every time a child does not want to play with her and remains upset for the rest of the day. Or a feeling of fear may spiral into a panic attack.

Every child will experience intense emotions from time to time and this, in itself, is not a cause of imbalance. However, when it happens on a frequent basis over a prolonged period, imbalance may arise. This is sometimes the case in a household which is full of emotional melodrama and where the only way to express emotion is with great intensity.

Any emotion that has become pathologically intense may bring about disorder of one kind or another in the child's *qi*. In an ideal world, the movement of *qi* brought about by the emotion will be short-lived and a state of equilibrium will soon be reached again. If the child is unable to do it on her own or does not get help to reestablish her equilibrium, or if the intense emotion or emotions come frequently, the *qi* remains disordered. A vicious circle arises whereby the child's intense emotions disrupt the movements of *qi* which in turn bring about more intense expression of the emotion. This may cause physical or psychological symptoms further down the line.

Sometimes a one-off incident in a child's life creates an intense emotion, echoes of which may stay with her for decades. This may also partly determine how the child responds to any future event which resonates with the original one. For example, if a mother and young child are separated for a prolonged period because the mother has to be in hospital, it may affect the child so strongly that she never really returns to a state of balance. The difficult feelings that the separation induced in the child are so profound that they almost become imprinted on her *qi*. Of course, exactly how it will affect her will depend on the nature of her emotional constitution.

Repressed emotions

A child may also repress an emotion rather than actually feel it. This may happen for various reasons which are discussed in Chapter 6. If an emotion is repressed, it disturbs the smooth flow of *qi* more than if it is expressed. If a child is discouraged from expressing anger, for example, it does not mean that the feeling goes away, it is usually just buried deeper within her. Instead of a temporary upwards movement of *qi* that accompanies the healthy expression of anger, the *qi* is likely to stagnate or become constrained. If a child is not able to verbalise worry and receive appropriate reassurance from a parent, the *qi* of her Spleen is likely to remain knotted. If a child suppresses her fear because she senses she may be ridiculed for expressing it, the *qi* of her Water Element will over time become depleted as a result. When any pathological movement of *qi* goes on for a lengthy period, it will often lead to psychological and/or physical symptoms developing.

There is, of course, a middle way between a child expressing every emotion at the moment she is feeling it, and repressing emotions to the degree that they are rarely expressed. Very few children (or adults) find this middle way but most are able to remain relatively healthy and happy if they do not veer too far from it. It is when a child's emotional life remains too close to one end of the spectrum or the other that disease and unhappiness are likely to arise.

Emotions affect the child's spirit

When the flow of *qi* in an Organ is disrupted by an emotion, it is likely to affect a child's spirit. This is in contrast to the disruption that results from an invasion by an External Pathogenic Factor, for example, which tends to affect the physical body. If a child has a bad cold that temporarily depletes Lung *qi*, it is likely to leave her with a physical ailment such as tiredness or a chronic cough. In contrast, if she experiences a loss or a sense of sadness that depletes the *qi* of her Lungs and/or Heart, it is likely to impact her spirit. *Su Wen* Chapter 5 clearly explains, 'The emotions of joy and anger are injurious to the spirit (*shen*). Cold and heat are injurious to the body.'[34]

This quotation only refers to two emotions and two External Pathogenic Factors. However, just as a particular Pathogenic Factor tends to affect a certain Organ, for example Damp affects the Spleen, different emotions also resonate with certain Organs (see the section 'The seven emotions' below).

Spirit means different things to different people. The words *shen* and *jingshen* are often translated as spirit. Larre described the *shen* as 'that by which a given being is unlike any other; that which makes an individual an individual and more than a person'.[35]

The practitioner may suspect that the child's spirit has been affected if, for example:

- he lacks the emotional and physical vitality that is usual in a young child

- he is agitated, hyperactive or cannot sleep

- he appears to have retreated into himself

- he has developed aggressive or out-of-control behaviour.

However, once a child's spirit has become compromised in some way, the body often responds with a physical ailment (see Figure 5.2). The *Dong Yi Bao Jian* states, 'The *shen* is the ruler of the whole body. It controls the seven affects. Harming the *shen* will result in illness.'[36]

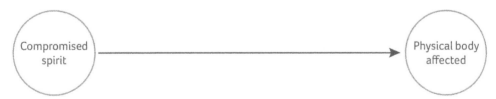

Figure 5.2 Interaction between the spirit and body

The seven emotions

Su Wen Chapter 39 describes the emotions and the effect they may have upon a person's *qi*. Although all emotions have an impact on the Heart, other Organs are affected too. *Su Wen* Chapters 4 and 5 set out the way in which particular emotions affect different Organs.

Joy (*xi le*)

The emotion of joy resonates with the Heart and the Fire Element. There are two key characters for this emotion. The first is *xi*.

This character conveys an image of singing and making music, giving the impression of people together enjoying themselves.

The second character is *le*.

This character depicts a person with internal harmony and unity and is also related to music.

Most references to joy in the classics of Chinese medicine relate to the harmful effects of excess joy. *Su Wen* Chapter 39 says that, 'When there is elation, *xi*, the *qi* becomes loose.'[37] Larre and Rochat de la Vallée explain that 'loose' in this sense means 'tiredness and over-emotionalism'. This is easily observable in young children who sometimes become out of control and agitated when they get over-excited. Most young children struggle to get off to sleep, wake up early or both in the run up to Christmas or a similarly exciting occasion. A child who is over-excited at her birthday party may suddenly switch to being unhappy and crying. The excess joy has become too much and the strong movements of *qi* have knocked her emotional and physical equilibrium.

However, excess joy rarely actually causes long-term illness. It is more likely in a child to cause a temporary upset. In contrast, an absence of joy (*bu le*) is a common cause of disease. A lack of warm relationships, happiness and fun often means that the Organs related to the Fire Element become deficient. Warmth and intimacy with other people create feelings of joy and happiness which feed the Fire Element. Feelings of joy and happiness enable the *qi* of the Fire Element and its associated Organs to remain vibrant and circulate properly. These feelings may be lacking in a child's life if she does not feel intimately connected with her family members or is neglected, or because the rest of the family are unhappy. It is very hard for a child to thrive in an unhappy household. As a child gets older, close connections with people outside the family become more important to her. It is hard for a child to remain vibrant and joyful if she has not found friends she feels close to at school.

 Lack of joy is a more common cause of long-term imbalance in children than excess joy (which is more likely to cause a temporary upset in the *qi*).

Sadness (*bei*)

Bei refers to a state of sadness and melancholy which, when intense, is akin to a feeling of heartbreak or devastation.

悲

The character conveys a sense of brutal sadness, desolation or loss.

This emotion tends to suppress the *qi* of the Heart and the Fire Element, but may also affect the Lungs and the Metal Element. The *Su Wen* states:

> When there is sadness, the *qi* disappears… When there is sadness, the system of the heart, *xin yi*, is tightened, the lung dilates and its leaves rise up. The upper heater no longer ensures its free communications, nutrition and defence are not diffused, the overheated *qi* is at the centre, *zhong*. This is how the *qi* disappears.[38]

A child may experience sadness for many reasons: for example, she has to leave her friends behind when she moves to a different school, or her parents no longer live together, or a friend, relative or much-loved pet dies. It is common to hear parents say that their child 'does not seem to be affected' by a move or a divorce. This perception that children are very adaptable may have some truth in it but it also means that the sad feelings a child has may not be acknowledged or recognised. They may then make themselves apparent through some kind of physical ailment because children often find it hard to articulate their feelings.

Older children and teenagers may experience sadness (*bei*) as they negotiate the turbulent world of best friends and first romances. Teenage girls especially may go through phases when they have a different best friend each week. The rollercoaster of feeling loved one minute and rejected the next, and the feelings of heartbreak and sadness that this induces, may take its toll on the robustness of her Heart or Lung *qi*.

Overthinking or worry (*si*)

Overthinking or worry is one of the emotions connected with the Spleen and the Earth Element. The character which depicts this state is *si*.

思

The character conveys the idea of both the brain and the Heart being involved in order for thinking to be focused and to avoid becoming repetitive.

Chapter 39 of *Su Wen* describes the effect on the *qi* of overthinking and worry, saying that 'when there is obsessive thought (*si*), the *qi* is knotted (*jie*)'.[39] Knotted *qi* has some similarities to stagnant *qi* in that the flow has become impaired. The child finds her thoughts become stuck or go around and around. It can become hard for her to translate thought into action. This is a very common situation in children who are prone to worry, and tends to worsen during times they are studying hard. If an event about which the child is preoccupied (such as an exam) is looming, her thoughts about it may become obsessive. Ironically, this preoccupation makes it hard for her to act in a way which would alleviate the worry – that is, revising. Overthinking or worry may also make it hard for a child to begin an activity or a piece of work. The knotted *qi* prevents her from being able to take the first step towards action.

Grief (*you*)

Grief is the emotion associated with the Lungs and the Metal Element. The character for grief is *you*.

> At the top of the character *you* is the head. In the middle is the heart, and beneath them are dragging legs with the idea of going along with troubles in the head and the heart. It means sadness, grief, sorrow or melancholy and oppression.[40]

However, *you* is sometimes also translated as oppression or worry and can be associated with other Elements too.

Grief is often less obvious in a child than sadness (*bei*) because it is usually carried very deeply and not expressed. A child who is experiencing grief may be sparkly and cheery on the outside because she is in denial of her grief or has buried it deep inside. As a result of this, her bright demeanour does not actually ring true or draw other children to her. She may come across as somewhat emotionally cold or inert, despite the cheerful facade. It is as if she is having to work hard to hold herself together so that she does not become overwhelmed by her feelings.

Sometimes in the English language, grief is only perceived as a response to the death of a loved one. However, grief may arise as a response to the same life events that produce sadness (as described earlier), and it is often associated with a painful separation as well as loss. There are many events and situations that could fill a child with grief. She may mourn the loss of a simpler time when she goes through puberty, or a time when her older sibling was happy to play with her. She may be sent off to boarding school and yearn to be at home with her family. Or she may desperately miss an older sibling when he has left home and she is the only one left. One child may go through childhood without any feelings of grief or sadness. Another, in part due to her constitutional tendency for the 'sad' family of feelings, may regularly respond to events with a feeling of grief.

> Sometimes grief is experienced as a strong yearning. One boy who came to the clinic with a chronic cough yearned constantly for his grandmother since she had died three years previously. Treatment of his Lungs enabled him to let go of the yearning and also stopped his cough.

Fear (*kong*)

The emotion of fear predominantly resonates with the Kidneys and the Water Element. The character which is used to describe fear is *kong*.

The character conveys the idea of fear causing a person to feel agitated on the inside, and frozen and paralysed on the outside.

The *Su Wen* says, 'When there is fear, *kong*, the *qi* descends... When there is fear, the essences withdraw; withdrawing, the upper heater closes; closing, the *qi* leaves; leaving, the lower heater is swollen. This is how the *qi* does not circulate.'[41]

This quote mentions two important effects of a child feeling fear. First, that it causes *qi* to descend; bedwetting in children is an example of this. It is common for a child to wet her bed if she has had an upsetting experience or is anxious about something. Second, it implies that there is a disruption of the flow of *qi* between the Upper and Lower Burners. This may manifest in asthma, for example, when it is caused by the Kidneys not grasping *qi*.

Fear may result from a one-off situation such as getting lost in a shop. It also describes chronic, low-grade anxiety. For example, a child may be afraid of a teacher because she shouts. She may experience feelings of dread about facing a child who has bullied her. Fear is generally focused on something that may (or may not) happen in the future about which the child has a tendency to create catastrophic fantasies. For example, she may become convinced that one of her parents is going to die. In some way, she has lost her innate sense of trust in the world.

Anger (*nu*)

The emotion of anger resonates with the Liver and the Wood Element. The character for anger is *nu*.

The character depicts a female slave, or a woman held down by the hand of a master.[42] This clearly conveys an image of anger that is being held in and repressed.

The *Su Wen* describes some of the effects of anger on the *qi*: 'When there is anger the *qi* goes into countercurrent... This is how the *qi* rises up.'[43]

This upward moving, *yang* emotion is often what enables a child to bring about a change in circumstances that limit or frustrate her. The very fact of being a child can produce a lot of frustration. A young child has very little power, either in her relationship with her parents or in the world in general. There are many things she would like to be able to do that she cannot yet do. She may not have the words to express what she would like to say or the physical ability to climb in the playground the way she sees older children doing. A toddler sometimes has such strong feelings of anger that they cause wide-ranging disruption. Tantrums are essentially an explosion of frustration and anger. The child may go red in the face, throw herself on the floor, scream and tense her body. A teenager may be either resentful or furious that her parents will not let her go out with her friends or that they will not buy her the kind of designer clothes her friends have.

The experience and expression of anger in appropriate circumstances is normal and does not necessarily generate problems. However, anger that is not recognised, expressed or resolved is likely to lead to an imbalance in *qi*. The natural movement of Liver *qi* is outwards. Unexpressed anger often leads the Liver *qi* to become constrained or stagnant.

Shock (*jing*)

The character for shock is *jing*.

The character suggests a person who is trembling on the inside but trying to appear still and self-possessed on the outside.

Shock makes the *qi* disperse and scatter, and suddenly depletes it. Zhang Jiebin said that with shock 'the spirits are frightened, and they disperse'.[44] In a young child, *qi* tends to scatter in a counterflow, upward direction. This may have severe consequences at a time when *qi* should ideally be gathered in and grounded.

Shock affects the Heart in the first instance. As the *Su Wen* says, after a shock 'the Heart no longer has a place to rely on'.[45] It is the suddenness of a shock which jolts the *shen* out of its resting place in the Heart. The child no longer feels steady in the world. When severe or prolonged, shock may also reach the Kidneys. This is because the body then reaches into its reserves, in the form of Kidney Essence, in an attempt to compensate for the sudden depletion of *qi*. When this happens, the balanced flow of *qi* between the Heart and the Kidneys becomes disrupted.

Most young children are particularly susceptible to the effects of shock. Their vulnerable and volatile *qi* are not yet robust enough to withstand sudden and strong influences from the external environment that would not even register in the consciousness of an adult or indeed another child. For example, there may be something about a character in a book or a film that is shocking to a child. Shock left untreated in a child may have harmful consequences for years to come.

> An eleven-year-old girl came to the clinic because she was having repeated panic attacks. These had begun after she had fallen off her bike into the road and only narrowly avoided being hit by a car. Her panic attacks were clearly traceable back to this shock. Simple treatment on her Heart stopped the panic attacks.

SUMMARY

» Emotions may affect the flow of *qi* in an Organ and Element and cause it to become pathological.

» This may happen only when an emotion is either habitual, prolonged, particularly intense or repressed.

» It is likely to manifest initially as a pathology in the child's spirit.

» A compromised spirit often leads to the physical body being affected.

» Joy tends to affect the Heart and the Fire Element and makes *qi* loose.

» Sadness tends to deplete the *qi* of the Heart and the Fire Element, and/or Lungs and the Metal Element.

» Overthinking or worry tend to knot the *qi* of the Spleen and the Earth Element.

» Grief is often hidden deep within a child and tends to impact the *qi* of the Lungs and the Metal Element.

» Fear tends to affect the Kidneys and the Water Element, and makes *qi* descend.

» Shock causes the *qi* of the Heart to scatter and may also affect the Kidneys.

• Chapter 6 •

THE ROLE OF THE FAMILY

The emotional environment of the family plays an enormous role in shaping the emotional and physical life of the growing child. A baby's cry is just as likely to be related to a disturbance in the functioning of the family as it is to physical discomfort. This chapter's discussion of the role of the family in shaping the child's emotional life is divided into the following sections:

- Imbibing the mother's emotional state

- Absorbing the wider atmosphere

- Unacceptable emotions in the family

- Over-parenting

- Lack of parenting

- The fit between the parents and the child

- The family under strain

- The family needing the child to be ill

Imbibing the mother's emotional state

 'Mother', in this context, refers to the main caregiver. This of course could be any male or female adult. I have used the word 'mother' because in the past, and still in the majority of cases today, the mother is the main caregiver for most babies and young children.

In most cases, the mother and child function largely as a unit for the first years of the child's life and their *qi* is therefore intertwined. As Fromm wrote:

> The effect [of the mother's emotions] on the child can hardly be exaggerated. Mother's love for life is as infectious as her anxiety is. Both attitudes have a deep effect on the child's whole personality; one can distinguish indeed, among children – and adults – those who got only 'milk' and those who got 'milk and honey'.[46]

Most parents recognise that their mood on a particular day is often reflected in the mood of their child. When they are stressed and irritable, the baby may be fractious and hard to settle. When they are tired and feel like they have nothing left to give, their young child may be clingy and demand even more than usual. On days when they feel happy and relaxed, the child tends to follow suit. If children so clearly mirror the internal state of their parents from moment to moment, then it is no surprise that the same thing also happens on a longer-term basis.

Novelists, doctors and psychologists have long recognised the link between the emotional state of the mother and that of her child. In the 19th-century American novel *The Scarlet Letter*, Hawthorne writes of the protagonist Hester Prynne and her baby Pearl:

For the child; who, drawing its sustenance from the maternal bosom, seemed to have drank in with it all the turmoil, the anguish, and despair, which pervaded the mother's system. It now writhes in convulsions of pain, and was a forcible type, in its little frame, of the moral agony which Hester Prynne had borne throughout the day.[47]

This idea has also been a part of Chinese medicine at least since 600 AD. Sun Simiao talks in *Essential Prescriptions Worth a Thousand in Gold for Every Emergency* (*Bei Ji Qian Jin Yao Fang*) of the effect of the mother's emotional state on the child: 'If a mother is angry and nurses a baby in this condition, the results [in the baby] are a tendency to fright…while also causing qi ascent and dian insanity and kuang mania.'[48]

Of course, it is not only the mother's anger that may impact the child. There are many other possible emotional events that have a similar effect. For example:

- the mother's emotional life during pregnancy

- shock or trauma that the mother experiences during childbirth

- post-natal depression in the mother

- parents having a blazing row in the presence of the baby or toddler

- the mother being very agitated or anxious

- the mother feeling unloved, alone or unsupported.

> The connection between mother and child is concerned with *qi*. It describes situations where subtle imbalances of *qi* in the mother cause subtle imbalances of *qi* in the young child. It is certainly *not* the case that these dynamics come about with any conscious intent. Nearly all parents do the best for their children that they possibly can, but harmful dynamics arise nevertheless. Life is imperfect. It is hard for parents to witness their child not thriving, especially if they sense that their best is not in some way good enough for their child. As practitioners, our role is to support and inform, and *never* to blame.

Absorbing the wider atmosphere

It is not only the mother's state which has an influence in the first months and years of life. Young children are like delicate shoots that are at the mercy of their environment. They are, to a large degree, moulded by the external world with which they come into contact. A child is deeply affected by the people and atmosphere around him.

Every family or household has a certain emotional tone or flavour, which results from the mix of people who form a part of it. For example:

- There may be lots of jollity and happiness in the family.

- There may be a predominance of unhappiness in the household.

- There may be lots of worry, agitation and anxiety.

- One or both parents may be chronically angry.

The child may absorb any of these emotions, and others, as if he were a sponge and begin to reflect them himself. In many cases the emotional mood of the family is reasonably harmonious and happy, but, if it is not, it will deleteriously affect the movements of *qi* within the child. The way in which a child's *qi* becomes disrupted depends on his emotional constitution. For example, one child may express the anger he senses around him in his behaviour, becoming aggressive and argumentative. Another child may respond by becoming very fearful and retreating into his shell. And another may feel responsible and seek to mediate between other family members.

Children often reflect the environment in which they grow, in the same way that plants and trees do. For example, the spiky and hard exterior of a cactus is a reflection of the harsh desert environment in which it has grown.

> A forty-four-year-old mother brought her baby to the clinic because he was fractious and not sleeping. It seemed to me he was reflecting the state of his mother, who was struggling to make the switch to motherhood after spending two decades in a 'big' job in the corporate world.

The impact of the mother's state and the emotional environment on the child

Absorbing an emotion from a parent or the family environment can adversely affect the movement of *qi* just as it would if the emotion arose in the child. For example:

- If there is a lot of sadness (*bei*) and grief (*you*) in the household, then the *qi* of the child's Lungs and/or Heart may 'disappear'.

- If there is a lot of worry (*si*) in the household, then the *qi* of the child may become 'knotted'.

- If there is a lot of anger (*nu*) in the household, then the *qi* of the child may become constrained or he may develop aggressive behaviour.

The presence of a strong emotion in the atmosphere may flood the child and cause havoc in his spirit, in the same way that an invasion from a climatic External Pathogenic Factor may do in his body. The Organ most affected may be the one that is associated with that particular emotion. For example, the Liver is most prone to being affected by anger, the Heart by a lack of joy and the Lungs by sadness. However, it is not quite as straightforward as this. Any emotion may impact the movements of *qi* in any Organ. It is sometimes the Organ that is most vulnerable in a particular child, due to the child's constitutional imbalance, that will become the most dysfunctional.

Of course, the fact that a child imbibes his emotional environment need not cause a pathology. Indeed, a child who is surrounded by relative happiness and a balanced expression of a wide range of emotions is in a fortunate position. He is a child who, to use Fromm's phrase, got the milk and the honey too.

Unacceptable emotions in the family

A child may pick up the message from his parents that certain emotions are disapproved of, or taboo.

> You find that in each family some emotions are regarded as 'good' and some as 'bad'. The bad ones get put behind the screen and the entire family has a kind of unspoken but very powerful agreement that the feelings behind the screen mustn't be noticed. Everyone in the family pretends they're not there. So each new child learns to put the same things behind the screen too. The habit of screening them off gets passed on, like the measles, quite unintentionally, without anyone knowing that it's happening.[49]

For example, a child may find that, when he is angry, his parents give him the message that he is 'wrong' to feel that way. They may shame him, punish him or become emotionally distant.

Broadly speaking, there are two possible responses a child may have to screened-off emotions within the family:

- suppression of the unacceptable emotion
- expression of the unacceptable emotion.

> A five-year-old once came for treatment for hay fever. Whilst chatting to him, he began telling me how cross he was. Whenever he squabbled with his younger sister, she would run crying to his parents and he would get the blame. His father interrupted him by saying, 'Don't be angry, there is no need to feel angry.' This was a good example of a young child learning that expressing a certain emotion will bring him disapproval.

Suppression of the unacceptable emotion

A young child depends on his parents for his survival. Therefore, the most common response to the sense that a particular emotion is strongly disapproved of is to suppress it. This suppression may begin in childhood and go on for a lifetime. It takes place without the child, or the parents, having any conscious idea that it is happening.

This denial of an emotion has a strong effect on a child's *qi*. If anger, for example, is suppressed, it will have a stronger and more lasting impact on the *qi* than if it is expressed and discharged. The natural upward surge of *qi* will be inhibited and may become constrained as a result. This may eventually cause physical symptoms and will predispose the child to a more imbalanced expression of anger in the future.

As a child goes through adolescence, the picture may become more complicated. If an emotion has been taboo in the family, and consequently suppressed, he may feel he is 'wrong' to have such a feeling and even be shameful about it. He may develop behavioural strategies to avoid feeling that emotion. For example, self-harming in some cases may be an expression of a child 'punishing himself' for having a particular feeling. Or he may find that if he exercises compulsively he no longer feels so tense and angry. These behaviours may in themselves become causes of disease.

Another way for a child to deal with an unacceptable emotion is by replacing it with a more acceptable one. For example, if neediness is taboo, the child may become grumpy or irritable instead because that is better tolerated within the family. Or, if the parents are not comfortable with sadness and similar emotions, the child may replace those feelings with angry ones instead.

Expression of the unacceptable emotion

The opposite reaction to repressing a taboo emotion is for a child to express the emotion on behalf of the family. There are a couple of aspects to this:

- A child may express something that is unexpressed in one or both of the parents or in a sibling.
- He may manifest a silent dynamic that exists between the parents, or between a parent and a sibling, for example underlying resentment or rage.

To return to Hawthorne's mother and child, Hester and Pearl: 'Pearl…betrayed…the emotions which none could detect in the marble passiveness of Hester's brow.'[50]

Ironically, because the repressed emotion is often one that the parent has tried to deny, seeing it expressed by his child may mean his tolerance for it is particularly low. He finds that it presses his buttons and he reacts especially strongly. If a parent has partially created an identity around being always cheerful and sparkly, he is likely to have little tolerance towards a child who has a melancholic nature. His tendency may be to jump in with statements like 'Don't be sad' or 'You really need to cheer up', which he may express with a degree of crossness. Other examples:

- A child may be prone to outbursts of anger, which makes the parent feel uncomfortable and so the child gets punished for it.

- A child may be prone to anxiety and worry, which touches into the parent's own suppressed feelings of anxiety. So the parent responds with statements such as 'Don't be silly, there is nothing to worry about'. The child is left feeling he is wrong to have the emotion or is somehow inadequate for feeling it.

Over-parenting

Over the past few decades, parents have become ever more heavily involved in all aspects of their children's lives. Whilst there is no perfect way to parent, and every approach has its potential pitfalls, a heavily involved style of parenting may in some cases contribute to both physical and psychological ill health in children.

Many children today live as if they are under a permanent microscope. There are many possible reasons for this. For example:

- Most families have fewer children than in the past. There are fewer children on whom parents may place their hopes and dreams.

- For some couples, their quest to conceive has been fraught with difficulty and a cherished child comes after years of frustration and disappointment.

- The world outside is perceived, rightly or wrongly, to be a far more dangerous place than it once was.

- There is increased competition for school places.

- In many parts of the world, unemployment rates have increased, meaning there is more parental anxiety about whether their children will find work as adults.

All of these factors have shaped the way that many people parent today, leading to concepts such as the 'tiger mum' and 'helicopter parent'. There are various aspects of this parenting style, all of which may place a physical or psychological burden on a child. These are:

- over-attentiveness

- pressures and expectations

- excessive criticism

- spoiling and over-indulging.

Over-attentiveness

It is very difficult as a parent to achieve an appropriate level of care for a child. There are probably few children who do not feel either neglected in some way or excessively fussed over at times. Some children, however, have their lives micro-managed for them. Decisions about every aspect of their lives are made by their parents. Minor scrapes and sniffles are given much more attention than they warrant. With mobile phones, there is the potential for anxious parents to be in constant contact with their children and to know what they are doing and where they are at all times. Parents often consider it too dangerous for children to go out to play on their own, either because of 'stranger danger' or traffic. So children are accompanied by adults until a much older age than they would have been a few decades ago. In an effort to ensure their child eats a good diet, everything that a child puts into his mouth is controlled by the parents.

Over-attentiveness may lead a child to feel he is living under a microscope. The mid-19th-century healer Wang Fengyi stressed that the focus of parents should not be on the child, but on harmony within the family. Too much focus on the child, particularly when it is critical, prevents a child from being happy and independent.

This over-attentiveness will affect children in a variety of ways. For some, it leaves them feeling constrained and is likely to cause their Liver *qi* to become imbalanced. For others, it creates a kind of anxiety as they unconsciously fear they are not meeting their parents' expectations. On a psychological level, children who have been given little autonomy often grow up with a fundamental sense of being inadequate and are less likely to grow up with strong self-confidence. They unconsciously interpret their parents' micro-management of their lives as a sign that they are not capable of managing it themselves.

Pressures and expectations

Parents generally want their child to do well in life. Sometimes, however, a parent's desire for his child to succeed may overshadow all else. A study published in June 2013 from the University of Utrecht concluded that 'some parents deal with their unfulfilled ambitions…by transferring them onto their successor – their child. Parents may thus desire their child to redeem their broken dreams.'[51] The study identified that this was especially the case when 'the parent identified the child as part of themselves, more so than as a separate individual'. The ways in which a parent exerts this pressure may be very subtle and the process is usually unconscious.

Children breathe in pressure as if it is the air. A few children may see it as a challenge and thrive as a result, but for many there is a negative impact. When parents have an inflated, rather than realistic, expectation of what their child can achieve, it usually leads to considerable unhappiness in the child and conflict in the relationship between them.

One area of pressure may be the need for a child to reach developmental milestones when he is not yet ready. It can cause understandable anxiety in a parent if her child is not, for example, walking, talking or reading at the expected time. This anxiety is fuelled by the fact that the Western medical model allows little space for the child whose way of doing things differs from the norm.

This kind of pressure may start very early on in a child's life, when the parents are using tactics to coerce their child into walking or talking before he is ready for it. An infant of this age is too young to know what pressure is, but he will unconsciously pick up that there is a lot of emotional charge attached to these activities. The pace of development in a child is determined by his *jing*. A child may need to dig deeply into his reserves of *jing* to meet the expectations that are being put upon him.

I once treated a six-year-old girl who had childhood arthritis. She had begun having extra tuition in several subjects at the age of three as her parents wanted her to 'get ahead' before she begun school. Then, when she was at school, she had an hour of extra tutoring each day, followed by various musical and sporting activities. Weekends and holidays were a time for her to do extra music practice and learn another language. I saw the arthritis as her body's way of 'screaming' that she needed a break.

Children respond to this often unspoken pressure in different ways. A child may push himself to strive ever harder in order to please his parent. Or he may rebel. His rebellion may be external or may be kept hidden inside. In the latter case, the child may have a great deal of internalised anger. He may behave in a passive-aggressive manner. In some children, behaviour that is labelled 'difficult' may derive from this pressure and is a sign that on some level he is not coping. Another child may develop a physical symptom when he is not able to verbalise that he feels this pressure.

The pressure to do well may be focused on different areas of the child's life, such as music, sport or academic achievements. In the case of the latter in particular, this is likely to increase in the teenage years when exam results become more important and a child's future is considered more seriously. A child may have coped with the expectations placed upon him up until then. As the pressure increases further, at a time when he is trying to ride the many changes taking place in his body and psyche, problems may rise to the surface. These may be either physical or psychological. For example:

- depression

- anxiety and/or panic attacks

- eating disorders

- self-harming

- increasing retreat from the real world (often into the world of video games or social media)

- escape into drink and drugs

- reckless behaviour.

Excessive pressure* rarely promotes health in a child, but the way it affects each child will vary. In one child, pressure may knot the *qi* of the Spleen as it causes him to worry. In another, it may deplete Lung *qi* as the child is constantly striving to reach an unattainable goal of perfection. In another child, the Organs of the Fire Element may be affected as the child feels he is unlovable unless he is achieving highly.

Excessive criticism

Over-parenting may come in the form of an overly critical parent, usually for reasons that stem back to her own childhood. She may have overly high expectations of her children and be prone to finding fault with what they do. Children have varying degrees of resistance to criticism. One sibling may be relatively 'thick-skinned' and not perceive his parent as critical, whilst another in the same family may take the most minor criticisms to heart.

The manner in which a child responds to criticism very much depends on his emotional constitution. Being frequently criticised may lead a child to become inhibited and lack spontaneity. Before doing or saying anything, he is weighing up whether it will meet with the approval of his parents. A child may also internalise this critical voice and become very critical of himself. In Freudian terms, overly critical parenting may lead to a highly developed superego. The child will often feel that he has not lived up to the expectations put upon him.

---

* In some children, the pressure to succeed comes from within. A child may have a naturally strong drive and sense of competitiveness. Her desire to achieve and be the best means that she has a natural inclination to work hard.

Spoiling and over-indulging

Another form of over-parenting is to spoil or over-indulge a child. Psychologists universally agree that it is the job of the parent to keep 'boundaries' for a child, and this often means saying 'no'. Although in the short term this may cause the child unhappiness, in the long term it is crucial for the child's psychological and emotional growth, and also creates a better parent–child relationship.

> If the parents never assert their own rights as individuals, but invariably submit to the wishes of the child, the latter comes to believe either that he is omnipotent, and that his every passing whim must immediately be gratified, or else that all self-assertion is wrong, and that he has no justification at all in seeking satisfaction for himself.[52]

A child who is given everything he wants may respond in a variety of ways. A school-age child who is over-indulged may develop physical symptoms as a means of avoiding school. He is not used to an environment where he is not always going to get his way and where he is not thought of as special. Another child may struggle to move towards independence in his teenage years. He may become depressed or develop a physical illness as a way of avoiding having to leave home. Another may become bitter and resentful when he discovers that the rest of the world does not treat him in this way. Ironically, many children who have been spoilt become furious with their parents. As the doctor and psychoanalyst Anthony Storr points out, 'the more a person remains dependent on others the more aggression will be latent within him'.[53] Strong or prolonged anger has a deleterious effect on the child's *qi*, which may lead to all manner of physical and emotional symptoms, such as headaches or digestive problems.

> A ten-year-old girl came to the clinic because of a constant headache, which had meant she had been off school for almost a year. It became clear to me that she was over-indulged by her parents, who answered her every whim. I felt her headache, although real, was a way that she could avoid school, where no doubt she was not indulged in the same way.

Lack of parenting

It is probably not possible for parents to meet every need that their child has, and not desirable either. However, when a child's basic physical and/or emotional needs are repeatedly not met over a long period of time, the effect on the child is damaging. There are many widely recognised forms of neglect, such as the following:

- children who are not provided with the basic necessities such as food

- children who are left to fend for themselves physically and emotionally from an early age

- babies who are regularly left in soiled nappies for hours.

There are also many more subtle ways in which a child does not get his needs met, even in well-off, middle-class families where children have everything they need for physical survival. They may possess a surplus of material goods, but at the same time be lacking in emotional care. Children in these families may, for example:

- rarely see their parents

- be largely brought up by a string of nannies or au pairs, and not have the opportunity for a long-term bond with any of them, or their parents

- have emotional needs that their parents are unable to meet due to the parents' own emotional limitations, work commitments or illness

- be sent to boarding school.

For a baby or young child to thrive physically, let alone emotionally, he relies on the *qi* of his main caregivers as well as on milk and food. The younger the child is, the truer this is. A newborn baby is incomplete and finds his equilibrium only in relation to those around him, particularly the mother. His *shen* and *qi* are not rooted and therefore easily become disordered. Part of the mother's role is to bring the baby to a state of balance where he feels comfortable. Her very presence helps him to establish internal harmony. Up until the age of seven or eight, the child relies on his surroundings to support and feed him in order that he may grow and develop. The *qi* of a child who has grown up in an environment where there is a lack of either physical or emotional care is likely to become compromised in one way or another.

> A seven-year-old boy came for treatment for chronic loose stools. His mother had become very ill during her pregnancy with him and had spent much of the boy's life in hospital. Despite the best efforts of his father, who also had his two older siblings to look after as well as the responsibility for earning a living, he had spent much of his time on his own or in front of a screen. I suspected it was a result of this that he had become chronically *qi* deficient.

Just which Organs and Elements are particularly affected by neglect will depend to a large degree on the constitutional make-up of the child, as well as on the exact nature of the neglect. One child may thrive when sent off to boarding school, whilst another may be left with a lifelong sense of rejection, whilst yet another may struggle to let go of the anger towards his parents for sending him there. Some examples of ways children may respond to emotional neglect are:

- feeling uncared for and having an internal sense that something he needs is lacking

- feeling fearful of the world and lacking confidence in his ability to cope with it

- being full of anger and resentment at the perceived failings of his parents

- displaying a degree of autonomy and responsibility far in excess of his years.

The fit between the parents and the child

If siblings raised in the same family are asked to describe their family life as a child, very often their answers will be strikingly different. This may of course be because they did have very different experiences. For example, a sibling who comes along many years after the other children in the family may be parented very differently to his older siblings. However, often the children's different versions of their childhood are a result of their emotional nature and how that influenced their experiences of their family. Difficulties may arise as a result of the fit between the child and his parents and siblings. This may take many different forms. For example:

- A child who needs a lot of independence may feel constrained by a mother who tends to worry and overprotect.

- A child who is fearful may struggle to thrive with parents who make him go climbing and kayaking.

- A child who requires clear structure and boundaries will probably flounder in a family who have a chaotic lifestyle and little routine.

- A child who is self-contained and not prone to displays of affection may be misunderstood by family members who only feel loved when there is lots of physical affection.

These clashes between a child and his parents need not become a cause of disease. When parents are aware of any incompatibilities and are secure enough to truly support their children in being their unique selves, the child can thrive. However, most parents know how incredibly difficult this is. As Solomon writes, 'Though many of us take pride in how different we are from our parents, we are endlessly sad at how different our children are from us.'[54]

When a child is given the message, either overtly or subliminally, that he is not right in some way, it will shape how he feels about himself at his core. If, because of his unique nature, he does not receive the love, understanding, acceptance and approval he needs, the balance of the Five Elements will be disturbed. This may be the root of many physical and emotional conditions, and will be discussed at length in Part 2.

> I once treated a woman in her seventies, and also her daughter who was in her forties. The mother talked at length about how much she had always adored her daughter. She had spent many years sad and confused as to why their relationship had not been better and why her daughter seemed constantly angry with her. The daughter used to talk at length about how unloved by her mother she had always felt. The mother was an intellectual who, I suspect, expressed her love in a way her daughter, who was an exceptionally sensitive and soft woman, did not recognise.

The adopted child

Adoption does not necessarily generate *qi* pathologies, but there are often areas of emotional vulnerability for adopted children. They commonly feel abandoned by their birth parents or carry within them a deep feeling of unlovability. Some adopted children describe feeling like an outsider because they do not have a feeling of kinship with the rest of the family. It is unwise to make assumptions about how being adopted may have affected a particular child. However, practitioners should be aware that the *qi* of a child is often affected by the fact of her adoption and her response to it.

The family under strain

Most parents in the developed world parent largely in isolation. It is no longer the norm for a child to be brought up in a community that in the past often included aunts, uncles, grandparents and others. Also, in many families both parents need to work and there is a big increase in the number of single-parent families. An old proverb says that 'it takes a community to raise a child', yet today that community rarely exists.

There are many reasons why a family may be strained. For example:

- A parent may be depressed or preoccupied with work.

- A parent may be struggling with her own health, or there may be a sibling in the family who requires extra care. Some families cope well until a child falls ill, but the illness brings extra strain which they cannot manage.

- A parent may be overstretched by having to care for an elderly parent as well as a young child.

- A parent may feel lonely and unsupported.

- The family may be stretched by a lack of financial resources or inadequate living conditions.

- One parent may work away from home.

- There may be many children in the family, so they may have to fend for themselves to a degree that is not appropriate for their age.

The consequences of strain in the family for the child may be profound. Whatever kind and size of family a child lives in has a finite amount of *qi* within it. The smaller the family or the network of support, the less *qi* is available. There is only so much time, energy and love that parents can give to their children, especially when they are juggling many other demands. Strain in one aspect of life or in one family member may mean a disproportionately large amount of the family's *qi* is consumed by that and another part of the family suffers.

One way in which a child may express that he is not getting what he needs is through developing a physical or psychological symptom. He will usually be unaware that he is struggling to get his needs met but his body is expressing it. Sometimes, coming for acupuncture treatment is a way for a child to get the *qi* that he is not, for whatever reason, getting from within his family unit.

> One boy came to the clinic because of persistent stomach aches. They had begun six months after his elder sibling had been diagnosed with cancer. I felt his stomach aches were his way of trying to claim back some of his share of the attention, which had largely been directed towards his brother since he had been ill.

The family needing the child to be ill

The notion that a child who is chronically ill is serving some purpose for the family as a whole has been prevalent in psychotherapeutic fields for decades: '[There is the] idea that everyone in the family may be trying all the time to get rid of their nasty feelings by playing "pass the parcel" with them – [this] could manifest in a child with an illness.'[55] It is often the most vulnerable or emotionally sensitive member of the family who takes on this role. He is essentially acting like a sponge to soak up the problems within the family, whilst other members are not ready to face up to these issues. This child becomes the scapegoat and his illness is what enables the other members to keep functioning and remain healthy. Of course, this process goes on at an unconscious level. At the conscious level, the parents will generally be concerned for their ill child and desperately want him to get better.

Sometimes a child's illness serves the purpose of uniting the parents. Focusing their energy and worries on the child can be a way of avoiding having to face the unresolved problems in their relationship. A child may unconsciously sense that if he gets better, his parents' relationship will fall apart. If there is rising tension between them, he may unconsciously believe that a flare-up of a chronic condition will divert his parents' attention away from their relationship, which he feels is about to disintegrate.

FAMILY CASE HISTORY WHICH ILLUSTRATES THE INTERCONNECTEDNESS OF THE MEMBERS

This case history illustrates the interconnectedness of family members. Just like the Five Elements, an imbalance in one affects all the others. It also shows how, when a family is under strain, different members may take up the strain to compensate for others at different times.

The Smith family was made up of Mum, Dad, five-year-old Dan and three-year-old Lucy.

Dan was the first family member to come for treatment. He had been suffering from a severe health condition since birth. Looking after such an ill child had left Mum and Dad feeling emotionally and physically depleted. Thankfully, Lucy had always been a healthy and 'easy' child.

After a few months of treatment, Dan's symptoms improved enormously and the strain on the family gradually reduced. They were all getting more sleep, the days were easier and the degree of worry diminished.

Just as Mum and Dad were beginning to relax, Lucy's behaviour seemed to go through a dramatic change. She began having tantrums, becoming hyperactive at times, and her sleep (previously not a problem) became disrupted. It was as if Lucy sensed that her parents, for the first time in her life, had some energy to focus on her and that she could express the sides of herself that she had been repressing.

Lucy began having treatment and, after a few weeks, she seemed to settle down and her behaviour became easier. She also began sleeping better.

Dan and Lucy's dad had found the past five years a great strain, and his response to this had been to retreat into himself. His long-standing diabetes had become unstable. Seeing how well his children had responded to acupuncture, he began coming for treatment himself. He found that he gradually began to feel 'more like his old self'.

Finally, with Dad, Dan and Lucy all relatively well, Mum had an emotional and physical 'crash'. The years of strain, through which she had valiantly battled, finally got to her and she unconsciously sensed that the rest of the family could cope if she did not for a while. She needed a few months of treatment to begin feeling replenished.

SUMMARY

- » The pathology of *qi* in a child may be a direct result and manifestation of the emotional state of the mother.

- » Young children are like sponges who absorb the emotional tone of their family and wider environment.

- » Emotions that are unacceptable in the family are particularly likely to become imbalanced in the child.

- » Over-parenting, such as 'helicopter parenting', may be a cause of imbalance in a child. The exact manifestation will depend on the constitutional nature of the child.

- » On the other hand, a lack of parenting is equally likely to cause an imbalance.

- » A child may develop a *qi* pathology because his unique nature is at odds with that of the parent.

- » Illness may arise in a child when the family is under strain and there is not enough *qi* to go around.

- » Sometimes illness in a child serves a purpose for the family unit as a whole.

• Chapter 7 •

THE CHALLENGES OF LIFE

· ·

The topics discussed in this chapter are:

* Overstimulation

* School

* Relationships

* The online world

* Sexuality

Introduction

The aspects of life discussed below are often important contributory factors in the decline of a child's well-being. They may also be a trigger for physical complaints, either directly or indirectly. For example, a child may unconsciously develop an illness as a way of avoiding school or as a justification to retreat from life which has become too painful or difficult to face.

There is often an unhelpful perception that psychosomatic complaints are in some way not as valid as those which have an organic cause. This perception has many consequences for the sufferer, who is driven to point to an external agent as the cause of her suffering. She may push for a diagnosis (which may be inaccurate) and medical treatment (which may be unhelpful). The perception that her physical complaint is not 'real' means she often will not get the support she needs. Appropriate support would enable her to face the difficulties that originally led to the emergence of the physical symptom.

It is vital when treating children to be aware of the issues in their lives that may be causing them stress. Sometimes treatment means they are able to respond to that part of their life in a different way. Sometimes the treatment room is a place where these worries and difficulties can be aired, and possible solutions may begin to emerge.

Overstimulation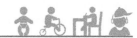

Sun Simiao wrote:

> The reason why the disease of intrusive upset exists in very early childhood is that an outside person has come [into the home] whose *qi* and breath has caused the upset. Another name is 'striking the person'. This is what intrusive upset means.[56]

He went on to talk about somebody returning home bringing in on their clothes the *qi* of cattle or horses, or a wet nurse who has been intoxicated. Our concerns today are no longer drunk wet nurses or the *qi* of farm animals, but the point that Sun Simiao was making is that babies and young children are extraordinarily sensitive to external influences. The barriers that protect them from external stimuli have not yet developed. Therefore, they should be shielded, to some degree, from strong or sudden stimuli, things that are unfamiliar to them or too many external stimuli at the same time. The nervous system of a baby is easily agitated and it is possible he may become overstimulated by an environment that, to an adult, seems relatively peaceful or unexciting.

A mother brought her three-year-old child, who was a twin, to the clinic for sleep problems. If she took her twins into the city from the quiet village where they lived, one would love the excitement and be transfixed by everything going on around him. The other, in contrast, would cry much of the time and need to be carried to prevent her from becoming too distressed. This shows the different levels of resilience children have to external stimuli.

Interestingly, Sun Simiao goes on to suggest that the impact of these external influences is to affect the *shen*. He says, 'The various treatments above generally all have the intention of calming [the patient's] heart. This is what is called the doctor's intention.'[57]

Sensory overload

The world today can be noisy, fast and bright. The most common place for a baby to be born in the West is in the maternity unit of a hospital, which is often full of lots of people, noisy machines and artificial lighting. Babies are then taken to homes where the television may be on all day. Emails, text messages and phone calls arrive with an array of often loud and abrupt sounds. The background noise of cars creates a constant drone, and motorbikes and trains may roar past intermittently. Classrooms may have thirty or forty children in them, so they may spend their day in a chaotic din. Leisure time is spent looking at screens, sometimes with the television on in the background too!

This is the reality of life, especially urban life, in the 21st century. Some babies and children take life in their stride, but for others the assault to their senses becomes a major cause of disease. They feel bombarded by stimuli coming at them from every angle. An extreme case of this is an autistic child, who is not able to cope with, for example, a trip to a noisy, busy shopping mall. But many neurotypical children come away from a day in the city or a fairground hyped up, ragged and miserable too.

Loud noises, bright lights and a constant background hubbub can act on the Liver in a similar way to external Wind, aggravating it and making it agitated. The Liver in children has a propensity to be in excess and is vulnerable to anything that makes it 'flare up'. Many children who come to the clinic today have conditions which involve an aggravated Liver. Some of the most common ones include food allergies, autistic spectrum disorders and behavioural problems such as ADHD. Finding ways to counterbalance this external aggravation often helps to soothe the Liver.

One girl who came to the clinic with chronic fatigue syndrome had an imbalance in her Liver. She was easily able to go for a long walk without her symptoms worsening. However, if she went to London for the day, she would be set back for weeks afterwards. The multiple stimuli of the city aggravated her Liver imbalance.

Over-scheduling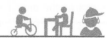

It has become the norm for many children in the West to have their daily lives scheduled from minute to minute. Gone are the days when children were sent out of the house in the morning and told to entertain themselves and not return until evening. From an early age, days are often filled with groups and activities, leaving little time which is not planned in advance.

A hectic and over-scheduled life is like an adult working two jobs. Babies and toddlers are constantly exposed to new experiences and stimuli that need to be absorbed and processed. The very fact of growing faster than at any other time of life is stimulating and exhausting enough. School-age children are still growing fast, and also have to meet the academic and social expectations that are put upon them. Teenagers, especially, may not thrive in an over-scheduled life, as their rate of growth is almost as great as that which takes place in the first few years of life. Instead of increasing their commitments, teenagers ideally would do less in order that their *qi* may be concentrated on the important tasks of growth and development.

Relentless routine

For some children, over-scheduling may have a negative impact on their Wood Element, the *qi* of which becomes constrained by the 'go, go, go' nature of life. There is little opportunity for them to explore their imagination or fantasy world. If given the opportunity, many young children will spend long periods of time in a kind of reverie. This is an important counterbalance to all the thinking and doing that makes up so much of life. It allows their Ethereal Soul (*hun*) to wander and explore sides of life which are otherwise not given enough expression.

Even though much of the planning and decision making is being done by the parents, the child will often feel harassed and nagged by the parent who needs to make sure she gets to the next activity on time. A child may become tense in anticipation of this, which may have the effect of further constraining her *qi*. She may also pick up on the parent being tense as she tries to keep to time in her busy schedule. For Liver *qi* to flow freely, children need time to unwind and relax.

Lack of rest

A child's *yin* is insubstantial and can therefore easily become depleted. For a child's *yin* to grow firm and strong, there needs to be a balance between rest and activity. Many children become very tired when they begin school. Yet at the same time they also start several extra-curricular activities too, so that there are very few hours of the week which are not scheduled.

As well as the short-term impact of an overly scheduled routine, there can be longer-term consequences too. If a child becomes habituated to being on the go most of the time, then it becomes harder for her to know how to stop and be still. This is a habit that may become lifelong and have long-term consequences for her health.

Too much out and about

The most important source of security for a young child is to be with his primary caregiver, but by the toddler years, the home also becomes more important to a child. Psychologists recognise that toddlers may go through a phase of 'separation anxiety from the home'. The developing *qi* and Organs of a child who is out and about for much of the time may suffer from the lack of a consistent physical base. A balance needs to be found, as always, between time at home and time outside. A child may go through times when he needs to just stay at home. Whilst of course this may sometimes come from laziness, at other times it is because a child is going through a growth spurt and needs to gather his energy.

Digital media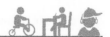

Using a screen, whether it be the television or a computer, has a very particular effect on the *qi* of a child. First, it encourages a child to be 'in her head', and therefore her *qi* to rise. This is a tendency that is already inherent in children, so anything that encourages it further can be detrimental. If a lot of screen time is combined with a lack of physical exercise, it leads to the combination of a mind that is overstimulated and a body that is underused.

Second, competitive computer games will often adrenalise the child. This explains why a child may be irritable or even aggressive when she finishes a long stint on the computer, and why so many children develop an addictive relationship with computers. They crave the adrenaline rush and clamour for more time on the computer to avoid the inevitable comedown when the adrenaline wears off.

Being adrenalised will, over time, deplete the child's Kidney *yin*, which is still insubstantial and therefore more susceptible to overstimulation. Frenetic and fast-moving computer games are the antithesis of the calm, still environment that encourages a child's *yin* to become strong.

Lastly, too much screen time agitates the Liver in some children. Fast-moving images of some video games aggravate and unsettle Liver *qi* (the eyes being the sense orifice of the Liver). When combined with lack of physical movement, too much screen time can exacerbate the tendency of the Liver to become excess in children.

Overall, whatever the specific effect on the *qi* of each Organ, spending time on a digital device leads a child to become more tense and tight. This colours the way in which a child responds and reacts to everything else she comes across in the world. It lures her further away from a state of calmness and relaxation, and hampers the growth and flow of her *qi*. In extreme cases, the real world begins to feel slow and uninteresting compared with the digital world and the child cannot resist the lure of the latter.

One five-year-old boy was an extreme example of a child whose symptoms (severe insomnia) had been caused by over-exposure to digital media. When he first came to the clinic, he made no eye contact and only spoke when he was allowed his mother's phone. He started talking to the characters in whatever he was watching on the phone as if they were real people. Advising the mother that he should not be allowed any time on screens at all in the short term, as well as acupuncture to resolve Phlegm-Fire harassing the Heart, enabled him to sleep better. He also gradually 'returned' to living in the real world.

School

After the family, school life probably has more influence on a child than any other factor. If school goes well, it can have an enormously positive effect on a child's health and well-being. When it does not go well, it may have significant consequences.

There are various aspects of school which may become a cause of disease for children. These are:

- separation from the mother and family
- the physical routine
- social dynamics
- academic/intellectual strain
- worry
- the fit of the child and the school.

Separation from the mother and family

In most countries, children start school at an age when they are still very linked to their mother. If a child has been used to spending most of her time with her mother, going to school means a sudden loosening of the symbiotic relationship that has given her great security. Of course, gradual separation from the mother is necessary, but starting school can mean it happens suddenly. Even if the child was in daycare, it is likely that the ratio of adults to children will have been higher and there would have been more adult *qi* available to help the child regulate her emotions.

Ironically, a child who has been well nurtured by her mother will probably find separating from her easier than one who has not. She has been able to build up an internal sense of home. A child who struggles to leave her mother at the start of the school day may also be unconsciously picking up on the mother's worry or anxiety about leaving her child.

The physical routine

A child may have been quite physically robust in her first three or four years of life but the routine of going to school five days a week may begin to cause depletion. Whilst one child may take the transition to school in her stride, another may find it a strain. Having to leave the house at a certain time five days a week and spend the school day engaged in activities exhausts some children, especially those who tend towards deficient pathologies.

> A five-year-old boy came to the clinic because he had constant coughs and colds, he wet the bed and he had lost his appetite. All these problems had started after he began school. Before that, he had been vital and robust. He loved school, had made lots of friends and enjoyed learning, but the exertion of the routine was just too much for him.

Social dynamics

Depending on the constitutional make-up of a child, the arena of social dynamics and friendships may present many challenges. The simple fact of being surrounded by so many other children may be tiring and stressful for a more introverted child, or for one who finds interpreting the unspoken social cues somewhat baffling.

Difficulties with friendships may become a source of worry. Rejection, whether perceived or real, may deplete the Organs related to the Fire Element. The ability of young children to be cruel to each other is renowned. For a girl in particular, one day she can be somebody's 'best friend', the next day the supposed friend refuses to talk to her or be seen with her. One day she is 'in' the group or clique; the next day she is 'out'. Most children will not find this easy and some will find it devastating. A bad phase with friendships at school can be the root of psychosomatic illness and, in teenagers, the trigger for serious mental health issues such as depression, anxiety and self-harm.

Social dynamics generally become more complicated in the teenage years, as teenagers increasingly identify with their peer group and separate from their family. Being part of the group, therefore, takes on great significance for the teenager. If she fails to find a group where she feels she fits in, she may feel alienated and alone. The particular effect this has on an individual will, in large part, depend on her constitutional imbalance. The Fire Element may suffer if she feels that she is not liked by her classmates. The emotional rollercoaster of feeling liked and included one minute, disliked and rejected the next, may take its toll on the Heart. A child with an already weak Metal Element may feel increasingly isolated and unable to connect with others.

Academic/intellectual strain

Going to school involves a child using her brain to acquire new skills. As Figure 7.1 shows, several different Organs are involved in this process. The brain is made strong by the *jing* and Marrow which come from the Kidneys. The *yi* of the Spleen is involved in concentration. The *shen* of the Heart plays a key role in thinking and memorising facts. This extra intellectual strain, on top of the other aspects of school life, may therefore have the effect of depleting one or more Organs in a young child. A child of this age is still growing and developing at a fast rate. Whilst that is almost her only task, there is less chance of deficiencies arising. With these extra demands, the *qi* that a child has available may be spread too thinly, so that some aspect of the child begins to suffer.

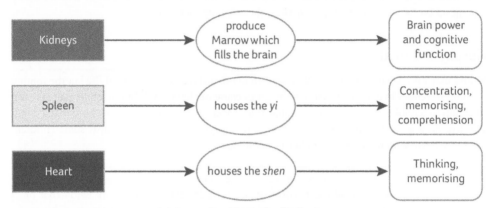

Figure 7.1 Organs involved in learning

The first years of school are not the only time that academic strain may be a cause of illness in a child. This may be the case during any period where the demands on the child exceed her stage of development, or when they coincide with big developmental leaps or growth spurts. This is especially likely during adolescence. Children have often moved to secondary school at this time, with an increase in workload and academic expectations. In the UK, there has been a shift in recent years away from the arts and sports towards 'hard' subjects such as sciences and social sciences. For many children, this also creates more pressure. The rate of physical, mental and psychological growth during this time is second only to that which happens in the first year of life. To navigate these changes whilst coping with this added pressure may create imbalance. The nature of the imbalance will depend on the constitution of the child and her energetic state as she enters adolescence.

Worry

Worry, a state that depletes Spleen *qi*, may become a part of a child's emotional world for the first time when she starts school. She may worry about who to play with, about having a teacher she does not like or about learning something that she finds difficult. An increase in intellectual activity, together with worry and separation from the mother and home, may all place a strain on the Spleen and the *yi*.

A six-year-old girl, who had an Earth constitutional imbalance, had begun worrying all the time after starting school. She was very conscientious and often chose to practise her spellings and maths at home. She was also a precocious reader. All of these things meant that her Spleen was under great strain. Her worry was both a cause and a symptom. Treatment to support her Spleen helped to moderate her worry.

The fit of the child and the school

A child may attend a school where she feels that she just does not fit, or where some aspects of it suit her and others do not. Few adults would probably look back at their schooling and say it was perfect for them. But when there is a pronounced mismatch, the impact on the developing child may be significant. Placing a child in a school that is not right for her is the equivalent of planting a cactus in waterlogged soil. The child will simply not be in an environment where she can grow and thrive.

Ideally, a child will go to a school that is a good match for her academic capabilities. If she struggles with intellectual work, she is unlikely to thrive at a school which places a lot of store in academic achievement. She is likely to feel pressured and perhaps tired out by always having to run to keep up. A child who does not enjoy or excel at sport may feel out of place at a school that prides itself on its sporting achievement.

A child may be at a school where the approach to discipline and structure does not suit her. Adults who were sent to liberal, progressive schools sometimes say that they wished they had gone to a more 'regular' school with more structure and routine. Conversely, a child who attends a very strict school may feel stifled by a lack of opportunity for personal expression and creativity.

It may be that a child finds herself at a school without another like-minded soul. This may lead her to feel dejected. These feelings may damage the Fire Element and the *qi* of the Heart and the Pericardium, which are fed by feelings of warmth and connection with others. This may be a problem for a child who goes to a very small school, where the pool of children is simply not big enough for her to find one who she feels is a friend.

Relationships

 Relationships and the online world tend to become causes of disease particularly in the approach to or during adolescence. Times of transition and change are always accompanied by an 'opening up' of the child's *qi*. This means there is an increased vulnerability and any cause of disease may have a stronger impact than it would at another time. Therefore, children of this age would ideally be shielded from these pressures to some degree.

Connections with others are, for most people, what make the world go round. The health and happiness of most children and teenagers is enhanced by stable and warm relationships. The subject of friendships and social dynamics at school has already been discussed under the section 'School'. This section will focus on the foray into romantic relationships that usually begins during the teenage years.

During adolescence, there is a surge of *yang* energy in the body. This is a driving force to help the child cross the bridge from childhood to adulthood. This crossing takes place on a physical, emotional and psychological level. One of the consequences of this surge of *yang* is that everything the child feels is magnified and felt with more force than it was before.

This has important implications when it comes to relationships. This *yang qi*, which derives from the Kidneys, may surge upwards and reach the Heart. The Heart and the *shen* are what drive our feelings towards and connections with others. In this heightened state, a teenager may experience feelings of love towards a potential girlfriend or boyfriend that are of an intensity they have never felt before. These crushes, characterised by powerful feelings, are commonplace.

Whilst there is the potential for this to lead to reckless behaviour or hasty decisions, on the whole when things are going well it is not too problematic. The problems arise, however, when the feelings are not reciprocated or the relationship ends. The feelings of rejection are likely to be felt as strongly as the feelings of passion were. A rejection when in this heightened state can be experienced as a shock, which is likely to have a deleterious impact on the Heart. It may also affect any other Organ that is not constitutionally robust. A teenager may also experience strong feelings of anger, worthlessness or anxiety after a rejection. As discussed in Chapter 5, these emotions, when either intense or prolonged, may become a cause of disease.

 The Grant Study, a seventy-five-year study on adult happiness carried out at Harvard University, found that the one factor that has more of an impact on the long-term physical and mental health of adults is the quality of their relationships with others.[*]

The online world

Adolescence is a time of heightened self-consciousness, lived out under scrutiny from parents, teachers and society, and now the online world. Teenagers are either 'liked', 'unfriended', adored, reviled or ignored on a moment-to-moment basis. Whenever a child looks at her phone, she may learn of parties she has not been invited to or see pictures of her friends doing things which do not include her. The photos and videos that people choose to post online are a filtered version of real life; anything that is not aesthetically pleasing or is boring is omitted. It can easily look as if everybody else is having far more fun and is thinner and more beautiful. When a child spends hours online every day, the impact of this on her mental health can be devastating.

For some, adolescence is in a kind of tortured drama. Negotiating it under this intense scrutiny can have a profound impact on the movements of *qi*, and the development of the Organs and Elements.

The way in which a child will be affected by the world of social media will depend on her individual nature. However, some common ways in which its impact is seen are the following:

- Instead of developing an internal sense of being loveable, the child becomes reliant on external validation. How she feels about herself fluctuates with how she feels about her standing on social media.

- The child feels she is 'not good enough' and that she cannot live up to the idealised world that is portrayed online.

- Online bullying, fear of a sexual encounter or an embarrassing, drunken exploit being exposed on social media may all have a corrosive impact.

The online world also provides a mass availability of news. Childline report that they receive an increased number of calls during major world events, such as after a terrorist attack, the Brexit referendum or the 2017 US presidential election.[58] They report that knowledge of these events, without the power to do anything about them, can make teenagers very fearful for their future.

An eleven-year-old girl, who was being treated for migraines, told me that she was taking a long time to get to sleep each night because she was worried about her parents dying in a terrorist attack. This began just after a spate of terrorist attacks in different cities across Europe.

---

[*] Robert Waldinger gave a TED talk on the results of this study which can be found at www.ted.com/talks/robert_ waldinger_what_makes_a_good_life_lessons_from_the_longest_study_on_happiness/transcript (accessed December 2017).

It is ironic that, in an age of increased connectivity, teenagers' reports of feeling socially isolated are more widespread than before. For some adolescents, an abundance of 'online' friends comes in lieu of real friendships.

Sexuality

Sexuality is a central component of most teenagers' lives. Sexual desire usually emerges around the time of puberty, and issues related to it can occupy the thoughts and feelings of an adolescent much of the time. For a few, the transition to becoming a sexual being can be a smooth path, but for many, it entails angst and difficulty. Some of the most frequent problems teenagers face are the following:

- There are the worries and risks of pregnancy, sexually transmitted diseases and also of sexual habits being exposed on social media.

- The loss of virginity may spark feelings of shame or powerlessness. In girls especially, it may bring feelings of rejection if not followed by increased emotional intimacy.

- A teenager may have a sense of inadequacy about not losing his or her virginity when many of his or her peers have done.

- Boys are especially prone to performance anxiety during adolescence.

- Societal pressure, and the influence of online pornography, mean that many teenagers feel coerced to behave in a certain way sexually. This may create much fear, angst and shame.

- Confusion or shame over sexual or gender orientation may lead to enormous levels of emotional turmoil.

Any of the above factors may add an extra layer of confusion to an already turbulent time, bringing about strong movements of *qi*. Existing imbalances may become stronger and new ones may arise.

A fifteen-year-old came to the clinic because he had become depressed, spending day after day in his bedroom and losing connection with his friends. During treatment, he revealed that he had become agonised about his sexuality, and felt an enormous pressure that he should know now whether he was gay, bisexual or heterosexual. Treatment of his constitutional imbalance (which was Metal) as well as space to discuss his worries helped him to accept that it was all right for him to have some uncertainties about who he was.

Conclusion

The aspects of life discussed in this chapter are, undoubtedly, the ones which the children who come to our clinics struggle with. They often place strain on a child, either physically or psychologically, or both. Treatment can help a child to withstand these strains better, and the treatment room may be a place for families to reflect upon the balance of their lives and perhaps decide to make small adjustments.

SUMMARY

» Babies and young children are particularly susceptible to their external environment. In older children, sensory overload, over-scheduling and digital media all have the potential to overstimulate.

» The social, emotional, academic and/or physical aspects of school all have the potential to cause imbalance in a child.

» Romantic relationships may strain the Organs of the Fire Element during adolescence.

» Over-dependence on the online world may be a cause of imbalance in a vulnerable child or teenager.

» A teenager's struggle with his or her sexuality may evoke strong emotions, which trigger imbalances in *qi*.

• Chapter 8 •

MISCELLANEOUS CAUSES
OF DISEASE
· · · · · · · · · · · · · · · · · · · ·

The topics discussed in this chapter are:

- Food and eating

- Lack of sleep

- Physical exercise

- Sexual activity

- Medications and vaccinations

- Recreational drugs and alcohol

Food and eating

Diet has long been considered one of the main causes of disease in children. *A Study of Chinese Medicine Paediatrics* (*Zhong Yi Er Ke Xue*) says, 'Children's transportation and transformation is not fortified and complete. Therefore, they are easily damaged by food.'[59] This is particularly true in children up to the age of three or four.

In practice, we commonly see children in the clinic who could benefit from a change in their diet. However, whilst food and eating should not be dismissed as an important cause of disease in children, neither should it be given overdue prominence. There is a perception that almost every problem in a child can be attributed to food. One of the roles of the practitioner may sometimes be to help the parent shift some of her focus away from the child's diet and towards other factors, such as emotions, which the practitioner deems to be a more important cause of the child's imbalance.

> A three-year-old girl was brought for treatment for what her mother described as multiple food allergies. The girl had had comprehensive food allergy tests at the most progressive children's hospital in the country and all of them had come back negative. Yet her mother was convinced the problem was food. My feeling was that the child had a strong digestive system and that her symptoms (sleep disturbance and anxiety) were actually due to the fact that her parents seemed to be permanently at war with each other.

Eating environment

The Chinese consider the entire process of eating to be sacred. Food should be eaten regularly and slowly, and is to be shared. It is a social event, and not something to be done in solitude.

The environment in which a child eats has an impact on how well her digestive system functions. A child's digestion is vulnerable and easily becomes imbalanced. The Spleen and the Liver are the two most important *yin* Organs involved. Worry or excessive thought knots the *qi* of the Spleen, and any emotion on the anger spectrum causes Liver *qi* to stagnate. If these emotions are present at mealtimes, a child's digestion is likely to become imbalanced.

Orthodox medicine also recognises this, but explains it from a different perspective. In her book *Gut*, the doctor Guilia Enders says:

> …mealtimes, for example, should be enjoyed without pressure, at a leisurely pace. The dinner table should be a stress-free zone, with no place for scolding or pronouncements like 'You will remain at the table until you've finished the food on your plate!', and without constant TV channel hopping. This is important for adults, but it is vital for small children, whose gut brain develops in parallel with their head brain. The earlier in life that mealtime calm is introduced, the better. Stress of any kind activates nerves that inhibit the digestive process, which means we not only extract less energy from our food, but we also take longer to digest it, putting the gut under unnecessary extra strain.[60]

It is common for children to be fed separately from the rest of the family. Life goes on around them as they eat, rather than the whole family stopping and the meal being a communal activity enjoyed by everybody. Some mothers have become so adept at breastfeeding that they can do it whilst their baby is being carried in a sling. Whilst this is convenient and practical, it may not always be the ideal, calm environment that promotes a healthy digestion.

In older children, the environment may be compromised by doing other things whilst eating. Reading, whether it be a book or on a screen, means that Spleen *qi* is diverted to digesting the reading matter, leaving less available for the digestion of food. Watching television or playing a computer game whilst eating has a similar effect.

Every child will have a slightly different ideal eating environment. Some children eat much better in a group, whilst others need a calm environment with no distractions for them to be at all interested in their food. Twenty-first-century living rarely allows for the ideal of long, leisurely meals that Enders alludes to. It is important nevertheless to look at the eating environment as a possible cause of disease in children.

Babies and toddlers

One of the main challenges for a child up to the age of about three is to consume and digest enough food to support the rapid growth during this phase. It is very easy for the digestive process to become imbalanced when it is dealing with large quantities of food in comparison to the child's size and development.

Too much food

The importance of not overfeeding a baby has been stressed in Chinese medicine for many centuries. Even when breastfeeding, it is possible to overfeed a baby. Sun Simiao said:

> Whenever you are breastfeeding a baby, you never want them to eat until they are too full. Overeating results in retching and vomiting. Every time you encounter the symptom of vomiting in babies, it means that they are over-satiated on breast milk. Nurse them on an empty breast, to make the already ingested milk disperse.[61]

Some children do not know when to stop eating. Scott explains that this is a particular characteristic of children who have very strong *qi*. A child of this nature often consumes more food than his digestive system can cope with, which may lead to Accumulation Disorder (see Chapter 27). It goes against the instinct of most parents to refuse a young child food, but this may sometimes be necessary.

It is also difficult for adults to know how little food a child needs. Young children have tiny stomachs, and what may look like a small snack to an adult is a full meal for a child. If he is teething or poorly, he may need to consume even less (see Chapter 66). Mothers have an instinct to make sure their children are well fed, so they may coax a child into having food that he does not really want or need. Children have an innate instinct for survival, and a healthy child will eat when he is hungry.

Too-frequent feeding or eating

It is not only the quantity of food that is important but also the breaks between eating. For a parent who has chosen to feed on demand, it is very hard to 'deprive' a baby of a feed if he is crying. Not only is it easy to assume that he is crying from hunger, but putting a baby on the breast is sometimes the only way to comfort him. The views of Chinese medicine here may conflict with the parenting style of many parents in the West. Wang Fengyi was very clear on this topic:

> It is essential that you manage the number of feedings properly. It is best to feed four times during the day, and you must not exceed three feedings at night, so even if you deviate from this norm a little bit, you cannot deviate too much. If you can follow this rule, the child will have a healthy appetite, and a healthy Spleen and Stomach.[62]

Whilst this advice may be rather too prescriptive for most parents, the pertinent point is that feeding too often and without breaks will weaken the digestive system of most babies. The Spleen is insufficient in babies and young children, and if it is required almost continually to digest food (even if purely breast milk), Spleen *qi* will become depleted. Therefore, breaks between feeds are important.

Once a baby starts solids, the same thing applies. Constantly snacking strains the *qi* of his Stomach and Spleen. Spleen *qi* deficiency is at the root of many common childhood illnesses. It also begs the question of whether food is being used to fulfil an emotional need. This could set up a dynamic that becomes a lifetime struggle.

The state of the baby and mother when breastfeeding

Chinese medicine stresses that both mother and baby should be in a calm state when breastfeeding. It is important that the baby does not start a feed whilst distressed, though this can be difficult to achieve as a hungry baby is usually not a happy baby. If a baby starts feeding when she is upset, the flow of her *qi* is already compromised. There is normally a pathological upwards movement of *qi* in a baby who is screaming and has a red face. Stomach *qi* needs to descend to avoid digestive symptoms such as reflux or vomiting.

Even more important, however, is the state of the mother when breastfeeding. Many mothers will recognise that a feed does not usually go well if they are tense or upset. A strong emotion may stagnate the flow of milk to the breast, so the baby cannot feed smoothly and usually he will not be able to digest the milk easily either. Wang Fengyi wrote that 'when your disposition is stirred or your body fatigued, never nurse a baby. When the heart is balanced and the Qi harmonious, this is best.'[63]

Inappropriate foods

COLD AND RAW FOODS

The Spleen loves warmth. Foods which are either physically or energetically Cold require more Spleen *qi* to digest them efficiently. Cold drinks and those with ice will also lead to a cold and deficient Spleen. Ice cream, whilst usually loved by children, is not loved by their Spleens. It is one thing to have the odd ice cream in the height of summer but quite another to have it every day for dessert. A child who is already *xu* and Cold will struggle with a cold diet more than a child who has a naturally strong and Hot disposition.

WHOLE FOODS

Some parents, particularly those who tend to bring their children for acupuncture, wean their children on whole foods in the belief that they are healthier than processed foods. This may be true for adults who benefit from having more roughage in their diet, but whole foods need more digesting than those which contain less roughage. For many babies, this is simply more than they can handle and it creates either Spleen *qi* deficiency or Accumulation Disorder. Lightly cooked vegetables and fruit will provide a baby with all the roughage he needs. Too much brown rice and pasta, wholemeal bread and cereals may strain his delicate digestive system.

DAIRY FOODS

Cow's milk products are not well tolerated by some children and may create mucus. For other children, goat's and sheep's milk products are also not easily digested. Dairy foods tend to be energetically cool, but it does not follow that children who are constitutionally Cold are the only ones to not tolerate them. It is sometimes only through trial and error that it becomes clear whether an individual can tolerate dairy products. If a child does not react well to milk in his diet, a suitable substitute needs to be found. Soya milk is Cold in nature, so also not suitable for many young children.[*]

> A six-year-old boy came to the clinic because he had a permanently snotty nose. His mother said that they had tried cutting out dairy foods but it had made no noticeable difference. I suggested they try again, whilst having acupuncture treatment. The combination of the two meant that his symptoms vastly improved.

Many parents are concerned that if their child does not drink lots of milk, she will not get enough calcium in her diet. However, there are many other sources of calcium which may be better tolerated than milk.[**]

School-age children

Sugar

Prior to the 18th century, sugar was a luxury in Europe, but nowadays is consumed in one form or another at every meal by many people. In addition to the obvious dental problems it causes, high sugar consumption in children may be a cause of several different internal imbalances.

The taste associated with the Spleen is sweetness. The Spleen likes a little sweetness, but too much is detrimental to its functioning. High sugar consumption means the Spleen is less able to transform and transport, leading to the accumulation of Damp and Phlegm. Considering that a child's Spleen is strained already, eating too much sugar only strains it even further.

Some children react to sugar by becoming hyperactive, and a relatively small amount of sugar may have this effect. For many, an occasion where they consume more sugar than usual may make them over-excited and slightly out of control. Some children become temporarily aggressive when they eat too much sugar. For children who already have a tendency to Heat in the Liver, sugar agitates their Liver *qi* further. Chocolate, which is energetically Hot, has a strong tendency to do this.

As well as these temporary effects of sugar, of course there are many long-term effects too. High sugar consumption is fuelling an epidemic of obesity and diabetes, and is increasingly being linked to a host of chronic diseases, such as heart disease, hypertension and certain types of cancer.

A child who has a strong craving for sugary foods may have an inherent Spleen weakness. The craving is both a symptom and a cause. For some children, eating sweet things is an attempt to fulfil an emotional need for more love, attention, warmth or understanding.

---

[*]   Rice, oat, hemp or almond milk are all possible alternatives which may be more easily tolerated.

[**]   For example, broccoli, kale, tofu, figs, oranges, sardines and salmon all have a relatively high calcium content. Many foods are also fortified with calcium.

Processed food

Processed food has fewer vital nutrients than fresh food. It will not nourish the *qi* and Blood of a growing child in the way that fresh food will. Much processed food is 'empty calories' which will fill a child up, but not truly feed him.

Additives

Many artificial additives, used to preserve, flavour or colour food (amongst other things), are not well tolerated by young children. Commonly, they create temporary Heat in the body which disrupts the Liver. Children who have a tendency towards being hyperactive may benefit hugely from excluding certain food additives from their diet.

> When my daughter was three, she was given a brightly coloured sweet that fizzed up in her mouth, which must have contained many insidious additives. For the rest of the afternoon, she became uncharacteristically aggressive and grumpy. Some children eat these kinds of sweets every day.

Lack of variety

Many children have a very limited diet despite the abundance of foods from all over the world that are widely available for most people. This seems to be more the case in the UK than it does in some other European countries. A special children's menu is found in most restaurants, pandering to the idea that children cannot eat what adults eat. In some families it is the norm for the children to eat one thing for a meal and for the parents to eat something different. It is probably true that a child would struggle to digest very rich food and that foods with tough textures may be difficult for him to chew. But many children's diets have become so limited that they are a cause of imbalance. Chapter 22 of the *Nei Jing* supports the notion that a varied diet is healthy when it says, 'The five grains act as nourishment; the five fruits from the trees serve to augment; the five domestic animals provide additional benefit; the five vegetables serve to complete the nourishment.'[64]

Generally speaking, a child who does not eat a wide enough variety of foods is likely to become *qi* and Blood deficient. The effect of a limited diet will depend on what foods it contains. If a child eats pasta, pizza and little else, she will be susceptible to the accumulation of Damp. If she eats nothing but fruit, she may tend towards being *yang* deficient. Being a picky eater can be both a symptom and a cause of Spleen deficiency. Treatment to strengthen the Spleen may help the child out of this vicious circle.*

Teenagers

Particular problems arise with diet during the teenage years.

Vegetarianism

As well as making a decision for ethical reasons to become vegetarian, it can be one of the many ways children may find of asserting their difference and independence from their parents. A good vegetarian diet containing a wide variety of vegetables, grains, fruit, nuts and pulses is probably not detrimental. A bad one, however, may not sufficiently nourish the Blood at a time when this is especially important. Vegetarians and, particularly, vegans are potentially susceptible to a deficiency of vitamin B12, and may well need to consume B12-fortified foods or B12 supplements. For some teenagers, a vegetarian diet consists mainly of pasta, bread and cheese, which is Damp forming and lacking in nourishment for *qi* and Blood.

---

* Of course, for some children, fussing over food is nothing to do with the state of their Spleen but is more related to the dynamic between them and a parent. Sometimes children choose the arena of food to play out their battles.

Fad diets

Trying out fad diets is common amongst teenage girls (although boys may of course do the same). In addition to the fact that it is depressing that so many girls (many of whom are not remotely overweight) feel the need to do this, it can have serious physical consequences. Most diets suit some people but not others. A teenager with a Cold and weak Spleen will not benefit from a raw food and juice diet. The Paleo diet, which involves consuming a large amount of meat, may not suit a teenager who has a degree of Full or Empty Heat. The 5:2 diet, which includes two days of near fasting a week, is probably not suitable for growing teenagers with exacting schedules.

A worrying trend, particularly amongst middle-class teenage girls, is an obsession with healthy eating. This is termed 'orthorexia' and is classified as an eating disorder. What starts out as an attempt to become healthier ends up with a life dominated by the attempt to eat only 'pure' and healthy foods. This may become a cause of disease if the child's range of foods eventually becomes very restricted.

> I once treated a fifteen-year-old girl for alopecia. My diagnosis was Blood deficiency. The girl had decided to become a 'fruitarian' six months earlier, around the time the alopecia started. After trying a more subtle approach and getting nowhere, I resorted to telling her that she had a choice between having alopecia or eating a more varied diet. Sadly, she chose the former and my treatment was not enough to help her whilst she continued with the same diet.

Lack of sleep

Sleep is the nourishment and food of a sucking child.

Thomas Phaer, 16th century

Babies and toddlers need an enormous amount of sleep. Modern research has confirmed that sleep has a direct impact on physical, mental and emotional development. The Sleep Council summarises the main reasons why children should get enough sleep as follows:

> As far as children are concerned the main benefit of sleep is the release of growth hormone encouraging normal growth and bodily development. Secondly, the brain benefits, by aiding the process of concentration – the making sense of the day's events, the things they learn at school and the skills they are developing as they grow up. Thirdly, the healthy brain development and emotional/mental health are encouraged by the 'de-toxifying' benefits of good sleep.[65]

During sleep, a child's *qi* is nourished as it is not being used for any activities for which it is required in the day. Blood returns to the Liver where it can be replenished. Sleep helps to nourish the child's *yin* as the stillness and calm it brings provide a balance to the *yang* activity of the day. The work of growing is so great that even a small deficit in sleep can make an enormous difference to both the emotional equilibrium and physical health of a young child.

Babies, toddlers and sleep

There are two main reasons a baby or toddler may not be getting enough sleep. The first is an imbalance in an Organ or the presence of a Pathogenic Factor. For example, a baby with too much Heat will often have disrupted sleep. Heat may rise up and disturb the *shen*, waking him up, whenever he tries to sleep. His mother may believe that her baby just does not need as much sleep as other children. When awake he is being fuelled by the pathological Heat in his system, so appears to have lots of energy. Yet it may be that, over time, this chronic lack of sleep brings about a depletion. Some babies make up for lost sleep at night by sleeping more during the day. Babies who are *qi* and Blood deficient often find it easier to sleep in the day than at night.*

The second reason children do not get enough sleep is that the sleeping environment is not right for them. It may be that the parents take the baby wherever they go in the belief that the child will become adaptable and learn to sleep in lots of different places. This may work for one child, but for another it means he is constantly overstimulated, so does not get enough sleep and becomes chronically depleted. One child will sleep better if he shares a bed or a room with his parents, whilst for another this is too stimulating and the presence of his parents nearby wakes him.

It is particularly important for young children that they sleep during the evening. This is the time when *yin* takes over from *yang* and brings about rest and replenishment. The old adage about an hour before midnight being worth two hours after midnight really applies to young children. Many parents find that if their child goes to bed later than usual, he will not sleep as well during the night. This is because he becomes adrenalised and overstimulated. His insufficient *yin* becomes too depleted if he missed the opportunity earlier in the evening when it is strong enough to bring the *yang* energy down into the body ready for sleep.

School-age children and sleep

The first few years of school are a demanding time for a child. She is still growing at an extraordinary rate and becoming accustomed to being around lots of other children, as well as learning new skills. Getting enough sleep, therefore, remains of vital importance.

The sleep of some children who may have slept well as toddlers deteriorates when they start school because they are overstimulated, or because they are unsettled by worries about school life.

A lack of sleep may bring about depletion in a child of almost any Organs or substances, and will depend on the child's constitution and other factors in her life. The dark circles under the eyes of a child who is chronically tired reflect a deficiency of Kidney *qi*. The Liver and Spleen are also susceptible to deficiency when a child does not get enough sleep.

> One distraught father brought his one-year-old baby to the clinic because the baby was grizzly all day long and wanted to be held all the time. On questioning, it became apparent that the baby was put to bed at 11pm when the parents went to bed, and woke up at 7am every morning, and was not given the opportunity to sleep during the day. He was getting eight hours' sleep a night, rather than the required twelve!

Teenagers and sleep

Sleep is the time when hormones needed for a teenager's growth spurt are released. Many teenagers struggle to have a rhythm and regularity to their sleep pattern. They may prefer to stay up very late but then struggle to get out of bed in the morning. The National Sleep Foundation recommend that teenagers get eight to ten hours' sleep a night.[66]

---

* This is because there is more *qi* available during the day, so they do not need to wake up to boost their *qi* by contact with an adult as they often do at night.

There are many changes taking place in the mind and body of an adolescent, all of which may cause difficulties with sleeping that were not present before puberty. For example, a teenage girl may become relatively more Blood deficient when she begins menstruating. This may affect her Heart, making it difficult for her to drop off to sleep. Liver *qi* stagnation often increases around this time too (see Chapter 68) and may lead to Heat which disturbs sleep, particularly in the middle of the night.

Apart from these physical changes, sleep in teenagers is often disturbed by the use of digital social media. Having phones and computers in the bedroom may mean that a teenager is adrenalised around the time he is meant to be heading towards sleep. Or he may be hyped up (or upset) by communication with his friends on social media.

A lack of sleep during the teenage years may cause deficiency in the same way that it might during the baby and toddler years. At this age, a deficiency of various Organs and substances may lead to any number of physical and emotional complaints.

Physical exercise

Ge Hong wrote, 'The body should always be exercised…yet even in exercise do not go to extremes.'[67] Not so long ago, physical activity was woven into the fabric of life in a way that it is not in the modern, developed world. Nowadays, parents are required to create opportunities for exercise for their children. Otherwise they spend much of their time being driven from place to place, remaining sedentary for most of the school day and spending much of their leisure time on some form of screen. As a result, exercise often becomes an 'issue' over which parents and children have a power struggle. Rather than it taking place naturally as a part of daily life, it has become something which needs to be artificially constructed. An outcome of this is that many children lose the ability to sense what level and type of exercise their body needs. It sometimes becomes about feeling an adrenaline rush, gaining some kind of satisfaction from having pushed oneself to the limit, or the impact the exercise has on how the child looks.

For many children, exercise is inextricably linked with competitive sport, meaning that only those who are naturally competitive or particularly talented take part. It has become something a child is either 'good at' or 'not good at' and yet another thing that has the potential to affect negatively their self-esteem. This seems to be particularly the case in boys. Significantly, it means that many children do not exercise in a balanced manner, either doing too much, or not enough.

Too much physical exercise

Young children are doing a lot of growing. Their Organs, channels, flesh and ligaments are not yet fully formed and 'firm'. Children have a strong need to move and run around, but too much exercise diverts their *qi* away from the process of growth and development, which suffers as a result.

This of course begs the question of what constitutes 'too much' exercise, to which there is no simple answer. Every child has a different constitution and can handle different types and amounts of exercise. For the first six or seven years of life, walking, running around, climbing and generally larking about is probably enough.

Problems of too much exercise may arise when a child is talented in a particular sport. A child who is required to train, week in week out, and who therefore has to 'dig deep' to get through it, is probably depleting herself in the process. Another common scenario is children whose parents' identity is bound up with exercise, sport and fitness. They often expect their children to participate in their sporting activities as soon as they are physically able to do so. Many young girls, in particular, do a lot of dance which may strain their growing tendons. During the teenage years, girls may over-exercise because they want to lose weight, and boys may over-exercise because they want to build muscle. Figure 8.1 shows the key Organs and vital substances that may be depleted by excessive exercise.

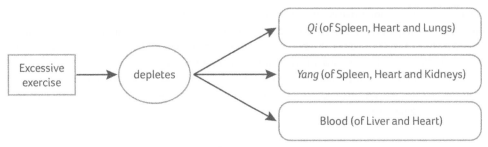

Figure 8.1 Possible effects of excessive exercise

The pernicious effect of too much exercise often begins to make itself known in older children and teenagers, who may develop musculoskeletal problems due to over-exercise. For a girl who may have recently begun menstruating, her Blood now goes to the Uterus and does not sufficiently nourish the tendons and sinews. Liver Blood deficiency may underlie problems of the tendons, such as tendonitis, and also more systemic problems such as fibromyalgia. For a boy, a lot of sport at the same time as rapidly growing means that his Kidney *qi* is easily depleted. As well as underlying musculoskeletal problems such as osteochondritis dissecans or Osgood-Schlatter disease, Kidney deficiency may also compound the natural tendency of some teenagers to lethargy, a lack of motivation, or even depression.

Dr JHF Shen talked of the particularly detrimental effect of exercising too much during the adolescent phase. He noted that it easily disturbed the balance of the gynaecological system in girls as they go through menarche, causing a mix of both deficiency and stagnation of Blood. Dr Shen also believed that excessive exercise during puberty could have a profound impact on the emotions which could last a lifetime. This is because of the tendency for prolonged excessive exercise to diminish the Heart, which houses the *shen*.[68]

> A fourteen-year-old told me that she could not understand why she always felt tearful in the few hours after she had been on a run, when others said they felt good for exercise. She was Heart Blood deficient, either as a result of the running or made worse by it. Her tearfulness confirms Dr Shen's view that excessive exercise diminishes Heart *qi*.

Inappropriate forms of exercise

One of the primary motives for teenagers to exercise is to remain slim (in the case of girls) and have well-developed muscles (in the case of boys). Many are also chasing an adrenaline rush, perhaps because society is often so focused on eliminating risk that humans have had to create other ways of feeling alive. This means that their exercise of choice is often very intense, maybe running or a hard workout in the gym. During puberty, children grow and develop nearly as quickly as in the first two years of life. Therefore gentler forms of exercise, such as yoga and walking, may be more appropriate and health enhancing.

Not enough physical exercise

There are swathes of children for whom not getting enough exercise is a big problem, so much so that the UK government, for example, has implemented initiatives such as Change4Life Sports Clubs which aim to get more children participating in sports. There is a crisis in many parts of the developed world of childhood obesity, diabetes and lack of fitness. This does not bode well for the health of these children as adults.

Children who are not active enough may develop certain imbalances as a result (see Figure 8.2). Some children may become Spleen *qi* deficient. The Spleen controls the muscles, and exercising muscles helps to keep the Spleen strong. A lack of movement may lead to a build-up of fluids in the body in the form of Dampness. Movement is also important to keep Liver *qi* flowing.

There are of course many emotional and psychological benefits of exercise too. The sense of doing something well can enhance a child's self-esteem, and playing team sports may help a child feel a sense of camaraderie.

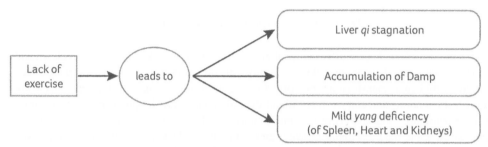

Figure 8.2 Possible effects of a lack of exercise

Sexual activity

Pre-pubescent sexual activity

Chinese medicine texts are clear that sexual intercourse pre-puberty in girls is harmful. Maciocia states, 'Excessive sexual activity (or indeed, any sexual activity) at an early age seriously weakens the Kidneys and injures the Directing and Penetrating Vessels.'[69] The reason is that there are great changes taking place in both the Directing Vessel (*ren mai*) and Penetrating Vessel (*chong mai*) at this time. Penetrative sex may therefore cause damage and stagnation in these vessels when they are at their most vulnerable.

The emotional impact of having sexual intercourse pre-puberty is likely to be just as damaging however, for both girls and boys. Sex pre-puberty will have taken place against the child's will. Children will find themselves unequipped emotionally to deal with the enormous and far-reaching consequences. It is likely to shape how they feel about themselves, their body and sexuality for many years to come. Hammer goes so far as to say that sex for a woman during the years surrounding puberty is a severe shock.[70]

Adolescent sexual activity

There is often a mismatch during adolescence between the maturity of the physical body and the relative immaturity of the psyche and the emotions. Even when consensual, there may be deep ambivalence in an adolescent who engages in sexual activity. The pressure a teenager feels from a romantic partner or from peers may mean he or she has sexual intercourse without truly wanting it. This may induce intense feelings that have a profound effect on the balanced movements of *qi*.

One of the reasons that sexual activity has such a strong impact on the emotions is the presence of the *bao mai* and the *bao luo*. The *bao mai* connects the Heart and the Uterus, and the *bao luo* connects the Uterus and the Kidneys. During sexual activity, the *qi* in these channels is stirred. Therefore, there is a physiological explanation for the fact that sexual activity has such a strong impact on a child's emotional world.

An added pressure for teenage girls in the 21st century is the fact that the boys are more likely than ever before to have accessed pornography. Much of the pornography that boys view portrays women as compliant partners whose primary purpose is to please men. This could not be more at odds with classical Chinese texts which focused heavily on the priority of sex being to heighten female pleasure.[71]

Sexual intercourse during menstruation in girls

Fu Qing Zhu wrote, 'If sperm is ejaculated into the uterus when the menstrual flow is surging and gushing out, the blood will retreat and contract…and the sperm will gather and transform Blood.'[72] As this passage illustrates, sex during menstruation is considered to impede the natural downward flow of Blood, giving rise to stagnation. This applies to women of all ages, but is particularly pertinent for teenage girls, in whom the menstrual flow is still trying to find its rhythm.

Sexual intercourse or masturbation in boys

Chinese medicine has long held the view that excessive sexual activity exhausts Kidney *yang* and depletes Kidney *yin* in men. This is because ejaculation of sperm is a direct loss of Kidney Essence.

> But if a man does not control himself and emits semen every time he sleeps with a woman, it is as if he were taking away oil from a lamp already nearly burnt out… Young men do not know this rule and those who know it do not practise it. (*The Classic of Su Nu*, 3rd century CE)[73]

The rise of Kidney *yang* during male puberty often causes a huge surge in libido. However, excessive sexual activity, especially in a boy who is already somewhat Kidney deficient, may curtail aspects of his growth. It may also lead to an imbalance between Water and Fire, between the Kidneys and the Heart. The Kidney *qi*, having become depleted, is no longer able to control the Heart. This may lead to emotional symptoms such as agitation, insomnia and lack of concentration.

In contrast, a boy who has grown up in a culture or family where masturbation is taboo may struggle in a different way. If he refrains from masturbation entirely out of a belief that it is somehow wrong, it may lead to a constraint of *qi*. If he masturbates but feels guilty for doing so, this will also be a cause of conflict which may bring about disruption in his *qi*.

Medications and vaccinations

Before any discussion of the possible role of medication in causing disease in children, it should be acknowledged that the lives of many children are saved by access to medications that now exist in the developed world in the 21st century. Antibiotics mean that most bacterial infections need not be life-threatening. Insulin means that a child who has Type 1 diabetes is now likely to live a long and active life. Fever-reducing medication means that children now only rarely die from a febrile illness. Modern medicine is responsible for a colossal reduction in human suffering.

However, the availability of drugs to treat all manner of childhood diseases has also led to their misuse. A grouchy baby may be given a dose of infant paracetamol because it is perceived that it will cheer her up or calm her down. I have heard three-year-olds refer to 'my Calpol' as if it is their friend, a kind of sugary comfort that can be turned to if they feel under the weather or unhappy. A bad cold caused by a virus may be treated with antibiotics (which do not affect viruses). There is often such a great deal of anxiety about a child being ill, even when the illness is mild, that it feels unbearable to the parent to do nothing. Children end up taking medication that does not help them but rather helps to allay the parents' anxiety about their child's illness. The lives of many families are so stretched and fast-paced that there is sometimes simply no time for a child to be ill. Parents feel that they cannot take time off work to nurse their child through a commonplace illness. So the child is medicated in order that she can keep going to daycare or school.

Medication has a role and a place in the treatment of children. It can also, however, be a cause of disease. In the traditional categories of causes of disease, this falls under 'wrong treatment'.

Ideally, before a child is given any form of medication, the potential benefits should be weighed up against the potential negative effects.

Below is a discussion of the energetic effects of some of the most commonly used medicines in children. As with every other cause of disease, the constitution and existing imbalances in a child will play a part in determining their response to medication. These are, therefore, only guidelines.

Topical corticosteroids

These are commonly used in the treatment of moderate-to-severe eczema. Doctors recognise the potential adverse effects of their long-term use, which include thinning of the skin, disturbance of the skin microbiome and even suppression of growth. However, it is generally thought to be good practice to prescribe them in order to gain control of the condition at the outset.

Steroid creams suppress the symptoms of eczema, rather than treating the root imbalance. It may be, therefore, that their use leads to a Lingering Pathogenic Factor as the pathogens involved in eczema are pushed deeper into the body.

Antihistamines

Antihistamines are frequently prescribed to children with allergies, hay fever and sleep problems. The medical view is that there are no long-term side effects of these drugs and that they do not lead to a worsening of the condition, even though symptoms may return once they are stopped. Antihistamines may have the following energetic effects:

- subduing Heat or Phlegm, which may lead to these pathogens manifesting at a mental level instead of a physical one, in the form of agitation or restlessness

- damage to the Kidney and/or Heart *yin*, suggested by the fact that they often lead to a dry mouth and palpitations.[74]

Laxatives

Three types of laxatives are commonly used in the treatment of constipation in children. The first is a bulk-forming laxative, such as Fybogel, which contains natural fibre. The second, such as Movicol, is one which softens the stool. The third is a stimulant, such as senna, which speeds up the action of the bowel.

None of these laxatives addresses the root of the problem. The child may become reliant upon them, and the condition may return or even worsen when they are withdrawn. In particular, the bowel may become dependent on stimulant laxatives. This would suggest that they deplete *qi* in the long term.

> An eight-year-old girl came to the clinic who had been constipated and taking a range of laxatives for four years. Every time she came off the laxatives, the constipation would return. With treatment to strengthen the *qi* of her Spleen and Intestines, she was able to come off the laxatives without the constipation coming back.

Fever-reducing medication

The most commonly used fever-reducing medicines in children, ibuprofen and paracetamol, have the short-term effect of clearing Heat from the exterior. Paracetamol has a medically recognised tendency to cause liver and kidney damage, suggesting that it depletes *yin* when used over the long term.

Whilst in a few cases of very high fever these medications are invaluable, they tend to be overused. In Chinese medicine, it is seen as a physiological aspect of childhood development for the child to need to expel Heat that arose in the womb (see Chapter 3). There may be subtle but significant consequences to the fact that an entire generation of children are medicated throughout even the mildest fever. A possible consequence would be that children become more deficient. However, it may also be that the child's ability to expel Heat is impaired, which leads to an LPF.

Please see Chapter 70 for suggestions of how to support children through a fever.

Vaccinations

 It is *not* within the professional scope of an acupuncturist to advise parents whether or not to vaccinate their children.

At the time of writing, children who follow the regular vaccination schedule in the UK are given nine vaccinations, involving seventeen different injections, between the ages of eight weeks and fourteen years old. The schedule for girls includes one vaccination on top of this, given at the age of fourteen. There are also an additional four vaccinations which are optional. The list of diseases that the regular vaccination schedule aims to protect children against are:

- diphtheria

- tetanus

- pertussis (whooping cough)

- *Haemophilus influenzae* type b (Hib)

- poliomyelitis

- *Meningococcus* serogroups ACWY

- *Meningococcus* serogroup B

- pneumococcus (*Streptococcus pneumoniae*)

- rotavirus

- measles

- mumps

- rubella (German measles)

- human papilloma virus (HPV).[75]

According to the conventional medical establishment, there are two main reasons for vaccinating children. The overriding one is an attempt to significantly reduce or even eradicate the occurrence of a particular illness. The second is to decrease the incidence of disease in individuals, particularly those who are deemed 'at-risk' because of, for example, a pre-existing health condition.

It is not within the scope of this book to debate the merits or otherwise of this ever more wide-reaching vaccination campaign. There is an overwhelming, as well as confusing and contradictory, plethora of information available on both the merits and dangers of vaccinations. Parents will often feel strongly pressurised by healthcare professionals, family members and acquaintances to make a decision one way or the other as to whether to vaccinate their child. It can be hard for many to come to a decision that they are able to live with comfortably.

On top of this, there simply do not exist many 'facts' about the possible adverse effects of specific vaccinations. Virtually the only facts we can be sure of are that many lives have undoubtedly been saved as a result of vaccinations and that they also carry risks of adverse reactions in a small number of children who receive them.

The role of the acupuncturist

It is inevitable that any paediatric acupuncturist will be asked time and again by concerned parents, all of whom want to do the best for their baby or young child, whether or not they should vaccinate. It is also likely they will be asked their opinion on whether a parent should give specific vaccinations and on the timing of vaccinations too. Practitioners will also see some children whose ill health arose within days, weeks, sometimes even hours, of having received a vaccination. Nevertheless, regardless of the strength of feeling a practitioner has on this issue, there is one point that should be remembered: it is *not* within the professional scope of an acupuncturist to advise parents whether or not to vaccinate their children. What we can do, however, is the following:

- treat any presenting pathologies before a child has a vaccination in order to minimise the chances of the child having an adverse reaction to it

- treat the child after a vaccination if he does have an adverse reaction

- treat the child through a childhood disease he contracts

- suggest to parents only to vaccinate when the child is healthy, for example not when he has a cold or is particularly run down.

Pathologies caused by vaccinations

From the Chinese medicine perspective, vaccinations may leave any of the following imbalances. Sometimes these imbalances manifest with relatively mild symptoms, such as recurrent earache. Occasionally, a child's life is irrevocably changed as a result of a vaccination, such as when it leads to epilepsy or convulsions.

- **Heat:** This may manifest as recurrent fevers, hot-type allergic symptoms, insomnia, behavioural problems or any sign of *shen* disturbance.

- **Phlegm:** This may manifest as a chronic cough, intermittent vomiting of phlegm and the child's character being subtly altered in some way, such as becoming spaced out or more irritable.

- **Qi deficiency:** This may manifest as a poor appetite, listlessness, tiredness and a pale face.

For a more detailed discussion of the particular effects of individual vaccines, the reader is referred to Chapter 19 of *Acupuncture in the Treatment of Children* by Scott and Barlow (1999).

Antibiotics

Antibiotics are energetically Cold and bitter, hence their ability to cool the Heat involved in infections. They commonly lead to digestive disturbances and diarrhoea, suggesting that they weaken Spleen *qi*. This often engenders the accumulation of Damp and/or Phlegm.* Maciocia[76] notes that they may cause peeled patches on the tongue, suggesting that in some cases they may deplete Stomach *yin*.

---

* In some cases, antibiotics may trigger anaphylactoid allergic reactions, suggesting that they create Toxic Heat.

Many children take antibiotics for recurrent infections of, for example, the ear or throat. Although they may be effective in terms of alleviating symptoms during the acute phase of the illness, they may leave the child further depleted and with more Damp, so therefore more susceptible to future infections. Teenagers may take antibiotics for acne, which is often a manifestation of Damp-Heat. They may help the Heat aspect but, in the long run, create more Damp.

Antibiotics also raise the chances of an LPF being left after an illness (see Chapter 27). Dr JHF Shen created a wonderful analogy about the effects of antibiotics. If a burglar breaks into your house, you have two options as to how to handle the situation. The first is to muster all your *qi* and wrestle the burglar out of your house. In the short term, this takes a lot of hard work, but in the long term entirely resolves the situation. The second is the path of least resistance, to simply shoot the burglar dead. This solves the short-term problem but creates a long-term problem of what to do with the dead body that is now in your house. Taking antibiotics is analogous to shooting the burglar dead. It does not require effort to do it and gets rid of the short-term problem of the infection. However, it often leads to an LPF in the child's body (analogous to the burglar's dead body). The consequences of an LPF may be recurrent illnesses, depletion and even subtle changes in character.

When antibiotics are necessary, ideally the child is supported by treatment to supplement the Spleen and Stomach, and possibly to clear Damp too. Dietary advice is obviously important in this respect.

Bronchodilators

Bronchodilators are commonly given to asthmatic children because of their ability to relax the smooth muscle of the airways. Their ability to do this can be explained by the fact that they mimic the effect of adrenaline in the body. Parents often notice that their child becomes hyperactive after using his bronchodilator. Adrenaline is *yang* in nature and creates movement. Therefore, the effect of bronchodilators in the short term is often to boost Kidney *yang* and move stagnant *qi*.[77]

Whilst this can be invaluable during a severe, acute asthma attack, in the long term there can be negative consequences. The short-term boost of Kidney *yang* is at the expense of the long-term strength of the Kidneys, which become depleted. The Lungs and Heart may also become depleted because the bronchodilators artificially stimulate these organs. The child may come to depend on the boosting effect of the bronchodilator as he becomes more depleted.

Inhaled corticosteroids

Inhaled steroids are also commonly used in the management of chronic asthma in children. They tend to create a temporary surge of *yang* and strong movement of *qi*, which enables the Lungs to function more effectively. As with bronchodilators, in the long term, their effect is to weaken the *qi* and possibly the *yin* of the Kidneys and Lungs.

At the same time, inhaled steroids also seem to subdue Heat and Phlegm. However, rather than ridding the body of these Pathogenic Factors, they tend to suppress them. This means that more Heat and Phlegm may arise when the drugs are removed. Heat which is suppressed also tends to deplete *yin* over time.[78]

Contraceptive medication

Teenage girls may take a variety of contraceptive medication. Although in most cases this is for the purpose of preventing pregnancy, they may also be prescribed if the girl's period is particularly painful or her menstrual bleeding excessively heavy. In a rather worrying trend, some teenagers use contraceptive methods that mean they do not have a monthly bleed, in a desire to avoid what they perceive as an inconvenience.

Different contraceptive medications have a variety of energetic effects on a girl's *qi* and Blood. As with most medications, they may cause severe side effects in one girl and be tolerated well by another. This is most likely determined by the pre-existing patterns of imbalance. For example, a medication that tends to cause an accumulation of Damp is likely to be less well tolerated by a child who has a pre-existing Spleen *qi* deficiency than by one who has a strong Spleen.

High doses of progesterone

This is given to the girl either in the form of an injection which may last between one and three months, or as an implant under the skin which may last up to three years. These high levels of progesterone prevent ovulation from occurring. Many girls experience the short-term side effects of weight gain and mood changes. Therefore, the energetic effects of progesterone-only contraceptive methods are likely to be an accumulation of Damp, stagnation of Liver *qi* and, in the long term, Kidney deficiency.

Slow-release and low-dose progesterone

The intrauterine progesterone-only system (IUS), otherwise known as the Mirena coil, is placed inside the uterus and releases a steady amount of progesterone. In some women this method vastly reduces their menstrual bleeding. However, in others it causes their periods to be more painful. It is possible that having a foreign body in the uterus creates a significant amount of local Blood stagnation.

The progesterone-only pill (otherwise known as the mini pill) contains a low dose of progesterone and is taken daily. Unlike the high-progesterone methods, this does not necessarily stop ovulation but, by changing the quality of the cervical mucus, prevents the implantation of a fertilised ovum. Common side effects of the mini pill include weight gain, acne and mood changes. Therefore, like the high-dose progesterone, this method of contraception also appears to create the accumulation of Damp and stagnation of Liver *qi*.

> One fifteen-year-old who came to the clinic had been prescribed the progesterone-only pill because her periods had been very heavy. Since taking it, she had developed mood swings and suffered from headaches, both of which may be symptoms of Liver *qi* stagnation.

Combined oral contraceptive pill (COCP)

Usually referred to as 'the pill', this is taken daily for twenty-one days of a twenty-eight-day cycle. During the days when the pill is not taken, the girl bleeds, but this is a 'withdrawal bleed' rather than a true period. The COCP both inhibits ovulation and affects the quality of the cervical mucus, which makes implantation impossible.

There are some known, long-term side effects of the COCP, such as an increased risk of thrombosis and of both breast and cervical cancer. However, many girls also experience short-term but unpleasant side effects. The most common of these are acne, mid-cycle spotting, nausea, mood changes, weight gain and headaches. Therefore, the energetic effects of the COCP are likely to be similar in nature to those of the progesterone-only pill, but perhaps more severe.

Stimulant drugs

Stimulant drugs, including amphetamines and methylphenidate, are often used in the treatment of behavioural conditions such as ADHD. They are thought to have a calming and focusing effect. In the short term they powerfully move Phlegm. In order to do this, however, they draw heavily on the *qi* of the Heart and the Kidneys which then become depleted in the long term.[79] Table 8.1 summarises the possible energetic effects of medications commonly prescribed to children.

Table 8.1 Possible energetic effects of medications commonly prescribed to children

Medication	Possible energetic effect
Topical corticosteroids	Create a Lingering Pathogenic Factor
Antihistamines	Subdue Heat and Phlegm Damage Heart and Kidney *yin*
Laxatives	Deplete *qi*
Fever-reducing medication	Prevents expulsion of foetal toxins (see Chapter 39) Depletes Liver and Kidney *yin* in the long term
Vaccinations	Create a Lingering Pathogenic Factor Deplete *qi*
Antibiotics	Create a Lingering Pathogenic Factor Deplete Stomach and Spleen *qi* Create Damp
Bronchodilators	Deplete Kidney *yang* Deplete Lung and Heart *yang* in the long term
Inhaled corticosteroids	Deplete *qi* Deplete Kidney and Lung *yin* Subdue Heat and Phlegm
Progesterone-only and combined oral contraceptive pill	Create Damp Stagnate Liver *qi* Deplete Kidneys
Intrauterine device	Stagnates Blood
Stimulants	Deplete Heart and Kidney *qi*

Conclusion

When treating a child who is taking long-term medication, or one who has in the past, it is important to attempt to ascertain what effect the medication has had on the child's *qi*. Of course, the medication may have hugely benefited the child. In some cases, it may even have saved her life. However, at the same time it will often have created other imbalances.

Treatment can help to negate any short- or long-term side effects of medication. It is helpful for the practitioner to be clear, when possible, about which imbalances are a part of the illness and which are a result of medication taken for the illness. For example, many children with asthma do not start out with a Kidney deficiency but they develop one after years of being reliant on bronchodilators and inhaled corticosteroids.

Differentiating between what is a part of the core, underlying imbalance, rather than a result of medication, helps the practitioner to direct treatment to the root of the condition. However, this is not always easy to do. The effect of each medication on a child's *qi* as described above is not set in stone. They are guidelines. Each child may respond differently to the same medication. It can be helpful to view either past or current medication as one of the many aspects of a child's life that will influence her health and well-being. Medication, just like, for example, diet and school life, has the possibility to both enhance and detract from a child's overall health, and sometimes to do both at the same time.

Recreational drugs and alcohol

The decision to have a section on recreational drugs and alcohol in a book about children may be somewhat sad but is, without doubt, necessary. In certain areas, they are prevalent and cause a multitude of problems, many of them severe.

Acupuncture can be useful to help deal with the negative physical and psychological effects of drugs and alcohol. It is more important, however, that an acupuncturist tries to understand what has led to the problem in the first place. The root problem, which may be feelings of pressure, loneliness or low self-esteem, may be partially helped with treatment too.

Alcohol

Although it may temporarily move *qi* and Blood (hence easing emotional inhibitions), in the long term alcohol creates more stagnation in the Liver. Stagnation often leads to Heat or Fire, and regular consumption of alcohol is therefore likely to exacerbate existing Liver Fire. This is what causes the red eyes and face of heavy drinkers, and the tendency towards anger or aggression. The movement of Liver *qi* in pre-teens and teenagers tends to be especially volatile, so they are particularly vulnerable to the effects of alcohol. This is beside the fact that early consumption of alcohol is thought to have irreversible effects on the developing brain.[80]

Marijuana

Smoking marijuana also has a strong impact on the Liver. Although it may temporarily heat up the Liver, its impact in the long term is to deplete Liver Blood and *yin*. This means the *hun* (Ethereal Soul) has no place to reside and is what causes the person to lose his sense of direction and focus, and to become less dynamic.

As with alcohol, marijuana consumption in the pre-teen or early teen years has been shown to strongly affect the developing structure of the brain. Young people are also known to have a higher risk than adults of becoming dependent on the drug. Also, it has been demonstrated that smoking marijuana has subtle effects on the expression of emotions and reasoning.[81]

Hallucinogenic drugs

Hallucinogenic drugs include LSD, psilocybin mushrooms, ketamine, MDMA and mescaline. This category of drugs, whilst not physically addictive, causes changes in the person's thoughts, perceptions and emotions. Whilst alcohol and marijuana tend to exacerbate familiar states, hallucinogenic drugs create states that are outside the person's regular consciousness.

The energetic effect of hallucinogenic drugs is to agitate the *hun*, causing it to 'come and go' to excess. Repeated use often leads to Heat in the Liver, and *yin* deficiency, particularly of the Liver and Heart.

Stimulants

Stimulants are mostly used by people who are seeking a 'high' or who want to stay awake all night (meaning their use amongst students is very common). The less desirable effects they commonly bring about are feelings of anxiety, paranoia and restlessness. Some stimulants, particularly cocaine, are highly addictive.

Repeated use of stimulants tends to deplete the *yin* of the Heart and Kidneys, leaving the person with chronic feelings of agitation and anxiety, often accompanied by severe insomnia.

> A sixteen-year-old boy came to the clinic for insomnia. He had taken stimulant drugs when revising for his exams in order to stay awake, but had seemingly lost his previous ability to sleep well since. His pulse revealed Heart *yin* deficiency. Nourishing Heart *yin* meant he began sleeping well again. We spoke about his obvious sensitivity to stimulants and that it would be wise for him to stay away from them in the future.

Conclusion

The aspects of life discussed in this chapter are some of the most commonly seen causes of disease in children who come for acupuncture treatment. Sometimes, lifestyle advice is all that is needed. At other times, advice and treatment is needed. There are times when, for a multitude of possible reasons, the child or the family are not ready to take on the advice that we give them, which we believe to be crucial to the child's recovery. It may even feel as if treatment is purely enabling the child to continue an activity which is detrimental to him. However, as flawed human beings we all know that what compels us to continue a bad habit may be stronger than the voices that tell us to stop it. As long as the child is still coming for treatment, there is still a possibility for ongoing dialogue which may, eventually, bring about the desired change in lifestyle. Furthermore, as treatment brings about more harmony, the desire to exercise to excess or take drugs, for example, may diminish.

SUMMARY

» Children have a delicate digestive system which is easily disrupted by the type and amount of food they eat, as well as when and how it is eaten.

» A lack of sleep is detrimental to all aspects of a child's health, especially in the first three years of life and during adolescence.

» Either too little or too much exercise may be a cause of disease in children.

» Pre-pubescent sexual activity in girls may affect both the body and the *shen*. Excessive sexual activity in boys during puberty may deplete the Kidneys.

» Medications, whilst sometimes necessary, may also cause imbalances of *qi*.

» It is not within the professional scope of an acupuncturist to advise a parent whether or not to vaccinate her child.

» When treating a child for the effects of drugs and alcohol, it is equally important to attempt to address the feelings that led the child to take them in the first place.

• Chapter 9 •

EXTERNAL CAUSES OF DISEASE

The external causes of disease discussed in this chapter are:

- Climatic factors

- Falls, physical trauma and accidents

Climatic factors

External Pathogenic Factors have been discussed as a cause of disease since the 2nd century BCE, for example in *Su Wen* Chapter 5. They broadly describe a range of both chronic and acute diseases, including what we now term as 'infectious diseases'.

Historically, infectious diseases were a common and much feared cause of illness and death in children and adults alike. In developing countries, infectious diseases are still one of the leading causes of death in children. In the developed world, with the advent of antibiotics and vastly improved living conditions, a very small number of children now die from an infectious disease.

However, invasions of External Pathogenic Factors are still the cause of illness and unhappiness in children and their parents. Babies and young children are more susceptible because their defensive (*wei*) *qi* is not strongly developed. Some children seem to have almost permanent colds. Moreover, a baby or young child may not have the strength of *qi* to fully expel a pathogen once it has invaded, which commonly leads to residual Damp, Cold or Heat lingering in the child's system. These lingering pathogens may then contribute to many chronic illnesses. Therefore, it is important to protect young children from external invasions. This involves, amongst other things, making sure they are appropriately dressed when they go outside.

The determining factor of whether a child succumbs to an External Pathogenic Factor is the strength of the pathogen in relation to the strength of his defensive (*wei*) *qi*. Some pathogens, such as the measles virus, are strongly infectious and a child is less likely to be able to defend himself against it than, for example, mumps.

However, because a child's defensive *qi* is relatively immature, even a mild wind, or being out on a summer's evening when the temperature suddenly drops, can be enough to cause illness.

It should be mentioned, however, that protecting a child against exposure to External Pathogenic Factors is not the same thing as keeping him inside. Fresh air is crucial for a child to develop strong Lung *qi*. Sun Simiao stressed that going out in the fresh air had many benefits for young children:

> Whenever the weather is mild and warm without wind, have the mother take the baby out into the sun to play. Frequent exposure to wind and sun congeals the blood, firms up the qi, and makes the flesh shut and tightly sealed. As a result, such babies are able to withstand wind and cold instead of falling ill.[82]

It is beneficial for a child's health, therefore, to be outdoors, but he should be well wrapped up and not allowed to become chilled.

In addition to the ability of External Pathogenic Factors to cause acute illnesses, climatic factors may also be a cause of chronic illness in children. Prolonged exposure to Damp, for example, may cause the gradual onset of a chronic condition. This may manifest in many different ways. For example, it may cause allergic symptoms that are worse in the winter, or digestive symptoms such as chronic loose stools.

I have not included Dryness because, working in the UK, I have never seen this in a child.

The individual climatic factors

Wind

Wind is known as 'the spearhead' of disease and will often carry another pathogen (such as Damp, Cold or Heat) with it into the body. Being a *yang* pathogen, it tends to cause a sudden onset of symptoms. It attacks the outer part of the body first and so tends to cause symptoms such as chills, fever and shivering. Children are particularly susceptible to invasions of Wind, because of their relatively weak defensive (*wei*) *qi*.

Wind can affect children in another way too. They have a tendency to be especially hyperactive and 'wild' on windy days. The Liver is affected by wind and may be aggravated by it, producing this agitated behaviour.

> The mother of a seven-year-old boy who suffered from attention deficit hyperactivity disorder said that she dreaded windy weather because she knew it always made her son's symptoms worse.

Cold

Children have a rather complex relationship with cold. A young child rarely notices the cold. He is quite happy to run around on a cold day with few clothes on and will often complain when asked to put on more clothes. Suddenly, and somewhat predictably from the parent's point of view, he will begin crying with pain because his fingers and toes are very cold. His exuberant *yang qi* seems to initially make him oblivious to the cold temperature but, because he does not have substantial and strong *yin* underlying, it will suddenly 'run out', leaving him vulnerable to the cold temperature. It is generally not disastrous these days in the modern world, as most children live in warm houses with heating, hot water and a kettle, so there are many ways of warming up again.

Although a young child may not feel the cold, that does not mean that he is not affected. Sun Simiao wrote that 'the reason why small children cannot yet be exposed to frost and snow is so that they do not fall ill with cold damage'.[83] It is common to see a child in the clinic who has gone down with a head cold or a stomach 'bug' or has started wetting the bed after he has become chilled. His weak defensive (*wei*) *qi* means that external Cold easily penetrates the interior.

Cold may also arise in the body because of dietary factors and medication (see Chapter 8).

Damp

For some young children, it is a continuous struggle to prevent the accumulation of Damp in their systems. The Spleen has to work hard in children to transform and transport the enormous amount of food they must eat in relation to their size. One result of it not working efficiently is that fluids remain in the body in the form of Dampness. It is easy to see the manifestation of this in young children, some of whom have a constantly runny nose, glue ear or a phlegmy cough.

> The mother of a four-year-old girl said that her daughter had had a snotty nose her entire life. The one exception to this was the family's two-week annual holiday in southern Europe. The dry climate meant that her Damp receded temporarily, only to return when they came home to the UK.

External Damp may invade the body with Wind and temporarily cause a type of head cold or it may cause chronic problems if a child lives in a damp house or in a particularly damp area. Damp is heavy and lingering, tending to cause symptoms which stay around for a long time.

A common cause of invasions of external Damp in children is swimming. For a child who is already prone to Damp, being in the damp and often cold environment of a swimming pool may make her susceptible to invasions of Damp, particularly in the Bladder and Intestines.

Damp may also arise in the body because of dietary factors (see Chapter 8).

Heat, Summer Heat and Fire

Heat may invade on its own, for example if the child is out in the sun too long. It may arise in the body if a child eats foods which are too hot in nature. It may also invade in combination with Wind and cause fever, rashes and potentially severe illnesses. Young children are prone to fevers because of their abundance of *yang*. Heat may have a rapid and severe impact on a child's body because his insubstantial *yin* is not able to keep it in check. He may go from being perfectly all right to burning up with a high fever in a matter of minutes.

Adapting to seasonal changes

Sun Simiao said, 'A rule for treating patients in early childhood: At the end of summer and beginning of autumn, you should constantly watch the weather and temperature.'[84] Children are particularly susceptible to invasions of External Pathogenic Factors during the changes between seasons, and at times when the weather is unseasonable. A sudden cold spell after the weather has begun to warm up in spring, for example, or a warm spell in the middle of winter, may leave a child vulnerable. The Triple Burner is responsible for regulating the temperature of the body. As with all the other Organs, in children it is immature and may not be able to adapt quickly enough to sudden changes in temperature.

At what age do children build up resistance to invasions of External Pathogenic Factors?

Without doubt, the first seven or eight years of life are often characterised by repeated bugs and infections, both respiratory and digestive. When a child starts playgroup or school, she may have a period when she succumbs with even more frequency to coughs, colds and digestive infections. Being in an enclosed space with many other children means that she is exposed to an unusually high number of pathogens. On top of this, the very fact of starting school, with all its inherent stresses and strains, may injure her *qi* and mean that she is more susceptible to pathogens.

However, from the age of about eight onwards, much to the parents' relief, most children will have stronger defensive (*wei*) *qi* and have built up some immunity. Moreover, when a child does catch a cough or cold, it does not have such far-reaching consequences as it does for a baby or toddler. It is unlikely to disturb her sleep or appetite to such a degree, and the ability to blow one's nose that most children of this age begin to master is a huge advantage. Generally speaking, a child's *qi* is much stronger by this age and her ability to fully expel a pathogen has greatly improved.

Falls, physical trauma and accidents

Children are particularly susceptible to physical trauma because they have not yet grown strong and robust. A bang to the head in a young child, for example, is more likely to lead to deeper stagnation of *qi* and Blood than it is in a twenty-year-old. It may not always cause immediate symptoms, but the cause of headaches that begin at the age of eight may be traced back to a particularly nasty bang on the head at the age of four, for example.

Physical trauma may be especially deleterious to young children because the imprint that it may leave on their *qi* means that subsequent development goes awry. It is as if it knocks them off course and, without treatment, they sometimes have no way of getting back on course. The pathological impact of the trauma then becomes set in, possibly for good, and may manifest in many ways throughout their life. For example, some cases of Parkinson's disease are thought to be due to a previous physical trauma.[85]

Some traumas, such as a car accident, can leave psychological scars too. The *shen* of a child is fragile and can be strongly impacted by a traumatic event. As seen in Chapter 5, shock makes Heart *qi* scatter and can, over time, disturb the movements of *qi* between the Heart and the Kidneys.

SUMMARY

» Young children have less ability than adults to withstand climatic factors.

» When an invasion of a Pathogenic Factor occurs, the consequences may be far-reaching and long-lasting.

» Physical traumas may imprint themselves on the *qi* of the child and be a cause of illness in either the short or long term.

Part 2

DIAGNOSIS OF CHILDREN

Chapter 10

INTRODUCTION TO THE DIAGNOSIS OF CHILDREN

The topics discussed in this chapter are:

- Diagnosis of the child
- Diagnosis of the illness
- Applying the different diagnostic frameworks

Introduction

Different practitioners will approach the treatment of children according to the style, or styles, of acupuncture they practise. In this section on diagnosis, I describe the approaches that I use in my clinic. It is desirable when treating children to have a variety of different methods with which to deliver treatment (e.g. needles, laser, *shonishin* tools) and it is also useful to employ different diagnostic frameworks. Children of different ages, and with differing conditions, benefit from a variety of approaches. This chapter is a brief outline of the various diagnostic frameworks that may be used with children of different ages.

Diagnosis of the child

Babies and infants

It is hard to separate physiology and character in a baby or a very young child. What is going on in his body, to a large degree, determines his mood. This is because his consciousness is very rudimentary and so experiences the world primarily through his body. For example, if his stomach is over-full, he will be physically uncomfortable. This will most likely be expressed with tears, moaning or fractiousness.

Excess or deficient constitution or Phlegm-type child

Young babies and infants may be categorised in three ways. Diagnosing whether a child has an excess or deficient constitution, or is a Phlegm-type child, is particularly pertinent up to the age of approximately three (although it may also come into play with older children too). This approach is important and unique to paediatrics. In itself, it is not necessarily something that needs treatment. However, knowledge of a child's constitution will strongly inform the practitioner's approach to treating the child and the lifestyle suggestions given to the parent. See Chapter 13 for a description of these three types.

Movements of qi

This is a very simple level of diagnosis that is most useful in the treatment of babies and infants but may also be relevant in children up to the age of approximately seven or eight. It describes a tendency within the child for his *qi* to flow in a particular way. This tendency may mean that he is susceptible to particular physical and emotional conditions. An imbalanced movement of *qi* may be treated with any technique described in Part 3. However, *shonishin* is particularly useful. See Chapter 13 for a description of the four different movements of *qi*.

School-age children and teenagers

Five Element constitutional imbalance

Nobody knows for sure whether a particular individual is born with his Five Element constitutional imbalance, or whether it develops over the first years of life. Whichever is the case, in most children it does not become apparent until at least the age of three and often not until the age of approximately seven or eight. A baby or young child can be likened to a flower bud which has not yet opened. His true nature is held within and gradually unfolds over the first years of life.

Once the practitioner is able to discern a child's Five Element constitutional imbalance, this can be treated with any method that stimulates acupuncture points. Treating the Five Element constitutional imbalance touches the very core of a child. It helps him to be the best he can, both physically and emotionally. In many cases, this treatment on its own may be enough to eradicate symptoms, physical or psychological. Sometimes, treatment of the Five Element constitutional imbalance is combined with treatment of Organ and non-Organ patterns. See Chapters 14 to 20 for a description of diagnosing and treating a child's Five Element constitutional imbalance.

Diagnosis of the illness

Organ and Pathogen patterns

Pattern diagnosis, which includes both Organ and non-Organ patterns, may be used when treating a child of any age. It is especially useful in the treatment of complex or long-standing physical conditions. Any method of stimulating acupuncture points (e.g. needling, laser, acupressure) may be used to treat patterns. Paediatric *tui na* may also be used in younger children.

Applying the different diagnostic frameworks

Below are examples of how the different diagnostic frameworks may be used and combined:

- A six-week-old baby with reflux is diagnosed simply as having 'counterflow *qi*'. Employing gentle techniques such as *shonishin*, to encourage her *qi* to flow downwards, may be enough to cure her of her reflux.

- An eight-month-old baby who is pale, quiet and uninterested in solids may be diagnosed simply as having an empty constitution. Needling a point such as St 36 *zusanli* with the tonification technique may be enough to awaken her interest in solid foods.

- A three-year-old child who has had a barking cough for the last six months will require a more detailed diagnosis. She may have a retained pathogen of Phlegm-Heat in the Lungs, possibly against a background of Spleen *qi* deficiency.

- An eight-year-old child, who seems overly defiant and unable to cooperate either at home or school, may be diagnosed as having a Wood constitutional imbalance. Treatment focused on bringing harmony back to the Wood Element may mean her behaviour changes significantly.

- Another eight-year-old child with recurrent urinary tract infections may be diagnosed with a Lingering Pathogenic Factor of Damp-Heat in her Bladder. The fact that she comes down with an infection whenever her 'best friend' tells her she is never going to be friends with her again may point to the fact that she has a constitutional imbalance in her Fire Element (see Chapter 16). Treatment of both the Lingering Pathogenic Factor and the vulnerability of the Fire Element may be necessary to prevent future recurrences of urinary tract infections.

In every situation, the practitioner must decide which diagnostic framework is the most relevant and whether it is necessary to combine two or more. This will partly depend on the practitioner's own background and way of working. This issue is not about choosing the right or the wrong diagnostic framework. As practitioners, we all know that different approaches can have similarly spectacular outcomes in the treatment of the same condition. We each have only one pair of eyes through which we can see the child in front of us. Figure 10.1 summarises the main diagnostic frameworks used in the treatment of children.

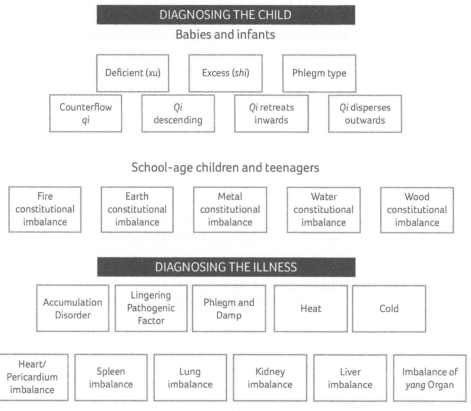

Figure 10.1 Summary of diagnostic frameworks

• Chapter 11 •

BUILDING RAPPORT WITH CHILDREN

The topics discussed in this chapter are:

- What is rapport?
- Why is rapport important?
- Techniques to help achieve rapport
- Gaining rapport with teenagers

What is rapport?

Rapport describes a relationship between the child and practitioner that is harmonious and that promotes trust and communication. It describes being 'in sync' with or on the 'same wavelength' as the child. It is often an unconscious aspect of human interaction, but one which profoundly affects relationships of all kinds. Gaining rapport means entering the child's world and getting a sense of what it is like for the child.

Although conversation is one aspect of rapport, there is a non-verbal aspect to it which is, of course, especially important when working with babies and very young children.

Why is rapport important?

Having a deep understanding of a child, gained through achieving rapport, helps the practitioner to diagnose more effectively. Many acupuncturists feel that their treatment achieves more when rapport is good. This is particularly important if the pathology lies at the level of the spirit.

When working with children, rapport serves another purpose. It means that the child is more likely to feel comfortable letting the practitioner carry out treatment. A child who does not trust or feel relaxed with her practitioner will rarely allow her to deliver the treatment. Rapport allows the child to feel relaxed, open and at ease whilst in the treatment room.

Achieving rapport with some children is easy. It arises naturally and spontaneously. With other children, the practitioner must work hard to gain rapport.

Techniques to help achieve rapport
Mirroring

Mirroring describes the process of the practitioner trying to match the child in as many different ways as possible. For example, she may match the child's body movements, voice tone or emotional state. This helps the child to feel connected to the practitioner and will engender a feeling that he is understood. It may sound strange to think of a baby or toddler having an awareness of whether or not he is understood. Of course, this process goes on at an unconscious level. It will be something that he feels rather than thinks. In fact, mirroring is probably the most important part of the rapport-building process in a pre-verbal child, with whom it is not possible to converse. It will, in turn, help the child to relax and trust the practitioner.

The practitioner may need to match a child's playfulness, or get down on the floor with her and join in her play. It may involve games of peek-a-boo or making funny noises which amuse the child. With an older child, the practitioner may match the child's enthusiasm when he talks about something that interests him.

Commonality

Commonality is the process of finding something that the practitioner and child have in common. This is an extremely important part of building rapport with a child from the age of around three. It means that the practitioner must try to become familiar with things that may be important to the child. This may be a book or series of books that the child enjoys reading, a film he has recently seen, a hobby or something that he enjoys at school. This gives the practitioner an opportunity to connect with her 'inner child'.

Every child should have something in her life that makes her come alive. It is the challenge of the practitioner to find what it is. A child usually lights up and opens up in front of the practitioner's eyes when she starts talking about it. Seeing the practitioner is interested in hearing about it can hugely help the process of rapport building.*

 A prerequisite to being a paediatric acupuncturist is to keep abreast with the current trends in children's books, films, computer games and crazes. An in-depth knowledge of the Harry Potter stories, for example, may be a valuable asset.

Acceptance

A child needs to feel truly accepted in order for rapport to develop between her and the practitioner. This means that the practitioner must work to deepen his feelings of compassion and must avoid judgement and blame. A child usually has a sixth sense for whether she is being judged. True compassion will be reflected in the practitioner's body movements, speech and manner. As André Gide said, 'True kindness presupposes the faculty of imagining as one's own the suffering and joy of others.'[1]

Acceptance of the child does not, however, mean acceptance of any behaviour. The art of placing limits on the child's behaviour in the clinic, whilst at the same time remaining compassionate, is one that the practitioner will most likely need to continually work at.

A clear and calm emotional state

Chapter 2 described how easily influenced children are by the emotional states of those around them. This is especially true of a child who is ill. The state of the practitioner's *qi* is of crucial importance. It could be argued that it is even more important than the treatment she actually gives to the child. Even a young baby is a highly tuned social being and will not truly 'receive' a treatment if she senses she is not being related to from the heart. If the practitioner is preoccupied, cross about something or generally fed up and tired at the end of a long day, it will be hard to gain intimate rapport with the child. There is no place to hide when we are in the presence of children. Children are like lie detectors. They will not be fooled by a pretence of cheeriness.

A three-year-old boy I had treated every week for two months came for his treatment. He had always been a joy to treat as he never protested at being needled and always seemed to really enjoy his treatments. This time, however, things were different. I went to needle him as I usually

---

* Some of the areas of life I am grateful to have learned about from the children and teenagers I treat include bicycle polo, Victorian gothic fashion, owls, palaeontology and the history of the dustbin lorry.

did and he looked at me with a very stern face and simply said, 'No needles today!' Despite my and his mother's efforts, he remained absolutely adamant and I treated him with laser acupuncture instead of needles. I was initially rather bemused by what had happened. That evening, I thought back over my day and realised that I had felt quite cross with the parent of the child in the previous appointment. I hadn't managed the feeling very well and it had got stuck inside me. The boy had sensed my crossness and knew instinctively he did not want to be needled by me. The next time I saw him everything was back to normal and I happily proceeded with needling!

A suitable ambience in the clinic and treatment room

It will be hard to gain deep rapport with a child if the general atmosphere in the treatment room is one of chaos and disorder. Furthermore, anything too sudden, strong or harsh may be experienced by the child as frightening. Children often come for treatment with one or more siblings in tow. A sibling may not like it when his brother or sister is the focus of attention, so may resort to devious methods to get everybody in the room to shift their attention to him. Similarly, an anxious parent may vie for the practitioner's attention. The practitioner needs to keep the focus of her attention on the child who is coming for treatment. To gain and keep rapport, the child must feel that the practitioner is directing her energy towards him.

Babies and young children also hate to feel rushed. A child will reveal less of who she is and be more likely to resist treatment if she senses the practitioner is rushing the process and she is being put under pressure.

Gaining rapport with teenagers

Everything already discussed about gaining rapport applies equally to teenagers as to younger children. Yet there are other complexities involved when working with teenagers. For example, in the UK, practitioners are required by their professional body to have the parent or guardian in the room throughout the entire case history and treatment if the child is sixteen or younger. In many cases this inhibits the teenager, who does not feel that he can say what he really wants to say. Since there is no way around this, the best thing is for the practitioner to try to turn around the parent's presence in the room to her advantage.

Observing the parent–child interaction

One way of doing this is to very closely observe the interaction, verbal but most importantly non-verbal, that takes place between the teenager and his parent and to use this information diagnostically. For example, there may be flashes of anger towards the parent or a sense that the teenager feels responsible and worried about his parent. The practitioner may notice that the parent answers every question she directs to the teenager on his behalf, or that parent and teenager contradict each other repeatedly. Observing the nature of the dynamic between the two may give the practitioner a valuable insight into the nature of the teenager's *qi* and, in particular, to the imbalance of his emotional state.

One thirteen-year-old girl was warm, friendly and open when addressing me. Whenever she spoke to her mother, on the other hand, her voice became clipped, a snarl came over her face and her eyes became hard. This showed me much about her internal world.

Summoning acceptance and compassion

It is very important for most teenagers that they do not feel disapproved of, especially if they suffer from a condition, for example self-harm or anorexia, for which they may already have met with disapproval. A teenager may also feel that everyone is 'getting on her case' all the time. She may have her parents, healthcare professionals or teachers telling her she needs to eat more or eat less, go out more or go out less, or do more exercise or stop exercising so hard, amongst many other admonitions and reproaches. The treatment room should ideally be a safe haven, where the teenager is entirely accepted as she is, warts and all.*

In order to gain rapport with teenagers, it is often helpful for the practitioner to familiarise herself with some aspects of teenage culture. An adolescent will connect much more easily with someone who can chat to him about the things that are most important to him.

Balancing gleaning information with maintaining rapport

It is usually a mistake to put any pressure on a teenager to open up about his internal world. The practitioner may hope that he does this in due course, once rapport has been established. Trying to force it, however, may mean that he closes down. It is easy to forget that a sullen and monosyllabic teenager may, at his core, be racked with feelings of vulnerability and inadequacy. Pressurising him to open up may result in a short-lived and pyrrhic victory for the practitioner.

For information on how to build rapport with a child according to her constitutional imbalance, please see the chapter on the relevant Element.

SUMMARY

» Rapport between practitioner and child is essential in order to diagnose accurately and treat effectively.

» The practitioner may try to 'match' a child's body movements, voice tone and gestures as a way of establishing rapport.

» Finding areas of common interest is also an effective rapport-building technique.

» Wholeheartedly accepting the child and interacting from a place of compassion will help the child to gain trust in the practitioner and to relax.

» The practitioner should endeavour to maintain a clear and calm emotional state and a suitable ambience in the treatment room.

» It is rarely fruitful to attempt to force information from a teenager who does not want to give it.

---

* Of course, this does not mean that the practitioner should not give a teenager advice, or urge her to go to bed earlier or eat more vegetables. But the advice will be better received if the teenager feels accepted and respected as a human being.

Chapter 12

THE DIAGNOSTIC PROCESS

. . . .

The topics discussed in this chapter are:

* The aim of diagnosis

* The process of diagnosis

* Pulling it all together

Introduction

Once some degree of rapport has been established, the diagnostic process may begin. Ideally, the practitioner will continue to deepen rapport during this process.

The discussion below focuses on how to go about the diagnostic process. It also includes some basic interpretations of the signs that the practitioner finds, especially where these are specific to children. Otherwise, the assignment of various symptoms and signs to Organ/Pathogen patterns or a Five Element imbalance should be made by consulting the relevant chapters. Interpreting signs in isolation can be useful but ultimately is of limited value.

The aim of diagnosis

Broadly speaking, the purpose of diagnosis is to answer the two following questions.

Who is the child?

The practitioner needs to find out who the child is. What is the nature of her spirit? How does it feel for her to be in the world? What tiny seeds of her personality are already beginning to sprout and what do they tell the practitioner about what the child needs from her? Which of the Five Elements is at the root of her imbalance? The aim is to get as clear a sense as possible of her true essence. Without this, it may be possible to treat her illness but it will not be possible to treat her. As the great physician William Osler said, 'Don't tell me what type of disease the patient has, tell me what type of patient has the disease.'[2]

In my opinion, the most effective method for treating the whole child is via her Five Element constitutional imbalance. This will often guide a practitioner in how she relates to the child. There is a discussion on building rapport with children of different constitutional imbalances at the end of each of the chapters on the Five Elements.

What is her illness?

Once the practitioner has begun to get a good sense of who the child is, the next question to address is the nature of her illness. For example, is the child ill because she does not have sufficient *qi* to cope with the demands of being in the world? Is there a pathogen that is blocking the smooth flow of her *qi*? Is she too hot or too cold? Or is the distribution of Heat and Cold in her body imbalanced?

The process of diagnosis

Traditionally, the process of diagnosis has been divided into the following areas:

- looking
- asking
- palpating
- smelling
- hearing.

When working with children, as well as 'asking', 'looking' and 'palpating' are particularly important. The reason for this is obvious in a pre-verbal child. However, even an older child or teenager may find it difficult to describe how she is feeling in any great detail. Even if the verbal acuity is there, the presence of a parent in the room may be another barrier to open expression.

Before describing how to undertake the traditional areas of diagnosis mentioned above, it is important to mention two preliminary stages that are essential if a full and accurate diagnosis is to be made: emptying the mind and opening the heart, and getting an initial 'hit'.

Emptying the mind and opening the heart

One of the many things that can be learned from a child is his ability to be in the moment. A young child very rarely has in his mind something that occurred a few minutes ago, let alone yesterday or a few weeks ago. A practitioner should endeavour to emulate this state. Anything in her mind that is not related to the child she is currently treating will hinder the process of diagnosis. An ongoing problem with a family member, or an anxiety about something happening later on that day, means that less of her *qi* is available to pick up everything that is in front of her now. Furthermore, the practitioner should aim to be in a state of openness in which she is able to receive all the information that the child presents. This includes the many sensory signs and signals but also something else that is harder to articulate. As Confucius said:

> It is better to listen with your mind than listen with your ears but better still is to listen with your *qi*. The ears only record sounds, the mind can only analyse and categorise but the *qi* is empty and receptive.[3]

As practitioners, it is easy for our minds to be full of theory and, indeed, it is important that we know the theory of the medicine we practise. However, it is equally important to ensure that theory does not lessen our sensitivity to the nature of the child in front of us.

In Antoine de Saint-Exupéry's children's classic *The Little Prince*, the fox tells the Little Prince, 'Here is my secret. It's quite simple: One sees clearly only with the heart. Anything essential is invisible to the eyes.'[4]

The practitioner must endeavour, therefore, with her *qi* and her heart, to become a skilled detective. She should be vigilant every second she is with the child so that she does not miss any vital clues as to the nature of the imbalances. It is in this state that the practitioner should embark upon the more formal diagnostic process described below.

Getting an initial 'hit'

Diagnosis should begin from the moment the practitioner and child meet.

Response to the surroundings

One child may appear excited and curious on arriving at the clinic and want to explore every corner of it. Another may be intimidated or nervous at being in this new place. One child will make her presence strongly felt as soon as she arrives. Her voice or cries can be heard even through the wall separating the treatment room and the waiting room, and she has taken out every toy by the time the practitioner appears. Another will sit as quietly as a mouse and not be tempted by any toys.

Response to the practitioner

A child may run up and greet the practitioner that he has never met before as if she is a long-lost friend. Another child may hide behind his parent's legs and refuse to look at or make eye contact with the practitioner. A child may start out the appointment nervous and shy but by the end be sitting on the practitioner's lap and not wanting to be parted from her.

Whilst observing all of these aspects of the child and his behaviour, it is crucial for the practitioner to begin gaining rapport with the child. Her way of being with the child must be shaped by her observations. It is up to the practitioner to meet the child at his level, rather than expecting the child to come to hers.

 POSSIBLE CLINICAL SIGNIFICANCE OF THE CHILD'S RESPONSE TO THE PRACTITIONER AND HER SURROUNDINGS

» Shy, nervous, reticent – deficiency

» Bold, loud – strong *qi*

Interaction with the parent

It is of course quite normal and healthy for a baby or toddler to be almost exclusively focused on her parent, especially when in an unknown situation. However, much useful information can be gleaned by observing the interaction between the two. A toddler may insist on doing everything herself rather than letting her parent help. She may cling to her parent for dear life throughout the entire appointment. She may get cross with her parent and push her away, or she may find ways to constantly vie for the parent's attention.

 POSSIBLE CLINICAL SIGNIFICANCE OF THE CHILD'S INTERACTION WITH HER PARENT

» Clingy – either Heat or deficiency

» Independent – strong *qi*

I describe below the process of traditional diagnosis applied to children.

Looking

Stature

Whether a child looks strong and robust, or small and delicate, gives us important information about the state of his underlying *qi*. The practitioner should also look at the child's limbs, which may be chubby and solid, or thin and fragile looking.

 POSSIBLE CLINICAL SIGNIFICANCE OF BODY STATURE

» Robust stature – strong *qi*

» Weak or thin stature – deficient *qi*

» Chubby, podgy stature – Damp and Phlegm

Body movements

Part of the observational process should involve noting how a child moves. In a young baby, this might involve simply with what degree of force she moves her legs and arms. With a toddler, it may involve looking at how quickly or slowly she moves, and whether she moves hesitantly or fluidly.

 POSSIBLE CLINICAL SIGNIFICANCE OF BODY MOVEMENTS

>> Fast body movements – Heat

>> Slow body movements – deficiency or Damp/Phlegm

Facial colour

Facial colour is one of the easiest things to observe in a young child and provides some crucial information. In children more reliable diagnostic information is available in the face than on the tongue.[5] The practitioner should note whether or not the complexion is pale or red. If there is redness, the depth and degree of redness is also significant. It may be that the entire face is red, or just the cheeks or just the lips, for example. Some children have a subtle, blue colour between the upper lip and nose, or on the bridge of the nose.

 POSSIBLE CLINICAL SIGNIFICANCE OF FACIAL COLOURS

>> Both cheeks red – Heat, often from Accumulation Disorder

>> Pale – *qi* deficiency

>> Yellow – Dampness

>> Blue colour on the bridge of the nose – shock and/or weak digestion

>> Green around the mouth – Accumulation Disorder

In order to clarify a Five Element diagnosis, other facial colours should also be noted. For example, there may be a green hue around the mouth or a yellow colour in some or all parts of the face (see Chapter 15).

Eyes

The eyes tell us a lot about the state of a child's spirit.

 POSSIBLE CLINICAL SIGNIFICANCE OF EYES

>> Vibrant eyes with sparkle – strong spirit

>> Dull eyes – weak spirit

>> Veiled eyes – Lingering Pathogenic Factor

Tongue

It is obviously not possible to ask a baby to hold her tongue out. The practitioner may be able to sneak a quick look at it whilst she happens to have her mouth open. Toddlers, on the other hand, are often experts in copying. If the practitioner sticks out her own tongue, or asks the parent to stick out his, the toddler will often follow suit. Even then, the practitioner has to get what he can from the tongue in the limited time he may have.

Tongue diagnosis is easier to carry out on a child once she reaches an age where she is able to put her tongue out and hold it out for a few seconds. There may be the odd child who will refuse to do it, either through defiance or embarrassment or else because she has been given the message that it is something she should never do. Telling the child that you are going to ask her to do something that she is only allowed to do whilst she is at the clinic often appeals to her mischievous side and raises the likelihood of compliance.

The most important aspects to look at are the colour, moisture and coating. A 'normal' tongue in a child is a few shades redder than the 'normal' tongue of an adult. This is because, as explained in Part 1, a child has an excess of *yang* and her *yin* is insubstantial. Bearing this in mind, other tongue signs have the same significance as they do in adults. The only exception to this is the tongue coating. It cannot be relied upon to be clinically significant in a baby or young child. This is particularly true in a milk-fed baby, where the milk itself means the tongue coating always looks thick and white. If there is something consistently striking about the tongue coating, then it should be noted and assessed for its significance in the context of all the other signs and symptoms.

Finger vein

This is a diagnostic method, dating back to the Tang dynasty, which is used exclusively with children up to the age of approximately three years old. The practitioner must observe the dorsal surface of the hand in the area between LI 4 *hegu* and LI 3 *sanjian*. In a healthy child, there should be no vein or one which is only very dimly visible. If a vein is present, the practitioner should look at the following aspects:

- **Length of the vein:** If the vein extends to the metacarpal-phalangeal joint (known as 'wind gate'), the disease is thought to be mild and at the exterior level. If the vein extends to the first interphalangeal joint (known as '*qi* gate'), the disease is thought to be severe and in the channels. If the vein extends to the distal interphalangeal joint (known as 'life gate'), the disease is said to be extremely serious, possibly even life-threatening, and is at the Organ level. (The wind, *qi* and life gates are shown in the diagram below.)

- **Width of the vein:** The wider the vein, the more virulent the pathogen is thought to be.

- **Colour:** A red vein indicates a Hot Pathogenic Factor.

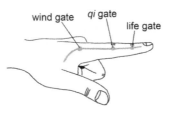

Asking

How to ask

TALKING TO THE PARENT

In a baby or pre-verbal child, it is obviously the parent who will provide most of the verbal information needed about the child and her symptoms. Whilst noting down this information, there are several other things to do. It is important to work on gaining rapport with the parent. The parent needs to feel that she is being listened to and being asked the right questions. If she is going to trust the practitioner to treat her child, she needs to feel she is trustworthy. The parent may be rather anxious about bringing her child for treatment in the first place. Sensing confidence, compassion and professionalism in the practitioner helps to allay her fears.

INTERACTING WITH THE TODDLER

Whilst taking the case history from the parent and observing the child, it is also wise to work towards interacting with the toddler at this stage. A child, especially one who is deficient in nature, needs time to slowly warm to the idea of interacting with an unknown adult. Simply picking a toy from the basket and offering it or mirroring his delight at the sound a toy makes when he squeezes it may be a good place to start. For one child making eye contact may be too much too soon, whilst for another not responding to his chat will be taken as a slight. The key thing is to be led by the child and to follow his cues. There are some young children who are so keen to interact that the struggle is being able to get all the information needed from the parent.

The following three aspects need to be borne in mind when taking the case history of a toddler:

» gaining the necessary information from the parent

» observing the child and beginning to gain some rapport with the child

» gaining rapport with and instilling confidence in the parent.

SCHOOL-AGE CHILDREN

Depending on how articulate the child is, and how willing or not he is to talk, it is likely that as the child gets older, he can be more and more involved in the process of taking the case history. It can be helpful for the practitioner to tell the parent and child that she is going to ask questions and she does not mind who answers them. It can be either the parent or the child, or both. It is also worth adding that sometimes parent and child might have different answers to the same question and that this is all right too. The practitioner may then use her own judgement as to whose answer is closest to the mark, or whether the truth lies somewhere between the two.

If the child is willing, then the more that he is able to be involved in taking the case history, the better. It can help him to feel that his thoughts and feelings are being listened to and respected. It can also give a child a sense of empowerment to be involved in this way, and the knock-on effect is often that he is happier to consent to the treatment that follows. Conversely, if a child would rather sit and play with a toy whilst the practitioner talks to his parent, then it is usually counter-productive to pressure him to become more involved. That is not to say that it might not be worth gently attempting to draw him into the conversation at times.

TEENAGERS

Once a child has reached the teenage years, it is reasonable to expect that she will be able to answer all the necessary questions herself, at least about her current health, if not her health history. This may be straightforward. Contrary to popular opinion, many teenagers are delightfully communicative and open. Some, however, are not. A teenager may feel ambivalent about telling the practitioner anything about herself, especially with a parent sitting in the corner of the room. As mentioned in the previous chapter, the practitioner always needs to balance the importance of getting certain pieces of information compared with remaining in rapport with the teenager. It is usually worth forgoing finding out a little more about, for example, the nature of the teenager's bowel movements if getting that information means she closes down and no longer feels comfortable.

Fortunately, this situation is far from being disastrous. One of the wonders of Chinese medicine is that diagnosis should be based more upon what the practitioner sees, feels and senses than on the content of what is said. The manner in which a patient talks is often far more important than the words she chooses. The information that is gained through the senses, together with the tongue and the pulse, will enable the practitioner to make a diagnosis and begin treatment.

An imbalance in *qi* may lead to an imbalance in the emotions. Therefore, once the imbalance in *qi* begins to be corrected with treatment, the practitioner may find that the teenager begins to talk more about how she feels. Obviously, the process of time and increasing familiarity between patient and practitioner also aid this process.

The practitioner might sometimes find herself in the middle between the parent and teenager. Whilst of course rapport with the parent is important (she is the legal guardian of the teenager and is usually bringing her to the treatment as well as paying for it), the teenager herself is the patient and the practitioner's primary focus should be on her and her needs. There may even be occasions when the practitioner feels the teenager is absolutely fine but the parent is insisting she is not. The practitioner must be mindful never to treat purely because the parent wants something about her child to be different.

> I once treated a fifteen-year-old girl who always came to the clinic with her mother. Her main complaint was painful periods. From the start, they vehemently disagreed with everything the other one said. If the girl said she slept badly, the mother said her daughter slept well. If the girl said she had a good appetite, the mother said that actually she did not eat nearly enough. Eventually, I had to ask the mother not to speak and let her daughter answer my questions on her own. I suspected that the endless conflict between them, and the mother's belief that she knew her daughter better than her daughter knew herself, was also a part of the aetiology.

LENGTH OF TIME

Obviously young children have a far less involved case history than an adult who has lived for decades. The practitioner needs to weigh up the importance of getting all the relevant information against keeping the baby or toddler happy. It is sometimes worth cutting short the case history and getting on with the treatment if the child is becoming agitated and restless. It will make the treatment much more difficult if she is unsettled by the time it starts. As long as all the key information has been gained, it is always possible to go back and fill in the gaps later on.

What to ask

What to ask during the taking of the case history depends on two key factors. First, the age of the child is significant. The older the child, the less detail is needed about her early life. When treating a teenager, knowing how well she slept when she was six months old may be of very little or no value.* Second, the nature of the child's symptoms will also influence what questions need to be asked. For example, if she is coming for treatment because of a sports injury, less time needs to be spent enquiring about her emotional life.

The areas defined below are a guide and should not be slavishly followed. The practitioner must use her common sense as to when certain areas need not be questioned, and when more detail is needed in others.

 When booking in a child for the first appointment, I always mention to the parent that she is welcome to email me any information she feels is important that she does not want to talk about in front of the child.

---

* Having said that, seeing a 'thread' throughout the child's life can be of value. The practitioner may notice that Spleen *qi* deficiency was present in babyhood (manifesting as waking every hour or two at night), then in toddlerhood (manifesting with picky eating) and then at eight years old (manifesting with excessive worry). Or, conversely, that a certain imbalance developed at a particular time but was not there beforehand. This can help to indicate a particular aetiology. For example, there may have been no signs of Spleen *qi* deficiency until the child started competitive sport when she was nine years old.

PHYSICAL SYMPTOMS

- **Main complaint:** nature of the symptoms; when they started; when most aware of symptoms; what makes them better or worse; what they stop the child from doing.

- **Digestion:** frequency of bowel movements; nature of the stools; any associated pain or discomfort; any nausea; vomiting; stomach aches; belching or flatulence.

- **Appetite:** details of breastfeeding or bottle feeding; process of taking to solids; quantity of foods eaten; variety and range of foods eaten; degree of thirst; intolerance or allergy to food.

- **Sleep:** sleep pattern including daytime sleeps; manner of waking in the night; how long it takes her to go to sleep; any tendency to wake up early or late; crying out whilst asleep; dreams or nightmares; sleeptalking or sleepwalking.

- **Vitality:** energy levels; stamina; what happens when tired; general vitality and vivacity.

- **Allergies:** the presence of any respiratory or food allergies; the age of onset, nature and severity of symptoms.

- **Chest and nose:** tendency to mucus, and if so, what colour and consistency; frequency of coughs and colds; runny nose; blocked nose; chronic phlegm on chest.

- **Ears:** blocked ears; hearing; ear infections.

- **Bladder:** urinary infections; bedwetting.

- **Temperature:** wants to be tucked up or throws the covers off at night; sweats at night; daytime sweating.

- **Skin:** rashes; temperature; itching; clamminess; puffiness.

- **Eyes:** vision; conjunctivitis.

HEALTH HISTORY

- **Childhood illnesses:** febrile diseases; febrile convulsions; respiratory infections; gastric infections. Anything out of the ordinary.

PREGNANCY, BIRTH HISTORY

- **Conception and pregnancy:** IVF baby; any significant health problems during pregnancy; medication during pregnancy; how the mother felt then, both emotionally and physically; any particular stresses during pregnancy.

- **Birth:** length of labour; vaginal or caesarean delivery; ventouse or forceps; antibiotics or anaesthetics during labour.

POST-NATAL PERIOD

- **First weeks of life:** how settled as a baby; jaundice; how feeding went; colic; how the mother was emotionally and physically.

- **Vaccinations and childhood diseases:** normal vaccination schedule; any childhood diseases.*

---

* Asking about pregnancy, birth and the post-natal period is of great importance in babies and young children, and becomes less important with older children. It may still have played a role, but other factors that influence the child's health have probably become more significant.

FAMILY HISTORY

- **Mother and father:** any significant history of health problems; any health problems around time of conception; any current health problems; any history of congenital family problems.

- **Siblings:** health of siblings.

FAMILY LIFE

- **Home life:** who lives at home; one or both parents; family set-up; number of siblings.

- **Stresses and strains:** relationship with siblings; parental relationships; one or both parents working; strains in the family.

- **Daily life:** how and where the child spends her day (e.g. home, nursery, school).

- **School life:** ease of separation from mother; degree of tiredness after a school day and at the end of term; ease with which the social side of school is managed; ability to concentrate in class and doing homework.

Palpating

Palpation of babies and toddlers

Touch is one of the most reliable ways to gain information about the nature of a baby's *qi*. A few babies and toddlers will resist being touched by somebody they do not yet know. However, most babies are very happy to be touched. It is important to approach touching a baby or toddler with confidence, yet to avoid any sudden or surprising movements. Ideally, touch should feel to the baby like an organic part of a growing interaction and a natural progression from the rapport building that began whilst taking the case history.

More diagnostic clues can be gained from touching a baby without clothes on. However, because the priority is to keep the baby in a calm and happy state in the lead-up to the treatment, the practitioner should be flexible about this. If a baby hates to have her tummy exposed, it is probably wiser to palpate the abdomen through clothes. Next time may be different, and the very fact of her resistance may in itself be diagnostically significant.[*]

ABDOMEN

The practitioner should use the palm of the hand to palpate the child's abdomen. Depending on the nature of the child, the pressure used should be firm but gentle. The important aspects to feel for are:

- the presence of any hardness or distension in the abdomen

- the temperature, specifically in relation to the other areas of the body.

● POSSIBLE CLINICAL SIGNIFICANCE OF ABDOMINAL FEATURES

» Hardness or distension – full condition

» Feels hot – Heat

» Feels cold – *qi* or *yang* deficiency, Cold

---

[*]   A strong resistance to have her tummy touched, for example, may indicate the presence of a full condition.

BACK

Placing the palm of the hand flat on the child or baby's back can reveal information about the state of the Kidney energy.

 POSSIBLE CLINICAL SIGNIFICANCE OF THE BACK

> » Strong, firm and upright back – strong Kidney *qi*
>
> » Weak, concave or cold back – deficient Kidney *qi*

LIMBS

Holding the baby's legs and arms will provide a lot of general information about the nature of the child's *qi*.

POSSIBLE CLINICAL SIGNIFICANCE OF LIMBS

> » Kicks in response to legs being held – strong *qi*
>
> » Does not move in response to legs being held – deficient *qi*
>
> » Soft, squishy, puffy limbs – Damp or Phlegm

Palpation of school-age children

Young children are usually happy to undress and allow us to palpate them. From the age when a child can first understand (which is usually before he can talk), the practitioner should always tell him what she would like to do before doing it. From the age of about five onwards, the practitioner should be aware that a child may begin to feel self-conscious about his body and this should always be respected.

The abdomen and back are the key areas to be palpated in a school-age child, as well as any area of the body where there is pain.

Palpation of teenagers

Palpation of a teenager is carried out in the same way as with an adult. The practitioner should always be sensitive to the fact that a teenager may be particularly self-conscious about her body. Just as the practitioner should avoid asking questions that may alienate the teenager, the same applies for palpation. It is always wise to weigh up the balance of possible benefits of palpating on a particular part of the body and the possible awkwardness it may engender.

Pulse

TAKING THE PULSE IN BABIES AND TODDLERS

Most authors agree that pulse diagnosis is of little value before the age of three.[6] This is for two reasons. First, because of the disparity in size between the practitioner's fingers and the child's wrist, it is not usually possible to differentiate the three different pulse positions. Second, the pulse in a child of this age is extremely variable depending on whether she has just had a feed or a sleep, or even simply what kind of mood she is in. As well as this, the practicalities of taking the pulse on a wriggly baby are also challenging. Luckily, there are so many other ways of diagnosing that this tends not to be too problematic.

If the practitioner does decide to take the pulse of a baby and succeeds in doing so, it should be remembered that the normal pulse rate is much faster than that of an adult.

From the age of about three upwards, pulse diagnosis becomes much more valuable. The size disparity between the practitioner's hand and the child's wrist is less, so the positions are easier to distinguish. The pulse is less variable from minute to minute than it is in a baby or toddler. Most importantly, the child should be able to stay still for long enough for the practitioner to make a reasonable assessment of the pulse picture. It can be helpful to explain to the child what you are doing when you are taking her pulse. An explanation along the lines that you are 'listening in' to what is going on in her body usually does the trick.

 It is easy to forget as an adult that five seconds of being still can seem like an eternity to an energetic three-year-old. Asking the child to focus her attention on something whilst she is having her pulse taken may help her to stay still. For example:

>> Ask her to count up to ten (or an age-appropriate number).

>> Ask her to see how many of something she can see from where she is sitting/lying in the treatment room (I hide tiny china pandas around my room for this purpose).

>> Ask her to see how many names of children in her playgroup or class she can come up with.

The normal pulse rate of a school-age child is still faster than that of an adult. The normal rate decreases slowly up until the age of about ten, by which time it will be the same as that of an adult. Table 12.1 shows the normal pulse rate at different ages.

Table 12.1 The normal ranges for pulse rate in children[7]

Age (years)	Rate (beats per minute)
< 1	110–160
2–5	95–140
5–12	80–120
> 12	60–100

Palpating the lymph nodes

A crucial part of diagnosis in a baby or young child is to feel the lymph nodes in the neck. This provides information about the presence or otherwise of a Pathogenic Factor.

NORMAL LYMPH NODES

Lymph nodes in the neck can always be felt, even when a child is healthy. They are not something that goes away. A 'healthy' lymph node is about the size of a pea or a baked bean (no more than half an inch across), and has a similar consistency to a pea.

PATHOLOGICAL LYMPH NODES

There are various ways in which a lymph node may manifest as pathological:

• It may be too big (i.e. more than half an inch across). It is helpful to compare the size of the node on one side of the neck with the equivalent one on the other side. If one is significantly bigger than the other, the practitioner can assume it is swollen.

• The node is very tender or painful on palpation.

• The lymph node feels hard, like a stone, and does not move when palpated.

RED FLAGS: LYMPH NODES
The following are signs that the child may be severely unwell and should immediately be referred to an orthodox medical practitioner:

✓ A lymph node is preventing the child from breathing, swallowing or drinking.

✓ The node becomes much bigger over a short period of time (i.e. less than six hours).

✓ The skin over the lymph node is red.

✓ The node limits moving the neck or head.

CLINICAL SIGNIFICANCE

Swollen or tender lymph nodes may indicate two pathologies:

- **Active Pathogenic Factor:** The lymph nodes will usually be swollen, and sometimes painful too, when the child is in the acute phase of an illness caused by an External Pathogenic Factor. This will, of course, usually also be evident because the child will have other symptoms of an acute invasion, such as fever, feeling unwell and sore throat.

- **Lingering Pathogenic Factor:** The lymph nodes will also be swollen and/or hard if the child has a Lingering Pathogenic Factor (see Chapter 27). The practitioner may go back to palpate the lymph nodes at various stages throughout the course of treatments. This is one way to assess the child's progress.

LOCATION

The nodes which are most important to examine in a child are:

- sub-mandibular nodes: underneath the length of the jaw.

- cervical nodes: these are in a z-shaped pattern along the sides of the neck. They are deep to the *sternocleidomastoid* muscle, and shallow to the scalene muscles. The tonsillar lymph node is especially important and is just behind the angle of the jaw (in the area of SI 17 *tianrong*).

- auricular nodes: the pre-auricular nodes are anterior to the tragus of the ear. The post-auricular nodes are behind the pinna of the ear.

It can also be helpful to palpate the lymph nodes under the armpits and in the groin.

METHOD

Lymph node examination, when done by an orthodox medical practitioner, is usually carried out whilst standing behind the person. When examining the lymph nodes of a child for the first time, however, it is advisable to stand in front. A child may not feel comfortable with things being done to her that she cannot see.

The practitioner should explain to the child beforehand what she is going to do (providing the child is old enough to understand). The flats of the fingers should then be placed in the relevant areas and should be used to move the skin over the underlying tissue in each area.*

Smelling

It is important when taking the case history to ask about the smell of the child's breath, urine and stools. If the child has been vomiting, then the practitioner should enquire as to the smell of the vomit too. The reader is referred to the chapter on the relevant conditions for the further clinical significance of the smell of urine, stools and vomit.

---

* There are many videos online which demonstrate this process. The reader is advised to find one connected with a respected medical institution of the country they are in.

CLINICAL SIGNIFICANCE OF SMELL

» Strong smell – Heat

» Absence of smell – no Heat

Practitioners of Five Element constitutional acupuncture, in particular, distinguish between different body odours in order to help make a diagnosis (see Chapter 15).

Most of us do not use our sense of smell to any great degree in our daily lives. We may notice whether odours coming from the kitchen smell good to us or that something needs to be chucked out of the fridge. Yet we are often oblivious to subtle smells. Therefore, to use the olfactory sense in the clinic takes much honing and practice. It is beyond the scope of this book to write a detailed account of how to go about doing this. The reader is referred to Chapter 25 of *Five Element Constitutional Acupuncture* by Hicks, Hicks and Mole (2011) for this purpose.

Hearing

Both the cry of a baby and the voice of a child can be useful diagnostically. The main information they give concerns whether the child tends towards deficiency or excess. Interestingly, Maciocia notes that if a baby moves his head from side to side whilst crying with a high pitch it denotes Accumulation Disorder.[8]

CLINICAL SIGNIFICANCE OF CRY AND VOICE

» Loud cry that cannot be ignored – strong child

» Quiet, whimpering cry – deficient child

» High-pitched cry with head moving from side to side – Accumulation Disorder

Pulling it all together

As can be seen, the diagnostic process is one which involves many different aspects of the practitioner, including her head, heart, senses and intuition. It may be that, after the end of the first meeting with parent and child, the practitioner feels overwhelmed with diagnostic information, some of which may be conflicting. Or she may feel she still has many questions and gaps in what she needs to know.

Whichever of those two possible scenarios most fits her experience, the most helpful question the practitioner may ask herself is 'Where is the best place to start?' When she feels overloaded with information, answering this question helps to gain focus and to ensure that she begins treatment with a clear plan in mind. If she feels she has lots of gaps and questions, this helps the practitioner to choose one thing she *is* clear about as a starting point.

SUMMARY

» The practitioner should aim to diagnose the nature of the child as well as the imbalance causing her illness.

» The practitioner should aim to be in an open and present state before starting the diagnostic process.

» The traditional methods of diagnosis may all be employed with children, but looking and palpating have greater importance.

» The aspects of the child that should be observed are: the way she responds to the practitioner and the surroundings; the way she interacts with the parent; her facial colour; eyes; stature; body movements; tongue; finger vein.

» The way of asking for information is determined by the age of the child. The practitioner needs to balance the need for information with the importance of establishing and maintaining rapport.

» The older the child, the less detail may generally be needed about the pregnancy, birth and early life.

» The key areas to palpate on babies and young children are the abdomen, back and limbs.

» The pulse is not reliable until the age of about three.

» If the information gained is confusing and conflicting, two helpful questions to ask oneself are:

  − What am I *sure* about?

  − Where is the best place to start treatment?

• Chapter 13 •

DIAGNOSING BABIES AND INFANTS

This chapter describes diagnostic models that tend to be used primarily, although not exclusively, on babies and infants. The models discussed are:

- Excess and deficiency
- The Phlegm-type child
- Movements of *qi*
  - Counterflow *qi*
  - *Qi* descending
  - *Qi* retreats inwards
  - *Qi* disperses outwards

Excess and deficiency

One method of diagnosing a child is according to whether he is constitutionally excess (*shi*) or deficient (*xu*). This is not so much a description of a pathological state but of the child's nature or constitution. It does not involve differentiating Organ or Element imbalances or the nature of pathogens. It is simply a statement concerning whether the child has too much *qi*, or not enough *qi*.

There are four key reasons that this differentiation is important and useful:

- It strongly guides the practitioner as to whether he should employ treatment principles which tonify or which clear pathogens from the child.
- It gives valuable information as to the nature of illness to which the child is likely to succumb, and also the course that the illness is likely to take.
- Even if the practitioner knows only whether the child is excess or deficient, she can still administer useful treatment.
- It enables the practitioner to give some simple but beneficial lifestyle advice to the parent which can make the difference between a baby who thrives and one who does not.

Characteristics of an excess (*shi*) child

- strong and robust-looking
- red cheeks
- big appetite
- cries loudly
- prone to high fevers

- strong pain

- inquisitive and interested in the world

- determined

- strong reactions

- strong presence.

Excess children are prone to:

- Accumulation Disorder

- Heat

- Phlegm.

Treatment of the excess type of child is usually focused on clearing Phlegm, Heat and/or Accumulation Disorder.

When an excess child comes to the clinic, he will most likely see it as an opportunity to explore a new place and meet new people. He will probably make his presence strongly felt. He may have a confident air to him, babble or talk loudly and have firm ideas about what he does or does not want to do.

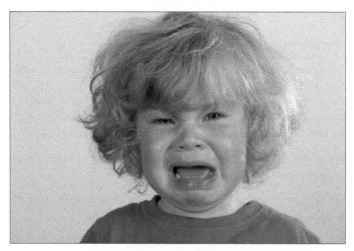

An excess child

Characteristics of a deficient (*xu*) child

- pale face

- poor appetite

- soft, whimpering cry

- mild, long-lasting illnesses

- prefers to stay with Mum rather than explore the world

- may not fully assert his presence in the world

- mild reactions

- thin and possibly frail-looking body.

Deficient children are prone to:

- deficiencies in any Organ. In young children, the Organs which most commonly become deficient are the Spleen, Lungs and Kidneys. However, any Organ may become deficient.

- Lingering Pathogenic Factors.

Treatment of a deficient (*xu*) child involves strengthening *qi*. The practitioner should decide on which Organs the treatment should primarily focus.

When a deficient child comes to the clinic, he may be apprehensive about coming to a new place and meeting new people. He may be shy or timid, and cling to his mum. He may need time to 'warm up'. He is also likely to be compliant and not to make a fuss about anything.

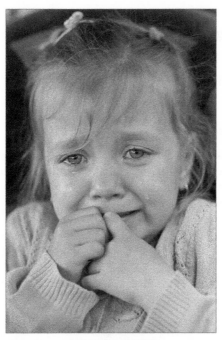

A deficient child

AN EXAMPLE OF HOW AN EXCESS OR DEFICIENT DIAGNOSIS MAY INFLUENCE TREATMENT

Two children come to the clinic, both suffering from a chronic, phlegmy cough. In both cases, there is undeniably retention of Phlegm in the Lungs.

Bill: Bill bounces into the clinic with a loud cough which is hard to ignore. He has red cheeks and has taken every toy out of the play box before the practitioner even reaches the waiting room. He makes immediate eye contact with the practitioner and enjoys leaping on and off the couch whilst the parent and practitioner are talking.

Ben: Ben is sitting on his mother's lap when the practitioner goes to the waiting room to call him in. He has a weak cough, although the phlegm on his chest is audible. His face is pale and he sits quietly as the practitioner talks to the parent.

Bill is an excess child. He has an abundance of *qi*. It is likely that the best treatment principle to use in order to clear his cough is to resolve Phlegm. In order to do this, the practitioner will need to use a sedation needle technique.

Ben is a deficient child. It is unlikely that resolving Phlegm will help his chronic cough. The practitioner will most likely need to use a tonification needle technique. Strengthening his *qi* will help him to throw off the phlegm on his Lungs.

The Phlegm-type child

A third category of basic constitution is the Phlegm-type child. Some babies are born with lots of Phlegm in their system. This overshadows everything else. All it is really possible to say about these children is that they are full of Phlegm. They will not necessarily have snotty noses and coughs. The Phlegm is often so thick that it blocks the channels and does not move.

The main characteristics of a Phlegm-type child are:

- chubby body
- may be puffy looking
- sleeps very well
- very contented and happy
- rarely complains
- may be slightly dulled and unresponsive.

As can be seen from the list of symptoms, parents often feel they have been blessed with an amazingly 'good' baby. Phlegm-type babies tend to be much easier to look after than either the excess or deficient type. However, if the baby is not able to throw off the Phlegm as he gets older, it may go on to cause problems and underlie many illnesses.

 The Phlegm-type child describes a constitutional tendency, rather than an inherent pathology. See Chapter 27 for a description of the non-Organ pattern of Phlegm/Damp.

Treatment involves loosening the Thick Phlegm so that it can then be expectorated, resolving phlegm and strengthening the Stomach and Spleen (see Chapter 27).

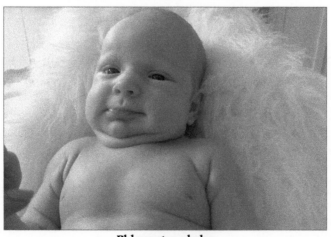

Phlegm-type baby

Movements of *qi*

In clinical practice, diagnosis according to movements of *qi* is most useful when treating babies and toddlers.

As mentioned in Chapter 2, the main channels only become 'activated' after the child is born. In the womb, the eight extraordinary channels determine the flow of *qi* in the foetus. Therefore, after birth and in the first weeks and months of life, the channel system is establishing its balance and rhythm. Rather like a toddler taking his first steps, it is unstable and can easily be knocked off its path.

Some symptoms that occur in young babies are simply a reflection of the fact that the flow of *qi* in this immature channel system has become disrupted. This idea has been given emphasis at various times during the history of paediatrics in TCM. For example, Qian Yi, often considered the grandfather of paediatrics, stressed the importance of promoting the ascending and descending functions of the Spleen and Stomach.[9] Sun Simiao stressed the propensity of *qi* in babies to rise upwards and that an important treatment principle in nearly all cases was to gently bring *qi* downwards. For example, he suggests that if a baby is too hot (during a transformation and steaming) the best treatment is to 'induce a mild downward action'.[10]

In clinical practice, there are four broad pathologies of *qi* that are commonly seen in babies and toddlers.

Counterflow *qi*

Counterflow *qi* involves an ascension of *qi* which then leads to physical or emotional symptoms. It may be caused by shock or overstimulation. The *qi* of babies and toddlers may be prone to ascending because *yuan qi* is immature and cannot yet strongly root *yang qi*. As can be seen in Parts 4 and 5, the majority of conditions for which parents seek treatment for their children involve an element of counterflow *qi*. Some of the most common are:

- reflux
- regurgitation of milk and vomiting
- sleep disturbances
- easily overstimulated
- red face, agitation and an inability to settle
- tendency towards fevers, or, in severe cases, febrile convulsions and seizures
- anxiety.

The treatment for counterflow *qi* is to gently bring *qi* downwards. There are various ways of achieving this. Using points which encourage the downward flow of *qi* or which root the *qi*, such as St 36 *zusanli* or Ki 1 *yongquan*, is one method. The stroking technique used in *shonishin* is another way (see Chapter 35). There are also various paediatric *tui na* moves which promote the descending of *qi* (see Chapter 34).

The aim of treatment is simply to encourage and support the immature *qi* of the baby or toddler to find its proper path and movement once more. The intervention normally needs to be light and delicate.

A baby who came for treatment for reflux had counterflow *qi*. I taught the mother a paediatric *tui na* routine to descend *qi*. She did this twice a day and it kept the baby's reflux at bay.

Qi descending

Qi descending arises from a deficiency of the Spleen which is often under strain in babies. Symptoms which may reflect *qi* descending are:

- diarrhoea
- loose stools and frequent bowel movements
- lethargy
- lack of physical vigour
- difficulty toilet training
- bedwetting (in older children).

The treatment of *qi* descending is to strengthen the Spleen, which is the Organ responsible for raising *qi*. Points on the Spleen channel or other points which affect the Spleen, such as Ren 12 *zhongwan*, may be used to do this. Paediatric *tui na* massages (see Chapter 34) are also useful. Sometimes, minor changes to feeding patterns and diet are enough in themselves.

> A two-year-old had loose stools since a gastric bug six months ago. Six acupuncture treatments, all of which used points to strengthen and raise Spleen *qi*, were enough to make his bowel habits healthy again.

Qi retreats inwards

In health, there will be a balanced distribution of *qi* both inwards in order to fuel the internal Organs which determine the baby's growth, and outwards in order to form a defensive layer between the baby and his environment. Sometimes the *qi* of a baby or toddler appears to have retreated inside. This may manifest in the following ways:

- struggle to make eye contact
- difficult to reach
- a strong sense of the child being in his own world
- delayed speech
- perhaps very agitated
- clingy
- fearful of new people, places and situations.

This pattern may occur because the *shen* of the child is weak and engaging with the world is overwhelming for him. It may also arise because of a shock either in the womb or early in life, when the *qi* and *shen* are immature and fragile.

Treatment of *qi* retreating inwards is to strengthen the *shen* of the child. The best way of doing this is to treat the Heart with points such as He 7 *shenmen* or He 1 *jiquan*. *Shonishin* techniques may also help to gently draw more of the child's *qi* to the surface of the body.

A three-year-old boy came to the clinic because his parents were concerned that he was not speaking yet. He made no eye contact with me and spent a lot of time trying to hide behind his mother. He did not respond to any of my attempts to interact with him. I had the sense that he was hiding inside himself and it did not feel safe for him to 'come out'. His mother told me that she had witnessed her father suddenly dying of a heart attack when she was seven months pregnant, and she wondered if this was why her son did not communicate. Treatment of the boy's Heart gradually enabled him to engage with the world more.

Qi disperses outwards

Sometimes the *qi* of a baby or young child appears to be too much on the surface of the body. This may mean that there is not enough *qi* available for the growth that needs to take place. This may manifest in the following ways:

- highly reactive to external environment and stimuli
- overstimulated or hyperactive much of the time
- hard to settle and always on the go.

The aim of treatment with a baby or toddler whose *qi* is dispersed outwards is to encourage the *qi* towards the centre of the body, and to strengthen the *yuan qi* so that it holds *qi* inwards more effectively. Using a tonification needle technique on points along the *ren* channel which runs along the midline at the front of the torso is one way of doing this.* *Shonishin* techniques may also be helpful. It is important for a baby or toddler with this pathology to avoid being in an overly stimulating environment.

A seven-year-old boy came to the clinic because he was very anxious and lacking in confidence. He had a rather thin and frail body and it seemed that his *qi* was concentrated on the surface of his body. He would constantly ask questions about the acupuncture charts on the wall of the clinic and was hyper-focused on the external environment. It was very hard for him to lie still. I always began treatment by using a point or points on the *ren* channel. This would enable him to settle enough for me to do the rest of the treatment.

SUMMARY

» Describing a baby as excess or deficient is not to say he has a pathology. It describes a constitutional tendency.

» A Phlegm-type child may not have any obvious mucus. The Phlegm is often thick and blocks the channels.

» Babies and young children may have a tendency for their *qi* to flow in a particular direction. Counterflow *qi* is especially common.

---

* It is interesting to note that many babies and young children with a tendency for their *qi* to disperse outwards naturally like to lie on their tummies to calm themselves down.

• Chapter 14 •

FIVE ELEMENT CONSTITUTIONAL ACUPUNCTURE APPLIED TO CHILDREN

The topics discussed in this chapter are:

- The internal causes of disease are emphasised
- Defining the level of treatment
- The primary constitutional imbalance
- Strong emphasis on inter-relationships
- Minimum intervention
- Preventive treatment
- Treatment of chronic conditions
- The importance of rapport
- Use of points
- Outcomes of Five Element constitutional treatment
- Blocks to treatment

Introduction

At the heart of Five Element constitutional acupuncture is the understanding that the whole person, rather than the symptom, should be at the heart of acupuncture treatment. This echoes the insight of the great 17th-century physician Xu Dachun, who explained, 'Illnesses may be identical but the persons suffering from them are different.'[11]

Although Five Element constitutional acupuncture is firmly rooted in the Han-dynasty classics of Chinese medicine, the underlying values of the style described below are set out in the *Nei Jing*, *Nan Jing* and other classics. This style was developed in the 1960s and 1970s by an Englishman named JR Worsley and has subsequently been taught, and continues to be taught, to thousands of acupuncture students and practitioners in the UK and the USA, and to a lesser extent in some other European countries and Canada.

The core understanding of this style of acupuncture is that the symptom and the person are indistinct from one another. Rather than only asking how a particular symptom can be relieved, it first asks how a particular person can be treated. Whilst the importance of relieving symptoms is embraced, it is considered even more important to bring about a positive change in the *overall* health of the person. The treatment of the person will, in many cases, also bring about an improvement in, or resolution to, physical and emotional symptoms.

I have laid out below the other most important distinguishing factors of this style of acupuncture, and have highlighted how they relate to the treatment of children. The reader will see how many aspects of this style are especially apt for children. However, what follows should by no means be seen as the definitive description of the style, which would be beyond the scope of this book. For the reader who is not trained in this style and who would like to understand it further, I refer them to the book *Five Element Constitutional Acupuncture* by Hicks et al. (2011). For readers whose training has been in Five Element constitutional acupuncture, I ask them to forgive what may read as a somewhat basic introductory synopsis.

The internal causes of disease are emphasised

Working in the developed world in the 21st century, most children who come to my clinic live in houses with central heating and have warm clothes to wear. If they get chilled, they are able to warm up at home with a hot bath and a bowl of warm soup. If they get a fever, they have access to medication which can usually control it. They are (arguably) well nourished and have access to a wide range of foods.

Without doubt, most of the chronic conditions for which children come for treatment have arisen at least in part as a result of an internal cause of disease. The stresses and strains that most children in the developed world face today are not primarily of a physical nature. They do not have to toil in the fields and are no longer sent up chimneys. The biggest strains in their lives are usually of an emotional and psychological nature. The illnesses from which they suffer, in many cases, arise from the impact of these strains on the child's emotions and consequently their spirit.

Whilst not discounting the external and miscellaneous causes, practitioners of Five Element constitutional acupuncture place a high degree of emphasis on the internal causes of disease. This is because emotions predominantly affect the spirit, compared with external causes of disease which are more likely to affect the body. *Su Wen* Chapter 5 clearly explains, 'The emotions of joy and anger are injurious to the spirit (*shen*). Cold and heat are injurious to the body.'[12]

Chen Yen, in the *San-yin Fang*, described seven internal causes of disease (*qi qing zhi bing*). These are:

- anger (*nu*)
- joy (*xi le*)
- sadness (*bei*)
- grief (*you*)
- overthinking or worry (*si*)
- fear (*kong*)
- shock (*jing*).

Please see Chapter 5 for a discussion of how emotions cause disease.

Defining the level of treatment

A practitioner of Five Element constitutional acupuncture will prioritise observing and experiencing the state of a child's spirit. In particular, she will endeavour to get a sense of how emotions have affected the spirit. Whilst the physical symptoms also need to be understood and diagnosed, these are often considered to arise as a result of an imbalance affecting the spirit of the child.

There are many varied views on the meaning of the word 'spirit' (*shen*). The best definition of the Chinese medicine view of the spirit is summed up by Claude Larre as follows: 'The *shen* are that by which a given being is unlike any other; that which makes an individual an individual and more than a person.'[13]

A dysfunctional expression or repression of an emotion may, over months and years, become etched in the very being of a child and define the nature of her *shen*. Once the spirit has become affected in this way, it begins to play a part in defining how a child responds to life. It may be that certain situations feel stressful for a child. Her ability to learn may become impaired or her relationships may be coloured by a difficulty with a certain emotion. For example, she may habitually feel easily rejected or unloved in her friendships. Treatment addressed at correcting this imbalance in the spirit is therefore considered of the utmost importance for the long-term emotional and physical health of the child.

The primary constitutional imbalance

One of the most important concepts of Five Element constitutional acupuncture is that every person has a fundamental, possibly innate, constitutional imbalance in one of the Elements. Chapter 64 of the *Ling Shu* contains an exploration of this idea of Five Element constitutional types, even though it is based on different criteria than those used in Five Element constitutional acupuncture. The constitutional imbalance is considered to be the root (*ben*), which may give rise to manifestations of dysfunction (*biao*), in any of the other Elements. Both diagnosis and treatment are focused on this constitutional imbalance. Treatment on the channels of the Organs related to whichever Element the imbalance is deemed to lie in may resolve symptoms which manifest in other Organs and Elements. It is also considered to be good preventive treatment, in order to ensure that symptoms and illnesses do not return and new ones do not form.

The question of when a person's constitutional imbalance is formed remains a much-debated one amongst practitioners of this style. Some babies are born with their constitutional imbalance already established, whilst in others it is formed due to their response to circumstances in the first years of their lives. This is the acupuncturists' version of the great 'nature versus nurture' debate which is ultimately unresolvable.[*]

Children up to the age of seven or eight years old are a 'work in progress'. Many aspects of them are not yet fully formed and set. Even if the seeds of a child's constitutional imbalance are present, they have rarely sprouted forth in the first few years of life. Therefore, up to this age, the practitioner cannot be sure that the predominating imbalance will be the one that remains for life but it is still the one that should be treated. After the transition to the second cycle, which has normally taken place by about the age of eight or nine, the child has become more formed and the constitutional imbalance that will most likely remain for the rest of the child's life comes to the fore.

Strong emphasis on inter-relationships

The reason that treating a child's fundamental constitutional imbalance in a particular Element may be enough to bring about overall health can be explained by the interconnectedness of all the Elements via both the Generating (*sheng*) and Controlling (*ke*) cycles (see Figures 14.1 and 14.2). This concept was discussed at length in the great classic of Chinese medicine, the *Nan Jing*. Oriental culture is steeped in the idea that relationships between things are more fundamental than the 'things' themselves. Oriental cooking, gardening and *feng shui* all reflect this concept. However, it is one which Westerners tend to struggle with, as it is so alien to the way that we have been brought up to understand the world. The practice of contemporary TCM does not place this much emphasis on the interconnectedness of the Elements.

---

[*] Loo puts forward a theory that childhood can be divided into four developmental stages, each of which correlates with one of the Five Elements. Please see her text *Pediatric Acupuncture* (2002).

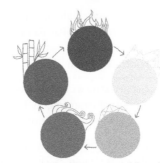

Figure 14.1 The Generating (sheng) cycle

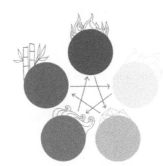

Figure 14.2 The Controlling (ke) cycle

The Elements are not discrete entities but phases in a cycle. The whole will only work well if each of the individual parts are balanced. A change in one Element will bring about a change in all the Elements. For example, using sedation points of the Liver and Gallbladder channels may mean that the *qi* of the child Element, Fire, increases. Or it may mean that the *qi* of the Wood Element stops 'invading' the Earth Element, which is the next Element in the *ke* cycle from Wood. The goal of Five Element constitutional acupuncture is to bring about harmony between all of the Elements. Even if the *qi* of all the Elements is somewhat deficient, as long as there is an equilibrium between them, the situation is considered preferable to large discrepancies in the *qi* of each Element.

This style of acupuncture is particularly suited to the treatment of children. At a time of life when growth, change and development are so extraordinarily rapid, imbalances frequently occur. Acupuncture treatment to ensure a consistent, fundamental harmony between the Elements vastly lessens the chances of this happening. It is akin to taking great care that the foundations of a house are laid correctly and strongly. If this happens, then the house is better able to withstand storms and extreme weather and will remain robust for many years.

Minimum intervention

The impact of these inter-relationships on treatment is that it means minimum intervention is required. The concept of the least intervention to bring about the maximum change is one that is threaded throughout the history of Chinese medicine. The great physician Hua To, for example, was renowned for the fact he successfully treated patients by using just one or two needles.[14] Just one or two points along the channels of the Organs related to the Element of the child's constitutional imbalance may be enough to affect the *qi* of all the other Elements and bring about a harmony between them. After each point is needled, the practitioner must take great care to observe any subtle changes in the child, in terms of her demeanour, colour, voice, odour and pulse. The experience of practitioners of this style is that the most profound changes often occur after a minimalist treatment.

This has particular advantages when treating children, who may neither like nor tolerate a large number of needles being used in each treatment. Paediatric practitioners who practise other styles of acupuncture also recognise that it is easy to 'over-treat' young children. Stephen Birch, a renowned practitioner of Japanese acupuncture, writes:

> Because everything is in a more accelerated state we can also see a quicker response to treatment. This makes it necessary to use lower doses of treatment, to do less, in order to trigger the same degree of change that we trigger in an adult using larger doses of treatment.[15]

Julian Scott, who practises TCM acupuncture on children, writes that 'great care should be exercised with respect to the number of points chosen'.[16] The fact that a child's *qi* is so dynamic, and that the rate of physiological change is so great, means that the minimalist approach of Five Element constitutional acupuncture suits paediatric practice remarkably well.

Preventive treatment

The idea of preventive treatment is one which runs through the classics of Chinese medicine. Chapter 1 of the *Su Wen*, for example, says:

> When medicinal therapy is initiated only after someone has fallen ill, when there is an attempt to restore order only after unrest has broken out, it is as though someone has waited to dig a well until he is already weak from thirst, or as if someone begins to forge a spear when the battle is already underway. Is this not too late?[17]

The idea of seeking treatment as a preventive measure is an alien one to most people in the West. Even though most of us unquestioningly go to the dentist for check-ups, few rarely think of giving their mind, body and spirit the same care. Five Element constitutional acupuncture places a high value on preventive treatment. Patients often say that, because they feel so much better in themselves, they would like to have occasional treatments to ensure that they stay that way. Preventive treatment is of particular benefit to children. Our experience of childhood strongly informs how we respond to and cope with life as an adult. Contentment and wellness as a child does not guarantee a trouble-free adult life but it is certainly 'credit in the bank'. Therefore, treatment that helps a child to achieve this contentment is incredibly valuable.

Treatment of chronic conditions

TCM paediatrics has traditionally been very heavily slanted towards the treatment of acute diseases. For example, *The Essentials of Traditional Chinese Pediatrics* (Cao, Su and Cao 1990) lists the treatment of twelve 'common' diseases and twelve 'seasonal' diseases. Of the twelve 'common' diseases, five of them could be acute or chronic but the differentiation is heavily weighted towards the acute form of the disease. All the 'seasonal' diseases are acute (e.g. whooping cough, measles, rubella). Of course this is because historically acute febrile diseases were a grave cause for concern and one of the leading causes of infant mortality. They are still a cause for concern today in many parts of the world but, largely due to antibiotics, can be much better treated by orthodox medicine. Acupuncture can also be extremely effective at helping children through acute diseases.

However, in the West, most children who come to paediatric acupuncture clinics come with chronic diseases. Most children with a severe, acute condition are taken to see a medical doctor. Parents may even cancel their child's acupuncture appointment if they have an acute condition.* Five Element constitutional acupuncture is particularly suited to the treatment of chronic diseases,

---

* However, we can of course educate parents about the ability of acupuncture to help a child through an acute condition such as a fever, asthma attack or cough.

especially those which have at their root a weakness in the child's constitution or an emotional dysfunction. It is less suitable for treatment of acute conditions.

The importance of rapport

A key characteristic of Five Element constitutional acupuncture is the importance that is placed on gaining rapport with the patient. The better the rapport the practitioner is able to gain, the more she will understand the nature of that patient's internal world, in particular the state of the key emotions within the person. This will then lead to a more individually tailored and effective treatment. Even though emotions tend to be less hidden in children than they are in adults, understanding the *child*, rather than just the physical symptoms, only comes from having gained rapport with her.

For a discussion of rapport, see Chapter 11.

Use of points

Any point on the relevant *yin* and *yang* channels may be used to treat a Five Element imbalance. However, emphasis is placed on the category of the point as laid out in the Han-dynasty classics. Points most commonly used to treat the constitutional imbalance are:

- *yuan* source points
- tonification points
- sedation points
- junction points
- horary points
- Element points
- back *shu* points
- front *mu* points.

Please see Chapter 30 for a table of these points and others that are commonly used to treat the spirit of each Element.

Most commonly, a 'pair' of points is used to treat both the *yin* and the *yang* Organs of the Element which is being targeted. For example, if the practitioner deems that the child's constitutional imbalance is in the Water Element, she may choose to needle the *yuan* source points of the Kidney and Bladder channels, Ki 3 *taixi* and Bl 64 *jinggu*. Providing treatment of this Element brings about the required changes to both the pulses and the child, a variety of points on these two channels will then be used during each subsequent treatment. This may be combined with another treatment principle, for example resolving Damp or calming the *shen*.

Outcomes of Five Element constitutional treatment

In Five Element constitutional acupuncture, treating the root imbalance which lies in the spirit of the child is believed to be the most effective way of bringing about improvements in the symptoms, which are often the manifestation of a deeper imbalance. Crucially, however, focusing treatment on the spirit usually helps the child to feel better in herself, rather than just to be rid of a particular symptom or symptoms.

A child who feels 'good in herself' often has a very different experience of life compared with one who does not. Moreover, her family will experience her very differently. She may eat better, sleep better and have more energy. She may be happier to spend periods of time playing on her own or, conversely, be more willing to join in with other children. Her friendships may go more smoothly or a relationship with one of her parents may become closer.

Treatment of the constitutional imbalance helps to keep a child's development 'on track'. Children are forever changing and developing. This has both advantages and disadvantages. On the one hand, it means that there is a greater possibility of bringing about any change that is desired. On the other hand, it means that things can more easily go astray. Just as a potter must keep his hands on the clay as it turns around the wheel in order to help shape the form of what he is making, so must the circumstances of a child's life support her growth and development. Acupuncture treatment of the child's constitutional imbalance is one way of helping to ensure the child keeps 'on track'. It is like the potter's hands around the emerging pot.

When the root imbalance is treated in an adult, she may notice that she worries less or feels less sad or has a more even temper. However, this may occur after decades of worry, sadness and bad temper. Many years of emotional imbalance, as well as affecting most key areas of life, also have a lasting impact on a person's *qi*. Years of feeling chronically sad, for example, will deplete Lung *qi*. Lung *qi* deficiency may lead to many and varied physical symptoms too, such as breathlessness or frequent coughs and colds. Emotions also become somewhat habituated and hardwired into the brain if a person experiences them over a long period of time.

Therefore, if this primary emotional imbalance is treated during childhood, the benefits of doing so can hardly be overstated. Treatment of the child's spirit during times of change or stress can prevent a particular emotion becoming distorted in some way and that distortion becoming the 'norm' for the child, possibly for decades to come. Distorted emotions lead to imbalances of *qi*. Imbalances of *qi* lead to emotions becoming more distorted and also, of course, to a multitude of physical symptoms.

Blocks to treatment

JR Worsley taught that there are four important ways that the *qi* of a person may become pathological which are distinct from the usual disharmony between the Elements. He called these 'blocks' to treatment and taught that, unless they are cleared, treatment of the underlying constitutional imbalance is unlikely to be effective. The four blocks are:

- Aggressive Energy
- Husband–Wife imbalance
- Possession
- Entry–Exit blocks.

These blocks may all occur in children, although some of them tend to do so less commonly than in adults. It is beyond the scope of this book to describe the diagnosis and treatment of the blocks in detail. However, there is a short description of those most commonly seen in children in Chapter 30.*

---

* The reader is referred to Section 4 of *Five Element Constitutional Acupuncture* by Hicks et al. (2011) for a full description.

SUMMARY

» The internal causes of disease are emphasised in Five Element constitutional acupuncture and are those frequently seen in children.

» The Five Element acupuncturist distinguishes different levels of treatment, namely that of the body and that of the spirit.

» Each person is born with a constitutional imbalance in one Element, or develops this in the first years of life.

» This style of acupuncture emphasises the importance of the inter-relationships between the Elements and, for this reason, treatment on the Element of the constitutional imbalance may bring about harmony in all the Elements.

» There is a strong focus on preventive treatment, based on the belief that it is easier to keep somebody healthy than to make him better once he has fallen ill.

» Five Element constitutional acupuncture is particularly suited to the treatment of chronic conditions and is less adept at treating acute conditions.

» Rapport is considered an important part of treatment.

» The categories of points laid out in the Han-dynasty classics are often used. In particular, one point on each of the *yin* and *yang* channels related to the Element of the imbalance are often paired.

» Patients often have an increased sense of well-being and vitality after receiving Five Element constitutional acupuncture.

• Chapter 15 •

DIAGNOSIS USING FIVE ELEMENT CONSTITUTIONAL ACUPUNCTURE

The topics discussed in this chapter are:

- Diagnosing the level of the imbalance
- Diagnosis is based primarily on signs rather than symptoms
- The importance of the emotional imbalance
- How to diagnose the emotional imbalance
- Colour, sound and odour
- The pulse

Diagnosing the level of the imbalance

Some problems have clearly arisen in the body. If a child comes to the clinic with a sprained wrist which occurred when she fell out of a tree, treatment clearly needs to be focused on the body. Another child may come because he has stopped seeing his friends and will not get out of bed in the morning. In this case, the problem is most likely to lie in his spirit, his *shen*.

The above examples are very clear cut and the reality is not always this simple. In many cases, the problem lies in the body and the *shen*. The job of the practitioner is to decide where the *primary* imbalance is and direct the treatment accordingly. Some problems have a clear physical origin, yet the fact that they do not heal as they are expected to is because of an underlying imbalance in the *shen*. A child may respond to a physical problem in a way which indicates that his *shen* is not healthy. In both these cases, purely treating the body is unlikely to resolve the problem. *Su Wen* Chapter 25 explains, 'In order to make all acupuncture thorough and effective one must first cure the spirit.'[18]

Some 'clues' that may point towards the child's problem being predominantly at the level of the *shen* are:

- **Interaction with others:** The child struggles to interact well with people. The practitioner will either observe this in relation to herself or the way the child interacts with his parent. Or the parent may report that the child struggles to make friends or get along with other family members.

- **Eyes:** The child struggles to make eye contact, or the eyes reveal an inner state of lifelessness or agitation.

- **Body language:** The child's body reveals an imbalance in the spirit. She may carry herself as if she has 'given up'. Her body is slumped and she drags herself around. She may, conversely, reveal an agitation of her spirit in her body. She may find it hard to be still or her body may be extremely tense and tight.

- **Speech:** She may not be able to express herself in an age-appropriate way or the language she uses may reveal an unhappy spirit.

- **Responses to life:** The normal events of a child's life, such as having a new teacher at school or going to another child's house to play, may evoke extreme emotions in a child that seem out of proportion with the event.

- **Emotional reactions:** Whilst in the treatment room, the practitioner notices that the child either has very extreme emotional reactions or, on the other hand, does not respond at all when some expression of emotion would be expected.

- **Emotional and psychological development:** The child is failing to meet the expected milestones in his emotional and psychological development by quite some way.

The practitioner needs to make a decision before beginning treatment about what 'level' the imbalance lies at. There are two main reasons for this. First, it enables the practitioner to have the right intention (*yi*) when she carries out the treatment. Second, it will inform the point choice that the practitioner makes. If the practitioner deems that the primary level of imbalance is in the spirit, then points which are particularly effective at addressing this level may need to be incorporated into the treatment (see the section 'Use of points' in Chapter 14 and Chapter 30).

Diagnosis is based primarily on signs rather than symptoms

A distinguishing feature of Five Element constitutional acupuncture is the emphasis on making a diagnosis based primarily on signs rather than symptoms or behaviour.

> Attempting to diagnose a child's constitutional imbalance by behaviour alone is flawed and usually ineffective. This is because it relies on speculating about the reason behind a particular behaviour. For example, a child who consistently misbehaves at school may be seen to be angry and defiant (normally related to a Wood imbalance). In reality, she may be behaving this way because she is fearful (stemming from a Water imbalance) or because she is displacing grief (stemming from a Metal imbalance). Sensory acuity has, throughout the history of Chinese medicine, been understood to be a superior method of diagnosis. It helps the practitioner to look beyond superficial behaviour and symptoms and to diagnose the imbalance that has led to that behaviour.

When an imbalance in a person's *qi* in any of the Five Elements arises, it will cause a change to take place in the physical body, mind and spirit. This change will 'resonate' with the Element in which the imbalance occurs. Chapter 34 of the *Nan Jing* gives an in-depth description of the Five Element resonances, which are shown in Table 15.1. The resonances convey to the practitioner which Element the disharmony has arisen in and also the particular nature of the disharmony. The 'key' resonances are the ones that most reliably inform the practitioner in this way.[*]

Table 15.1 Key Five Element resonances

	Fire	Earth	Metal	Water	Wood
Colour	red	yellow	white	blue	green
Sound	laughing	singing	weeping	groaning	shouting
Emotion	joy	sympathy/worry	grief	fear	anger
Odour	scorched	fragrant	rotten	putrid	rancid

In order to diagnose by signs, the practitioner must hone her senses in order to *feel* the *qi* of the child. The four key signs used for diagnosis are:

---

[*] The 'supporting' resonances provide further information which is not usually used to fundamentally inform the diagnosis but still helps the practitioner to build a more complete picture of the disharmony.

- the colour on the face

- the sound of the voice

- the odour

- the predominant inappropriate emotion.

These are considered more reliable forms of diagnosis than the answer to questions or the nature of the patient's physical symptoms.

Diagnosis based on signs rather than symptoms is a skilled art that takes practice. Relatively speaking, making a diagnosis by asking a person about her symptoms is easy. Fortunately, however, diagnosis based on signs is easier in children than it is in adults. First, there are usually fewer layers of pathology and thus less complexity than in adults. Second, a child's *qi* is much more alive and less hidden than that of an adult.

Once mastered, diagnosis by signs particularly lends itself to the treatment of children because it is hard to get an accurate verbal description of their physical symptoms. It is often not until the teenage years (and in some people much later than that) that a child is able to describe in any great detail how she feels. The parent is able to fill in some of the gaps but cannot himself truly know how his child feels. He may also have his own bias when describing to us the nature of his child's symptoms.

The importance of the emotional imbalance

The most useful sign in diagnosing a Five Element imbalance in the spirit is the emotions. This is because an emotion can be both a symptom of an imbalance and a cause of disease. When treating adults, the emotion that is most imbalanced may be difficult to detect. However, when treating children, emotion is usually less hidden. Whilst those practitioners with a training in Five Element constitutional acupuncture may employ colour, sound, odour and emotion in the diagnosis of children, all practitioners may incorporate diagnosis of Five Element emotional imbalance into their treatment of children.

The practitioner needs to walk a fine line between understanding that every child is unique and therefore will have her own emotional norm, and at the same time spotting which emotions have weakened the child and are not helping her to thrive in the world. One child may be perpetually angry and in conflict with her parents and teachers in a way that is hindering her relationships and her ability to do well at school. It would serve her well to find a way of lessening her anger. Another child may allow her siblings and classmates to walk all over her and never stand up for herself. She, conversely, would thrive if she were able to be more assertive in the world. The more that the practitioner is able to tune in to who the child is, the more he is able to have a vision of how that child would be if she were living according to her true nature. It could be said that the goal of treatment is to help the child to become closer to her true nature.

Chapters 16 to 20 describe the different ways in which the key emotion related to each Element may become imbalanced, and what this looks like in a child. In broad terms, when an emotion is imbalanced within a child, it may happen in one of the following ways:

- **One emotion predominates:** A child may be prone to one particular emotion much of the time that does not seem to be appropriate in the context of her life. For example, she may live in an almost permanent state of fear and anxiety.

- **The child avoids an emotion:** A child may *not* express an emotion when it would seem appropriate that she does. For example, she may talk about the death of a beloved pet yet not admit to or seem to show any feelings of sadness.

- **There is an incongruence between the words spoken and the emotion conveyed:** Sometimes a child will say something about how she feels, yet to the practitioner it does not ring true. For example, she may say that she is really excited about going to a new school but neither her voice nor body language convey joy and excitement. Her voice may groan as she says it, and a groaning voice, resonant with the Water Element, may reveal that her primary emotion related to the new school is fear.

How to diagnose the emotional imbalance

Evoking emotions

Hicks et al. describe an effective way of working with adults that involves 'testing' an emotion.[19] This involves creating an opportunity for the patient to reveal the state of a particular emotion, usually by talking about an event in her life where the practitioner would have the expectation of a particular emotion being present. Hicks et al. stress that this should only be done once good rapport has been created with the patient.

When working with children, it can also be useful to steer the conversation to certain areas in order to evoke an emotion, so that the practitioner can then observe whether or not the expression of that emotion is balanced or not. However, children are much less prone to 'hiding' their emotions than adults.

It is of crucial importance when evoking any emotions that the practitioner does not try to get the child to talk about a particular event or subject which may be too disturbing for her. Whilst with an adult this may sometimes be a crucial part of the dialogue, with children it is rarely fruitful and at worst can be damaging. Children have much less control over their emotions than adults do, and experiencing an emotion strongly can disturb the child's *qi* and mean that the practitioner loses rapport.

Therefore, the most effective way to gain a good picture of the state of each of the five key emotions in a child is simply to relate to the child about the aspects of his life that are most relevant and important to him. Exactly what these aspects are will depend on the age, circumstances and nature of the child. They may include the following:

- pets
- sports
- friends
- siblings/relatives
- hobbies
- birthdays
- presents
- outings
- holidays
- favourite books/TV programmes/films.

It should appear to the child that we are merely chatting to her in a way which puts her at ease and helps us to get to know her. This is, in fact, a beneficial part of what we are doing, but at the same time we should be closely observing the child and making a mental note of moments in the conversation when an emotion seems to be imbalanced in some way. For example, we may observe that, when telling us about a recent outing to a theme park, the child does not seem to be able to 'raise' her joy at all. Conversely, she may get what appears to us to be overly excited and agitated when talking about it but immediately after slump into a state which is characterised by a deep lack of joy.

It may become apparent to the practitioner that, even when the child tells us about the fact that her pet hamster died, or that her best friend has just moved to a different school, she has done so with a big smile on her face. In this situation, the practitioner would be wise to ask herself which emotion the smile is hiding. Is she sad or angry or both? Might she be feeling hurt and rejected? If the child is unable to express any of these more 'difficult' emotions, it may point towards an imbalance in the associated Element.

Observing emotions

It is often the case when treating children that the practitioner does not actually need to evoke any emotions. She just needs to be vigilant in observing the wide range of emotions that the child naturally expresses. She might steer a conversation in a particular direction on occasion and then closely observe the flow of emotions in the child. The practitioner should attempt to have a 'conversation' with all the emotions of the child in order to glean a better sense of her state of health or otherwise.

What does the child need from the practitioner?

The child needs to be able to relax and be himself in the treatment room. In order for this to happen, practitioners find that they need to bring different aspects of themselves to the fore when they are with different patients. It is useful for the practitioner to ask herself how a child most needs her to be during the treatment. For example, one child may light up in front of her if she gives him lots of warmth and is playful. Another might relax and become more at ease if the practitioner gives him lots of sympathy for a physical symptom or something he is finding difficult in his life. Reflecting on how she needs to be in order for the treatment to go well will often reveal useful diagnostic information about the state of each of the Elements.

For further discussion on rapport, see the sections on building rapport at the end of Chapters 16 to 20.

Observation of the parent–child dynamic

Carefully watching the nature of the interaction between the parent and child can also give the practitioner clues as to the primary emotional imbalance in the child. The child may have a need to challenge everything the parent says, indicating a possible imbalance in the Wood Element. Or she may be constantly asking the parent for reassurance which may indicate an imbalance in the Water Element. Depending on the upbringing and age of a child, she may be 'on best behaviour' with the practitioner, especially during the first few treatments, and therefore attempt to hide the parts of herself that she perceives are not 'polite' or acceptable. These sides of the child will most often reveal themselves when she is interacting with the parent.

> During the initial appointment with an eleven-year-old boy, I was struck by how poised and confident he appeared when answering my questions. It took me a while to realise that every time I looked away to write something down, he would look at his mother with a very anxious expression, as if seeking her reassurance. This was revealing of the underlying emotion.

Information from the parent

A parent may simply tell us about her child's temperament and emotional life in a way which provides us with information as to the primary emotional imbalance. The practitioner needs to take into account the fact that parents are not in a position to be objective in this matter. Also, a parent will perceive her child through her own particular lens. This is bound up with her own constitutional imbalance and her hopes and desires for her child, which are virtually impossible to totally relinquish. However, if the practitioner puts together what the parent says with his own observations, then this information can be of value.

Colour, sound and odour

Colour

The colour resonant with an Element will often be present on a child's face. It is most reliably present by the side or under the eyes, in the laugh lines and around the mouth. Sometimes the practitioner will notice that the colour is permanently present. At other times, the child will show momentary 'flashes' of a colour, particularly when the emotion resonant with the same Element has been evoked in her. In the case of the Fire Element, the practitioner may also diagnose the absence of red, the colour resonant with this Element, on the child's face. Sometimes the practitioner will notice more than one colour on a child's face. When this is the case, this information must be put together with all the other diagnostic features in order to make sense of the complete picture.

In order to effectively see and label colours on the face of a child, practitioners must train themselves to increase their visual acuity. These colours tend to be subtle hues rather than obvious blocks of colour. They may be seen equally on children with all different skin tones. On a practical level, it is important to make sure that there is good, natural light in the treatment room. Artificial lighting may distort the colours.

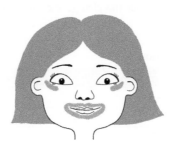

Sound

In health, the voice will contain each of the five sounds and will move between them depending on the emotion that the child is experiencing at any one time. If the sound resonant with an Element is nearly always present in the child's voice or, conversely, is absent from the child's voice, it may indicate an imbalance in that Element. Similarly, if the emotion being expressed and the voice tone are incongruent, this alerts the practitioner to an imbalance in this particular Element. For example, if the child is talking about the delights of her recent birthday party, the practitioner would expect her voice tone to contain laughter which resonates with the Fire Element. If this is not the case, then it points towards an imbalance in the *qi* of the Fire Element.

Most practitioners find that, when a child is speaking, their primary focus is the content of what she is saying. However, in order to become adept at diagnosing from sound, practitioners need to hone their auditory acuity and recognise *how* something is being said more than *what* is being said.

A ten-year-old girl told me all about her school residential trip from which she had just returned. Her words conveyed excitement, but her voice tone was a lack of laugh, suggesting that in reality she had not found it a fun and joyful experience. Presumably the expectation that she *should* have had a great time made it hard for her to reveal her true feelings about it.

Odour

The odour resonant with an Element may be detected on a child. Actually, parents often notice when their child's smell is different to normal. In a state of health, a child will not have a particular odour, so if one is detected it indicates an imbalance in that Element. The odour may only be present momentarily. Not all practitioners are adept at noticing and defining an odour because they may not be very olfactorily oriented. However, if the practitioner naturally has that ability, or can develop it, it can be a very useful diagnostic tool. Odour is often easier to detect on a child than on an adult. This is partly because children do not wear deodorant or perfumes and tend not to use so many body lotions or creams. Even if the practitioner cannot distinguish which Element a child's smell is related to, she may still notice when it changes or becomes particularly intense, both of which can be useful diagnostically.

The pulse

Practitioners of Five Element constitutional acupuncture place great emphasis on pulse diagnosis. However, the way in which they do this is somewhat different to practitioners of other styles of acupuncture. The strength of the different pulse positions is considered more important than other qualities, as shown in Table 15.2. This is because it helps to reveal the state of balance between the different Elements. The other twenty-eight classical pulse qualities are not considered relevant when discerning the harmony or otherwise of the Five Elements. Second, the changes in the various pulse positions that occur during treatment are an indication to the practitioner whether or not her treatment has brought about the change she has required, or whether she needs to do more.

Table 15.2 Example of pulse notation

	Left		Right		
SI/He	–	–	–1	–1	Lu/LI
GB/Liv	+1	+1	–2	–2	Sp/St
Bl/Ki	–2	–2	–2	–2	Pc/TB

The dash in the Heart and Small Intestine positions symbolises a pulse that is neither excess nor deficient. The + symbol on the Liver and Gallbladder pulse indicates that it is excess. All the other pulse positions, prefaced with a – symbol, are deficient to one degree or another (–2 being more deficient than –1).

For reasons mentioned in Chapter 12, it is difficult to discern the subtle differences in strength between the different pulse positions on a baby or young child. From the age of four or five onwards, depending on the particular child, pulse diagnosis may become a more central part of the way a practitioner monitors treatment. Up until this age, the practitioner must rely mostly on colour, sound, emotion and odour.

SUMMARY

» The Five Element constitutional acupuncturist will decide whether or not the child's imbalance lies in his spirit or his body, or a combination of the two.

» The signs of colour, sound, emotion and odour are used to diagnose over and above a description of symptoms.

» Emotional imbalance is considered particularly important.

» An emotional imbalance is diagnosed by observing that a child has difficulty expressing a particular emotion or seems to be 'stuck' in that emotion.

» Diagnosing the emotional imbalance may be helped by the practitioner sensing what the child needs from her, and also by observing the interaction between parent and child.

» Five Element constitutional acupuncturists place more emphasis on the strength of the child's pulse than on the other qualities.

Chapter 16

THE FIRE ELEMENT

This chapter is divided into three sections:

- Factors that challenge the healthy development of the Fire Element
- Manifestations of an imbalanced Fire Element
- Gaining rapport with a child who has a Fire constitutional imbalance

KEY RESONANCES OF THE FIRE ELEMENT

> » Colour: Red
> » Sound: Laugh
> » Emotion: Joy
> » Odour: Scorched

SUPPORTING RESONANCES

> » Season: Summer
> » Power: Growth
> » Climate: Heat
> » Sense orifice: Speech and tongue
> » Body part: Blood and blood vessels
> » Taste: Bitter

ORGANS PERTAINING TO THE FIRE ELEMENT

> » *Yin* Organs: Heart and Pericardium
> » *Yang* Organs: Small Intestine and Triple Burner

SPIRIT OF THE FIRE ELEMENT

Shen: associated with inner vitality; alertness of the mind; calmness of mind; the ability to pay attention; emotional resilience; sleep; short-term memory; clear consciousness; oversees the other spirits.

CHARACTER FOR FIRE

火

The character for Fire is *huo*. It represents a fire that would have been used both for cooking and for providing warmth. It evokes an image of people congregating to keep warm and have social contact.

Introduction

The Fire Element is concerned with a child's ability to feel joyful and happy, particularly when this is associated with contact with other people. It also determines the ease with which a child is able to form healthy, appropriate and satisfying relationships of different kinds as he grows. From around the time that the baby first smiles, he begins to develop his relationships primarily by means of his *shen*, which is the spirit housed in the Fire Element. The Fire Element must be in balance in order for a child to feel connected to others as opposed to lonely. When the Fire Element is healthy, a child will experience joy as a result of his interactions with others. He will also emit warmth and joy which will touch the lives of those he meets. He will be able to love and be loved, both one-to-one and in groups. He will know who to trust emotionally, and when and how to protect himself from harmful emotional engagement.

 KEY THEMES RELATED TO THE FIRE ELEMENT

Appropriate levels of joy; relationships; intimacy; speech; enthusiasm; excitement; emotional vitality; emotional stability.

Factors that challenge the healthy development of the Fire Element

- A lack of love, warmth, attention, intimacy and communication
  - Lack of motherly love
  - Lack of love of family, friends and peers
  - The 'wrong' kind of love
  - Neglect
  - Lack of communication and intimacy
- Rejection, abandonment and betrayal
- A depressed environment
- Shock and melodrama

Before considering these factors it is important to remember that parents generally want the best for their children. Nevertheless, parenting skills are rarely perfect. The quality of the parents' own *qi* is affected by their history and circumstances, which may compromise their ability to do as good a job as they would wish to.

A lack of love, warmth, attention, intimacy and communication
Lack of motherly love
The Fire Element is nourished and sustained by healthy contact with other people. There are very few people who can maintain a sense of joy in life without feeling connected to others. For a child to grow up with this feeling of connection, she needs an abundant supply of ongoing love and warmth.

A child's first experience of this ideally comes when she bonds with her mother. A present, warm and loving mother will nourish the Fire Element of the young baby in the earliest days of her life. The best possible start to life in the emotional realm that a baby can have is that she feels loved for who she is and simply because she is.

A baby whose mother is absent, depressed or who struggles to bond with her may begin life without receiving the essential nourishment that her Fire Element depends on to be strong. Her first feeling experience is one of aloneness rather than welcome.

Lack of love of family, friends and peers

The love from a mother or a mother figure is obviously crucial. However, on its own it is not enough. As she grows, a child's life opens up and gradually includes contact with more and more people. This will typically involve the father, siblings, extended family and then peers at nursery and school. The more heartfelt contact a child has with all those around her, the more sustenance her developing Fire Element will receive. She will imbibe the feeling that she is essentially loved and lovable. Although having this feeling as a child does not guarantee it continuing into adulthood, it is a good start. On the other hand, if a child's default position is that she is unlovable, this may permeate all her adult relationships.

The 'wrong' kind of love

It is a curious discrepancy that the vast majority of parents love their children, yet many children feel unloved by their parents. If a mother is not thriving because she, for example, has post-natal depression, feels unloved in her relationship or is beleaguered by the stresses of her life, she may struggle to communicate her love to her child. The same goes for a child's father and other extended family members. Martyrdom, overprotection, high expectations and material gifts are rarely experienced as a sign of love by a child. What really feeds and nurtures a child's Fire Element is focused attention and genuine encounter.

Sometimes, a child's need for love, warmth and attention does not fit with the personalities of her family members. She may feel that she has been 'born into the wrong family'. If she is someone for whom having heartfelt connections with others makes the world go round, she is unlikely to feel loved enough if she is born into or adopted by a family of thinkers, who place the highest value on intellectual discussions. If she is a sensitive and creative child, she may not thrive in a family who spend their leisure time watching sport.

The wrong kind of love also includes inappropriate physical or sexual touch with a sibling, older child or adult. This may, of course, seem like 'good' love to the child, but is actually abusive and is likely to confuse her compass regarding relationships.

Neglect

The Organs of the Fire Element are fed through healthy and nurturing interaction with others. Neglect, therefore, is perhaps one of the most damaging childhood experiences for the healthy development of the Fire Element.

Neglect may be overt, as is the case when a child is largely left to fend for himself both physically and emotionally. A child may also feel neglected when he is brought up by a nanny and does not see much of his parents. He may have all his physical needs tended to but have little emotional input. He may feel that his parents are not really interested in him and what makes him tick. He may crave his parents sometimes playing games with him or initiating conversations. The feeling that he may be left with is essentially that he must not be lovable. This is hugely detrimental to the Organs of the Fire Element.

A teacher who had worked both in schools in a severely deprived area and in one of the most elite private schools pointed out that she saw children who suffered from neglect in both. Neglect has little to do with economic status.

Lack of communication and intimacy

It is not only warmth and loving attention that feed a child's Fire Element. Authentic communication will also help a child to feel that she is connected to the people in her family. This involves family members showing each other who they really are, rather than interacting with a mask of joviality or superficiality, or maintaining distance or excessive privacy. A family who co-exist but do not truly communicate may mean a child is deprived of real intimacy and closeness. Her Fire will not be getting the daily nourishment it needs in order to develop robustly.

Rejection, abandonment and betrayal

If a child is rejected, abandoned or betrayed by somebody whom she relied upon to feel loved, it will be deleterious to the health of her Fire Element. A child who has been adopted may feel enormously loved by her adoptive parents but at the same time carry within her a deep feeling of rejection or abandonment that comes from the knowledge that she was given away by her birth mother. We hear adults talk of the enormous and lasting pain resulting from one of their parents leaving the family home when they were young.

An eight-year-old boy came to the clinic with recurrent tummy aches. Despite my best efforts, he neither smiled nor laughed as I talked to him. He looked as if his internal Fire had completely gone out. His tummy aches had begun after his father left home. Even though the Fire Element is not directly related to his symptom, it was by tonifying his Fire Element that he got better.

Good family relationships are perhaps the most fundamental basis for the development of a healthy Fire Element. However, as a child grows, she has to negotiate relationships outside her immediate family. Being rejected by a friend or excluded from a group of friends may be a strong blow to a child's Pericardium (also known as the Heart Protector). The school playground can be perceived by a child as a place where she needs to survive, rather than one where she can thrive.

Every child with a Fire constitutional imbalance is different. Louis Pasteur's famous phrase 'Le terrain est tout' (the terrain is everything) is applicable to the emotional as well as the physical body. Some children seem to survive emotional blows relatively well. Others may tend to perceive rejection and abandonment everywhere.

A depressed environment

As well as enabling a child to experience close and loving relationships, the Fire Element also gives her *joie de vivre*. It is the source of much of a child's joy and happiness. Therefore, living in an environment where there is a dearth of joy and laughter can negatively impact a child's Fire Element. A child will tend to absorb her emotional environment and the moods of those around her. If there is a lack of laughter in the family, and one or both of the parents are depressed, then the child may grow up internalising this low mood. In many families, the parents are not clinically depressed but they are worn down by the mundanity and drudgery of their daily lives. They have forgotten how to have fun, be spontaneous and laugh.

A three-year-old girl with sleep problems always responded well to treatment on her Fire Element. However, every few weeks the problem would return and the pulses related to the Fire Element would feel low again. Her mother, with much sadness, told me that life at home was difficult as her husband was depressed and she was struggling to cope trying to hold the family together. I suspected that this was why the girl's Fire Element kept being knocked.

Sometimes, being an only child can mean there is a dearth of vitality, especially if the only child's parents are rather serious and there are few other children around to play with. Adults need joy and laughter in their lives, but the development of a child's emotional and physical health absolutely depends on it.

Shock and melodrama

The balance of all of the Organs within the Fire Element is easily disturbed by shock (*jing*). Chapter 39 of the *Su Wen* states:

> When there is starting with *jing* the Heart no longer has a place to rely on. The *shen* no longer has a place to refer to, planned thought no longer has a place to settle. This is how the *qi* is in disorder.[20]

Shock may come in the form of a one-off event or may be a more chronic situation. A one-off, deeply traumatic event – such as a parent leaving – may have such an impact on the child's Heart that she never really recovers from it. An environment where there is constant melodrama can have a similar effect. A parent who is repeatedly threatening to leave, or a family where every week there is some kind of crisis which evokes intense emotions, can lead to a child's Fire Element receiving repeated blows. These will gradually erode the *qi* of the Heart and the Pericardium. If the external environment is like an emotional rollercoaster, her vulnerable Fire Element will find it hard to maintain internal constancy.

A note about teenagers and the Fire Element

The very fact of being a teenager tests the health of the Fire Element. Most people experience feelings of intense vulnerability during their adolescence as they try to create a truly independent identity for the first time.

As a teenager tries out new ways of presenting herself to the world, she must also inevitably cope with some degree of rejection. Teenagers may be ruthless in dropping friends overnight who no longer fit in with their new identity. There are also inevitable knocks that come when friendships change. Falling in (and out of) love for the first time (and perhaps repeatedly) will test the robustness of anyone's Fire.

Teenagers today also have the added stress of social media. A teenager may begin to equate whether she is lovable or not with whether she is 'liked' on Facebook, and how many 'friends' she has on Snapchat. Photos posted on Instagram of a party that she was not invited to may serve as confirmation that she is not lovable. Sometimes ignorance is bliss.

As if all of this were not enough, the relationship between a teenager and her parents may also become more distant. It is, of course, a necessary thing that adolescents become more independent from their parents. Many will strongly push their parents away during this time. Yet teenagers still need to feel loved. It takes an emotionally strong parent to keep acting lovingly towards his stroppy, defiant and cross teenager, who behaves as if everything her parent does is wrong. Whilst a teenager may be the one who has created much of the distance between her and her parents, that does not mean she may not simultaneously feel unloved when her parent withdraws.

A twelve-year-old girl came for treatment for depression. Prior to the appointment, her mother told me that she was deeply saddened by the deterioration in her relationship with her daughter who, she felt, was angered by everything she said and hated to be in her company. The daughter, on the other hand, told me that she felt her mother did not love her any more and that they no longer had fun together. I diagnosed the daughter as having a Fire constitutional imbalance. Treatment to strengthen the Organs of that Element helped her and her mother to feel closer again.

Manifestations of an imbalanced Fire Element

A child's constitutional imbalance is both a strength and a weakness. He is likely to possess both *qualities* that relate to the Element of the imbalance, as well as *pathologies*. This chapter focuses predominantly on the pathologies related to the Fire Element, because the practitioner will be seeing children who are in need of help in some way. In order to effectively treat a child, the focus must, of course, be on the pathology.

However, before looking at the manifestations of an imbalanced Fire Element, it is useful to be reminded of the *qualities* of Fire too. When the Fire Element is healthy, the child may:

- be very loving

- be very easy to love

- have strong *joie de vivre*

- be warm and sensitive

- be able to create and maintain relationships of all kinds

- be emotionally stable.

The manifestations of an imbalanced Fire Element considered below are:

- joy:
  - lack of joy
  - compulsively cheerful

- relationships:
  - closed off and unable to form friendships
  - desperate for contact
  - excessively vulnerable.

 The key to understanding the clinical relevance of a perceived emotional imbalance is when it begins to hamper the child's ability to thrive. It is then pathological.

Joy

One of the key ways in which a Fire imbalance manifests is in an imbalanced relationship with the emotion of joy. Please see Chapter 5 for a further discussion on the nature of joy.

Lack of joy

A child whose Fire is not thriving may lack enthusiasm for life. It is usual for young children to light up at the mention of a friend coming over, an outing or a treat of some kind. When the Fire

Element is deficient, a child will not be able to raise his joy sufficiently to either feel or show any enthusiasm for something. He may frequently say he is bored or sad if he does not have anybody to play with. As Roald Dahl wrote, 'it's impossible to make your eyes twinkle if you aren't feeling twinkly yourself'.[21]

> A five-year-old girl used to accompany her brother for his weekly treatments. My focus and that of the mother would inevitably be on the boy. Every time, within five or ten minutes the five-year-old would start saying 'I'm hungry', even though she had eaten just before they came to the clinic. I observed that the girl had a constitutional imbalance in her Fire and her cries of hunger were really a sign that she needed someone to play with to stoke her internal Fire.

Compulsively cheerful

At the other end of the spectrum is a child who appears to be *always* cheerful. He is a child who often draws other children to him because everybody finds him funny and entertaining. His Fire may also be so excessive, however, that at times others (particularly adults) find him tiring or irritating to be around.

It is hard to say where the line is between healthy cheer and excessive jollity. However, even for a child, life involves a range of emotions. There are times when a child will necessarily feel sad, angry or fearful. Compulsive cheerfulness may be the response to feelings of vulnerability and a fear of rejection. It may also be a mask that helps him to avoid another, deeper emotion.

> A seven-year-old boy would always entertain me when he came for his treatments, with jokes, magic tricks and wonderful stories. Even though this was very beguiling, I sensed it was a mask for a deep feeling of vulnerability. As his Fire Element grew stronger through treatment, he was able to reveal his vulnerable side more easily.

A child with a Fire imbalance may oscillate between these two states. He is either flat and lacking in joy or excessively jolly, but rarely seems to inhabit a middle ground between the two. It may be that when he is with his friends he always plays the role of the clown. When he is at home, however, he is flat and unable to raise his joy. His parents and siblings may therefore experience a different side of him to the one his classmates see.

Relationships

Closed off and unable to form friendships

The Fire Element underlies a child's ability to form meaningful connections with other people. The Pericardium in particular plays an important role in this aspect of life. If a child is closed to the possibility of closeness with anybody, it may be that the 'door' to his Heart (i.e. the Pericardium) is locked too tightly shut. It may be that a young child whose Fire is imbalanced in this way finds real intimacy difficult even with his parents. He may become giggly or over-excited at bedtime, for example, which is normally a time when a parent and her child experience a closeness that is not possible amid the activities of the day. Managing this closeness which precedes the separation that bedtime entails just feels too scary for a child whose Pericardium is locked tightly shut and so he must find a way of fending it off.

A child whose Pericardium is locked tight may find it easy to be in a big group of friends, but not develop a close friendship with another child. He may be popular and have a large number of people he gets on with. Yet his connections with other children are relatively superficial. At some point in the lead-up to or during puberty, a child developmentally needs to have somebody outside the family to confide in. This is one tool amongst many that enables him to perform the necessary task of separation from his parents. If his Fire is not strong enough to risk this level of intimacy, he may experience feelings of disconnection and loneliness.

Desperate for contact

Young children often have an openness that, in adults, would be deemed inappropriate. For example, it is not uncommon for a toddler to approach another child or an adult who is not familiar to her and tell them that she is three years old, or that she has a dog called Patch, or to ask them what they are called. We would probably think it was odd if an adult did the same thing. It is arguable as to whether it is necessary or just sad that we lose this kind of openness as we grow up. However, maintaining this quality of openness as a child grows may become problematic. His enormous desire for contact means he may throw himself into friendships very quickly and with the whole of his being, only to feel let down or rejected when he finds this is not reciprocated. He may 'wear his heart on his sleeve'. His openness may be a beguiling quality but also lead to a lot of heartbreak. During the teenage years, it becomes even more important for him to understand the steps that two human beings must go through in order to form a healthy, close relationship. To jump in without going through all the necessary stages has high stakes for a teenager.

A young child whose Fire is not strong may only be able to sustain a feeling of being 'OK' when he is relating to others. He may seem needy of attention and feel easily hurt when this is not immediately forthcoming. If his parents or siblings are all busy doing something, he may start to moan. Or he may complain of a stomach ache in lieu of being able to say, 'I am not feeling good about myself because I need some contact with somebody.' This intense need for contact with others may also mean there is a danger that this intense need for contact with others may override the need to protect himself emotionally.

Some children with a Fire imbalance oscillate between being closed and unable to form connections one minute, and then inappropriately open the next.

Excessively vulnerable

A child without a strong Pericardium 'protecting' his Heart may appear to be excessively vulnerable in relationships. Big family gatherings where he is expected to interact with many extended family members may fill him with dread. At home, if his sibling tells him she does not want to play at the moment, he feels unloved and hurt by this. Parents, siblings and friends of a child who is excessively vulnerable may feel that they are constantly 'walking on eggshells' so as not to upset him. They may tell him that he needs to 'toughen up'.

However, it is not only perceived rejection that is difficult for an excessively vulnerable child to take. Even mild teasing that is meant affectionately may be perceived as hurtful. One minute the child is laughing and seemingly enjoying affectionate family banter. In the next moment, a family member has crossed an imaginary line between joking and teasing. The child becomes upset and feels exposed and vulnerable.

Gaining rapport with a child who has a Fire constitutional imbalance

A child with a deficient Fire may find relationships with people he doesn't know very well a source of difficulty. With this kind of child, the practitioner must be respectful of this aspect of his personality and attempt to build rapport with the child slowly and gently. If the practitioner starts relating to him too quickly or strongly, the child may retreat. As far as possible, the child should be allowed to lead the way.

A child with a Fire constitutional imbalance will usually respond well to genuine and gentle warmth from the practitioner. A little bit of fun and humour may help to stoke his Fire. Playing the fool, trying to turn the whole process into a game or generally adopting a jokey persona can light up a child's Fire and increase his level of compliance in the process.

Another child with a constitutional imbalance in his Fire Element will come to the clinic excited about a new person to meet. The challenge with this type of child is to engage with him but not to stoke his Fire too much. Whilst the child will respond well if the practitioner raises her sense of joy to match that of the child, there is a danger that the child may become over-excited if this goes too far.

A four-year-old with an excess Heart imbalance came to the clinic for the first time. By the time I came to meet him in the waiting room, he had already befriended the sister of my previous patient who had been sitting there. Even though she was a rather sullen teenager, he had managed to draw her into a conversation and get her to play a game with him. When we went through to the treatment room, he immediately came and sat on my knee and spoke to me with a rather beguiling openness as if we were lifelong friends!

 The behaviours and traits described are supportive evidence of a child's constitutional imbalance. They should not replace the key diagnostic methods of colour, sound, emotion and odour.

SUMMARY

» The Fire Element plays a key role in how a child relates to others, learns to speak and manages emotions.

» The love a child receives from the mother, other family members and friends plays a large part in the development of the Fire Element.

» The Fire Element is especially susceptible to neglect, abandonment, a lack of joy and shock.

» A child with an unhealthy Fire Element may either be lacking in joy or compulsively cheerful, or swing between the two.

» Such a child may struggle to form strong, close relationships with others.

» He may also feel extremely vulnerable to rejection.

• Chapter 17 •

THE EARTH ELEMENT
· ·

This chapter is divided into three sections:

- Factors that challenge the healthy development of the Earth Element
- Manifestations of an imbalanced Earth Element
- Gaining rapport with a child who has an Earth constitutional imbalance

KEY RESONANCES OF THE EARTH ELEMENT

- » Colour: Yellow
- » Sound: Singing
- » Emotion: Sympathy or worry
- » Odour: Fragrant

SUPPORTING RESONANCES

- » Season: Late summer
- » Power: Harvest
- » Climate: Humidity, damp
- » Sense orifice: Mouth and taste
- » Body part: Muscles and flesh
- » Taste: Sweet

ORGANS PERTAINING TO THE EARTH ELEMENT

- » *Yin* Organ: Spleen
- » *Yang* Organ: Stomach

SPIRIT OF THE EARTH ELEMENT

Intellect (*yi*): associated with clarity of thought, studying, intention, concentration, memorising, generating ideas.

CHARACTER FOR EARTH

The character for Earth is *tu*. The top horizontal line represents the surface soil, and the lower line represents the subsoil. The vertical line represents everything that is produced by the Earth. Altogether, the character conveys the impression of both nourishment and stability.

Introduction

The Earth Element enables a child to both give and receive physical and emotional nourishment and support. It also provides a child with a feeling of emotional security and stability. The Earth Element is often compared to a mother. It is sometimes said to signify 'the soil on which plants grow, but also the ability of the earth to be like a mother'.[22]

The health or otherwise of a child's Earth Element will depend to a large extent on the quality of mothering that she receives (from whatever source) as a child. This will, in turn, determine her ability to look after herself as she grows up and also to what degree she becomes able to nurture others.

 KEY THEMES RELATED TO THE EARTH ELEMENT

Needs; nurturing; feeding and food; mother and mothering; caring for oneself; caring for others; thoughtfulness; studying; concentrating.

Factors that challenge the healthy development of the Earth Element

- Lack of mothering
- Smothering/overly dominant mothering
- The 'wrong' mother for the child
- Lack of a stable home environment
- Worry in the family
- Too much intellectual stimulation

Before considering these factors it is important to remember that parents generally want the best for their children. Nevertheless, parenting skills are rarely perfect. The quality of the parents' own *qi* is affected by their history and circumstances, which may compromise their ability to do as good a job as they would wish to.

Lack of mothering

 The Earth Element is resonant with bodily needs, comforts and securities which are often associated with the home, domesticity and the mother. Apart from pregnancy, breastfeeding and childbirth, these needs may otherwise be met by an adult figure of either gender. Although traditionally it has usually been the mother or other female members of the extended family who meet these needs in a child, this is not so much the case in the 21st century. Wherever the word 'mother' or 'mothering' appears in the text, it should be taken to mean the 'mother figure' in the child's life, be that a male or female figure.

If a mother or substitute mother figure is not able to care properly for her child, the Earth Element of the child will not receive what it needs and will fail to thrive. A mother may go through the motions of giving her baby or child enough food, bathing him and getting him to bed on time. Mothering involves a lot more than this. A baby is sensitive to whether he is being held tenderly or mechanically. He can sense if the arms that hold him are offering only vague and disinterested support. If a mother is not emotionally equipped to nurture her child because of her own circumstances, the child may feel uncared for. If the mother is depressed, exhausted or preoccupied, the quality of her mothering is likely to be diminished.

A psychologist called Harry Harlow did some fascinating, if ethically dubious, research with monkeys to look at the impact mothering had on their ability to move into independence. He put them into four groups. One group were put with their mothers, one group had no mothers, a third were put with wire frames shaped like a mother and the fourth were put with a piece of furry cloth shaped like a mother.

He noticed that the group put with their mothers would happily go off and explore and then come back to their mother, and then go off and explore again. The group without any kind of mother did not play or explore and grew up unable to cope with social situations. The group with the wire-frame mothers acted in a similar way to those without any mother figure at all. The group with the furry cloth shaped like mothers did not do as well as the group who had their real mothers but did a lot better than the group with the wire mothers.

He concluded that the group with their mothers, and to some degree even the ones with the cloth mother, were given the chance to steady themselves after going off and exploring. The purpose of the mother was to help calm their anxiety that came from having experienced new things.

A strong Earth Element is like a child's internal mother. It is a place inside herself she can go to feel centred and stable.

An adult patient whose mother had been depressed for much of her childhood spoke of her realisation that she had a big hole inside her that, despite therapy and a family of her own, would never entirely go away. She said that, whilst she was able to 'live with the hole' fairly well most of the time, when she became ill she would revert to a childlike state in order to try to get her needs met, something that had not happened in her childhood. This shows the lifelong impact a lack of motherly care may have.

Smothering/overly dominant mothering

The ultimate role of parents is to bring up a child who is eventually capable of independence. As Fromm wrote, 'The very essence of motherly love is to care for the child's growth, and that means to want the child's separation from herself.'[23]

In order for this to be achieved, parents must endeavour to adapt constantly to the ever-changing capabilities of the child. It is necessary to help a two-year-old to get dressed, but to be still doing this when a child is seven is not normally appropriate. Whilst it is universally acknowledged that breastfeeding is best for a child, sometimes it is the mother's inability to let her child move to the next stage that keeps her breastfeeding well into the school years. The mother cannot bear to give up the maternal feeling that having a feeding baby provides for her.

Ideally, a mother's care will be a response to the needs of the child. Sometimes, however, a mother's need to care is so strong that it overshadows the needs of the child. As a child strives for independence, his mother unwittingly discourages this because of her strong need for her child to remain dependent on her. This may manifest as answering to his every whim or controlling every little detail of his life. In an older child, it may be that the mother does not allow him the emotional privacy and space that he begins to need. It could be that the mother has a need to keep her child physically close to her, so does not allow him to spend time with his friends. Whatever the manifestation, the child will likely feel smothered and will grow up without a clear sense of how to look after his own needs. He may indeed come to feel he has the burden of responsibility for some of his mother's needs: 'Certainly parents who are over-protective cause distress in their children, just as parents who cannot be reliable make their children muddled and frightened.'[24]

The 'wrong' mother for the child

In an ideal world, the 'fit' of the mother with her child would always be a perfect one. In the real world, sadly this is often not the case. This is possible with either a birth child or an adopted child. It may be that the mother values self-reliance very highly and has a deeply sensitive child who requires a degree of emotional acumen that the mother is not able to give. Or, conversely, the mother may be very effusive in her emotions and tactile but the child is very self-contained. In either case, it may feel to the child that she is not getting the 'right' kind of mothering and this will affect the way in which her Earth Element develops.

Lack of a stable home environment

The Earth Element is sometimes depicted as being in the centre of the other Elements. It symbolises stability. Earth within a person enables her to feel secure, stable and centred. For a child, the more stable her external environment is, the more she is able to internalise this sense of stability. Children with a constitutionally strong Earth Element will be better able to cope with external instability than others. As Maya Angelou wrote, 'the ache for home lives in all of us, the safe place where we can go as we are and not be questioned'.[25]

A child's security extends beyond a strong connection with her family and those she loves. It is also dependent on her home. If a child frequently moves house or even country, it may challenge the healthy development of her Earth Element. Similarly, school is a very big part of the lives of most children. Regularly changing school, and therefore friendships, perhaps even before they have had time to develop, may also make it challenging for a child to develop an internal sense of security. Community is also important to the developing Earth within a child. Being part of a group enables a child to feel supported.

A stable home environment is also one which is emotionally secure. If a child lives with a sense that life is about to change in some way, it will be difficult for her to remain internally centred and relaxed. Uncertainty of any form hanging over the family often has a profound effect on a child. The uncertainty may take the form of a marriage that is on the brink of breaking down or financial insecurity. A sibling with severe health problems can have the same impact.

A six-year-old boy was brought to the clinic with recurrent tummy aches which had come on after the family had moved house three times within two years. His mother said that he had simultaneously become much more clingy. Treatment on his Earth Element, which had been knocked by the house moves, rectified both issues.

Worry in the family

One of the emotions associated with the Earth Element is *si*, which is usually translated as overthinking, worry or obsessive thought. If a child is surrounded by worry, she will imbibe this and it will become her own. *Su Wen* Chapter 39 explains that 'when there is obsessive thought, the *qi* is knotted'.[26] Knotted *qi* is a form of stagnant *qi*. It often manifests with the child having thoughts and worries that become stuck, and which go around and around in her mind. If the *qi* of the Earth Element becomes knotted in childhood, this may become the child's habitual state that she carries into adulthood.

Living in an atmosphere of worry will make it hard for a child to grow up trusting that her needs will be met and that life will provide for her. It is common to hear adult patients who are prone to worry say that their mother used to be a big worrier.

Too much intellectual stimulation

Excessive intellectual stimulation was discussed as a cause of disease in Part 1. Here, it is discussed specifically in relation to the Earth Element.

The spirit housed by the Spleen and therefore related to the Earth Element is *yi* 意. The *yi* is responsible for 'applied thinking, studying, memorising, focusing, concentrating and generating ideas'.[27] If a child is either intellectually precocious or pushed too hard academically, it will place a strain on her tender Earth Element. During the first seven or eight years of life, this may mean that so much of the Earth Element's *qi* is being consumed by the *yi* digesting information and ideas that there is not enough for the child to establish a strong feeling of being centred and nourished. 'Tiger mothers' or families who prize intellectual achievement above all else may expect an enormous amount from a child in this sphere. This may become a cause of disease either in the short term or when the child is older. The same problem often arises in teenagers too. At the same time that a child is going through enormous physical changes around puberty, she is often called upon to use her intellect more and more as academic pressure increases.

Of course, every child and teenager is different. What constitutes too much studying for one child will be well tolerated by another.

A thirteen-year-old came to the clinic because she had weak, achy legs (often a symptom of Spleen *qi* deficiency). The symptoms had come on within a few months of moving to a new school. She was happy there but was under a lot more academic pressure than she was used to, and she had to study for several hours each evening in order to keep up. That meant there was not enough Spleen *qi* available to govern the limbs and muscles.

Manifestations of an imbalanced Earth Element

A child's constitutional imbalance is both a strength and a weakness. He is likely to possess both *qualities* that relate to the Element of the imbalance, as well as *pathologies*. This chapter focuses predominantly on the pathologies related to the Earth Element because the practitioner will be seeing children who are in need of help in some way. In order to effectively treat a child, the focus must, of course, be on the pathology.

However, before looking at the manifestations of an imbalanced Earth Element, it is useful to be reminded of the *qualities* of Earth too. When the Earth Element is balanced, the child may:

- be exceptionally good at empathising with others

- be very centred and grounded in herself

- be adept at looking after her own needs.

The manifestations of an imbalanced Earth Element considered below are:

- having a tendency to worry

- being excessively dependent and needy

- being overly independent

- having an unhealthy relationship with food

- being overly empathic or lacking in empathy.

The key to understanding the clinical relevance of a perceived emotional imbalance is when it begins to hamper the child's ability to thrive. It is then pathological.

Having a tendency to worry

One of the key ways in which an Earth imbalance manifests is a propensity to worry and overthinking. Please see Chapter 5 for a further discussion on the nature of worry and overthinking.

A child with an Earth imbalance is likely to have a strong tendency to worry. This is different to the anxiety that stems from the Water Element, which is often felt as a very physical sensation and which stems from the Lower Burner. Worry is obsessive, unfocused and unproductive thought. For proper thinking to take place, the brain and the Heart both need to be involved. Worry comes about when this connection with the Heart has been lost. The child's thoughts are liable to go around and around and become stuck. She is not able to translate thoughts into action.

Some worry in a child is almost inevitable. However, a child with an imbalance in her Earth Element may worry about many things. The worrying may focus on something that has happened in the family, such as an argument she has overheard between her parents. She may worry about school the next day because a child was unkind to her and it may happen again. Older children with an Earth imbalance typically worry a lot around exam time. Ironically, the extra study that usually goes on prior to exams further weakens the Earth Element and therefore exacerbates this tendency.

The worries a child has may become more pronounced at bedtime which, for most children, falls at a time when the *qi* of the Earth Element is at its lowest, between 7pm and 11pm. The more tired the child is, the more likely she is to become overwhelmed with worry.

Being excessively dependent and needy

In the womb, a child is physically connected to her mother by the umbilical cord. Every aspect of her care and survival is done for her. When she is born, her mother will continue to take care of most of her needs. As she grows, she will gradually take the first steps on the long journey of separating from her mother and beginning to care for herself. A child whose Earth Element is not strong may struggle to achieve a level of independence that is appropriate to her age. 'Appropriate independence' is obviously largely culturally defined. Even so, sometimes we see a degree of dependence in a child, particularly on her mother, which prevents her from thriving.

If a child is not able to look after her own needs in a way that would be expected at her age, it is often a sign that her Earth Element is struggling. A common manifestation of this is a child who routinely becomes very upset when she has to separate from her mother at the school gates in the morning. Another child may constantly try to interrupt her mother and get her attention when she is talking to another adult or on the telephone. She relies on her mother for her internal sense of security and has not yet found a way of developing it within herself. An older child or teenager may express this neediness by wanting constant contact with her mother, via texting or talking on the telephone, when she is not with her. She may experience a great deal of worry or anxiety prior to going away on an overnight stay, and feel homesick when she is away.

Young children have enormous needs. Babies usually require huge amounts of touch and to be held much of the time. Toddlers often seem to have an uncanny ability to sense when there is a free adult lap that could be sat upon. A child who is getting used to being at school and away from her mother for the first time will require her mother's full attention when she comes out of school. Some children may intermittently need a parent at some point during the night for many years. This is all part of the healthy development of a child. However, if a child is never able to be happy whilst away from her mother and is often clingy, this is likely to be a reflection of a weak Earth Element.

Some children with an Earth imbalance experience feelings of insecurity when they are not in their home. A child who does not feel 'at home' in herself has a strong reliance on her external home in order to feel secure. For some children, even a day trip may stress their Earth Element too much and they may become very unhappy and complain of wanting to go home all the time.

> One parent told me that they had decided to stop going on family holidays because her son was so unhappy whenever he was away from home. He would become very clingy and lethargic, and lose his appetite. Invariably, as soon as they returned from holiday, he would return to normal within a matter of minutes.

Being overly independent

At the other end of the spectrum is a child who is not able to accept any help. The Earth Element gives a child the ability not only to look after herself, but also to acknowledge when she needs help from others and to receive that help. This may derive from the fact that the child has not had her needs met in the past and either feels too vulnerable to ask for help and thus risk not getting it again, or has simply learned to get on without it.

A child who is overly independent may place very high expectations on herself about needing to 'be a grown-up'. Even if she is struggling, she may insist on doing her homework alone rather than ask for help. She may push herself to take up an opportunity to go away on a camp because she feels she should be able to do it. She may then become very upset and cross with herself if she finds she is not able to manage it.

> One eleven-year-old girl who was due to start boarding school told me, 'I know it will be really good for me as I need to learn how to be away from Mum and Dad', as if she was trying to convince herself of this fact. She was unable to admit to feeling scared and worried about it.

The road to independence is ideally a gradual and relatively smooth one, even though there is often a big leap in this direction in the teenage years. In many traditional cultures, puberty rites and ceremonies give a person the clear message that he is no longer a child. In our modern culture, the process often becomes confused and sticky. On the one hand, a teenager is being asked to be more independent and to 'grow up'. On the other hand, he is being told he is too young to go out late on a school night or make decisions about his future. A teenager whose Earth Element is out of balance may particularly struggle with this process of separation. He may totally reject his parents in the misguided belief that he should be able to cope wholly on his own. Or he may oscillate between being excessively needy of his mother one minute, and then rejecting of her the next.

> The mother of a nine-year-old girl spoke of her difficulty understanding her daughter's behaviour. It seemed to alternate between entirely rejecting her parents and any support they offered, and being excessively needy. This is an example of how a child with an Earth imbalance may struggle to find a balance between dependence and independence and will flip from one extreme to the other.

Having an unhealthy relationship with food

The relationship between food and mothering is a highly complex one. To eat is one of our most basic needs. The way that a child looks after herself in the realm of food may reflect the state of her Earth Element.

A child whose Earth Element is not strong may 'feed' off the *qi* of her mother as a substitute for eating. This is a relatively common dynamic in children up to the age of about four. However, if a child continues to have a poor appetite as she gets older, it may be a reflection of a deeper inability to nourish and look after herself. In its most extreme form, this may manifest as an eating disorder such as anorexia. (However, not all eating disorders indicate an Earth constitution – please see Chapter 41 for a more detailed discussion of eating disorders.)

On the other hand, a child who does not feel a strong sense of internal stability may overeat in a misguided attempt to create a feeling of security. As a baby, feeding was associated with being held close to her mother and it felt good. In an attempt to reproduce this feeling, she may begin to comfort eat. Food may also become a way of blocking out feelings that are painful.

Being overly empathic or lacking in empathy

Another manifestation of an imbalanced Earth Element in a child is a difficult relationship with empathy. This may manifest in several different ways. It may be that a child gets extremely wobbled by somebody else's distress. She is so empathic that she feels the pain of another as if it is her own. This may of course be a trait that can be put to good use as she gets older but it can also make life difficult for the child. If she sees another child at school in distress, she may be a wonderful friend and go to comfort that child. Yet she may herself be left with a feeling of upset because she has taken on the other child's feelings. As she grows up she may not develop the ability to understand what is her suffering or responsibility and what is someone else's. She may be inclined to 'rescue' people when they are in distress, sometimes at the expense of her own well-being.

A child who lacks internal stability may not cope with films or books that have a sad story line. She may feel the distress of a character so strongly that she loses her own sense of being grounded and centred. This feeling may even continue long after the film is over or the book has been finished.

> Whilst taking the case history of a ten-year-old boy, his mother told me how sensitive her son was. She said that if anybody else in the family was hurt or upset, she always seemed to end up needing to comfort her son because he would be distraught at the other person's upset.

One of the roles of a parent is to be an emotional rock to her young child. Many children are ill-equipped to cope with seeing one of their parents distressed. In particular this may be true for a child whose Earth Element is not in good shape. A more extreme case of this is a child of a mother who is emotionally unstable, chronically ill or depressed. In these situations there is often a role reversal and the child is required to look after the mother at a stage of her life where she needs her mother to look after her.

 The British TV sitcom *Absolutely Fabulous* was a great illustration of a role reversal between mother and child. The mother, Edina, is a heavy-drinking, drug-using, promiscuous PR agent who spent her time chasing fads in a desperate attempt to stay young and hip. She relies heavily on her sensible and conscientious daughter, Saffron, to look after her and pick up the pieces when she has created another disaster in her life. Having to look after a parent will invariably strain the Earth Element of the child.

A child without a sense of strong, internal security may find any change in her usual routine difficult to manage. Her external routine helps her to maintain a feeling of stability, so when the routine changes she is disconcerted. If the family's usual daily routine has to change for some reason, the child may develop physical symptoms whilst she struggles to cope with the change.

At the other end of the spectrum, children with an Earth imbalance can sometimes be astonishingly unempathic. An otherwise kind child may become involved at school in the exclusion of another child. She may taunt and tease a child who was previously a friend and be seemingly oblivious to the pain that it is causing. Although there are often complex psychological roots to why children bully, this ability to be blind to another's distress is often a manifestation of an underdeveloped or imbalanced Earth.

Gaining rapport with a child who has an Earth constitutional imbalance

A child with a constitutional Earth imbalance may thrive from the feeling that he is being looked after and cared for. Therefore, he often really enjoys coming to the clinic. He may feel particularly aggrieved if the practitioner turns her attention too much towards the parent or sibling during the treatment. This child needs to feel as if he is being metaphorically picked up and wrapped in a blanket. The practitioner must summon her *yi* in order to shower the child with a quality of attention which will mean he feels really well looked after. This child will respond well to genuine sympathy and understanding.

Another child with a constitutional Earth imbalance may appear to be asking for sympathy and understanding, but reject it when the practitioner tries to give it. For example, she may have been talking about how hard she finds it that her father is working abroad. If the practitioner responds with sympathy and understanding, the child may then quickly switch to saying that it is not really that hard.

Another child with a constitutional imbalance in the Earth Element may employ disruptive behaviour as a way of trying to get the attention and care he is seeking. A quite different approach is needed in this situation. The practitioner needs to make sure that she does not collude with the child's attempts to gain attention in a disruptive and indirect way. She needs to be really clear with the child about what is acceptable behaviour in the clinic and what is not, and to really mean it when she says 'no'. This child may kick up an enormous fuss about the prospect of being needled in order to get more attention from his parent. This is very different from the genuine fear that a child with a Water imbalance may experience. It may be necessary for the practitioner to help the parent realise this and to model a firm approach with the child.

 The behaviours and traits described are supportive evidence of a child's constitutional imbalance. They should not replace the key diagnostic methods of colour, sound, emotion and odour.

SUMMARY

» The Earth Element is involved in a child's ability to receive motherly love and also to meet her own needs to an age-appropriate degree.

» It plays a role in helping a child to separate from the mother, and also to develop empathy.

» The Earth Element is affected by and influences a child's relationship with food.

» A lack of mothering, an overly dominant mother or the wrong 'fit' of mother may hamper the ability of the Earth Element to thrive.

» The Earth Element of a child who moves homes or countries frequently during childhood may suffer as a result.

» Excessive worry, either in the child herself or the family, may deplete the *qi* of the Earth Element.

» Too much intellectual work and reading at too young an age may also compromise the Earth Element.

» A child with an Earth constitutional imbalance may have a tendency to worry excessively.

» Such a child may be either very needy or overly independent, or move between these two extremes.

» She may also sacrifice her needs for the sake of others, lack empathy for others or move between these two extremes.

• Chapter 18 •

THE METAL ELEMENT

· ·

This chapter is divided into three sections:

- Factors that challenge the healthy development of the Metal Element
- Manifestations of an imbalanced Metal Element
- Gaining rapport with a child who has a Metal constitutional imbalance

KEY RESONANCES OF THE METAL ELEMENT

- » Colour: White
- » Sound: Weeping
- » Emotion: Grief
- » Odour: Rotten

SUPPORTING RESONANCES

- » Season: Autumn
- » Power: Decrease
- » Climate: Dryness
- » Sense orifice: Nose and smell
- » Body parts: Skin and nose

ORGANS PERTAINING TO THE METAL ELEMENT

- » *Yin* Organ: Lung
- » *Yang* Organ: Large Intestine

SPIRIT OF THE METAL ELEMENT

Corporeal Soul (*po*): associated with physical movement, agility, balance, coordination, clear physical sensations, psychic protection.

CHARACTER FOR METAL

金

The character for Metal, *jin*, is composed of two short lines at the bottom which are covered by two longer horizontal lines and also a sloping roof. The two short lines represent something of value buried deep within the earth.

As a child grows, much of his self-esteem depends on being connected with something of value within himself. This connection enables him to feel that he is of value in the world and to appreciate the quality of other people and things.

Introduction

The emotions related to the Metal Element are grief (*you*) and sadness (*bei*). Grief is a response to the loss of or separation from someone or something which is precious. The most obvious manifestation of grief is the bereavement that we feel if somebody dies. However, grief may also be evoked by the passing of a particular phase in life – for example, the pre-school phase when we were at home with our mother every day. Or it may be evoked by the loss of an object that was dear to us. Grief is usually associated more with the middle and end of life than the beginnings, as elderly parents die, children leave home and physical health declines. Yet a child needs to begin learning how to let go of things as he passes through the different phases of life. Without letting go of the old, he is unable to fully take in the new and to be nourished by it.

 KEY THEMES RELATED TO THE METAL ELEMENT

Skin; touch; breathing; acknowledgement; nuggets of gold; loss; grief; letting go; taking in the new.

Factors that challenge the healthy development of the Metal Element

- Loss

- A distant or absent father or father figure

- Lack of positive acknowledgement or too much criticism

- Lack of inspiration

Before considering these factors it is important to remember that parents generally want the best for their children. Nevertheless, parenting skills are rarely perfect. The quality of the parents' own *qi* is affected by their history and circumstances, which may compromise their ability to do as good a job as they would wish to.

 As a child grows out of infancy, stops breastfeeding and is in less need of physical skin-to-skin contact, he begins to need more and more guidance on being 'out in the world' and becomes involved in matters of intellect and judgement. These needs have historically been met by the father but may of course be met by an adult of either gender. Therefore, wherever the word 'father' or 'fathering' appears in the text, it should be taken to mean a 'father figure', whether that person is male or female.

Loss

The emotion connected with the Metal Element is grief. Grieving depletes the *qi* of the Lungs. A child who suffers a great loss may be hugely affected by it because his inherently immature Metal Element does not have the resources to bounce back from it. A young child may appear to carry on with life after a bereavement as he always has done, yet he may still have been profoundly affected.

Many parents relate a problem for which they are bringing their teenager for treatment back to a bereavement suffered many years before.

Loss for a child may come in many forms. The most obvious loss is of someone the child loves. The first bereavement a child is faced with may be that of a grandparent or a pet. However, leaving behind a group of friends, a school or a community due to a house move may be a great loss for some children. A child may have to deal with the break-up of her family, her father moving out or an older sibling leaving home. A child also has to face the loss of his unquestioning belief in his specialness and being confronted by his ordinariness. For example, he will need to acknowledge that he will probably not, as he has dreamt, be scoring the winning goal for his team in front of thousands of adoring fans.

Of course, loss is a part of life and no child will escape some kind of loss throughout his childhood. In the 20th century, death and grief became taboo in Western culture. As a result, children did not often attend funerals. Thankfully, nowadays, in many families death is not quite such a taboo and a child who has suffered a bereavement is supported in dealing with his grief. The more this is done, the stronger the Metal Element will remain as a result. If a child has an unusual amount of loss early in life, however well supported he is, it may weaken the developing *qi* of his Metal Element. The philosopher Ernest Becker[28] suggests that, somewhere before the age of nine or ten, a child will begin to develop an awareness of the inevitability of death. He will realise that people are sometimes taken away from the world forever. For some children, even this awareness can be difficult to manage.

A boy of four was brought for treatment for a chronic cough. He had become ill when his family moved to Oxford from Ireland. As well as developing a cough, his mother said that she felt her son had been sad and withdrawn too. His Metal Element had become depleted by the grief he felt at leaving his old life and extended family behind.

A distant or absent father or father figure

A child needs another adult in his life whose role complements the 'mothering' role of nurture and comfort. A child who grows up without an appreciative and encouraging father or any kind of father figure may struggle to develop a strong inner sense that he is worth something. A child whose father plays a peripheral role in his life, because he works very hard, is ill or does not live in the same house, may struggle more than others to internalise a sense of quality and meaning.

A child obviously needs to feel loved and secure. He also needs to feel that he is respected and thought of as a valuable human being. The simple acts of listening to a child when he speaks, asking his opinion on something and taking him into account when family decisions are made all serve this purpose. A parent who is clearly a symbol of authority, and the arbiter of right and wrong, will enable a child to develop an internal framework which helps him to feel good about himself in relation to the world.

A child who has not had a close relationship with a father figure may grow up with a sense of longing. He may feel that there is always something missing. Children of single mothers sometimes crave contact with men who may serve as father figures. They may swarm around them as if driven by a primal need to internalise a sense of the father. In Enid Nesbit's classic novel *The Railway Children*,[29] the father of three siblings disappears from their lives for a number of years. Even though the children are much loved and well cared for by their mother, they spend a lot of time longing for their father to return and mourning his absence. To use Fromm's words again:

> The child, after six, begins to need [fatherly love,] authority and guidance. Mother[ing] has the function of making him secure in life, father[ing] has the function of teaching him, guiding him to cope with those problems with which the particular society the child has been born into confronts him.[30]

> A teenage girl with a Metal constitutional imbalance once articulately described to me how she loved her step-father, who had brought her up and to whom she was very close. At the same time, she had a very strong longing for her birth dad. She said the longing was more for the idea of him than the reality.

Lack of positive acknowledgement or too much criticism

For the Metal Element to develop strongly, a child needs to be supported in the process of connecting with his own internal sense of worth. Some children seem to be born never doubting their worth and value, whilst others spend a lifetime battling negative feelings about themselves. In order to help a child to know that he has worth, it is important that he receives positive acknowledgement from those around him. If a child is frequently put down, criticised or told he is not good at things, he will internalise this feeling of not being good enough and it may become his habitual state. A young child is not able to praise himself – so he needs it to come from outside.

A child may feel that whatever he does, it is not good enough. He can never live up to the expectations of one or more of his parents. All parents want their children to do well, but for some parents, their child's achievements are never enough. An adult patient of mine, an incredibly successful doctor, told me that his father's response to being told his son had had his first book published was: 'Anybody could get a book published in your specialism.'

> I once listened in disbelief as the mother of a teenager I was treating (for anxiety and insomnia) tried to reassure her when she was expressing her worries. She said it would be very hard for the whole family if she (the daughter) did not get all A stars in her exams but that they would 'somehow find a way of coping'.

Teachers are usually the other key authority figures in a child's life and they can also have an important influence. For a child who is thin-skinned, a year at school with a teacher who is prone to criticising him may have detrimental effects. Every child has a varying sensitivity to criticism and children have different needs for being praised. The right fit between the child, his parents and teachers is the key. A child who has a strong need to be praised and is very sensitive to criticism will cope less well with a parent or teacher who is frugal in their compliments.

It should be added that if a child is praised for *everything* he does, it becomes meaningless. Praise needs to be specific. It means much more to a child who is proudly showing a drawing he has done to his parents if they say 'I really like the colours you have chosen' rather than if they just say 'That's good'. Young children usually have sharp antennae for throw-away comments that are not truly meant. Integrity and authenticity are important for the Metal Element, and children will spot a fraud. False praise for what a child knows for himself to be second-rate is likely to undermine his sense of self-esteem.

Lack of inspiration

The Lungs are said to be 'the Receiver of qi from the Heavens'.[31] As well as inhaling *qi* in order for a child to be able to breathe, the Lungs also take in what may be described as 'inspiration'. A child may be inspired by a teacher, by music, by beautiful scenery or by talking about interesting ideas. The more that he is inspired, the more he will be able to connect with his own internal sense of quality and the more he will be able to remain vital. If childhood is lacking in anything that is inspiring, the child's Metal Element may not receive the nourishment it needs to grow vital and strong.

Manifestations of an imbalanced Metal Element

A child's constitutional imbalance is both a strength and a weakness. He is likely to possess both *qualities* that relate to the Element of the imbalance, as well as *pathologies*. This chapter focuses predominantly on the pathologies related to the Metal Element because the practitioner will be seeing children who are in need of help in some way. In order to effectively treat a child, the focus must, of course, be on the pathology.

However, before looking at the manifestations of an imbalanced Metal Element, it is useful to be reminded of the *qualities* of Metal too. When the Metal Element is balanced, the child may:

- have an ability to deal with sadness and loss without his spirit being compromised

- have an appreciation of quality

- be able to bring quality to what he does

- have a strong sense of his own worth.

The manifestations of an imbalanced Metal Element considered below are:

- relationship with sadness and grief:

  - chronic sadness

  - grief denial

- fragile sense of self:

  - cold, inert or withdrawn

  - arrogant or brittle

- constantly striving or being self-critical; being overly critical/dismissive of others.

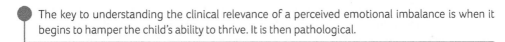

The key to understanding the clinical relevance of a perceived emotional imbalance is when it begins to hamper the child's ability to thrive. It is then pathological.

Relationship with sadness and grief

One of the key ways in which a Metal imbalance manifests is in a difficult relationship with the emotion of grief. Please see Chapter 5 for a further discussion on the nature of sadness and grief.

Chronic sadness

Many people feel uplifted around children because of their infectious happiness, laughter and *joie de vivre*. It feels as if it is almost going against the natural order of things when a child has a demeanour of chronic sadness. A child whose Metal Element has been depleted by sadness may appear as if he is carrying a heavy burden around. The character for grief, *you* 憂, shows a head at the top, a heart in the middle and at the bottom is a pair of dragging legs. A child who is burdened with sadness may struggle to feel inspired by anything he does in life. Most children would feel uplifted by a picnic with family and friends on a sunny day when they can run around and have lots of fun. A child who is full of sadness, however, may remain unmoved by the experience. He is not inspired and cannot connect with 'the *qi* of the heavens' because the sadness is blocking his ability to do this.

A fourteen-year-old girl came to the clinic with depression. She said that she did not understand why the things she had previously enjoyed doing, such as going for cycle rides and playing in

> a band with her friends, now held no pleasure for her at all. Her symptoms and signs pointed towards the fact that her Metal Element was deficient.

It is worth noting that, in the Five Element system, sadness (*bei*) associated with the Metal Element is different from the lack of joy that is associated with Fire. A lack of joy is usually 'cured' by warmth from others. A child who has a low Fire Element often sparks up when he is in the company of others. In contrast, a child who has a low Metal Element is not usually changed so much by being around others, and may in fact seem rather remote or cut off.

Grief denial

Whilst some children may be obviously sad, others may wear a mask of 'I'm OK'. In the same way that in many families a child is not allowed to be angry, he may not be allowed to be sad either. Children are often perceived as not really having strong feelings. Adults will say of a child that he is resilient or taking the loss in his stride. Whilst on one level this may be true, it may also be a reflection of the adult's own complex relationship with the emotion of grief. If she is uncomfortable with the emotion herself, it may mean she is reluctant to see the emotion in a child. If so, she is likely, in one way or another, to give the child the message that the feeling is not acceptable. The English, with their famous 'stiff upper lips', are particularly prone to this tendency.

Fragile sense of self

Cold, inert or withdrawn

In the same way that *wei qi* protects a child from invasions of External Pathogenic Factors, Lung *qi* also serves as a kind of 'armour' on a psychic and emotional level. If this aspect of a child's Metal Element is weak, it may mean that he feels particularly sensitive and vulnerable to the outside world. He may, for example, take any degree of criticism very much to heart and be easily offended by what his peers and family say to him. A throw-away comment by a tired and stressed parent of 'You are *so* slow at getting ready in the mornings!' may devastate him and leave him feeling worthless.

As a result of feeling so fragile, he may cut himself off from others as a way of protection. If he isolates himself, then he reduces the chances of further hurt (although of course isolation brings about other problems). He may only allow himself to connect with those that he feels he can entirely trust not to be critical of him. He may choose to have just one or two friends and to keep himself separate from big groups of children. He may even become a loner. It is not that he does not want to connect with others, and he may actually feel very lonely. It is just that he feels too vulnerable to take the risk of doing it.

Arrogant or brittle

A different response to feeling fragile is to defend oneself more strongly. A child may come across as being arrogant or a 'know it all' but underneath he feels the exact opposite of this. Rather than admit to his feelings of vulnerability, he develops a facade to hide the fact that he has these feelings at all. He may feel that if he admits to any feeling of weakness, he will be totally swamped by the feeling – so it is easier to push it away altogether.

> A ten-year-old boy who suffered from a chronic cough used to tell me at length and with great pride, at the start of every treatment, all of his achievements in the time since I had seen him. Although it is natural for a child to do this to some extent, I felt there was a desperation in him to be acknowledged and that he was almost trying to prove to himself that he was 'good enough'. This is typical of some children with a Metal constitutional imbalance.

He may also, therefore, appear to be somewhat cold or brittle and may not be a child who others easily warm to. There may be an aloof quality to him. A young child with a weak Metal Element may even spurn hugs and cuddles from his parents and family. 'Letting in' a cuddle involves temporarily removing the armour around him and this may make him feel too vulnerable.

Constantly striving or being self-critical; being overly critical/dismissive of others

A strong Metal Element enables a child to feel an inner sense of worth and to acknowledge his talents and abilities. Conversely, if a child does not feel that he is good enough, nothing he ever does will change this internal feeling. He may therefore push himself to do more and more in an attempt to feel good about himself. Yet this feeling is elusive for him. As a young child who does not get the acknowledgement he needs from his parents, he may try ever harder to win their praise. As an older child, he may push himself harder and harder at school to achieve the best results possible. However much he achieves, it never feels like enough.

> A girl springs to mind whom I treated for various different physical ailments on and off for a number of years. She achieved enormous academic success as well as excelling in music and art. At the age of seventeen, she reached what most would consider a pinnacle of achievement in being offered a place at a top university to read medicine, with a choral scholarship as the icing on the cake. When I congratulated her, her response was to say she had been berating herself ever since her choral audition. She knew that she had not sung to the best of her ability and therefore she could have done even better.

A child who has an imbalance in his Metal Element may, alternatively, develop the opposite behaviour and stop trying altogether. He may not bother to achieve anything because it is a way of avoiding intensely painful feelings of constantly failing. It is easier never to try than to deal with the feelings of disappointment if it does not work out.

Strongly related to constant striving is the fact that a child who has a weak Metal Element may have, to borrow a Freudian term, a very strong superego. He has an internal voice that keeps telling him that neither he nor his actions are good enough. He is his own harshest critic. It is considered part of normal development for a child, particularly in middle childhood, to occasionally say he hates himself or he is no good at anything. If this becomes a more chronic pattern, it may be as a result of an imbalance in his Metal Element.

As discussed, a child is likely to have low self-esteem if his own achievements and value have not been recognised or acknowledged. One way in which he might try to make himself feel better is by dismissing or putting down the achievements of others.

Gaining rapport with a child who has a Metal constitutional imbalance

A child with a constitutional Metal imbalance may feel easily bombarded by the external environment. He will often be 'thin-skinned'. For most children, noises, physical sensations and visual images are reduced in intensity by the outer, protective layer of *qi* which is related to the Metal Element. For some children with a Metal imbalance, everything feels magnified because this defensive layer is very weak. Therefore, even palpating a child to find a point can feel too intense for him. An effusive display of emotion may feel overwhelming. So the practitioner needs to approach the treatment of this type of child very gently and be sure to ask his permission before doing anything. Once rapport has been gained he may hugely benefit from gentle touch such as that involved in *shonishin* (see Chapter 35). This may stimulate his defensive (*wei*) *qi* and his *po*.

It is usually very important for an older child with a constitutional Metal imbalance to feel that he is being treated with respect and that his talents and qualities are acknowledged. Therefore, it can be helpful for the practitioner to find opportunities to compliment him, perhaps on something he mentions he has done at school or simply on the way he has behaved during the treatment. A child with a Metal imbalance tends to value order highly, so will also benefit from the treatment being carried out in a methodical fashion.

> A two-year-old boy came to the clinic because he suffered from almost constant coughs and colds. He was very pale and rather inert. His mother said, much to her distress, that he couldn't stand being cuddled. He hated baths and, unusually for a child of that age, also appeared to hate being outside. He wouldn't let me hold his hand to take his pulse, let alone perform any kind of treatment on him. I began by doing some acupressure through his clothing which he could stand if his mother read him a story to distract him. As his Lung *qi* grew stronger, we gradually progressed to acupressure directly on his skin, then *shonishin*, and eventually I was able to use needles on him.

 The behaviours and traits described are supportive evidence of a child's constitutional imbalance. They should not replace the key diagnostic methods of colour, sound, emotion and odour.

SUMMARY

» The aspects of childhood that particularly relate to the Metal Element are: skin-to-skin contact, touch, grief and loss, and acknowledgement.

» The lack of a father figure in childhood may hamper the development of the Metal Element.

» The Metal Element of a child who suffers a huge loss, or one who struggles to deal with a loss, may become imbalanced.

» A child who is heavily criticised and lacks acknowledgement may also struggle to develop a healthy Metal Element.

» A child with an imbalance in the Metal Element may either appear to be sad or avoid emotions related to sadness and loss.

» He may also appear arrogant or hard to warm to, but this is a mechanism to protect his fragile sense of self.

» Some children with an imbalance in the Metal Element constantly strive to do better but never feel that their best is good enough. Others avoid putting any effort into anything because of the fear of failing.

• Chapter 19 •

THE WATER ELEMENT

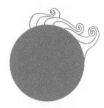

This chapter is divided into three sections:

- Factors that challenge the healthy development of the Water Element
- Manifestations of an imbalanced Water Element
- Gaining rapport with a child who has a Water constitutional imbalance

KEY RESONANCES OF THE WATER ELEMENT

- » Colour: Blue/black
- » Sound: Groan
- » Emotion: Fear
- » Odour: Putrid

SUPPORTING RESONANCES

- » Season: Winter
- » Power: Storage
- » Climate: Cold
- » Sense orifice: Ears and hearing
- » Body part: Bone, bone marrow and hair on the head

ORGANS PERTAINING TO THE WATER ELEMENT

- » *Yin* Organ: Kidney
- » *Yang* Organ: Bladder

SPIRIT OF THE WOOD ELEMENT

Willpower (*zhi*): associated with the drive to survive; will; determination; motivation; fear; wisdom.

CHARACTER FOR WATER

水

The character for Water is *shui*. The character shows a central current of water with whirls of water beside it.

Introduction

Water within a person enables movement and flexibility, both physically and emotionally. The Water Element is at its most replete in a baby. *Jing*, housed in the Kidneys, is a child's inherited constitution. It is the aspect of a person which powers growth and development, both physical and mental. *Jing* is a finite resource and everybody is born with a different quantity and quality of *jing*.

A balanced Water Element will ensure that a child is able to grow physically in a way that is fitting for her age. It will also mean that she is able to reach the key developmental milestones of childhood. The Water Element underpins a child's mental and cognitive development too. There is more rapid growth and development in the first seven or eight years of life than at any other time. Therefore, one of the goals of childhood should simply be to support this process, by providing all the essentials that a child needs and not asking too much of her in other ways.

The Water Element, and specifically the *zhi* which it houses, provides a child with the will and drive to survive. This will, to some degree, determine her ability to 'go for' what she wants and needs. It also provides her with an innate sense of trust in the world. If the Water Element becomes imbalanced, the child may be overly driven and squander her precious resources of *jing*. Conversely, she may lack the drive to engage fully in life, or feel too frightened to do so.

 KEY THEMES RELATED TO THE WATER ELEMENT

Growth; development; assessment of risk; trust; reassurance; potency; sexuality; drive and motivation; energy reserves.

Factors that challenge the healthy development of the Water Element

- An atmosphere of fear

- An imbalance between rest and activity

- Shock

Before considering these factors it is important to remember that parents generally want the best for their children. Nevertheless, parenting skills are rarely perfect. The quality of the parents' own *qi* is affected by their history and circumstances, which may compromise their ability to do as good a job as they would wish to.

An atmosphere of fear

The Organs of the Water Element, in particular the Kidneys, are depleted by intense or chronic feelings of fear. Growing up in an environment that induces chronic or repeated feelings of fear will mean that a child will habitually be 'on red alert'. A part of him is constantly under threat, waiting for the next frightening thing to happen. His habitual state becomes one of being on edge and he may struggle to find a sense of internal stillness.

There are obviously many different circumstances and events that may induce fear in a child. A parent who is unpredictable, aggressive or violent is one. Living in an unstable or war-torn society will do the same, as may being a member of a persecuted or oppressed social group. If the adults that surround a child are fearful, then the child will, to a greater or lesser degree, also internalise this fear. So if parents are frightened over a long period of time about their safety, financial predicament, or the health of one of their children, this will seep into the *qi* of the household and be absorbed by a young child.

A three-year-old boy came to the clinic with a series of very minor symptoms. His mother, who had a Water constitutional imbalance, catastrophised about her child's health and became convinced, whenever a new symptom appeared, that it was extremely serious. She verbalised her fears in front of her child, who became more and more anxious himself. He was being given the message that his body could not fundamentally be trusted.

Some parents perceive the outside world to be full of potential dangers. They may then become plagued by fantasies of the many catastrophes that could befall their children. If the parents verbalise their fears, or if the child picks up on them anyway, it may impede the healthy development of the Water Element in the child. Of course, it is a fine line between equipping a child to deal with the many, real hazards that life entails and instilling in him a sense of trust in the world and life, and in his own judgements and instincts. However, if a child is taught only that the world is full of dangers, the chronic fear that results from this will be detrimental to the development of his Water Element. If a toddler falls over and grazes himself, he usually looks straight to his parent when he sees the cut to gauge just how upset or frightened he should be. Strong, stable and internally calm parents help a child to feel the same.

Secrecy also induces fear in children. The *zhi* enables a child to respond instinctively to what is going on around him. If a child senses from a parent's body language or voice tone that something is awry but is told when asked that nothing is wrong, it may breed fear and confusion within him. A lack of age-appropriate openness and honesty leaves a dangerous opening for a child to begin catastrophising.

If a child is pushed into unknown situations too early for his stage of development and his individual personality, it is likely to induce fear in him. All growth involves uncertainty. Starting a new school, for example, naturally brings up questions in a child of what it will be like and whether he will like the teachers. However, if a child is given time to become familiar in his new surroundings and to build rapport with his new teacher, he is far more likely to embrace the new situation than if he is thrust into it without preparation.

An imbalance between rest and activity

Excessive physical activity as a cause of disease was discussed in Part 1. Below is a more detailed discussion of how it particularly affects the Water Element.

The spirit of the Water Element, the *zhi*, gives a child the wisdom to know when to be active and when to be still and rest. If he does too much of one or the other, it will compromise the *qi* of the Kidneys and the Water Element. A child who grows up in an environment where he and everyone around him are always on the go will not learn how to embody the quality of stillness that pertains to the Water Element. He may feel agitated when he has nothing to do and therefore crave constant stimulation. Conversely, if he grows up with a 'couch potato' lifestyle, the *qi* of his Water Element will stagnate.

It may be that the child's life is over-scheduled and that he has little time at home to just 'be' and to 'do' nothing. The only mode he knows is one of constant doing. In the first years of life, a child's activities are determined mostly by her parents. A mother may plan many outings because she feels lonely or bored at home. She may feel it is 'a good thing' for her baby to be exposed to lots of different environments and activities early in life. Whilst all of this is understandable, it may mean that the baby is programmed from very early on to be always on the go. Much of the *qi* needed for growth derives from the Water Element. If a child is also doing many activities and a lot is being demanded of him, the Kidneys will be strained and this will affect the development of the Water Element.

Alternatively, it may be that one or both of his parents are habitually adrenalised because of their personality or their lifestyle. The child then absorbs this adrenalised energy. Not being able to rest means the Water Element is constantly challenged and eventually weakened.

> A nine-year-old boy came to the clinic with symptoms of hyperactivity. He was brought by his father who was an exceptionally driven and successful man. During the appointment, the father made successive work calls, appeared adrenalised and paced around the treatment room. I suspected that at least some of his son's problems stemmed from having imbibed this edgy, hyper-alert state that was the norm for his father.

A child whose parents have extremely high expectations of him, whether spoken or not, will often live with a fear of failure and an internal feeling of pressure that makes it hard for him ever to truly relax, even though he may be exhausted. He may feel a combination of being depleted and internally agitated.

Another reason for a child to become depleted is that she may not be getting enough sleep. As any parent knows, there are two kinds of child: a rested child and a tired child. The fact that a child's ability to cope with life when she is tired is so profoundly altered is evidence of just how important sleep is to her. The aftermath of a sleepover (which could more accurately be called an 'awake over') is often an exhausted, grumpy and tearful child with dark circles under her eyes. Every time a child does not get enough sleep, it will compromise the delicate state of her Water Element. Although a loss of sleep is unavoidable at times, it should always be followed by an opportunity for the child to replenish her reserves.

At the opposite end of the spectrum is a child who has too little activity in his life. Although *yang* is depleted by too much activity, it also needs to be activated by some degree of movement. A child who sits inside all day doing very little may develop stagnation of *qi* which prevents the Water Element from developing properly.

Shock

Shock is defined in the Oxford English Dictionary as 'a sudden upsetting or surprising event or experience'. Nobody would argue with the fact that an intruder breaking into the home, a sudden bereavement or being involved in a car crash constitutes a shock. Yet we so easily forget, as adults, what it feels like to be a child. A baby, without the resources to keep himself alive, may feel profoundly shocked by his mother's absence. 'Stress for babies,' as Gerhardt writes, 'may even have the quality of trauma.'[32] A four-year-old who leaves his mother's side in a shop and cannot find her again for a minute or two may be shocked by the overwhelming sense of aloneness he is suddenly faced with. Of course, one child may laugh at what another may find traumatising, but we should never underestimate the power of a seemingly trivial event to shock a child.

> A six-year-old girl was brought to my clinic with insomnia, which had begun after she had been left alone for two or three minutes in a car with a dog. Even though she knew the dog to be friendly and placid, she had come away from the experience deeply shocked by the sense of being trapped for those few minutes.

In the first instance, shock affects the Heart and makes *qi* scatter. However, a very deep or prolonged shock may interrupt the flow of *qi* between the Heart and the Kidneys and consequently affect the Water Element.

Manifestations of an imbalanced Water Element

A child's constitutional imbalance is both a strength and a weakness. He is likely to possess both *qualities* that relate to the Element of the imbalance, as well as *pathologies*. This chapter focuses predominantly on the pathologies related to the Water Element because the practitioner will be seeing children who are in need of help in some way. In order to effectively treat a child, the focus must, of course, be on the pathology.

However, before looking at the manifestations of an imbalanced Water Element, it is useful to be reminded of the *qualities* of Water too. When the Water Element is balanced, the child may:

- be particularly adept at assessing risk
- be neither particularly fearful nor reckless
- provide others with a great feeling of safety
- show prudence in his approach to rest and activity.

The manifestations of an imbalanced Water Element considered below are:

- being overly fearful and anxious
- being reckless
- chronic agitation and being on 'over-drive'
- lack of drive and willpower.

 The key to understanding the clinical relevance of a perceived emotional imbalance is when it begins to hamper the child's ability to thrive. It is then pathological.

The emotion connected with the Water Element is fear (*kong*). One of the key ways in which a Water imbalance manifests is in an imbalanced relationship with the emotion of fear. Please see Chapter 5 for a further discussion on the nature of fear.

Being overly fearful and anxious

A child in whom the Water Element is compromised may perceive the world as a place full of potential dangers. He may imagine threats where there are none. New situations may induce feelings of anxiety in him. Most children will have some degree of nerves before, for example, starting a new school. A child with a weak Water Element may go one step further than that. He may become agitated and anxious leading up to his first day and find it hard to settle himself. His fear is different to the worry that comes from the Earth Element. It may even approach a feeling of terror. The spirit of the Water Element, the *zhi*, resides in the realm of the unconscious. If a child is fearful (rather than worried), he may not consciously know too much about it or be able to articulate how he feels. The fear may manifest as a physical agitation or as some other physical symptom.

When a child whose Water Element is not strong has been in a situation that makes him fearful, he may remain agitated for some time afterwards. For example, he may come out of school 'hyped up'. This is because he will have had to dig into his reserves of Kidney energy in order to get him through it. So it is hard for him to then come out of that adrenalised state and settle again.

A child who is fearful may respond by trying to avoid any situations that induce even more fear in him. When other children are busy cycling at full speed down steep hills and jumping into lakes, he may prefer to sit and watch. He may turn down opportunities to do a new activity or join a new club because the fear of the unknown only makes him feel even more anxious.

A child with a Water imbalance may became plagued by fear of future catastrophes. His fears may focus on being in an accident of some kind, on an intruder getting into the house at night or on a parent dying. Alternatively, he may become consumed by a fantastical imagined event, such as the sky falling in or a nasty character from a film he has seen coming to eat him up. Most children have fears of some kind, but a child with a Water imbalance will be prone to them, and it will be very hard to reassure him, if it is possible at all.

A child with an imbalance in his Water Element may have difficulty trusting other people and even the process of life in general. His default state when it comes to new people or situations may be one of suspicion. Words of reassurance from his parents will probably do little to ease his wariness.

> A twelve-year-old girl with a Water constitutional imbalance came for treatment. When she first arrived, she looked like a rabbit caught in headlights, almost paralysed by fear. She could not look at me and curled up in the chair holding her knees to her chest looking incredibly afraid. Over several visits, she gradually began to sense that it was a safe place to be and to relax. Reassuring words made little difference. She simply needed time to 'feel out' the situation.

Being reckless

It is not reasonable to expect young children to be able to judge what is safe and what is not, or to be able to foresee potential dangers. A parent will be the eyes, ears and sixth sense for her child entirely for the first few years of life. The child will gradually take over being able to do this more and more as he gets older. A two-year-old may not have the foresight to know not to put his hand in a flame. Most five-year-olds will have learned this is not a good idea. A child with a Water imbalance may, as he grows up, show an inability to assess risks appropriately in various different situations. As an eight-year-old, he may play with fire on a hot day outside. As a fourteen-year-old, he may drink to excess with little concept of the potential dangers.

Adolescence is the phase of a child's life when recklessness may become a big problem. There will no longer be a parent around all the time to watch what is going on. There is a thin dividing line between excitation and fear. Many teenagers are drawn towards scary fairground rides and horror movies, and activities that include an element of danger and thrill such as drug taking and driving too fast. The reckless behaviour of a teenager may have disastrous consequences. To some degree it is almost a rite of passage for teenagers to take some risks. Most adults shudder to some degree when they remember what they did as teenagers. For an adolescent with a Water imbalance, the degree of recklessness may be way beyond that of most of his peers.

> It is common for a child with a Water constitutional imbalance to be overly fearful in one area of his life, and reckless in another. For example, the mother of a nine-year-old boy who came to the clinic with abdominal pain told me that he became extremely anxious and agitated every day before school, even though he always enjoyed it once he was there. On the other hand, his favourite hobby was high-diving, an activity many would consider frightening.

Chronic agitation and being on 'over-drive'

A child with an imbalance in his Water Element may just not be able to stop. The *yin* energy of the Water Element enables him to be still, restful and calm. If a child has weak Kidney *yin*, it will be difficult for him to achieve this state. He may appear as if he has unlimited energy and does not need much sleep (in fact he may be a child who struggles to get off to sleep and wakes up early in the morning). Yet at some point, he has to stop and may have an enormous physical and emotional crash when this moment comes.

> The mother of a boy who was brought to the clinic told me that his nickname within the family was 'Duracell Bunny' (after the long-life battery), because he just kept going and going and going.

In an older child, there is a real danger of burn-out as he may not recognise when he needs to stop. In young children, to a large degree it is the parents who manage the balance between rest and activity. By the time of adolescence, parents have less and less say in the matter. The *zhi* gives a child the wisdom to know when to conserve resources and when to spend them. A child who enters adolescence with a weak Water Element will therefore be less able to make these decisions wisely.

A child with a constitutional imbalance in Water may live with a chronic, low-level state of fear and anxiety and find it hard ever to relax properly and feel calm. This child may be described as a 'live wire' or may appear as if he is perpetually on alert, or even 'ready for battle'. This is because he sees potential threats and dangers wherever he goes.

Lack of drive and willpower

At the opposite end of the spectrum is a child who lacks any drive or willpower. It is common for a young child to go through periods when he is tired and wants to have a more quiet and restful time than normal. This often coincides with a growth spurt or a major developmental leap, both of which require a surge of Kidney *yang* energy. However, if a child's habitual state is one of tiredness and a lack of drive, then it may indicate an imbalance in his Water Element. For this young child, going to school or even just going to the playground may feel like an enormous effort. He may groan at the thought of having to do anything that involves getting off the sofa and leaving the house. He may become very tired at the end of a school term. He will not be able to cope as well as other children might with a particularly busy time, or one where he does not get the sleep he needs.

> The parent of an eight-year-old girl told me that she had come to realise that, if her daughter were to avoid getting ill, she needed a few days off school in the middle of each term so she could rest. She simply did not seem to have the stamina to go through a whole term without getting ill.

A time when this commonly becomes noticeable is around adolescence. A lot is required of the Water Element at this time with so many major physical and psychological changes taking place. If a child's Water Element is deficient, then he may lose his drive to take part in life much at all. Although it is not a sign of imbalance for a teenager to need a lot of rest, neither is it a sign of health for him to be lacking the drive and motivation necessary to get on with and enjoy his normal life.

Gaining rapport with a child who has a Water constitutional imbalance

A child with a deficient Water Element may genuinely be exceedingly fearful of coming to a new place and meeting an unfamiliar person. Furthermore, he may be petrified at the thought of needles. The practitioner must summon his *zhi* and remain as calm and solid internally as he possibly can. The child may be particularly sensitive to picking up any emotion that the practitioner is feeling but trying to hide. The more solid the practitioner is able to be, the more the child will be reassured.

In verbal children, it is helpful for the practitioner to explain to the child what she is going to do as she goes along. The child's fears will be somewhat allayed by reassurance that there will be no surprises, nothing unexpected, and that he can say no at any time if he does not feel comfortable. Treatment may begin with moxibustion, paediatric *tui na* or a laser pen, giving the child time to build trust.

A child with a constitutional Water imbalance may be rather hyped up much of the time. This is a response to his feelings of fear. The approach to this child is the same as that described above. The practitioner needs to be as calm, solid and reassuring as possible. Sometimes a child who is hyped up may be mistaken for one who is angry, when fear is actually at the root.

> The behaviours and traits described above are supportive evidence of a child's constitutional imbalance. They should not replace the key diagnostic methods of colour, sound, emotion and odour.

SUMMARY

» The role of the Water Element during childhood is to govern growth and development.

» It also determines how a child will manage fears and assess risks.

» Living in an atmosphere of fear, either in the home or society, may bring about imbalance in the Water Element.

» A common cause of depletion in the Water Element is a child who is always 'on the go' and does not have enough downtime.

» Although shock initially affects the Heart, a severe or prolonged trauma may upset the balance between the Heart and the Kidneys, therefore impacting the Water Element.

» A child with a Water constitutional imbalance may be overly fearful or reckless, or swing between the two.

» Many children with a Water constitutional imbalance live in a chronic state of agitation and find it hard to relax.

» A few lack the drive and willpower that is normal in a child.

• Chapter 20 •

THE WOOD ELEMENT

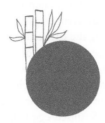

This chapter is divided into three sections:

- Factors that challenge the healthy development of the Wood Element
- Manifestations of an imbalanced Wood Element
- Gaining rapport with a child who has a Wood constitutional imbalance

KEY RESONANCES OF THE WOOD ELEMENT

- » Colour: Green
- » Sound: Shouting
- » Emotion: Anger
- » Odour: Rancid

SUPPORTING RESONANCES

- » Season: Spring
- » Power: Birth
- » Climate: Wind
- » Sense orifice: Eyes
- » Body part: Ligaments and tendons
- » Taste: Sour

ORGANS PERTAINING TO THE WOOD ELEMENT

- » *Yin* Organ: Liver – 'the planner'
- » *Yang* Organ: Gallbladder – 'the decision maker'

SPIRIT OF THE WOOD ELEMENT

Ethereal Soul (*hun*): associated with thinking; sleeping; consciousness; mental focus; strategising with insight and wisdom.

CHARACTER FOR WOOD

The character for Wood is *mu*, which represents a tree. On the top are the branches, in the middle the trunk and at the bottom, the roots. The horizontal line is the earth, showing that much of the tree is underground.

Introduction

A tree begins its life as a seed. Within the seed is contained the potential of the type of tree it may become. The seed will go through many different stages, from seed, to seedling, to sapling, and finally mature tree. If, at any of these stages, the environment that the tree is growing in does not suit it (the specifics of climate, temperature, moisture, soil composition, and so on), the tree will not thrive and it will not achieve the full potential that was inherent within the seed. As Fromm wrote, 'It is the surroundings that make it possible for each child to grow.'[33]

From the moment the sperm of the man and the ovum of the woman fuse in the fallopian tube, there is an inherent potential in the now fertilised egg that is unique. The degree to which this potential is realised will, to start with, depend on how well the environment of the womb is suited to that particular egg. After birth, much depends on how suitable the different aspects of a child's circumstances are. The degree to which she is able to be flexible, adaptable and to seek out people, places and paths that support her growth and development will also play a role.

KEY THEMES RELATED TO THE WOOD ELEMENT

Relationship to the emotions in the 'anger family', for example frustration or irritation; boundaries; power; constraint versus freedom; personal growth and development; compliance versus assertion.

Factors that challenge the healthy development of the Wood Element

- An overly repressive environment
  - Lack of freedom and independence
  - Emotional repression
  - Too much responsibility
- An environment lacking in boundaries, rules and guidance
- Living in an atmosphere of conflict or violence

Before considering these factors it is important to remember that parents generally want the best for their children. Nevertheless, parenting skills are rarely perfect. The quality of the parents' own *qi* is affected by their history and circumstances, which may compromise their ability to do as good a job as they would wish to.

An overly repressive environment

Lack of freedom and independence

A child learns that she exists in a world where there are rules that limit what she can and cannot do. A one-year-old begins to understand that it is all right to draw on paper, but not on the walls. He realises that at bedtime he has to stay in his bed. By the time he is four, he knows that he has to wait his turn to play with a toy, that his big brother is allowed to stay up later than he can and that, if he says rude words to his teacher, he will be told off or even punished. By the age of eight, he has learned that he has to wait until Christmas to get the new bicycle he so desperately wants and that, even though his classmate is allowed to watch the latest James Bond movie, his parents think he is too young for it.

Parents, teachers and society impose these rules, and a child slowly learns where his boundaries are. He learns when he needs to yield and when he can assert himself. If a child lives in a family where any attempt to assert himself is met with repression, over time he may either give up ever trying to assert himself or become either inwardly or outwardly chronically frustrated, angry or depressed. If the ethos of the family is that all decisions should be made by the parents and the children should automatically go along with whatever has been decided, a child may begin to feel powerless and grow up without learning how to make decisions for himself.

It may be that the family environment is conducive to the healthy expression of a particular child's Wood Element up until a certain age. One of the many challenges of parenting is to be able, constantly, to respond to the changing needs of the child. A parent may be quite happy to allow his nine-year-old the freedom that she demands. In a matter of just a few months, the balance may shift. Whereas previously she did her piano practice when she was asked to, now she wants to stop learning the piano altogether. Before, she was happy for her little sister to join in the game, now she wants her to keep out of the way. She wants to wear her headphones on car journeys rather than join in with family games or conversation. How a parent responds to these ever-changing demands for independence will determine not only the continued balance of the child's Wood Element but also the degree of harmony in the relationship between parent and child.

Sometimes the way in which a family is repressive may be subtle. Perfectionist parents, or ones with very high hopes for, or expectations of, their children, may unwittingly create an environment where their children feel repressed. If a child picks up early on in life that his parents have particular expectations of him, he subconsciously knows that they will be disappointed if he doesn't achieve them. Since a young child fears disappointing his parents, their expectations can feel to him like a constraint when he is starting to find out and express who he *really* is. When parents expect excellence or perfection, either in terms of behaviour or achievement, it leaves little room for a child to explore freely and make mistakes. 'There is no clear delineation between supporting and pressuring a child, between believing in your child and forcing your child to conform to what you imagine for him.'[34]

There are families where one sibling seems to thrive and yet another struggles. The nature of some children's Wood Element is that they will thrive in a more controlled and structured environment. Others will find the same environment restrictive and constraining.

Although for most children the home environment has more of an impact on their development than the school they attend, a school that is particularly badly suited to the unique nature of a child may also interfere with the healthy development of a child's Wood Element. For example, if a boy who is especially creative and independent goes to a school where obedience and exam results are prized most highly, it may be hard for him to thrive. A very strict teacher may mean that a child feels constrained in the classroom and is too inhibited to express his unique personality.

Emotional repression

Another way in which a child may be repressed is in the expression of his emotions. It is not considered acceptable in some families for a child to get cross with his parents or to squabble with his siblings. Many parents finds themselves saying 'Don't be angry' to their child. Anger (and its cousins, e.g. frustration, irritation and resentment) is not an emotion that it is possible to avoid, and ideally we should not be trying to avoid it. Yet it is one that in North European and North American culture is often seen as being negative. Learning how and when to express angry feelings is possibly one of the hardest challenges of being human.

Parenting inherently means having to frustrate a child on many occasions. A baby whose physical and emotional needs are not met quickly may cry or scream with frustration. A toddler who is seeking power and independence but does not yet have the ability to assess risk has to deal with being told 'no'. A school child may feel constrained by the lack of opportunity to move her body and run around. A teenager who wants more freedom may become furious as a result of the restrictions her parents impose. If a child is made to feel that he is wrong to have these feelings of frustration, or at least that he should not express them, it is likely that the health of his Wood Element will become compromised as a result.

In some families, a child suppresses her anger simply because there is an inherent power imbalance. She senses that if she gets into an argument, she will lose. She is no match for the force of Wood *qi* of her parent, or even an older sibling.

Too much responsibility

Too much responsibility at too young an age may feel like a burden. It may cause a child to be anxious or stressed. The responsibility may come in the form of helping to care for younger siblings, or even for parents who have health or social problems. Or it may come in the form of too many academic or extra-curricular commitments. For a two-year-old, even giving her the choice of what she wants to wear may feel like too big a decision to have to make and may cause her to end up in tears.

Responsibility involves decision making and having to make judgements about things. This leads to the Liver and Gallbladder, the Organs responsible for planning and decision making, becoming overly stretched at a time when they are tender and vulnerable.

A twelve-year-old girl came for treatment for depression, which I diagnosed as stemming from her Wood Element. Her mother had a degenerative neurological condition, and her younger sister had severe learning difficulties. Her father did not live with the family. She had taken on the role of 'mother' from an early age and I believed this, in part, to be what had caused the imbalance in her Wood.

An environment lacking in boundaries, rules and guidance

Whatever the current fashion for child-rearing, most experts, and certainly most parents, agree that young children rarely thrive without clear rules and boundaries. When he is very small, rules keep a child physically safe. As he gets older, rules take away the burden of endlessly having to make decisions for himself. Every time a child makes a decision, he relies upon the Wood Element to be able to do so. Too much of this means placing a strain on it. That is why children need adults to create clear boundaries and rules, and to provide guidance about what is acceptable in a certain situation and what is not.

A child whose parents can never say no to him, who is never made to wait or whose every whim is indulged is rarely a happy one. Rules and boundaries in themselves help to support a child's growth and development, just as a climbing plant needs a trellis to hold it up. A child left to his own devices may struggle to bring his plans to fruition and achieve his goals. He may meander in one direction and then another, never being able to find his true path. As one writer put it, 'permissiveness is the principle of treating children as if they were adults; and the tactic of making sure they never reach that stage'.[35]

Supporting a child's Wood Element may also come in the form of guidance. A child who does not get enough input from her parents may struggle to develop the resoluteness and creative drive associated with the Wood Element. Guidance may come in the form of being there to help when a child is trying to complete a task, whether it be making something or doing homework. It may also simply be provided by engaging the child in conversation, in order to guide him as he tries to express himself. Parents say and do many things every day, often instinctively, such as giving praise or suggesting a different way of doing something, which all help to guide a child in his growth and development.

> A thirteen-year-old Italian boy came to my children's school for a year in order to learn English. When he arrived, he was charming, polite and well behaved. Whilst here, he lived with a childless couple who indulged his every whim and gave him no rules. He was initially the envy of other children who saw he was allowed to watch movies until late every evening, have his own mobile phone and eat sweets whenever he wanted. After six months of being there, he began to get into trouble at school, to become aggressive with other children and to flout authority. This was a clear case of a child crying out for some rules and structure in his life.

Living in an atmosphere of conflict or violence

Just as the Liver is said to be the Organ that regulates and harmonises on a physical level, the Wood Element needs external harmony to be able to thrive. If a child grows up in an atmosphere where there is excessive conflict, either within the family or in the wider context in which she lives, it is likely to have a negative impact on her Wood Element.

Within families, and particularly within the parental relationship, conflict is dealt with in different ways. Some couples will openly and frequently argue and then make up. As long as there are periods of harmony between the arguments, and also a lot of love, a child will, it is hoped, not be negatively impacted by this. Problems arise when the conflict between the parents is extreme, constant or even violent. Equally problematic is an atmosphere of chronic, unspoken resentment and irritation. As Aristotle so succinctly put it:

> Any one can get angry – that is easy…; but to do this to the right person, to the right extent, at the right time, with the right motive, and in the right way, that is not for everyone, nor is it easy.

Of course, a child may be exposed to conflict outside the home too. He may have a teacher who is prone to getting cross and shouting. He may become involved in or witness ongoing and strong disagreements between his peers at school. A child may also experience conflict if he lives in a neighbourhood where there is racial tension or other conflicts within the community. Whatever the nature of an individual child's response, the Wood Element is particularly susceptible to imbalance when exposed to disharmony and conflict in the external environment.

Manifestations of an imbalanced Wood Element

A child's constitutional imbalance is both a strength and a weakness. He is likely to possess both *qualities* that relate to the Element of the imbalance, as well as *pathologies*. This chapter focuses predominantly on the pathologies related to the Wood Element because the practitioner will be seeing children who are in need of help in some way. In order to effectively treat a child, the focus must, of course, be on the pathology.

However, before looking at the manifestations of an imbalanced Wood Element, it is useful to be reminded of the *qualities* of Wood too. When the Wood Element is healthy, the child may:

- be creative in some way
- have strong organisational skills
- have a strong sense of right and wrong
- be capable of great benevolence
- show flexibility
- have a strong sense of adventure
- be a natural leader

- strongly express his individuality.

The manifestations of an imbalanced Wood Element considered below are:

- chronic anger:
    - aggressive and/or destructive behaviour
    - irritability
    - being spoiled, petulant and moody
- repressed anger:
    - being depressed and apathetic
    - being overly compliant and unassertive
- excessively strong drive towards independence
- inability to grow into independence.

 The key to understanding the clinical relevance of a perceived emotional imbalance is when it begins to hamper the child's ability to thrive. It is then pathological.

Chronic anger

The emotion connected with the Wood Element is anger (*nu*). One of the key ways in which a Wood imbalance manifests is in a difficult relationship with the emotion of anger. Please see Chapter 5 for a further discussion on the nature of anger.

Whilst it is convenient to translate the character *nu* with the single word 'anger', this is overly simplistic. Anger covers a relatively wide range of related emotions, including irritability, frustration, resentment, bitterness and rage.

Aggressive and/or destructive behaviour

One common way for this imbalance to manifest is for a child to behave in an overly aggressive way. What constitutes aggressive behaviour is somewhat dependent on the cultural norms in which the child is growing up. It also varies according to the age of the child. It may be considered acceptable for a three-year-old to sometimes roll around on the floor crying when she does not get what she wants, but most people would probably not deem this acceptable behaviour in a thirteen-year-old.

Strong outbursts of anger may arise because a child feels something is unjust or frustrating. They may also stem from another emotion, such as fear, jealousy or even sadness. Sometimes it is easier for a child to express a *yang* emotion such as anger than it is to admit to the more *yin* feelings of sadness or vulnerability. Angry feelings may also arise because a child feels overwhelmed or out of control. The *qi* of the Wood Element is *yang* in nature; it moves quickly and rises up. It may therefore feel to the child (and to other people) that the anger comes from nowhere and takes him over.

A child whose anger manifests in this way may get into trouble at school because he gets into fights with other children, or frequently challenges or contradicts his teachers. This often happens at moments when the child is feeling especially constrained, for example if he is waiting in a queue, has been sitting in a cramped classroom for too long, or has been asked to do something he perceives is pointless. Aggressive behaviour may take the form of violence towards a parent, friend or sibling. It may be that he has outbursts of screaming and shouting or smashing and breaking things.

Irritability

If a child is frequently or habitually irritable or frustrated, then it is an indication that her Wood Element is not thriving and that the *qi* of her Liver is not flowing smoothly. Constant teasing, squabbling between siblings and sarcasm are often a sign of underlying irritation. A child who rolls her eyes, huffs and puffs and sighs loudly when asked to do anything is also expressing her irritation and frustration.

Chronic irritation is an indication that a child is 'stuck' in her feelings. Children are usually a wonderful example of how *not* to get stuck in emotions. Whereas an adult may carry with her for days the feelings induced by a trivial disagreement with her spouse, a full-scale altercation between siblings over a toy is often forgotten in a matter of seconds.

Habitual irritation or frustration may be caused by circumstances in a child's life that would, to almost anybody, feel frustrating or irritating. In another child, chronic irritation may arise because of a pre-existing imbalance in his Wood Element, which means he is prone to finding almost anything frustrating. In either case, treatment can help him be more resourceful and respond to his circumstances differently.

Being spoiled, petulant and moody

Changing moods are a normal and healthy response to the complex nature of life. Life would be rather dull if we only ever experienced one emotion. However, a child with an imbalanced Wood Element may find it hard to have any consistency in her feeling world. The Liver regulates the emotions and, when in health, ensures the smooth flow of *qi* to this realm. A child whose Wood Element is strained may be constantly up and down. One minute she is incredibly enthusiastic, loving school and wanting to take part in every activity that is offered. The next, she may be saying that *everything* about school is awful. One moment, she plays harmoniously with her brother, the next everything her brother does is annoying and she wants nothing to do with him.

A child who is never satisfied, often labelled as spoiled, is manifesting an imbalance in her Wood. If she goes on and on, asking again and again over a period of days or weeks for her own computer, she is, on the face of it, simply expressing her deep desire for a computer. Another way of looking at it is that she is unable to contain this desire on her own and is asking her parents to help her with this. A firm and clear message – such as that she will not be getting her own computer until she is a teenager – gives her a definite boundary that she is not able to create for herself.

The natural movement of Liver *qi* is to spread outwards. However, it needs something to bump up against, something to contain it, to help the child get the measure of it, otherwise its spreading out will have no limits. Sometimes in a family one child begins to dominate to the detriment of everybody else. The nature of his Wood Element is such that, unless there are people around who are strong enough to contain him energetically, he will take up too much space.

> The character of Veruca Salt, in Roald Dahl's *Charlie and the Chocolate Factory*,[36] is a wonderful example of a spoiled and petulant child. Her father gives her everything she wants, and she wants many, many things. The Oompa Loompas decide to teach both Veruca and her father a lesson by throwing them down the garbage chute. By the end of the story, it is implied that her father has 'learned his lesson' and become less indulgent, which will change Veruca's life forever (for the better!).

Repressed anger

Being depressed and apathetic

Perhaps more upsetting than an angry or petulant child is to see one who is depressed and apathetic. Anger has been thought to play an integral role in depression since the early stages of psychoanalytic theorising about this disorder. The *qi* of the Wood Element should, in health, be directed outwards. If it becomes blocked for some reason, it may turn inwards and sink downwards. This will lead to the child feeling as if life is hopeless and has no point to it. The child may have a strong 'can't be bothered' attitude to life and lack an interest in the activities that her peers get enjoyment from. She may give up engaging in home or school life. Internally, she may be feeling powerless to change anything and make her life better. This kind of mood is most commonly, though not exclusively, seen in older children and teenagers.

A moderate amount of these feelings is part and parcel of being a teenager. Sometimes, however, the degree of hopelessness that an adolescent feels becomes more pronounced. At the most extreme end of the scale, it may manifest with mental health problems, including suicidal thoughts or tendencies. The child is usually unaware that this feeling is anger or frustration that has turned inward and will describe feeling very depressed and low. Treatment on the Wood Element to help promote the smooth flow of Liver *qi* can help the child to begin feeling hopeful and positive, and consequently to re-engage with life.

Being overly compliant and unassertive

Over-compliance is not generally something that parents complain about. Yet it is not a sign of emotional health for a child *always* to do what she is asked, or *always* to concede to the wishes of other children with whom she is playing. This pattern may arise because one or both of her parents are very over-bearing and the child's Wood energy is simply not a match for them. She may fear the consequences of asserting herself so much that she gives up ever doing it. Alternatively, the parents may not be particularly forceful or strict but the child is especially meek. An unassertive child may remain very dependent on her parents as she grows up. She does not have the force that derives from a strong Wood Element to separate herself and carve out her own identity and path in life.

A child who tends towards this kind of over-compliance may find that she is a target for bullying children at school. She simply does not have enough force in her Wood Element to stand up for herself. Unfortunately, bullies often seem to have a way of seeking out children whom they sense are not a match for them. Even if she is not bullied, this child may tend to shy away from conflict and arguments. She may also prefer to be a follower rather than a leader.

Whereas most of the imbalances described are thought of as being temporary imbalances of *qi*, a child who is rather timid, unassertive and overly compliant is described in Chinese texts as a personality type. The Chinese use the expression 'they have a small gallbladder' to describe somebody who is lacking in courage, or who is timid and fearful. There is no doubt that some children tend to be this way from birth, yet others become this way because of a combination of factors that are described in the previous section. Treatment on the Wood Element cannot change the fundamental constitution of a child, but it can enable her to make the most of her constitution.

Excessively strong drive towards independence

A child with an imbalanced Wood Element may feel a need to constantly defy the authority of her parents and/or teachers. There are times when it is appropriate for a child to rebel, in order to assert her independence. Some rebellion during the teenage years, for example, is healthy. However, a child who is compulsively defiant is expressing the fact that her Wood is not balanced.

A child may be adept at finding all sorts of wonderful ways to express defiance. It may be that she consistently refuses to comply with what seem to her parents like the most basic requests. It appears that she needs to say no to everything 'for the sake of it'. It may be that she always does the exact opposite of what is expected of her. She may be outraged at being asked to wear slightly smarter clothes than normal to a family gathering. She may be compelled to break the school rules whenever she can. Or she may show an intellectual defiance by compulsively arguing with and challenging the opinions of parents and others. Of course, this may just be that she is a politician in the making. It is when the degree of defiance begins to hamper a child's ability to thrive that it can then be seen as pathological. Treatment on the Wood Element can help a child to become more flexible, to know when to hold firm and when to concede.

> A parent told me about her battles with her twelve-year-old daughter to get her to wear her hair up, so it did not fall over her face. For months, she fought with her and endlessly told her how much better she looked when her hair was in a ponytail. Her daughter flatly refused to put it up. The mother then decided to begin complimenting her daughter on how lovely her hair looked when it was down. Within a week, her daughter had started wearing her hair up every day. This child just needed to defy for defiance's sake.

Inability to grow into independence

Another manifestation of an imbalance in the Wood Element is a child who struggles to achieve the independence that would usually be expected of her at each given age. This is most noticeable as a child gets older, especially during adolescence. The mother of an eleven-year-old boy described how he had to be 'coached' to do anything independently. It never seemed to come to him spontaneously, whether it be reading on his own, putting himself to bed or getting his own breakfast. Although this lack of independence could come from other imbalances, in this boy it came from the fact that he lacked the quality of Wood *qi* required to forge his own path in life and make his own decisions.

Gaining rapport with a child who has a Wood constitutional imbalance

One of the ways a constitutional imbalance in the Wood Element may manifest is that the child is rather timid and well behaved. The practitioner may look forward to him coming because he is so compliant and easy to treat. This kind of child requires the practitioner to be gentle, yet firm. He may feel anxious if the practitioner is too domineering. He may also find it difficult and stressful if he is given too many choices (such as 'Shall we do the moxa or the needles first today?'). However, as treatment improves his Liver *qi*, he may assert himself more strongly. He may begin to test the authority of the practitioner and his parents. Although this may be challenging in some respects, it is usually a good sign in terms of the progression of the treatment.

A constitutional Wood imbalance may also manifest in a very different way, with a child who is rather domineering and sometimes disruptive. This child needs to be given a really clear message about what behaviour is acceptable or not whilst he is having his treatment. 'Boundaries' is a much overused word, but a child with an excess Wood imbalance really does need to be given very clear boundaries. This does not mean the practitioner needs to be bossy or domineering, or convey her own frustrations. This will only add fuel to the fire and further stress the already struggling Liver *qi* of the child. Rather, the practitioner must endeavour to muster her own Liver *qi* so that she behaves in a way which leaves no doubt in the child's mind that she is commanding the situation. There may come a time when the practitioner needs to 'match' the force of Wood energy that the child is displaying. She must engage the child as best she can. She must be clear, very calm and lacking in any kind of hesitation.

 The behaviours and traits described above are supportive evidence of a child's constitutional imbalance. They should not replace the key diagnostic methods of colour, sound, emotion and odour.

SUMMARY

» The Wood Element underpins a child's personal growth and development, enabling her to express her individuality and carve out her individual path.

» The Wood Element will play a large part in determining the child's ability to manage emotions in the 'anger family'.

» The Wood Element may become imbalanced if the child is given too much or too little independence and emotional freedom.

» Too much responsibility may also harm the development of the Wood Element.

» An atmosphere of conflict or violence may also impact negatively on the Wood Element.

» A child with an imbalance in the Wood Element may be aggressive, irritable and/or moody.

» He may also be depressed and apathetic, or overly compliant.

» Another manifestation of an imbalanced Wood Element is an excessively strong drive towards independence, or a lack of ability to become dependent.

• Chapter 21 •

THE HEART AND PERICARDIUM

The topics discussed in this chapter are:

- The characteristics of the Heart particularly pertinent to children

- Common Heart Organ patterns seen in children

- The characteristics of the Pericardium particularly pertinent to children

THE HEART
The characteristics of the Heart particularly pertinent to children

- The Heart houses the *shen*

- The Heart enables a child to speak and to communicate

- The Heart governs Blood

The Heart houses the *shen*

For the first three months of a baby's life, the mother will often have a feeling that her baby does not recognise her or communicate with her in any way. Then, all of a sudden, the baby will smile at his first moment of awareness of his mother being a separate person to him. There will be a luminosity in the baby's eyes that was not previously there. This is the moment at which the *shen* first shows itself.

The *shen*, which resides in the Heart, gives a child her ability to connect with others. As a baby grows into a toddler, and a toddler into a young child, life becomes increasingly about relationships. For the first few years, relationships are formed primarily with family members. From the age of around four, friends become increasingly important. As the Heart and the *shen* mature, so does the child's ability to manage relationships.

The Heart is one of the Organs which regulate the emotions. During the first years of a child's life, whilst the Heart is still maturing, she will easily become destabilised by a habitual or intense emotion. Blood and *yin* being insufficient in that stage, the *shen* is not strongly rooted. When a child's *shen* is disturbed, it can affect her entire being. Chapter 8 of the *Su Wen* talks of the Heart as the Emperor. An Emperor quietly sits on his throne and his presence ensures order throughout the land. When the Emperor is knocked off his throne, everything is thrown into chaos. A child's reaction to an emotional upset may reveal this. She may become unreachable and cannot be calmed. She may shake, sweat, scream or withdraw. She may spontaneously develop a physical symptom such as a cough or diarrhoea. Time, gentle touch and the calm presence of a parent should ensure that tranquillity once again reigns.

The most extreme example of this function becoming imbalanced is when the child has had a shock. Chapter 39 of the *Su Wen* says, 'When there is starting with *jing* [shock], the Heart no longer has a place to rely on. The *shen* no longer has a place to refer to, planned thought no longer has a place to settle.'[37]

Of all the Organs, the Heart is the one that is usually most affected by shock. This is the case at any age, but a child is especially vulnerable to the effects of shock. Some events are obviously shocking to a child. However, a child may be shocked by something that is not recognised as shocking by most adults.

> One child who came to the clinic showed signs of severe shock that had come on after imagining a monster was hiding in the small gap between her bed and the wall.

Dechar describes the *shen* as 'the guiding light of our individual destiny'.[38] The *shen* of the Heart enables a child to communicate who she is to the world and to live in a way that reflects her true self. Many parents comment that their child 'came out of the womb that way'. Every baby is born with the seeds of who they are to become, and it is the role of the Heart to manifest that in the world.

The Heart enables a child to speak and to communicate

The Heart opens into the tongue and influences speech. As a child grows, language enables him to communicate his desires and to relate to the most important people in his world. The healthy development of a child's speech is a sign of strong Heart *qi* and Blood. A lack of desire to speak or a speech impediment such as a stutter may be a sign of an imbalance in the Heart *qi*.

> A three-year-old boy who once came to the clinic had stopped talking after being attacked by a dog. Treating his Heart over a period of a few weeks meant that he gradually began speaking again.

The Heart governs Blood

Along with Kidney Essence, Heart Blood goes some way to determining the robustness of a child's constitution. This is because the transformation of Food (*gu*) *qi* takes place in the Heart. When Heart Blood is replete, it circulates well and helps to keep a child warm. The propensity for young children's hands to become cold very quickly in the winter may be a reflection of their immature Heart not being able to circulate Blood sufficiently well. Strong Heart Blood will mean a child is full of vigour, both mentally and physically.

In teenage girls, Heart Blood also plays a role in menstruation. Via the *bao mai*, the Heart provides the impetus for the discharge of blood when a girl menstruates.

Teenage girls are prone to becoming Blood deficient when they start menstruating, for a variety of reasons which include a poor diet and excessive exercise and/or study. When this happens, the Heart Blood no longer houses the *shen* securely and they are liable to become *shen* disturbed.

● **SOME KEY SIGNS AND SYMPTOMS OF A HEART IMBALANCE**

>> Sleep difficulties

>> Hyperactivity or a lack of concentration

>> Excessively talkative or reluctant to speak, stuttering

>> Lacking in emotional and/or physical robustness

>> Emotionally volatile or excessively vulnerable

>> Red face or a pale, lacklustre complexion

Common Heart Organ patterns seen in children

The Heart is often said to be prone to excess in a child. This is because of the child's predominantly *yang* nature and the propensity of the Heart to be affected by Heat that rises up in the body. However, in practice, it is just as common to see children with a deficient Heart pattern as it is an excess one.

Of course, any Heart pattern may be present in a child. However, the ones discussed here are those most commonly encountered in a paediatric clinic. For a comprehensive list of all possible Heart patterns, see *The Foundations of Chinese Medicine* by Giovanni Maciocia.[39]

The following Heart patterns will be discussed:

- Heart *qi* and Blood deficiency

- Heart-Fire Blazing; Phlegm-Fire harassing the Heart

- Phlegm misting the Heart

> All Heart patterns involve a degree of imbalance in the *shen*. Therefore, although not explicitly stated under each pattern, the *shen* should often be treated when addressing these patterns in the clinic. This is done by choosing points which have a particular effect on the *shen* and may involve either the tonification or sedation needle technique, depending on the particular pattern.

Heart *qi* and Blood deficiency

0–3-year-olds

- easily unsettled and upset

- finds it hard to settle herself after upset

- needs a lot of contact with parents or to be around other people

- tendency to poor sleep

- reluctance to speak or stuttering

- pale complexion

- congenital heart problems

School-age children

- easily feels hurt and rejected

- anxiety

- may struggle with separation from family

- tendency to poor sleep in the first part of the night

- difficulty concentrating or tired after mental activity

- forgetful or absent-minded

- reluctance to speak or stuttering

- pale face

- congenital heart problems

Teenagers

Any of the symptoms already listed, plus:

- easily startled
- aware of heartbeat when tired or anxious

Pulse: thin or choppy in the Heart position

Tongue: may be pale or thin

Treatment principles: nourish Heart Blood

> One sign of Heart Blood deficiency often seen in the clinic is that the child is 'easily startled' when needled. He may 'jump' when the needle is inserted. This is different from when a child feels pain when needled. When using a guide tube, it is best to use several gentle taps to insert the needle with this child, rather than one, sudden movement.

Variation

Heart Blood deficiency may develop into Heart *yin* deficiency. The tendency for this becomes more marked as the child gets older and especially around puberty. The symptoms of Heart *yin* deficiency are similar to Heart Blood deficiency, with the following key differences:

- the agitation is greater with Heart *yin* deficiency
- the pulse will be floating and Empty
- the tongue may be especially red on the tip
- there may be signs of Heat, although these are generally not as pronounced as in adults.

Key aetiological factors

- inherited tendency
- shock (either pre- or post-birth)
- feeling unloved
- melodrama in the family
- difficult friendship dynamics
- overuse of social media
- anxiety and worry
- diet lacking in Blood-nourishing foods
- fevers (for Heart *yin* deficiency)

SUGGESTED TREATMENT

It is usually sufficient to use one or two of the following points per treatment.

Points

Any point on the Heart channel can be used to strengthen Heart *qi*, Blood or *yin*. The points chosen should depend on the nature and location of the symptoms, as well as the emotional state of the child. Some of the most commonly used points to tonify the Heart in children are:

He 1 *jiquan*
He 6 *yinxi*

He 7 *shenmen*
Pc 6 *neiguan*
Pc 7 *daling*
Bl 14 *jueyinshu*
Bl 15 *xinshu*
Bl 43 *gaohuangshu*
Bl 44 *shentang*
Ren 14 *juque*
Ren 17 *shanzhong*

Method: tonification needle technique

Other modalities: moxa may be applicable

Paediatric *tui na*

Heart *xinjing* (straight pushing tonification)
Spinal Column *jizhu* (pinching from bottom to top)
Heaven Gate *tianmen* (straight pushing)
Heart Gate *xinmen* (straight pushing)
Water Palace *kangong* (pushing apart)
Palace of Toil *laogong* (kneading)
Small Heavenly Heart *xiaotianxin* (tapping)

Heart-Fire Blazing

0–3-year-olds

- agitated and unable to settle
- wakes at night and needs help to settle
- clingy during the day
- hot temper
- strong emotional reactions
- tendency to strong fevers
- constipation with dry and possibly foul-smelling stools
- tendency to red, painful mouth and tongue ulcers
- red face

School-age children

- always on the go
- anxiety and agitation, which may be extreme
- impulsive
- restless sleep (throws off the bed clothes) or insomnia
- seems to be able to survive on little sleep
- hot temper
- strong emotional reactions

- hyperactivity
- talkative with loud voice
- tendency to high fevers
- constipation with dry and possibly foul-smelling stools
- tendency to red, painful mouth and tongue ulcers
- red face

Teenagers

Any of the previous symptoms, plus:

- panic attacks
- manic behaviour
- tendency to red acne
- heavy periods in girls

Pulse: overflowing Heart pulse, rapid

Tongue: red tip, yellow coating

Treatment principles: clear Heat; calm the *shen*; tonify underlying deficiencies (which may be in any Organ, especially those related to the constitutional imbalance)

> One six-year-old boy with Heart-Fire Blazing manifested this pathology in a very endearing way. He was incredibly open and affectionate, was talkative and had a wonderful laugh. He just seemed to ooze joy and happiness. He was the life and soul of the family and the classroom. Whilst these are obviously not, on their own, traits that one would necessarily want to change, in this case they were a reflection of an imbalance. The boy also only slept for a few hours each night and his family felt his behaviour was bordering on mania much of the time.

Variation: Phlegm-Fire harassing the Heart
Heart-Fire Blazing often leads to Phlegm-Fire harassing the Heart. The Fire condenses fluids, which leads to the creation of Phlegm. When this is the case, as well as the symptoms above, there may also be the following:

- the child being hard to reach and in her own world
- phases of extreme lethargy, alternating with periods of hyperactivity
- impaired speech.

Key aetiological factors
- inherited tendency
- womb Heat
- chronic and/or intense emotional difficulties (such as instability within the family or difficulties at school)
- chronic and/or intense anger and frustration (causing Liver Fire which transmits to the Heart)

- Phlegm-forming and heating foods (in the case of Phlegm-Fire harassing the Heart)

- external invasions of Heat (such as strong fevers)

- drugs and alcohol in teenagers

SUGGESTED TREATMENT

It is usually sufficient to use one point to clear Fire, and one to resolve Phlegm, in each treatment. On teenagers, more points may need to be used.

Points

To clear Fire:

> He 7 *shenmen*
> He 8 *shaofu*
> He 3 *shaohai*
> SI 5 *yanggu*
> Pc 8 *laogong*
> Ren 14 *juque*
> Bl 15 *xinshu*

To resolve Phlegm:

> Pc 5 *jianshi*
> St 40 *fenglong*

To calm the *shen*:

> Du 24 *shenting*
> M-HN-3 *yintang*

Method: sedation needle technique

Paediatric *tui na*

> Heaven Gate *tianmen* (straight pushing)
> Heart Gate *xinmen* (straight pushing)
> Water Palace *kangong* (pushing apart)
> Heart *xinjing* (straight pushing sedation)
> Liver *ganjing* (straight pushing sedation)
> Palace of Toil *laogong* (kneading)
> Small Heavenly Heart *xiaotianxin* (kneading)
> Milky Way *tianheshui* (straight pushing)
> Six *Yang* Organs *liufu* (straight pushing)

Phlegm misting the Heart

A baby or child with Phlegm misting the Heart may have a veil between her and the world. This may mean that her emotional responses and reactions to the world are dulled.

Babies

- sleeps a lot

- rarely perturbed or upset

- may not react to stimuli as would be expected

- may be unusually happy to be on her own

- there may be other symptoms of Phlegm, such as chronic cough or recurrent vomiting of mucus

School-age children

- withdrawn

- may be off in her own world and hard to reach

- speech may be impaired

- mental confusion

- there may be other symptoms of Phlegm such as chronic cough or recurrent vomiting of mucus

Teenagers

Any of the symptoms previously listed, plus:

- disengaged from life and people

- depressed

- lethargic

- lacking in initiative and motivation

Pulse: wiry or slippery

Tongue: swollen, thick sticky white coat

Treatment principles: resolve Phlegm, open the Heart's orifices

It may also be necessary to tonify any underlying deficiencies, which are likely to be of the Spleen, the Heart or the Organs related to the constitutional imbalance.

SUGGESTED TREATMENT

It is usually sufficient to choose one or two points per treatment.

Points

Pc 5 *jianshi*
Bl 15 *xinshu*
St 40 *fenglong*
Ren 14 *juque*
Du 24 *shenting*

Method: sedation needle technique

Points should be chosen to treat the underlying deficiencies depending on which Organ or Organs are involved.

Paediatric *tui na*

Heaven Gate *tianmen* (straight pushing)
Heart Gate *xinmen* (straight pushing)
Water Palace *kangong* (pushing apart)
Small Palmar Crease *zhangxiaowen* (straight pushing)
Hand *yin yang shouyinyang* (pushing apart)

Key aetiological factors

- inherited tendency

- extremely difficult circumstances in the first years of life (e.g. a lack of basic care or a very depressed family environment)

- excessive consumption of greasy, cold and raw foods

THE PERICARDIUM
The characteristics of the Pericardium particularly pertinent to children

- The Pericardium protects the Heart from pathogens

- The Pericardium protects the Heart during interpersonal interactions

The Pericardium has the important role of protecting the Heart. Many Chinese medical texts do not differentiate to any further degree between the Heart and the Pericardium. For example, *The Yellow Emperor's Classic*[40] normally refers to the six *yang* Organs but only five *yin* Organs. Therefore, there is virtually nothing written in paediatric texts specifically about the Pericardium. However, it is useful to differentiate the two Organs when thinking about the physical and particularly the emotional development of children.

The Pericardium protects the Heart from pathogens

Chapter 71 of the *Ling Shu* says that, 'if a pathogenic factor attacks the Heart, it will be deviated to attack the Pericardium instead'.[41]

Children have insubstantial *yin* and are therefore prone to invasions of Heat. This function of the Pericardium comes to the fore when a child is in the throes of a febrile disease. The *Ling Shu* states that, 'if the Heart is attacked by a pathogenic factor, the Mind suffers, which can lead to death'.[42] If a child has a very high temperature and is delirious, confused and aphasic, it indicates that pathogenic Heat has attacked the Pericardium and should be taken as a warning sign that the condition is potentially dangerous.

The Pericardium protects the Heart during interpersonal interactions

An adult with a healthy Pericardium will have an inherent sense of how much of her inner being it is appropriate to reveal to different people. She will know, for example, that to open up to the postman about her innermost thoughts and feelings would probably leave a rather shocked postman. Sometimes young children surprise us with their openness. Whilst this may be very endearing, it may also be a sign that the Pericardium has not yet developed enough to know when to stay a little more closed. On the other hand, there are children who struggle to truly make deep-level contact with anybody and who appear to be rather closed off. In a healthy child, some balance between these two extremes is achieved as they grow and mature.

SOME KEY SIGNS AND SYMPTOMS OF A PERICARDIUM IMBALANCE

Any of the signs and symptoms of a Heart imbalance may also be related to the Pericardium. In addition, the following are specifically related to the Pericardium:

» high fever with delirium and confusion

» an overdeveloped sense of fear of other people and acute shyness

» a level of emotional openness that is not appropriate to the age of the child.

Why are there no patterns associated with the Pericardium?

Patterns that are normally listed under the Heart in modern Chinese medicine texts may affect the Pericardium too. The symptoms are the same, whichever of these two Organs are affected. It is the pulse which usually determines whether the practitioner should predominantly use points on the Heart or the Pericardium channel. For example, in the case of Heart Blood deficiency, either the Heart or the Pericardium pulse may be thin. If the Heart pulse is the thinnest, the practitioner may choose to use a point such as He 7 *shenmen*. If the Pericardium pulse is the thinnest, she may choose Pc 7 *daling* instead. In chronic conditions, the Heart is more prone to Heat than the Pericardium. In acute conditions (i.e. fevers), the Pericardium is the more prone to Heat.

SUMMARY

» The following characteristics of the Heart are especially relevant in childhood:
  − the Heart houses the *shen*
  − the Heart enables speech and communication
  − the Heart governs Blood.
» In children, some of the most commonly seen symptoms relating to a Heart pattern are:
  − sleep problems
  − speech difficulties
  − difficulty concentrating
  − hyperactivity
  − emotional vulnerability
  − being excessively talkative or excessively withdrawn and shy.
» The most commonly seen Heart patterns in children are:
  − Heart *qi* and Blood deficiency
  − Heart-Fire Blazing
  − Phlegm-Fire harassing the Heart
  − Phlegm misting the Heart.
» Any of the patterns usually attributed to the Heart may affect the Pericardium too. The pulse should be the factor that determines which channel is best used to treat the pattern.

• Chapter 22 •

THE SPLEEN
. . . .

The topics discussed in this chapter are:

- The characteristics of the Spleen particularly pertinent to children
- Common Spleen Organ patterns seen in children

The characteristics of the Spleen particularly pertinent to children

- The Spleen is responsible for transportation and transformation of food
- The Spleen controls Blood
- The Spleen controls the four limbs
- The Spleen houses the *yi*
- The Spleen opens into the mouth and manifests in the lips
- The Spleen controls saliva
- The Spleen raises *qi*

The Spleen is responsible for transportation and transformation of food

The Spleen extracts the nutrients that the child needs from food and drink. It keeps food moving through the digestive system, so that blockage and stagnation do not arise. Considering the amount of food a baby eats compared to her size, this is indeed a Herculean task. Furthermore, as with the other Organs, the Spleen is not yet fully matured. It is therefore no surprise that this function can easily, and often does, become deficient. Many common childhood disorders have their root in a dysfunction of this aspect of the Spleen. Tummy pain, loose stools, constipation and permanently snotty noses are but a few examples.

 Some physical signs that are almost considered 'normal' in babies and toddlers are a sign of the transformation and transportation function of the Spleen being under strain. For example, a bloated tummy, regurgitation of milk after feeds and colic may all have this imbalance at their root.

The Spleen controls Blood

The Spleen plays a crucial role in the production of Blood. The Spleen extracts Food (*gu*) *qi* from food and drink and, along with *yuan qi* from the Kidneys, this is transformed into Blood in the Heart. This process is helped by the *yuan* (original) *qi* of the Kidneys. As Maciocia explains, 'this is another reason why it is called the Root of Post-Heaven *qi*'.[43] Much of the basic health and vitality of a growing child relies upon the state of her post-heavenly *qi* and Blood. It is also essential for her emotional well-being. The *shen* needs strong *qi* and Blood in order to remain rooted and vital.

The Spleen controls the four limbs

Part of the *qi* extracted from food by the Spleen goes to the arms and legs. This will enable a baby or toddler to learn to crawl, stand up, walk and hold things. As he grows up, a child will increase his level of coordination. He will be able to run without falling over so often or reach for a particular object and grab it. He will be able to ride a bike and kick a ball. As the Spleen matures, so the ability of a child to do these physical tasks that require strength and control of the limbs increases.

The three functions of the Spleen mentioned so far provide the foundation of a child's physical energy. If a child easily tires and lacks the inclination to run around and be physical, it often points to a deficiency of Spleen *qi*.

The Spleen houses the *yi*

Around the age of four or five, physical growth slows down a little and mental or intellectual development come more to the foreground.

The spirit of the Spleen is the *yi*, which is often translated as 'thought'. The *yi* gives a child the capacity for clear thought and studying. It enables her to stick with a task, to concentrate and to absorb information. When a child begins school, the *yi* plays a key role in her ability to understand concepts and learn. An inability to focus on a task and take in facts may point towards an imbalance in the Spleen, which is affecting the *yi*.

> A twelve-year-old girl, who was studying for the entrance exam for her secondary school, came for treatment for chronic stomach aches. She had also lost her appetite over the time she had been revising for her exams. Her Spleen *qi* (specifically, her *yi*) was being used to fuel all the studying she was doing. Worry about her exams was further depleting the Spleen. Consequently, there was less *qi* available for it to maintain a healthy digestive function.

The Spleen opens into the mouth and manifests in the lips

This function of the Spleen may in part determine how well a baby is able to latch on to his mother's breast and feed in the first months of life. Mothers often report differences in the ability of each of their children to do this. For some babies, it seems easy. Others struggle and don't seem to have quite the same mastery of their mouths.

This function of the Spleen also has an impact on how a child approaches the task of eating solid foods. Chewing prepares food for the Spleen to then carry out its task of transforming and transporting food essences. Taste is also a Spleen-related function. It is striking how children differ in their willingness to try to eat a wide variety of foods. Whilst some of this inevitably stems from the differing approaches parents take to introducing solid foods and eating in general, it is also partly determined by the nature of the child's Spleen.

The lips are a reflection of the state of the Spleen. A tendency towards dry and cracked lips may be a sign of a Spleen imbalance in a child.

The Spleen controls saliva

Saliva (*xian*) is the fluid related to the Spleen. Excess saliva, manifesting as drooling, is a relatively common pathology in children and may be a sign that the Spleen is deficient and Cold.

The Spleen raises *qi*

There are two aspects of this function which are particularly relevant to children. The first is that if the Spleen is not effectively raising *qi*, then *qi* may sink downwards. This may be a contributory factor in bedwetting and also chronic diarrhoea. Second, the Spleen sends *qi*, food essences and fluids upwards to the Lungs. If this function is impaired, then it may mean that Lung *qi* becomes deficient as a result.

 SOME KEY SIGNS AND SYMPTOMS OF A SPLEEN IMBALANCE

>> Problems with eating and appetite

>> Tendency to loose stools

>> Tendency towards digestive symptoms

>> Easily tires

>> Clingy and whiny

>> Lack of strength and control of limbs

>> Pale face

Common Spleen Organ patterns seen in children

The Spleen is often said to be prone to deficiency in a child. This is because of the degree of Spleen *qi* constantly called upon by the body to digest food and drink. However, in practice, it is common to see mixed conditions of the Spleen too.

Of course, any Spleen pattern may be present in a child. However, the ones discussed here are those most commonly encountered in a paediatric clinic. For a comprehensive list of all possible Spleen patterns, see *The Foundations of Chinese Medicine* by Maciocia.[44]

The following Spleen patterns will be discussed:

• Spleen *qi/yang* deficiency

• Spleen *qi* deficiency with Dampness

• Damp-Heat in the Spleen

Spleen *qi/yang* deficiency

In some children, Spleen *qi* deficiency may manifest with only physical symptoms. In others, it will manifest with predominantly emotional symptoms. In others, there will be a mix of physical and emotional symptoms.

 The Spleen's function of digestion is weak and immature in children. Therefore, every young child has some degree of Spleen *qi* deficiency. However, if the circumstances of the child's life (in particular, diet) are good, this will not necessarily manifest as symptoms. The symptoms discussed below occur when the inherent weakness in the Spleen has gone one step further and led to an imbalance.

Symptoms in any age group

• frequent bowel movements

• unformed stools

• undigested food in stools

• easily tired

• pale face

0–3-year-olds

Physical symptoms

- struggles to go for long gaps without feeding or eating
- wants to 'snack' little and often
- eats a narrow range of foods
- is reluctant to try new foods
- appetite decreases when tired or upset
- sleeps a lot during the day
- wakes up frequently at night
- muscle tone feels weak or spongy
- pale or clear nasal mucus

Emotional tendencies

- clingy and whiny
- unsettled by others' distress
- may want to be near Mum a lot of the time
- will need to 'recharge' by contact with parent after a time of playing on own
- tends to be on the quiet side

School-age children

Physical symptoms

- eats a narrow range of foods
- reluctance to try new foods
- appetite may decrease when tired or upset
- pale or clear nasal mucus
- easily feels tired by school, intellectual or physical activity
- struggles to concentrate when tired

Emotional tendencies

- sensitive and easily upset
- unsettled by others' distress
- may find moment of separation at start of school day difficult
- tendency to worry
- needs a lot of sympathy for minor hurts

Teenagers

Any of the symptoms listed above, plus:

PHYSICAL SYMPTOMS

- tends to eat a lot of carbohydrates and sugary foods
- irregular appetite
- picky with food

EMOTIONAL TENDENCIES

- tearful and 'emotional' especially in the evening when tired
- may struggle to get off to sleep because of worries
- may alternate between being very needy and then rejecting help or sympathy

Pulse: deficient

Tongue: pale, wet, swollen

Treatment principles: tonify Spleen *qi*

Key aetiological factors

- inherited tendency
- lack of nurture and support
- depleted mother
- poor diet
- excessive studying
- excess exercise
- worry
- lack of stability at home

SUGGESTED TREATMENT

It is usually sufficient to use one or two of the following points per treatment.

Points

Any point on the Spleen channel can be used to strengthen Spleen *qi*. The points chosen in each particular case should depend on the nature and location of the symptoms, as well as the emotional state of the child. Some of the most commonly used points in young children are:

St 36 *zusanli*
Ren 12 *zhongwan*
Sp 3 *taibai*
Sp 4 *gongsun*
Sp 6 *sanyinjiao*
St 25 *tianshu*
Bl 20 *pishu*
Bl 21 *weishu*

Method: tonification needle technique

Other techniques: moxa may be applicable

Paediatric *tui na*

Spleen *pijing* (straight pushing tonification)
Stomach *weijing* (straight pushing tonification)
Three Passes *sanguan* (straight pushing)
Knead Ren 12 *zhongwan* (kneading anti-clockwise)
Spinal Column *jizhu* (pinching from the bottom to the top of the back)
St 36 *zusanli* (kneading)

Variations

- Spleen *qi* deficiency may also include an element of *yang* deficiency. In this case, the above symptoms may be stronger and may be accompanied by feelings of cold. It is essential to use moxibustion.

- Spleen *qi* deficiency may include Spleen not controlling Blood. As well as the above symptoms, there may also be mild nosebleeds or heavy, long-lasting periods in teenagers. Sp 1 *yinbai* should be added to the point prescription.

- Spleen *qi* deficiency may include Spleen *qi* sinking. In this case, as well as the above symptoms, there may be a tendency to bedwetting in young children, a tendency to loose stools or frequent bowel movements, and heavy, long-lasting periods in teenagers. Points that raise *qi*, such as Du 20 *baihui* or Ren 6 *qihai*, should be added to the point prescription.

Spleen *qi* deficiency with Dampness

As with all mixed conditions, in every case the practitioner should assess whether the emphasis of treatment should be on clearing the excess (in this case Damp) or tonifying the underlying deficiency.

Symptoms common to all age groups
Any symptoms of Spleen *qi* deficiency, plus:

- mucus in the stools

- bloating

- tendency to sleep a lot

- catarrh

- glue ear

- chronic cough

- tendency to eczema

- puffy face

School-age children

- tendency to lethargy

- difficulty concentrating and taking in information

- tummy pain

- nausea

- muzzy head

- difficulty getting going in the morning

- tendency towards being overweight

Teenagers

Any symptoms previously listed, plus:

- vaginal discharge

- tendency to acne

- craves sugar and/or carbohydrates

Pulse: deficient, slippery or soggy

Tongue: pale, thick white coat

Treatment principles: resolve Damp; tonify Spleen *qi*

> **SUGGESTED TREATMENT**
>
> It is usually sufficient to use one point to resolve Damp, and one to tonify the Spleen (when necessary), per treatment.
>
> **Points**
> To resolve Damp:
>
> > Sp 9 *yinlingquan*
> > Sp 6 *sanyinjiao*
> > Ren 12 *zhongwan*
> > St 8 *touwei*
>
> **Method:** sedation needle technique
>
> To tonify Spleen *qi*:
>
> > St 36 *zusanli*
> > Sp 3 *taibai*
> > Bl 20 *pishu*
>
> **Method:** tonification needle technique
>
> **Other techniques:** moxa may be applicable
>
> **Paediatric *tui na***
>
> > See Spleen *qi* deficiency

Key aetiological factors

Any of the causes of Spleen *qi* deficiency, plus:

- a diet with too many damp-forming foods

- living in a damp environment

Damp-Heat in the Spleen

This pattern may be acute or chronic. The description below is of the chronic pattern. There is nearly always an underlying deficiency in Spleen *qi*, which has been a precursor to this pattern. The presence of the Damp and Heat then strain Spleen *qi* further, so a vicious circle begins.

Symptoms

- chronic loose stools or diarrhoea with smelly stools
- in severe cases, blood in the stools
- sore or burning anus
- poor appetite
- low-grade fever
- grouchy
- tired
- tendency to eczema
- yellow complexion with red cheeks
- may have a diagnosis of Crohn's disease or ulcerative colitis

Pulse: slippery, rapid, deficient

Tongue: sticky yellow coat

Treatment principles: resolve Damp; clear Heat; tonify the Spleen

> **SUGGESTED TREATMENT**
> It is usually sufficient to use one or two points per treatment.
>
> **Points**
> To resolve Damp and clear Heat:
>
> St 25 *tianshu*
> Sp 9 *yinlingquan*
> Sp 6 *sanyinjiao*
> LI 11 *quchi*
> Bl 25 *dachangshu*
>
> **Method:** sedation needle technique
>
> To tonify Spleen *qi*:
>
> St 36 *zusanli*
> Sp 3 *taibai*
> Bl 20 *pishu*
>
> **Method:** tonification needle technique
>
> **Paediatric *tui na***
>
> Spleen *pijing* (straight pushing tonification)
> Stomach *weijing* (straight pushing tonification)
> Milky Way *tianheshui* (straight pushing)
> Six *Yang* Organs *liufu* (straight pushing)

Seven Bound Bones *qijiegu* (straight pushing sedation)
Knead Ren 12 *zhongwan* (kneading anti-clockwise)
Spinal Column *jizhu* (pinching from the bottom to the top of the back)
St 36 *zusanli* (kneading)

Key aetiological factors

- any of the causes of Spleen *qi* deficiency

- Accumulation Disorder

- contaminated food

SUMMARY

» The following characteristics of the Spleen are especially relevant in childhood:

 − the Spleen is responsible for transportation and transformation of food

 − the Spleen controls Blood

 − the Spleen controls the four limbs

 − the Spleen houses the *yi*

 − the Spleen opens into the mouth and manifests in the lips

 − the Spleen controls saliva

 − the Spleen raises *qi*.

» In children, some of the most commonly seen symptoms relating to a Spleen pattern are:

 − clingy and whiny

 − lacking in energy or easily tires

 − problems with eating and appetite

 − tendency to loose stools

 − catarrh

 − tendency to phlegmy coughs

 − glue ear

 − lack of control or strength in limbs

 − pale face.

» The most commonly seen Spleen patterns in children are:

 − Spleen *qi/yang* deficiency

 − Spleen *qi* deficiency with Dampness

 − Damp-Heat in the Spleen.

• Chapter 23 •

THE LUNGS
. . . .

The topics discussed in this chapter are:

- The characteristics of the Lungs particularly pertinent to children
- Common chronic Lung Organ patterns seen in children

The characteristics of the Lungs particularly pertinent to children

- The Lungs are responsible for *qi* and respiration
- The Lungs protect a child against invasions of External Pathogenic Factors
- The Lungs control the descending of *qi* and body fluids
- The Lungs house the Corporeal Soul (*po*)

The Lungs are responsible for *qi* and respiration

The combination of the air a child breathes, and the food and drink she consumes, creates the post-natal *qi* that enables her to do everything her daily life entails. If a child's Lung *qi* is deficient, she will tire easily. Lung *qi* also governs respiration. Up until the moment of birth, the foetus receives oxygenated blood from the mother via the umbilical cord. After birth, the Lungs must immediately start taking over this role. A baby's first cry is often the sign that the Lungs' job of respiration has kicked in.

The Lungs protect a child against invasions of External Pathogenic Factors

'Children's exterior defensive *qi* is not secure. Therefore, external evils easily enter the exterior and assail the lungs.'[45]

Defensive (*wei*) *qi* is stored in the Lungs and is dispersed to the surface of the body in order to prevent pathogens from entering. The defensive (*wei*) *qi* of a baby or young child is not fully developed and therefore she may succumb to Pathogenic Factors more easily than an adult. As well as Wind, the Lungs are particularly susceptible to Cold. Sun Simiao wrote that 'the reason why small children cannot yet be exposed to frost and snow is so that they do not fall ill with cold damage'.[46] Parents may notice that their child only coughs when she goes outside in the cold weather.

Every time a child succumbs to an invasion of an External Pathogenic Factor in his Lungs, it will weaken his Lung *qi* a little more. The Organs of a child are immature and therefore more easily damaged. This will leave him more vulnerable to further invasions and a vicious circle may ensue.

> One boy who came to the clinic illustrated perfectly the way in which the Lungs loathe cold. In mild weather, he had no symptoms at all. If the weather became cold, he would become breathless and would start coughing immediately he went outside. Treatment with moxa and needles to warm the Lungs made him much better able to withstand the cold.

The Lungs control the descending of *qi* and body fluids

The Lungs are also responsible for descending *qi* and body fluids. When this function is working well, it helps to prevent the accumulation of fluids in the Lungs.

A child is particularly susceptible to the accumulation of fluids in the Lungs, in the form of mucus, after the invasion of a Pathogenic Factor. A small child does not have the ability to blow her nose or cough productively. Therefore, when her nose and chest are blocked with mucus, it often leads to discomfort and unhappiness. Sleep is interrupted, she is distressed a lot of the time and she may lose her appetite.

> A seven-year-old girl with a constitutional Metal imbalance came for treatment because she always felt 'bunged up' in her head and nose. She had no symptoms of Damp anywhere else in her body. It was a simple case of her inherent Lung deficiency meaning that body fluids did not properly descend. Strengthening this function of the Lungs with acupuncture eased her symptoms.

The Lungs house the Corporeal Soul (*po*)

So much of a baby's world is experienced through the *po*. In the first weeks of life, when her vision is blurry and there is an onslaught of new sounds to get used to, it is largely through touch that a baby feels comforted and secure. Skin-to-skin contact after a baby is born is now recognised to be beneficial in many ways, for example more stable breathing and heart rate, less crying and better uptake of breastfeeding. The fundamental processes in the body that are carried out without the assistance of the conscious mind are all regulated by the *po*.

As she grows, a child's agility and movement are influenced by the *po*. Whilst in the first two or three months of life a baby's body seems to move in an involuntary manner, as he grows, he will gain an increasing awareness of his body and control over it. A healthy *po* will mean that the child's body moves rhythmically. The Corporeal Soul 'gives the capacity of movement, agility, balance and coordination of movements'.[47]

The internal Organs will also find a balanced rhythm. Breathing will be easy, and bowel movements will be regular.

● SOME KEY SYMPTOMS AND SIGNS OF A LUNG IMBALANCE

- » Frequent coughs and colds
- » Chronic cough
- » Tired by physical exertion
- » Respiratory allergies
- » Wheezing
- » Blocked nose
- » Constipation
- » Skin diseases
- » Pale (verging on white) complexion

Common chronic Lung Organ patterns seen in children

Some children are prone to chronic Lung deficiency. However, many others come to the clinic with mixed conditions in the Lungs too.

Of course, any Lung pattern may be present in a child. However, the ones discussed here are those most commonly encountered in a paediatric clinic. For a comprehensive list of all possible Lung patterns, see *The Foundations of Chinese Medicine* by Maciocia.[48]

The following Lung patterns will be discussed:

- Lung *qi* deficiency

- Retained Damp/Phlegm in the Lungs

- Heat in the Lungs

- Invasion of Wind-Cold (with or without Damp) or Wind-Heat in the Lungs

Lung *qi* deficiency

In some children, Lung *qi* deficiency may manifest with only physical symptoms. In others, it will manifest with predominantly emotional symptoms. In others, there will be a mix of physical and emotional symptoms.

Symptoms in any age group
PHYSICAL

- catches many coughs and colds

- prefers to be inside rather than running around outside

- easily tired by physical activity

- pale or clear mucus

- pale, white complexion

- respiratory allergies

- asthma

EMOTIONAL TENDENCIES

- quiet or even withdrawn

- may not like too many cuddles or too much physical touch

- may appear chronically sad

School-age children and teenagers

PHYSICAL

- tired at the end of the school day

EMOTIONAL TENDENCIES

- may choose to spend playtimes etc. alone or playing with one or two other children

- may have extremely high expectations of herself

- may struggle accepting not being 'the best' at something

- may appear arrogant or a 'know it all'

Lung *qi* deficiency may manifest predominantly with a defensive (*wei*) *qi* deficiency. This is common in children who are atopic (who have eczema, asthma and/or respiratory allergies from an early age). A deficiency of *wei qi* is often connected also to deficiency of Kidney *yang*, because *wei qi* derives from the *ming men*.

Pulse: deficient

Tongue: pale

Treatment principles: tonify and warm Lung *qi*

SUGGESTED TREATMENT

It is usually sufficient to use one or two of the following points per treatment.

Points

Any point on the Lung channel can be used to strengthen Lung *qi*. The points chosen in each particular case should depend on the nature and location of the symptoms, as well as the emotional state of the child. Some of the most commonly used points in young children are:

Lu 9 *taiyuan*
Lu 7 *lieque*
Lu 1 *zhongfu*
Bl 13 *feishu*

Method: tonification needle technique

Other techniques: moxibustion

Paediatric *tui na*

Lung *feijing* (straight pushing tonification)
Spinal Column *jizhu* (pinching from bottom to top)
Outer Palace of Toil *wailaogong* (kneading)
Wind Nest *yiwofeng* (kneading)
Three Passes *sanguan* (straight pushing)

Variations

Lung *yin* deficiency may also be present. This is particularly common in children who have had repeated invasions of Wind-Heat in the Lungs, or who are asthmatic and take inhaled corticosteroids or bronchodilators. Lung *yin* deficiency in a child often manifests with:

- chronic, dry cough

- dry and/or tickly throat.

Key aetiological factors

- inherited

- premature birth or complications at birth

- repeated invasions of External Pathogenic Factors

- lack of fresh air

- lack of running around

- over-exercise

- sadness and loss

Retained Damp/Phlegm in the Lungs

Phlegm in the Lungs may be acute or chronic. The description below is of the chronic version.

Symptoms

- chronic cough with bouts of coughing
- worse when lying down and first getting up in the morning
- mucus in the throat
- asthma
- wheezing or difficulty breathing

Pulse: slippery on the Metal and possibly Earth pulses

Tongue: swollen with a sticky coat

Treatment principles: resolve Phlegm in the Lungs; restore descending function of Lungs; tonify underlying deficiency (which may be of the Lungs, Spleen or the constitutional imbalance)

> **SUGGESTED TREATMENT**
> It is usually sufficient to use one or two points per treatment.
>
> **Points**
> To resolve Phlegm and restore the Lungs' descending function:
>
> > Lu 5 *chize*
> > Lu 7 *lieque*
> > St 40 *fenglong*
> > Ren 22 *tiantu*
>
> **Method:** sedation needle technique
>
> Points to treat the underlying deficiency will depend on which Organ or Organs are involved.
>
> **Paediatric *tui na***
>
> > Lung *feijing* (straight pushing sedation)
> > Spleen *pijing* (straight pushing tonification)
> > Eight Trigrams *bagua* (circular pushing anti-clockwise)
> > Small Palmar Crease *zhangxiaowen* (straight pushing)
> > Hand *yin yang shouyinyang* (pushing apart)
> > Central Altar *shanzhong* (pushing apart and straight pushing)
> > Breast Sides and Breast Root *rupang* and *rugen* (kneading)
> > Flanks and Ribs *xielei* (straight pushing)
> > Lung Transport *jianjiagu* (pushing apart)
> > Celestial Pillar Bone *tianzhugu* (straight pushing)
> > St 40 Abundant Bulge *fenglong* (kneading)
>
> ● Phlegm in the Lungs may be neutral in terms of temperature; it may be Cold-Phlegm or Phlegm-Heat. Symptoms will vary accordingly, and the treatment principles and points used should also be adjusted.

Key aetiological factors

Any of the causes of Lung *qi* deficiency, plus:

- diet of Damp-forming foods
- living in a damp environment
- vaccinations

Heat in the Lungs

Heat in the Lungs may be acute or chronic. The description below is of the chronic version.

Symptoms

- chronic, dry cough
- cough worse at night
- asthma or breathlessness
- dry skin
- red cheeks

Pulse: overflowing on Metal pulses, rapid

Tongue: red in the front third

Treatment principles: clear Heat from the Lungs; tonify the underlying deficiency (which may be of any Organ, for example those related to the constitutional imbalance)

SUGGESTED TREATMENT
Points

> Lu 5 *chize*
> Lu 10 *yuji*
> Bl 13 *feishu*

Method: sedation needle technique

Points to treat the underlying deficiency will depend on the Organ or Organs involved.

Other techniques: *gua sha* over the upper back

Paediatric *tui na*

> Lung *feijing* (straight pushing sedation)
> Lung Transport *jianjiagu* (pushing apart)
> Milky Way *tianheshui* (straight pushing)
> Spinal Column *jizhu* (pinching from top to bottom)

Key aetiological factors

- after-effect of an invasion of an External Pathogenic Factor
- vaccinations

Invasion of Wind-Cold (with or without Damp) or Wind-Heat in the Lungs

As mentioned, a child is particularly susceptible to invasions of external pathogenic Wind because her defensive (*wei*) *qi* is immature. This, combined with an inherently weak Spleen, means that an external invasion often leads to an accumulation of Phlegm and Damp. It is therefore especially worthwhile to treat a child suffering an acute external illness.

Symptoms

WIND-COLD

Cough, fever, stuffed or runny nose, clear mucus, sneezing, aversion to cold, occipital headache, earache.

With Damp: muzzy head, stuffy feeling in the chest, feeling of heaviness in the body, blocked ears

Pulse: floating, tight, slippery

WIND-HEAT

Cough, fever, blocked nose, yellow mucus, sneezing, headache, thirst, swollen tonsils, ear pain.

Pulse: floating, rapid

Treatment principles: expel Wind; expel Cold or Heat; resolve Dampness

SUGGESTED TREATMENT

It is usually sufficient to use two or three points per treatment.

Points

To expel Wind, release the exterior and descend Lung *qi*:

Lu 7 *lieque*
LI 6 *kongzui* (to open the water passages)
LI 4 *hegu*
LI 11 *quchi* (for Heat in the throat)
Bl 12 *fengmen*
Bl 13 *feishu*
Ren 9 *shuifen* (to open the water passages)
Du 14 *dazhui* (for Wind-Heat)
TB 5 *waiguan* (for Wind-Heat)

To resolve Damp and Phlegm:

St 8 *touwei*
Sp 9 *yinlingquan*
St 40 *fenglong*

Method: sedation needle technique

Other modalities

Moxa (in the case of Wind-Cold)
Cupping on the upper back
Gua sha on the upper back

Paediatric *tui na*

Two Panels Gate *ershanmen* (pinching or kneading)
M-HN-9 *taiyang* (kneading)
Bees Entering the Cave *huangfeng rudong* (kneading)
Wind Pond GB 20 *fengchi* (kneading)
Big Bone Behind the Ear *erhou gaogu* (kneading)
Fishing for the Moon in the Water *shuidi laoyue* (pushing) if there is fever

SUMMARY

» The following characteristics of the Lungs are especially relevant in childhood:

- the Lungs are responsible for *qi* and respiration

- the Lungs protect a child against invasions of External Pathogenic Factors

- the Lungs control the descending of *qi* and body fluids

- the Lungs house the Corporeal Soul (*po*).

» In children, some of the most commonly seen symptoms relating to a Lung pattern are:

- frequent coughs and colds

- chronic cough

- tired by physical exertion

- respiratory allergies

- wheezing

- blocked nose

- constipation

- skin diseases

- pale (verging on white) complexion.

» The most commonly seen Lung patterns in children are:

- Lung *qi* deficiency

- retained Damp/Phlegm in the Lungs

- Heat in the Lungs

- invasion of Wind-Cold (with Damp) or Wind-Heat in the Lungs.

• Chapter 24 •

THE KIDNEYS
· ·

The topics discussed in this chapter are:

- The characteristics of the Kidneys particularly pertinent to children
- Common Kidney Organ patterns seen in children

The characteristics of the Kidneys particularly pertinent to children

- The Kidneys store Essence and govern birth, growth, reproduction and development
- The Kidneys produce Marrow which fills the brain and nourishes the bones
- The Kidneys control the two lower orifices and keep the Lower Burner strong
- The hair and teeth are a reflection of the Kidneys
- The Kidneys open into the ears
- The Kidneys house the willpower (*zhi*)
- The Gate of Life (*ming men*) resides in the Kidneys

The Kidneys store Essence and govern birth, growth, reproduction and development

The ability to grow physically, develop mentally, reach sexual maturation and eventually produce his or her own offspring is largely determined by the nature of the Kidney Essence.

Kidney Essence plays an especially important role in the first year of a child's life, when his growth rate is phenomenal. A baby generally triples his birth weight by the time of his first birthday. His teeth begin to appear at around six months and by the end of his first year a baby may already have eight or ten teeth. All of this growth is fuelled by Kidney Essence.

Kidney Essence also controls the phases of heightened growth and development that happen in cycles of seven years for girls and eight years for boys. During the transition from one cycle to the next, robust Kidney Essence fuels the changes and ensures that the child remains healthy and steady whilst this flux occurs.

The Kidneys can be seen to fundamentally underpin the entire health and development of the child.

The Kidneys produce Marrow which fills the brain and nourishes the bones

A healthy child will grow in height and develop strong bones. At the same time, her mental faculties will expand so that she is able to speak and understand the world in an ever more complex way.

Sometimes, this process of the Marrow filling the brain and nourishing the bones of a child does not happen as smoothly as it might. For example, a child may be intellectually precocious but not very sturdy in his stature. Scott and Barlow[49] list a child being thin (or thin-boned) as one of the symptoms of Kidney deficiency.

It is as if the distribution of the Kidney *qi* has become imbalanced. Too much of it has been directed to the brain and not enough to the body. This may happen in a child who is very bright and so naturally tends towards a lot of mental activity. It may also happen in a child who is pushed too hard at school or home.

Conversely, if the Kidneys are not strong, then the brain may not be sufficiently filled by Marrow. This may result in a child having some degree of cognitive impairment. On a more subtle level, it often means a child seems to be 'away with the fairies' and unwilling to or incapable of fully engaging with the world in a way that is age appropriate.

> The condition of a seven-year-old girl who came to the clinic illustrated perfectly this kind of mal-distribution of Kidney *qi*. She was exceedingly tall for her age (she was the height of an average ten-year-old) yet had cognitive impairment. Her mental development was akin to that of an average four-year-old.

The Kidneys control the two lower orifices and keep the Lower Burner strong

A child's ability to gain control over his bladder is largely dependent on the Kidneys. If Kidney *qi* is either weak, or being used too much elsewhere (see above), then urine may leak out – meaning that the child either wets the bed or struggles to maintain bladder control during the day. The Kidneys also supply *yang* to the Bladder for transformation of urine.

Simply looking at and feeling a child's lower back provides some information about whether his Kidney *qi* is well rooted and strong. If the lower back is sturdy, it indicates that the Kidneys are robust and, consequently, the Lower Burner strong. If it is concave and weak, then it suggests a weakness in the Kidneys.

The hair and teeth are a reflection of the Kidneys

The first chapter of the *Su Wen* explains, 'If the Kidneys are strong, the teeth will be firm and hair grow well.'[50]

The Kidneys are responsible for 'pushing things out':

> The teeth are like the push towards the exterior of the same thing which internally makes the bones, and the hair is like the push to the exterior of the same thing which internally makes blood coming from essences and from the yin of the kidneys and so on.[51]

Therefore, a full head of hair may be a sign of strong Kidney *qi*.

Late teething or teeth which are prone to cavities (despite being looked after properly) may indicate weak Kidney *qi*. Teeth which are set wide apart may be suggestive of inherently weak Kidney *yin*.

> A six-year-old girl came for treatment for alopecia. This had begun after she had witnessed a violent intruder come into the house and her father trying to defend the family. Since that shocking event, she had also begun to wet her bed and was too fearful (understandably) to sleep on her own. The shock had affected her Kidneys and this was manifesting with her hair falling out.

The Kidneys open into the ears

Small ears are seen to be a reflection of weak Kidney Essence.

A child's hearing may also be a reflection of her Kidney *qi*. Rochat de la Vallée writes, 'The ear cannot hear from infinity but it hears everything that is going on all around, and it never stops working as there is no way to close your ears.'[52]

Poor hearing or deafness, when it is not due to the common childhood condition of glue ear, may be a sign of weak Kidney *qi*. The above quote also implies that hearing is not just a passive activity. It takes *qi*, specifically Kidney *qi*, for a child to absorb all the sounds he is surrounded by. This highlights the importance of a child having quiet surroundings.

The Kidneys house the willpower (*zhi*)

The *zhi* of the Kidneys provides a child with his most basic instinct to survive. Residing in the Lower Burner, the *zhi* is the deepest and most primal aspect of the spirit. If the *zhi* is well rooted in the Kidneys, then a child will want to be in the world and will feel that it is a safe place. He will feel secure and be relatively free of anxiety and fear. He will have an innate desire to explore and experience new things. There is a very fine balance though. Being exposed to something new, threatening or disturbing at too young an age when the Kidney *qi* is vulnerable will be like a jolt to this natural process of maturation. An image, idea or experience may become lodged in this deep, unconscious realm of the child and cause him to be fearful or feel disturbed.

> A mother told me about her nine-year-old daughter who had become very anxious and had developed problems going to sleep on her own since she had learned about the Second World War at school. She had begun dreaming about being separated from her family and taken to a concentration camp. The mother commented that she did not think any other of the children in the same class had reacted in a similar way. I knew her daughter to be an exceptionally bright but rather physically delicate child. I suspect that her intellectual precocity meant her Kidney *qi* was rather deficient and she was therefore more susceptible than her classmates to being disturbed in this way.

The *zhi* gives a child an innate wisdom which enables him to know when he needs to stop and replenish, and when it is all right to keep going. When left to his own devices, a child usually stops when he needs to, has a bit of time out and then starts up again when he is ready. It is easy for a parent to interpret a six-year-old who is flatly refusing to read another word as being lazy, unmotivated or reluctant to learn. This may, of course, be the case. However, it is equally likely that it genuinely feels to the child as if he has used up his quota of 'physical and mental development *qi*' for the day. He simply needs to stop. Sadly, as a child grows, he is usually encouraged more and more to override this innate ability.

The Gate of Life (*ming men*) resides in the Kidneys

The Gate of Life, sometimes known as the Minister Fire, has the role of providing warmth for all the other Organs. So, for example, it provides warmth to the Bladder in order that it may transport fluids, it warms the Stomach and Spleen so that they can perform their task of digestion and it sends warmth to the Heart. The Gate of Life is also the source of the *yuan qi*. It is, therefore, of crucial importance to all the Organs in a child develop strongly.

The Gate of Life in a child is, however, immature and vulnerable and may easily be injured by Cold. This is why, if a child becomes cold, it is often very difficult for him to warm up again. The Gate of Life may, conversely, easily burn out of control in a child and rise up to affect the Heart. This may manifest as a child becoming hyperactive, unable to sleep or developing a fever.

In a teenager, the Gate of Life fuels the sexual awakening that usually occurs as a child goes through puberty. She may feel sexual desire for the first time. This goes hand in hand with a more generally increased sense of power and potency. Young teenagers may have phases of feeling that they can do anything and everything that they want, and that they are indomitable. This is a reflection of the upsurge in power of the Gate of Life.

SOME KEY SIGNS AND SYMPTOMS OF A KIDNEY IMBALANCE

> » Hyperactive and adrenalised
> » Lethargic and unmotivated
> » Difficulty falling asleep or wakes early
> » Sleeps a lot and sleeps deeply
> » Dark circles under the eyes
> » Tendency to feel either cold or hot
> » Fearful or agitated
> » Lacks physical robustness
> » Tendency to bedwetting
> » Delayed development

Common Kidney Organ patterns seen in children

The Kidneys are generally said to tend towards deficiency in children. This is, of course, true of adults too. However, because they are responsible for so much of the rapid growth and development that takes place in the first years of a child's life, their tendency to become deficient is even more pronounced in children.

Of course, any Kidney pattern may be present in a child. However, the ones discussed here are those most commonly encountered in a paediatric clinic. For a comprehensive list of all possible Kidney patterns, see *The Foundations of Chinese Medicine* by Maciocia.[53]

The following Kidney patterns will be discussed:

- Kidney deficiency

- Kidney *jing* deficiency

Kidney deficiency

In some children, Kidney deficiency may manifest with only physical symptoms. In others, it will manifest with predominantly emotional symptoms. In others, there will be a mix of physical and emotional symptoms.

KIDNEY *YIN* OR KIDNEY *YANG* DEFICIENCY?

In a young child, Kidney deficiency rarely manifests as being particularly of *yang* or *yin*. A child may be Kidney deficient but not have any marked symptoms of Heat or Cold. As a child gets older, usually not before the age of seven or eight, the split between *yin* or *yang* deficiency tends to become more marked. By the time the child reaches the teenage years, it is usually possible to clearly distinguish whether the Kidney deficiency is predominantly of *yin* or *yang*.

Symptoms in any age group
PHYSICAL SYMPTOMS

- lack of physical resilience and robustness

- recovers slowly from illnesses

- weak lower back

- dark circles under the eyes

- some developmental milestones may happen slightly late

EMOTIONAL TENDENCIES

- fearful
- agitated
- easily overstimulated

0–3-year-olds

PHYSICAL SYMPTOMS

- late to toilet train
- tendency to bedwetting
- sleeps badly if overstimulated or overtired
- milk teeth come through late

Pulse: deficient Water pulses

School-age children

PHYSICAL SYMPTOMS

- tired by the school day and exhausted by the end of term
- tendency to bedwetting
- takes a long time to get to sleep (especially when overtired or overstimulated)
- adult teeth slow to come through

EMOTIONAL TENDENCIES

- may be either very driven or lacking in drive and motivation
- agitated and fearful

Pulse: deficient Water pulses

Teenagers

Any of the symptoms previously mentioned, plus:

PHYSICAL SYMPTOMS

- late onset of menstruation in girls
- late puberty in boys

EMOTIONAL TENDENCIES

- panic attacks
- finds it hard to stop and relax
- recklessness and risk taking
- lack of willpower and motivation

Pulse and tongue: pulse and tongue will depend on whether the Kidney deficiency predominantly affects *yin* or *yang*

> A girl of sixteen with autistic spectrum disorder came to the clinic to be treated for anxiety and aggressive behaviour that had worsened in the last year. A Kidney *jing* deficiency is often a part of the picture in autism and it was interesting to note that this girl had not yet begun her periods, which is another sign of Kidney deficiency.

Key aetiological factors

- inherited
- living in an atmosphere of fear
- shock
- chronic illness
- being pushed academically at too early an age
- lack of downtime and too busy a schedule
- excessive physical exercise

Kidney *jing* deficiency

Symptoms in any age group

- congenital diseases
- small in stature
- small ears
- may have a large head or large forehead
- little resilience or robustness

0–3-year-olds

- slow development such as late to be able to sit up
- milk teeth late to come through
- may be vacant and dulled
- sense that the child is not fully 'in the world'

School-age children and teenagers

- physically weak
- cognitively impaired
- late onset of menstruation in girls
- late puberty in boys
- struggles to mature through the change of the seven- or eight-year cycles either physically or psychologically

Pulse: deficient (may be deep and weak, or floating and empty if the deficiency is particularly of Kidney *yang* or *yin*)

Tongue: colour of tongue will depend on whether the deficiency is particularly of *yang* or *yin*

Treatment principles: nourish Kidney *Jing*

A NOTE ABOUT KIDNEY *JING*

The intention and prognosis when treating a child who is Kidney *jing* deficient are somewhat different to treating deficiency of other substances. A child is born with the quality and quantity of *jing* that he is born with. This cannot really be changed. However, particularly in the first seven or eight years of life, a child's *jing* is unfolding. Treatment during this time can maximise the way a child's *jing* manifests in the world. It is similar to feeding and nurturing a flower as it grows and matures before it fully blooms. It is not possible to make it a different kind of flower, but good food and the right kind of nurture will mean it can be the best that it possibly can.

Key aetiological factors

- inherited
- birth trauma

SUGGESTED TREATMENT FOR ANY DEFICIENT KIDNEY PATTERN

It is usually sufficient to use one or two points per treatment. More may overstimulate a Kidney-deficient child. Any point on the Kidney channel can be used to strengthen Kidney *qi* or *jing*. The points chosen in each particular case should depend on the nature and location of the symptoms, as well as the emotional state of the child. Some of the most commonly used points to tonify the Kidneys in young children are:

Ki 1 *yongquan*
Ki 3 *taixi*
Ki 7 *fuliu*
Ki 23 *shenfeng*
Ki 24 *lingxu*
Ki 25 *shencang*
Bl 23 *shenshu*
Ren 4 *guanyuan*
Ren 6 *qihai*

Method: tonification needle technique

Other techniques: moxibustion may be applicable

Paediatric *tui na*

Kidney *shenjing* (straight pushing)
Two Men Upon a Horse *erma* (kneading)
Outer Palace of Toil *wailaogong* (kneading)
Wind Nest *yiwofeng* (kneading)
Three Passes *sanguan* (straight pushing)
Winnower Gate *jimen* (straight pushing from knee to groin)
Lower Back – area around Bl 23 *shenshu* (strong rubbing)
Spinal Column *jizhu* (pinching)
Du 20 *baihui* (kneading)

SUMMARY

» The following characteristics of the Kidneys are especially relevant in childhood:
  - the Kidneys store Essence and govern birth, growth, reproduction and development
  - the Kidneys produce Marrow which fills the brain and nourishes the bones
  - the Kidneys control the two lower orifices and keep the Lower Burner strong
  - the hair and teeth are a reflection of the Kidneys
  - the Kidneys open into the ears
  - the Kidneys house the willpower (*zhi*)
  - the Gate of Life (*ming men*) resides in the Kidneys.

» In children, some of the most commonly seen symptoms relating to a Kidney pattern are:
  - hyperactive and adrenalised
  - lethargic and unmotivated
  - difficulty falling asleep or wakes early
  - sleeps a lot and sleeps deeply
  - dark circles under the eyes
  - tendency to feel either cold or hot
  - fearful or agitated
  - lacks physical robustness.

» The most commonly seen Kidney patterns in children are:
  - Kidney deficiency
  - Kidney *jing* deficiency.

Chapter 25

THE LIVER

· · · · · · · · · · · · · · · · ·

The topics discussed in this chapter are:

- The characteristics of the Liver particularly pertinent to children
- Common Liver Organ patterns seen in children

The characteristics of the Liver particularly pertinent to children

- The Liver ensures the smooth flow of *qi*
- The Liver stores Blood
- Liver Blood and *yin* root the Ethereal Soul (*hun*)
- The Liver is prone to excess in children
- The Liver is affected by Wind

The Liver ensures the smooth flow of *qi*

The Liver is responsible for the smooth flow of *qi* that strongly affects both the expression of emotions and the functioning of the digestive system. Children of all ages may suffer from Liver *qi* stagnation. There are several different possible causes of *qi* stagnation. In a baby or infant, it may arise because of stagnation in the digestive system. In older children, it is more likely to arise because of repressed feelings of anger and frustration or a lack of physical movement.

The effect of Liver *qi* stagnation on the emotions is very clear in children. A young child is often prone to huge fluctuations of mood and may struggle to manage her emotions, which may easily become out of control. The characteristic moodiness and changeability that are typical of the teenage years are also largely due to the uneven flow of Liver *qi*. A teenager may oscillate between rebellion and conformity, or hope and despair. She may be sweetness and light one minute, angry and obstinate the next.

The smooth flow of *qi* to the emotions also helps a child to be flexible. The ability to be able to handle the inherent frustrations of life, and to deal with plans not working out in the desired way, relates to this function of the Liver.

Children are also very prone to digestive upsets. Whilst this may be due to weak Spleen *qi*, it may also be a result of a lack of smooth flow of Liver *qi* in the Middle Burner. This may lead to a wide range of digestive symptoms, including belching, flatulence, constipation, diarrhoea and tummy pain.

The Liver stores Blood

The phenomenal rate of a child's growth means that the Liver has a lot of work to do. It is predominantly Liver Blood which nourishes the growing tendons so that they are both strong and flexible. Abundant Liver Blood also ensures the smooth movement of joints and muscles as the child becomes increasingly active.

Liver Blood is also necessary to root *yang*. When Liver Blood is deficient, *yang* has a strong propensity to rise. A little of this is not really pathological. It would be an unusual child who got through childhood without ever flaring with anger and going a bit red in the face. In some children, however, this tendency becomes an ongoing behavioural characteristic which begins to cause problems for her and her family.

In adolescent girls, the Liver's function of storing Blood also encompasses the menstrual function. When a girl begins her periods, Blood is diverted to the Uterus and so has an 'extra' job to do. If the girl does not have a good diet or if she is doing a lot of physical activity, it may mean that symptoms of Liver Blood deficiency arise for the first time.

 Many teenage girls suffer with migraines from Liver *yang* rising which begin with the onset of menstruation. This is an example of Liver Blood not rooting *yang*, which rises up to the head and causes the migraines.

Liver Blood and *yin* root the Ethereal Soul (*hun*)

The Liver Blood and *yin* also play an important role in housing the spirit of the Liver, the *hun* or Ethereal Soul. A well-rooted *hun* enables a child to be emotionally balanced, to remain focused and to be able to take in instructions. In China it is not uncommon to hear a mother say to her child 'What is the matter with you? Have you lost your *hun*?' when he does something impulsive or reckless.

Another aspect of the *hun* is to do with the realm of imagination. Children are often a wonderful example of a *hun* that is unencumbered by stagnation. When a child is lost in an imaginary game, which may go on for hours at a time, we are seeing the *hun* in action. A healthy child will be able to explore the imaginary realm and come back into the real world easily.

A well-rooted *hun* also contributes to a child having peaceful sleep which is not disturbed by bad dreams. Frequent sleeptalking or sleepwalking may be signs of an unstable *hun*. The *hun* may be unrooted either because of Liver Blood or *yin* being deficient, or by excess Heat in the Liver.

An eight-year-old once came to the clinic having been diagnosed with attention deficit disorder. Her mother (and teachers) said that she was a delightful child but that she seemed to live almost permanently in her imaginary world. She struggled to take in any instructions or commit herself to a task she was asked to do at school. This was not because she was being defiant. She simply was not present as she was living in another realm. Her pulse and tongue confirmed that she was Liver Blood deficient. Nourishing her Liver Blood with acupuncture and talking to her mother about diet made a big difference to her (although, happily, she remained a girl with the most wonderful imagination).

The Liver is prone to excess in children

Chinese texts abound with sayings regarding the propensity of the Liver to become excess in children. For example, Zhu Dan-xi, of the Jin Yuan dynasties, wrote that 'the Liver commonly has a surplus'.[54]

The constitution of a child is pure *yang*. This, together with the fact that Liver Blood and *yin* are insufficient, means that Liver *yang* will easily rise. This may lead to Liver Fire, which may in turn create internal Wind.

A six-year-old came for treatment for digestive problems resulting from an excess condition in her Liver. Treatment was progressing well and generally the appointments would run smoothly. One day, as I was about to begin treatment, she asked her mother for her soft toy, Tommy, who always accompanied her. Her mother told her that she had left Tommy at home. In a split second, the girl had turned red in the face, began screaming at the top of her voice and was hitting and

> trying to bite her mother. This was a vivid example of the propensity of the Liver to flare up quickly in a young child.

There are various possible ways in which Liver Fire in a child may manifest. One is febrile convulsions (see Chapter 62). Another is psychological and behavioural symptoms, such as a child being aggressive and/or hyperactive.

However, it should by no means be assumed that the Liver is *always* excess in a child. Many children, particularly in the 21st century, are constitutionally Liver Blood or *yin* deficient. These children may struggle to keep up with the demands of a busy life without developing physical symptoms as a result.

 It should always be the pulse that tells the practitioner whether a Liver imbalance in a child is from an excess or a deficiency, and consequently how to approach treatment. A child with a full condition, such as Liver *qi* stagnation, may be unassertive and compliant. Conversely, a child with Liver Blood deficiency may be irritable and angry. It is the pulse that determines the pattern and mode of treatment, not the symptoms.

The Liver is affected by wind

As previously mentioned, a child may develop internal Wind as a result of Liver Fire. However, a child with an imbalanced Liver is also likely to be strongly affected by climatic wind. Primary school teachers are often aware that, on a particularly windy day, the children tend to be more wild and excitable. Some parents even report that their child becomes unusually grumpy, hard to manage, erratic or angry in windy weather.

> A five-year-old girl came for treatment because she sleepwalked nearly every night. She responded well to treatment on her Liver and the sleepwalking stopped. About a year later, I had a call from her mother saying that her daughter had begun sleepwalking again totally out of the blue. On questioning, it turned out that the problem had returned whilst the family were in holiday in Spain in a town known for its extraordinarily windy climate! The Wind had agitated the girl's Liver and that is why she had begun sleepwalking again.

SOME KEY SIGNS AND SYMPTOMS OF A LIVER IMBALANCE

- » Flares with anger and aggression
- » Moody, irritable or depressed
- » Hyperactivity or agitation
- » Headaches
- » Irregular bowel movements
- » Food allergies

Common Liver Organ patterns seen in children

As mentioned previously, the Liver is often said to be prone to excess in a child. However, in practice, it is also common to see children with a deficient Liver pattern.

Of course, any Liver pattern may be present in a child. However, the ones discussed here are those most commonly encountered in a paediatric clinic. For a comprehensive list of all possible Liver patterns, see *The Foundations of Chinese Medicine* by Maciocia.[55]

The following Liver patterns will be discussed:

- Liver *qi* stagnation

- Liver Heat

- Liver Blood deficiency

- Liver Wind

Liver *qi* stagnation
Symptoms in all age groups

- symptoms get worse when stressed

- symptoms get worse with inactivity

- irregular bowel movements

- emotional volatility, moodiness and grumpiness

Babies and toddlers

In this age group, Liver *qi* stagnation usually manifests, and is treated, as Accumulation Disorder. Please see Chapter 27 for a discussion of this.

PHYSICAL SYMPTOMS

- prone to regurgitation of milk or vomiting

- grouchy and unhappy before a bowel movement

- green around mouth

EMOTIONAL SYMPTOMS

- tendency to strong, fluctuating emotions

- hates being physically constrained (e.g. in a buggy)

- easily cross and frustrated

School-age children

PHYSICAL SYMPTOMS

- flatulence

- tummy pain

- headaches

EMOTIONAL SYMPTOMS

- tense and wound up

- quick to anger

- depressed and low

Teenagers

PHYSICAL SYMPTOMS

- headaches

- period pain in girls

- pain and stiffness in the muscles

- strong desire to exercise

EMOTIONAL SYMPTOMS

- withdrawn

- angry or irritable

- tense

- pre-menstrual syndrome

Pulse: wiry on the Wood pulses

Tongue: may be normal, may be red on the sides

Treatment principles: smooth the Liver and move *qi*

Key aetiological factors

- inherited

- too much or the wrong kind of food in babies and infants

- lack of movement

- repressed emotions, particularly in the anger family

- feelings of constraint and pressure

- over-scheduled lifestyle

- food additives

- Lingering Pathogenic Factors (either inherited, or from illness or vaccination)

SUGGESTED TREATMENT

It is usually sufficient to use two points per treatment.

Points

Any point on the Liver and Gallbladder channels, when needled with the sedation technique, will move *qi*. The points chosen in each particular case should depend on the nature and location of the symptoms, as well as the emotional state of the child. Some of the most commonly used points in young children are:

Liv 3 *taichong*
GB 40 *qiuxu*
GB 34 *yanglingquan*
Liv 14 *qimen*
GB 24 *riyue*
Bl 18 *ganshu*
Bl 19 *danshu*

Method: sedation needle technique

When Liver *qi* stagnation manifests with digestive symptoms in a baby or toddler, and when it derives from overeating, the method of treatment is to prick the *sifeng* points of one hand.

Paediatric *tui na*

The paediatric *tui na* routine will depend on which part of the child the Liver *qi* stagnation is affecting, for example emotions, digestive system. Please see the relevant chapter in Part 4 or Part 5.

Variations

Liver *qi* stagnation may also develop into Liver Blood stagnation. This is uncommon in young children but begins to be more common around puberty. The main symptom in girls is strong period pain and clotted menstrual blood. In both sexes, Liver Blood stagnation may manifest as painful headaches. Points to move Blood should be added to the other points, for example Sp 10 *xuehai*.

Liver Heat

The Liver may become Hot and agitated but without the extreme symptoms usually listed under Liver Fire.

Babies and toddlers

- red cheeks

- cries very strongly and loudly

- disturbed sleep throughout the night

- strong-smelling stools and vomit

- hates to be constrained

School-age children

PHYSICAL SYMPTOMS

- hyperactivity

- constipation

- food intolerances

- asthma

- poor sleep

- dream-disturbed sleep

- sleepwalking or sleeptalking

- nosebleeds

- headaches or migraines

- 'angry' skin conditions

- urinary tract infections

- red face
- symptoms worse when stressed or after inactivity

EMOTIONAL SYMPTOMS

- quick to flare with anger
- moody
- irritable
- withdrawn
- touchy
- agitated
- tantrums and flying off the handle

Teenagers

Any of the symptoms previously mentioned, plus:

PHYSICAL SYMPTOMS

- heavy periods in girls
- vaginal itching and yellow vaginal discharge

EMOTIONAL SYMPTOMS

- pre-menstrual syndrome in girls

Pulse: wiry and overflowing on the Wood pulses, may be rapid

Tongue: red sides

Treatment principles: clear Heat from the Liver

Key aetiological factors

- long-term Liver *qi* stagnation
- repressed emotions, particularly in the anger family
- lack of movement
- food additives
- Lingering Pathogenic Factor (from an illness or vaccination)
- too much screen time
- drugs and alcohol in teenagers

SUGGESTED TREATMENT
It is usually sufficient to use two points per treatment.

Points

Liv 2 *xingjian*

Liv 3 *taichong*

GB 38 *yangfu*

GB 34 *yanglingquan*

Liv 13 *zhangmen*

Liv 14 *qimen*

TB 6 *zhigou*

Method: sedation needle technique

Paediatric *tui na*

Liver *ganjing* (straight pushing)
Milky Way *tianheshui* (straight pushing)
Six *Yang* Organs *liufu* (straight pushing)

Other *tui na* moves will depend on where in the child the symptoms of Liver Heat are manifesting.

Liver Blood deficiency

Symptoms in any age group

- poor vision

- slightly restless

- light sleeper

- dry hair and skin

School-age children

PHYSICAL SYMPTOMS

- prone to injuring tendons if playing sport

- cramps and numbness

- dull headaches

- light-headedness

- brittle nails

- symptoms worse when tired or anxious

EMOTIONAL SYMPTOMS

- difficulty concentrating

- tendency to drift off

- vague and scattered

- slightly anxious

- tearful

- indecisive
- irritable

Teenagers

Any of the symptoms previously listed, plus:

PHYSICAL SYMPTOMS

- light periods, long cycle or no periods in girls

EMOTIONAL SYMPTOMS

- lacking in direction
- pre-menstrual syndrome

Pulse: thin or choppy

Tongue: pale, orange sides

Treatment principles: tonify the Liver; nourish Blood

Key aetiological factors

- inherited
- diet lacking in Blood-nourishing foods
- excessive exercise
- onset of menstruation, or heavy menstruation, in girls

SUGGESTED TREATMENT

One or two points per treatment is often sufficient.

Points

> Liv 3 *taichong*
> Liv 8 *ququan*
> Bl 18 *ganshu*
> Ren 4 *guanyuan*
> Sp 6 *sanyinjiao*

Method: tonification needle technique

Other techniques: moxa may be applicable

Paediatric *tui na*

> Liver *ganjing* (straight pushing tonification)
> Spinal Column *jizhu* (pinching from bottom to top)
> Knead the Navel *rou qi* (kneading anti-clockwise)

Other *tui na* moves may be added depending on which other Organs are deficient.

Variations

Liver Blood deficiency may co-exist with Liver *yin* deficiency. In this case, there may be a greater degree of restlessness and some symptoms of Heat too.

Liver Wind

Internal Liver Wind arises from Extreme Heat (i.e. high fevers), Liver *yang* rising or Liver Blood deficiency. In young children, Liver Wind most commonly arises from Extreme Heat. In older children and teenagers, Liver Blood deficiency may arise from Extreme Heat, Liver *yang* rising or Blood deficiency.

Extreme Heat generating Wind

SYMPTOMS

- febrile convulsions
- epileptic seizures
- high temperatures
- strong tremors
- loss of consciousness

Pulse: wiry, rapid, overflowing

Tongue: red, yellow coating, may be stiff

Treatment principles: cool Blood; clear Heat; extinguish Wind

> **SUGGESTED TREATMENT**
> **Points**
>
> Liv 2 *xingjian*
> Liv 3 *taichong*
> GB 20 *fengchi*
> Du 14 *dazhui*
> Du 16 *fengfu*
> Du 20 *baihui*
>
> **Method:** sedation needle technique
>
> **Paediatric *tui na***
>
> Heaven Gate *tianmen* (straight pushing)
> Heart Gate *xinmen* (straight pushing)
> Water Palace *kangong* (pushing apart)
> Wind Pond *fengchi* (kneading)
> Celestial Pillar Bone *tianzhugu* (straight pushing)
> Big Bone Behind the Ear *erhou gaogu* (kneading)
> Milky Way *tianheshui* (straight pushing)
> Thick Gate *banmen* (straight pushing)
> Eight Trigrams *bagua* (circular pushing anti-clockwise)
> Four Wind Creases *sifengwen* (pinching)
> Knead the navel *rou qi* (kneading clockwise)

KEY AETIOLOGICAL FACTORS

- acute febrile diseases
- vaccinations

Wind from Liver Blood deficiency

SYMPTOMS

- body or facial tics
- mild tremor
- numbness of limbs

These symptoms will be accompanied by symptoms of Liver Blood deficiency.

Tongue: pale

Pulse: thin or choppy

Treatment principles: subdue Wind; nourish Liver Blood

KEY AETIOLOGICAL FACTORS
See Liver Blood deficiency.

SUGGESTED TREATMENT
Points
To nourish Liver Blood:

Liv 8 *ququan*
Liv 3 *taichong*
Bl 18 *ganshu*

Method: tonification needle technique

To subdue Wind:

GB 20 *fengchi*
Liv 3 *taichong*
Du 20 *baihui*
LI 4 *hegu*

Method: sedation needle technique

The practitioner needs to decide at each treatment whether to nourish Liver Blood, subdue Wind or do both. Liv 3 *taichong* will nourish Liver Blood when needled with the tonification technique and subdue Wind when needled with the sedation technique. It should obviously only be used for one of these purposes in any one treatment. In most cases, tonifying the underlying deficiency is the key treatment principle.

Paediatric *tui na*
See Liver Blood deficiency.

SUMMARY

» The following characteristics of the Liver are especially relevant in childhood:

- the Liver ensures the smooth flow of *qi*

- the Liver stores Blood

- Liver Blood and *yin* root the Ethereal Soul (*hun*)

- the Liver is prone to excess in children

- the Liver is affected by Wind.

» In children, some of the most commonly seen symptoms relating to a Liver pattern are:

- flares with anger and aggression

- moody, irritable or depressed

- hyperactivity or agitation

- headaches

- irregular bowel movements

- food allergies.

» The most commonly seen Liver patterns in children are:

- Liver *qi* stagnation

- Liver Heat

- Liver Blood (and/or *yin*) deficiency

- Liver Wind.

» In particular with Liver patterns, the pulse rather than the symptoms should determine the diagnosis of the pattern.

• Chapter 26 •

THE *YANG* ORGANS

The topics discussed in this chapter are:

- Characteristics of the Small Intestine particularly pertinent to children
- Common Small Intestine Organ patterns seen in children
- Characteristics of the Triple Burner particularly pertinent to children
- Characteristics of the Stomach particularly pertinent to children
- Common Stomach Organ patterns seen in children
- Characteristics of the Large Intestine particularly pertinent to children
- Common Large Intestine Organ pattern seen in children
- Characteristics of the Bladder particularly pertinent to children
- Common Bladder Organ patterns seen in children
- Characteristics of the Gallbladder particularly pertinent to children
- Common Gallbladder Organ patterns seen in children

THE SMALL INTESTINE

In a child, there are two main reasons the Small Intestine may be imbalanced. The first is that the Spleen has not done a good enough job of digesting the foods that it then passed on to the Small Intestine, putting it under extra strain. The second is that the child's Kidney *yang* is not sufficiently warm and strong to fuel the Small Intestine. In both cases, the most likely symptoms are stomach ache and loose stools. However, because the Small Intestine and the Bladder work together to move fluids in the Lower Burner, the Small Intestine may also play a role in urinary symptoms.

Characteristics of the Small Intestine particularly pertinent to children

- The Small Intestine separates the pure from the impure on a physical level
- The Small Intestine separates the pure from the impure on a mental level

The Small Intestine separates the pure from the impure on a physical level

The Small Intestine receives partially digested food and fluids from the Stomach and Spleen. On a physical level, its key role is to divide what it receives into pure and impure. The pure is then passed on to the Spleen and is used to nourish all the tissues of the body. The impure is sent to the Large Intestine to be excreted as stools, and to the Bladder to be excreted as urine. Just like the Bladder, the Small Intestine relies on the *yang* of the Kidneys to perform this process.

The Small Intestine separates the pure from the impure on a mental level

A healthy Small Intestine will help a child to be able to discern 'good' from 'bad' in the many choices he has to make. If the Small Intestine is sorting efficiently, a child will discard things that are not nourishing for him, and accept those that are. This may apply to all sorts of things in his life – from friendships, to food, to courses of action, and even down to which websites to browse. Children probably have more choices today than they have ever had before. A child as young as four or five may go to look for a dress to wear to a party and be confronted by an enormous range from which to choose. When she watches television, she has dozens of channels to choose from. If a child has liberal parents who believe in her right to choose from an early age, she may be given a choice of what she would like to eat for supper each day. Each one of these choices requires work from the Small Intestine.

> A mother brought her five-year-old son to the clinic with chronic tummy aches which I diagnosed as stemming from a Small Intestine imbalance. She happened to mention that her son always seemed to choose to play at school with children who upset him and led him into trouble. This suggested to me that the boy's Small Intestine imbalance was manifesting at a mental level too.

Common Small Intestine Organ patterns seen in children

The following Small Intestine patterns will be discussed:

- Small Intestine *qi* pain
- Small Intestine deficient and Cold

Small Intestine *qi* pain

This pattern may be either acute or chronic. Below is a description of the chronic pattern.

Symptoms

- severe, twisting, lower abdominal pain
- distended abdomen
- cannot stand abdomen being touched
- flatulence which temporarily helps to relieve pain
- lots of gurgling noises in the abdomen
- lack of appetite
- intermittent nausea

Pulse: wiry

Tongue: may be unchanged

Treatment principles: move *qi* in the Small Intestine; promote smooth flow of Liver *qi*

> **SUGGESTED TREATMENT**
> **Points**
>
> Liv 3 *taichong*
> Liv 13 *zhangmen*
> Ren 6 *qihai*
> St 39 *xiajuxu*

Method: sedation needle technique

Paediatric *tui na*

> Seven Bound Bones *qijiegu* (straight pushing sedation)
> Thick Gate *banmen* (straight pushing)
> Eight Trigrams *bagua* (circular pushing anti-clockwise)
> Six Bowels *liufu* (straight pushing)
> Abdomen Stimulation *fuyinyang* (pushing apart)
> Knead Ren 6 *qihai* (kneading clockwise)

> One eight-year-old who came to the clinic had a gluten intolerance. If she ever unwittingly ate gluten, she would develop tummy pain from Small Intestine *qi* pain. The Liver was unable to digest the gluten and this put a strain on her Small Intestine.

Small Intestine deficient and Cold

This pattern nearly always appears against a background of Spleen *yang* deficiency.

Symptoms

- dull abdominal pain for which the child wants touch and warmth
- loose stools
- lots of gurgling noises in the tummy
- pain worse when tired or hungry
- feels cold

Pulse: deep, weak, slow

Tongue: pale

Treatment principles: expel Cold; warm the Intestines; tonify and warm Spleen *yang*

> **SUGGESTED TREATMENT**
> It is usually sufficient to use two points per treatment.
>
> **Points**
>
> > Ren 6 *qihai*
> > St 36 *zusanli*
> > St 25 *tianshu*
> > St 39 *xiajuxu*
>
> **Method:** tonification needle technique
>
> **Other techniques:** moxa
>
> **Paediatric *tui na***
>
> > Spleen *pijing* (straight pushing tonification)
> > Small Intestine *xiaochangjing* (straight pushing tonification)
> > Thick Gate *banmen* (straight pushing)
> > Three Passes *sanguan* (straight pushing)
> > Knead the Navel *rou qi* (kneading anti-clockwise)
> > Knead the Lower Abdomen *rou qihai* (kneading anti-clockwise)
> > Spinal Column *jizhu* (pinching from the bottom to the top of the back)
> > St 36 *zusanli* (kneading)

THE TRIPLE BURNER

The Triple Burner is a function more than it is an Organ. It is a division of the body into three separate parts, each of which is responsible for a particular aspect of the transformation process of food, drink and air. The Upper Burner contains the Heart, Pericardium and Lungs and is responsible for dispersing defensive (*wei*) *qi* around the body. The Middle Burner contains the Liver, Gallbladder, Stomach and Spleen and is responsible for the rotting, ripening, transformation and transportation of food. The Lower Burner contains the Kidneys and Bladder, and both the Large and the Small Intestine. It is responsible for separating the pure from the impure, storing and excreting urine and absorbing water.

Characteristics of the Triple Burner particularly pertinent to children

- The Triple Burner moves fluids through the three Burners

- The Triple Burner spreads *yuan qi* throughout the body

- The Triple Burner helps to regulate temperature

In young children, the Middle Burner is under great strain as it has the enormous job of processing the large amount of food that the child takes in relative to his size. Flaws goes so far as to say that 'almost all diseases or problems of the child or infant are related to the strength of their Middle Burner'.[56] It is certainly true that, up until the age of three, digestion plays a key part in their health.

The Triple Burner moves fluids through the three Burners

Su Wen Chapter 8 says, 'The Triple Burner is responsible for opening up the passages and irrigation. The regulation of fluids stem from it.'[57]

The Triple Burner plays a role in preventing the build-up of fluids in the form of mucus which is such a prevalent problem in children. Fluids need to be moving freely through each of the three Burners. It is possible to see in a baby or infant just from looking that he may have some form of stagnation in the Middle Burner (which may look out of proportion to the rest of him). If fluids are stuck in the Upper Burner, he may be prone to having a chesty cough, a snotty nose and blocked-up ears. If fluids are not moving properly, they may also sink and settle in the Lower Burner. This may lead the child to have urinary or bowel symptoms.

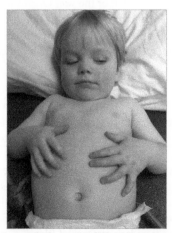

A disproportionately large Middle Burner in a young child

The Triple Burner spreads *yuan qi* throughout the body

In the same way that the Triple Burner moves fluids throughout the three Burners, it also spreads *yuan qi*. It takes *yuan qi* from the Kidneys, through the three Burners, to the channels and to the *yuan* source points that are located on the wrists and ankles. One of the functions of *qi* is to warm the body. By placing a hand on each of the three Burners of a child (the chest, the epigastrium and the abdomen) and noting the differences in temperature between them, it is possible to get a sense of whether or not the *yuan qi* is flowing smoothly throughout the body.

The Triple Burner helps to regulate temperature

A lesser-known role of the Triple Burner is to help maintain a balance of temperature within the body. The Japanese writer Sawada wrote, 'In what way can we describe the Triple Burner? The reaction of the burner is as heat. Heat is the fire; fire is the body temperature. Therefore, this also is the regulator of the body temperature.'[58]

This role of the Triple Burner in regulating body temperature is very relevant in children who are prone to suffer from fevers. In treatment, points along the Triple Burner channel can be used to help regulate a child's body temperature to stop it from going too high. Similarly, treating points along this channel can also help warm a child who has become cold.

> One girl who came to the clinic found it very difficult to ever be at the 'right' temperature. Her menopausal mother said her daughter was just like her in that she was always taking layers off or putting extra layers on! She had a constitutional imbalance in her Fire Element. Treating her Triple Burner (one of the *yang* Organs related to Fire) helped her to maintain a more stable temperature.

THE STOMACH
Characteristics of the Stomach particularly pertinent to children

- The Stomach receives food and drink
- The Stomach controls the rotting and ripening of food
- The Stomach controls the descending of *qi*

The Stomach receives food and drink

The Stomach is arguably the most important of the *yang* Organs in children because of the central role it plays in digestion. First, the Stomach receives food and drink. A poor appetite, particularly a reluctance to eat breakfast (which for most people is eaten around the time that the *qi* is at its highest in the Stomach channel, i.e. 7–9am), may be an indication of weak Stomach *qi* not receiving food.

The Stomach controls the rotting and ripening of food

The Stomach also controls the rotting and ripening of food. This is crucial in children, who have a small stomach and eat a large amount of food relative to the stomach's size. If this process of maceration does not work well, or the Stomach cannot keep up with the amount of food that enters it, then the common pattern of Accumulation of Food may result. This may involve digestive symptoms such as vomiting but can also lead to profuse, green mucus and a grouchy child.

A failure of the Stomach to rot and ripen food efficiently will also mean that not enough Food (*gu*) *qi* will be extracted from the food. Food (*gu*) *qi* is the basis of *qi* and Blood in the body. It is vital that a child builds up a good foundation of *qi* and Blood.

The Stomach controls the descending of *qi*

The *qi* of the Stomach should descend, enabling food to go downwards to the Small Intestine for further refinement. This may fail to happen either because the child has constitutionally weak Stomach *qi* or because she has eaten more food than the Stomach can manage at one time. A failure of Stomach *qi* to descend may result in reflux and regurgitation, belching, hiccuping, nausea and vomiting.

Common Stomach Organ patterns seen in children

The following Stomach patterns will be discussed:

- Stomach *qi* deficiency
- Stomach *yin* deficiency
- Accumulation of Heat in the Stomach
- Accumulation of Phlegm in the Stomach
- Cold invading the Stomach

Stomach *qi* deficiency

Stomach *qi* deficiency almost always goes hand in hand with Spleen *qi* deficiency.

Symptoms

- mild reflux in babies
- poor appetite
- no desire to eat breakfast
- tiredness which is worse in the mornings
- mild and dull ache in the epigastrium when hungry or if has overeaten

Pulse: deficient

Tongue: pale

Treatment principles: tonify Stomach and Spleen *qi*

> **SUGGESTED TREATMENT**
> One or two points per treatment are usually sufficient.
>
> **Points**
> Ren 12 *zhongwan*
> St 36 *zusanli*
> St 42 *chongyang*
> Sp 3 *taibai*
> Bl 20 *pishu*
> Bl 21 *weishu*
>
> **Method:** tonification
>
> **Other techniques:** moxibustion

> **Paediatric *tui na***
>
> Spleen *pijing* (straight pushing tonification)
> Stomach *weijing* (straight pushing tonification)
> Three Passes *sanguan* (straight pushing)
> Knead Ren 12 *zhongwan* (kneading anti-clockwise)
> Spinal Column *jizhu* (pinching from the bottom to the top of the back)
> St 36 *zusanli* (kneading)

Note: Stomach *qi* deficiency may manifest with an element of Cold too. This is especially likely when there is a background of Spleen *yang* deficiency. In this case, there will be additional symptoms of occasional vomiting of clear fluid and other general signs of *yang* deficiency.

Stomach *yin* deficiency

Although children these days rarely suffer from 'true' *yin* deficiency (due to the fact that *yin* rarely gets severely depleted by high fevers), Stomach *yin* deficiency is an exception to this.

Symptoms

- variable appetite

- sometimes very small and sometimes a voracious eater

- dull pain in the epigastrium

- slightly foul breath when hasn't eaten

- tends to be thirsty

- possibly slight lack of concentration and restlessness

Pulse: deficient, slightly floating

Tongue: may be redder in the centre

Treatment principles: nourish Stomach *yin*

> **SUGGESTED TREATMENT**
> One or two points per treatment are usually sufficient.
>
> **Points**
>
> Ren 12 *zhongwan*
> St 36 *zusanli*
> St 42 *chongyang*
> Sp 3 *taibai*
> Bl 20 *pishu*
> Bl 21 *weishu*
>
> **Method:** tonification needle technique
>
> **Paediatric *tui na***
> As for Stomach *qi* deficiency.

Accumulation of Heat in the Stomach

Symptoms

- reflux of food and milk
- vomiting
- epigastric pain
- sore throat
- tonsillitis
- constipation
- strong thirst
- insomnia
- bleeding and sore gums

Pulse: overflowing on the Earth pulses, rapid

Tongue: red in the centre, yellow coating

Treatment principles: clear Heat from the Stomach

SUGGESTED TREATMENT
Points
One or two points per treatment are usually sufficient.

St 44 *neiting*
St 21 *liangmen*
Ren 12 *zhongwan*
Pc 6 *neiguan*

Method: sedation needle technique

Paediatric *tui na*

Stomach *weijing* (straight pushing sedation)
Thick Gate *banmen* (straight pushing)
Knead Ren 12 *zhongwan* (clockwise kneading)
Milky Way *tianheshui* (straight pushing)

Accumulation of Phlegm in the Stomach

Symptoms

- intermittent vomiting of phlegm
- variable appetite which increases after vomiting
- nausea
- tendency towards a snotty nose and a congested chest
- greasy skin

Pulse: slippery

Tongue: thick, sticky coat

Treatment principles: resolve Phlegm

> **SUGGESTED TREATMENT**
> One or two points per treatment are usually sufficient.
>
> **Points**
>
> Ren 12 *zhongwan*
> St 40 *fenglong*
> Sp 4 *gongsun*
> Pc 6 *neiguan*
>
> **Method:** sedation needle technique
>
> **Paediatric *tui na***
>
> Spleen *pijing* (straight pushing tonification)
> Stomach *weijing* (straight pushing sedation)
> Thick Gate *banmen* (straight pushing)
> Eight Trigrams *bagua* (circular pushing anti-clockwise)
> Knead Ren 12 *zhongwan* (kneading clockwise)
> St 36 *zusanli* (kneading)

Cold invading the Stomach

This is an acute pattern, which is more common in young children than in adults.

Symptoms

- sudden and severe pain in the epigastrium

- often comes on after eating cold food

- vomiting of clear fluids

- feels cold

- desire for warm foods and drinks

Pulse: deep, slow, tight

Tongue: white coat

Treatment principles: expel Cold; warm the Stomach

> **SUGGESTED TREATMENT**
> **Points**
>
> St 21 *liangmen*
> St 34 *liangqiu*
> Sp 4 *gongsun*
> Ren 12 *zhongwan*
>
> **Method:** sedation technique
>
> **Paediatric *tui na***
>
> Spleen *pijing* (straight pushing tonification)
> Thick Gate *banmen* (straight pushing)
> Four Wind Creases *sifengwen* (pinching)

> Eight Trigrams *bagua* (circular pushing anti-clockwise)
> Three Passes *sanguan* (straight pushing)
> Knead Ren 12 *zhongwan* (kneading clockwise)
> Abdomen Stimulation *fuyinyang* (pushing apart)

Note: For a description of what is, in adults, called Retention of Food in the Stomach, please see Accumulation Disorder (Chapter 27).

THE LARGE INTESTINE
Characteristics of the Large Intestine particularly pertinent to children

- The Large Intestine controls the passage and conduction of stools
- The Large Intestine enables a child to 'let go' emotionally

The Large Intestine controls the passage and conduction of stools

Large Intestine pathologies, particularly loose stools and constipation, are very common in young children. In nearly all cases, however, the pathology stems from the Spleen or the Liver. The Spleen controls the transformation and transportation of food and fluids through the entire digestive system, including the Intestines. The Liver ensures the smooth flow of *qi* for digestion.

The function of the Large Intestine may also be impaired by deficient Lung *qi*, which may not provide the Large Intestine with enough *qi* for the act of defecation.

The Large Intestine enables a child to 'let go' emotionally

On an emotional level, the Large Intestine gives a child the capacity for letting go, something that needs to be continually done throughout childhood as each stage is passed through. In some children, a fear of letting go may manifest on a physical level as constipation.

> One four-year-old boy became constipated for the first time in his life after the death of his beloved dog. He had found it very difficult to accept that his dog was no longer there. Acupuncture that was focused on strengthening the *qi* of his Metal Element helped him to let go both emotionally and physically.

Common Large Intestine Organ pattern seen in children

The following Large Intestine pattern will be discussed:

- Large Intestine Cold

Large Intestine Cold

This pattern is essentially a component of Spleen *qi/yang* deficiency in which the key symptoms manifest in the Large Intestine.

Symptoms

- loose stools and frequent bowel movements
- dull tummy ache which is worse when tired and after cold food

- tired

- pale face

Pulse: deficient

Tongue: pale

Treatment principles: tonify and warm the Large Intestine and Spleen

---

SUGGESTED TREATMENT
Two points per treatment are usually sufficient.

Points

> LI 4 *hegu*
> St 25 *tianshu*
> Ren 6 *qihai*
> St 36 *zusanli*
> Bl 20 *pishu*
> Bl 25 *dachangshu*

Method: tonification

Other techniques: moxibustion

Paediatric *tui na*
As for Spleen *qi* deficiency.

Note: There is also a Full pattern of Damp-Heat in the Large Intestine. This equates with Damp-Heat in the Spleen (see Chapter 22) but the key symptoms manifest in the Large Intestine.

There is also a Full pattern of Heat in the Large Intestine. This almost always derives from and co-exists with Liver Heat (see Chapter 25). It is characterised by constipation.

THE BLADDER

The Bladder stores and excretes urine. Having received dirty fluids from the Small Intestine, the Bladder transforms these fluids into urine, stores them and excretes them. The correct functioning of this process helps to achieve a balance of fluids within the body. The Bladder relies on *yang qi* from the Kidneys to be able to carry out its functions.

Characteristics of the Bladder particularly pertinent to children

- The Bladder removes water by *qi* transformation

The Bladder removes water by *qi* transformation

In a child, the most common symptoms associated with the Bladder are recurrent urinary tract infections and bedwetting. Both of these symptoms are often brought on or exacerbated by the emotions of fear and anxiety, which pertain to the Kidneys. Some authors (e.g. Maciocia[59]) also note that an imbalance in the Bladder can lead to feeling states such as jealousy and suspicion. It is possible to surmise, therefore, that jealousy and suspicion could also bring about an imbalance in the Bladder. Jealousy, particularly between siblings, is a very common emotion for many children.

A six-year-old girl used to get what her mother referred to as 'jealousy attacks' every time her extremely clever sister got yet another award or amazing result at school. Sure enough, these would be characterised by urinary frequency and discomfort as well as huge outbursts of emotion.

Common Bladder Organ patterns seen in children

The following Bladder patterns will be discussed:

- Lingering Damp in the Bladder
- Bladder deficient and Cold

Lingering Damp in the Bladder

This pattern usually arises against a background of Spleen and/or Kidney *qi* deficiency in children.

Symptoms

- frequent urination
- difficulty urinating
- clouded urine
- discomfort or dull ache in the lower abdomen

Pulse: deficient, slippery

Tongue: pale, may have a sticky white coat

Treatment principles: resolve Damp in the Bladder

Note: Damp in the Bladder may be associated with either Cold or Heat. If Damp-Heat is present, it will be associated with more severe symptoms, such as very painful urination and blood in the urine.

> **SUGGESTED TREATMENT**
>
> It is usually sufficient to use one or two points to resolve Damp per treatment.
>
> **Points**
> To resolve Damp:
>
> > Sp 9 *yinlingquan*
> > Sp 6 *sanyinjiao*
> > Ren 3 *zhongji*
> > Bl 63 *jinmen*
>
> **Method:** sedation needle technique
>
> To tonify Spleen and/or Kidney *qi*:
>
> > St 36 *zusanli*
> > Sp 3 *taibai*
> > Ren 12 *zhongwan*
> > Bl 20 *pishu*
> > Ki 3 *taixi*
> > Bl 64 *jinggu*
> > Bl 23 *shenshu*
> > Bl 28 *pangguangshu*

Method: tonification needle technique

Paediatric *tui na*

Eight Trigrams *bagua* (circular pushing clockwise)
Winnower Gate *jimen* (straight pushing from groin to thigh)
Three *Yin* Meeting Sp 6 *sanyinjiao* (kneading)

Plus moves to tonify the Spleen and Kidneys.

Bladder deficient and Cold

This is another manifestation of Kidney *yang* deficiency but with most symptoms affecting the urinary system.

Symptoms

- frequent desire to urinate
- mild and dull ache in the lower abdomen
- tendency to bedwetting
- pale urine

Pulse: Water pulses deep and weak

Tongue: pale

Treatment principles: tonify and warm the Bladder

SUGGESTED TREATMENT

One or two points per treatment are usually sufficient.

Points

Bl 28 *pangguangshu*
Bl 64 *jinggu*
Ren 3 *zhongji*
Ki 3 *taixi*
Ki 7 *fuliu*

Method: tonification needle technique

Other techniques: moxibustion

Paediatric *tui na*
As for Kidney *yang* deficiency.

THE GALLBLADDER
Characteristics of the Gallbladder particularly pertinent to children

- The Gallbladder provides warmth to the digestive system
- The Gallbladder provides *yang* for the sinews and tendons to move
- The Gallbladder is important in decision making

The Gallbladder provides warmth to the digestive system

The Gallbladder stores and excretes bile which is needed for the digestive process. The Gallbladder, in communication with the Minister Fire, provides the *yang* energy necessary for the digestive process. Therefore, if a child has Cold in the digestive system, it may impair the workings of the Gallbladder. Conversely, if Gallbladder *qi* is Cold, it may impair the digestive process. As has already been mentioned, the digestive process is fundamental to a child's health, particularly in the first years of life. Every aspect of it is under strain. If one aspect of it is not working well, it will affect the entire process.

The Gallbladder provides *yang* for the sinews and tendons to move

The Gallbladder also influences the state of the sinews and tendons in the body. Whilst they rely on nourishment from Liver Blood, it is the *qi* of the Gallbladder which ensures their agility and movement. An imbalance in the Gallbladder should be considered one of several possible reasons that a child lacks the usual ease and flexibility of movement.

The Gallbladder is important in decision making

On a mental level, the Gallbladder gives a child the capacity to make decisions. It is often a strain for a young child's Gallbladder to be asked to make too many decisions. The reason a three-year-old may end up screaming or crying when she is asked which of ten ice cream flavours she would like is simply because it is too much of a strain for her Gallbladder to have to choose between them.

> Children who come to my clinic may choose one of several different panda stickers to take home with them after a treatment. One six-year-old girl used to find it so difficult, even stressful, to choose which one to take that it often drove her to tears. Her mother said this was the case with any decision she had to make. Treatment to strengthen her Gallbladder gradually meant that decisions became easier for her.

Common Gallbladder Organ patterns seen in children

The following Gallbladder patterns will be discussed:

- Damp in the Gallbladder
- Gallbladder deficiency

Damp in the Gallbladder

Symptoms

- jaundice
- discomfort around the lower rib area
- nausea
- frequent vomiting
- difficulty digesting fatty foods
- lethargic
- lack of appetite

Pulse: slippery and wiry in the left middle position

Tongue: thick sticky coat that may be unilateral or bilateral

Treatment principles: resolve Damp; promote the smooth flow of Liver *qi*

Note: Damp in the Gallbladder may also combine with Heat. In this case, there may be the following additional symptoms and signs:

- scanty, dark and strong-smelling urine

- thirst

- low-grade fever or a feeling of heat

- rapid pulse

- yellow tongue coating

SUGGESTED TREATMENT

One or two points per treatment are usually sufficient.

Points

> GB 34 *yanglingquan*
> GB 24 *riyue*
> Liv 14 *qimen*
> Ren 12 *zhongwan*
> Sp 9 *yinlingquan*

Method: sedation needle technique

Gallbladder deficiency

This pattern is often said to describe the character of a person, rather than being a pathological state.[60] It is commonly seen in children in the clinic. It may be constitutional, in which case it is often seen in a child with a Wood constitutional imbalance. It is also commonly seen in a child with domineering parents and/or older siblings. The child senses she is no match for the assertiveness or anger of the parent and, rather than fighting, becomes timid and overly compliant instead.

Symptoms

- nervous and shy

- struggles to make decisions

- lacking in initiative

- any symptoms of Liver Blood deficiency

Pulse: deficient

Tongue: pale or normal

Treatment principles: tonify and warm the Gallbladder; nourish Liver Blood

SUGGESTED TREATMENT

One or two points per treatment are usually sufficient.

Points

> GB 40 *qiuxu*

Liv 8 *ququan*
Bl 18 *ganshu*
Bl 19 *danshu*
Bl 47 *hunmen*

Method: tonification needle technique

Other techniques: moxibustion

SUMMARY

» An imbalance in the Small Intestine often results from a deficient Spleen or Kidneys.

» The key symptoms of a Small Intestine imbalance in a child are tummy ache and loose stools.

» The two most commonly seen Small Intestine patterns in children are:

  – Small Intestine *qi* pain

  – Small Intestine deficient and Cold.

» The Triple Burner's role of moving fluids is crucial in children to avoid the build-up of mucus.

» The Triple Burner's function of regulating body temperature is often immature in children.

» The Stomach is the most important of the *yang* Organs in children because of the key role it plays in the digestive process.

» Its functions of rotting and ripening, and descending *qi*, are particularly prone to imbalance in a child.

» The most commonly seen Stomach patterns in a child are:

  – Stomach *qi* deficiency

  – Stomach *yin* deficiency

  – Accumulation of Heat in the Stomach

  – Accumulation of Phlegm in the Stomach

  – Cold invading the Stomach.

» Large Intestine pathology usually stems from an imbalance in the Spleen and/or Liver.

» Constipation may also stem from a deficiency of Lung *qi*.

» The most commonly seen Large Intestine pattern in a child is Large Intestine Cold.

» The most commonly seen symptoms of a Bladder imbalance in children are urinary tract infections and bedwetting.

» Bladder symptoms often stem from a background of Kidney deficiency.

» Gallbladder *yang* provides warmth for the digestive system and also keeps the sinews and tendons supple and agile.

» The most commonly seen Gallbladder patterns in children are Damp in the Gallbladder and Gallbladder deficiency.

Chapter 27

NON-ORGAN PATTERNS

The non-Organ patterns discussed in this chapter are:

- Accumulation Disorder

- Lingering Pathogenic Factor

- Phlegm and Damp

- Heat

- Cold

Accumulation Disorder

 Accumulation Disorder is a condition that predominantly affects babies and children up to the age of approximately three years old.

Accumulation Disorder (*ji zhi*) describes blockage in the digestive system. The nearest equivalent pattern seen in adults is Retention of Food in the Stomach. However, Accumulation Disorder is seen much more frequently in children than Retention of Food in the Stomach is in adults. In fact, Accumulation Disorder is often referred to as 'the cause of 100 diseases' because it underlies so many of the most common childhood conditions, such as allergies, asthma, eczema, constipation and diarrhoea.

Accumulation Disorder is essentially stagnation in the digestive system. The transformation and transportation functions of the Spleen are impaired. Food is only partially expelled and lingers in the system, often fermenting. This build-up of food and stagnation often leads to Heat which may rise up and affect the *shen*. The Heat also condenses fluids and sometimes leads to the formation of Phlegm.

Although Accumulation Disorder is an excess pattern, it manifests differently depending on whether the child has an excess- or deficient-type constitution. Therefore, two types of Accumulation Disorder are described, namely the deficient type and the excess type.

Why is Accumulation Disorder common in babies and toddlers?

There are several reasons why babies and infants are prone to Accumulation Disorder:

- Compared to their size, babies have to eat a disproportionately large amount. The Spleen and Stomach are the key Organs that have the enormous task of dealing with all the food the baby eats. By the age of approximately two, growth will have begun to slow down and the child starts to eat less relative to his body weight. The strain on the Spleen and Stomach is then reduced. Accumulation Disorder becomes less common from about this age.

- At the same time as having to work so hard, the Spleen and Stomach in a child are immature and undeveloped. This means that they are more likely to develop an imbalance and for things to go awry. It is as if the digestive system is being asked to run a marathon when it has not had any training to build up its stamina, power and muscles.

- The type of food a baby is given and the manner of eating place yet another strain on the Spleen and Stomach. The key aspects of diet which may increase the chances of Accumulation Disorder developing are:

  - not enough time between feeds or meals (including breastfeeding on demand)

  - too many rich and fatty foods, a complex variety of foods in one meal or too many whole foods

  - too large a quantity of food.

There are two types of Accumulation Disorder, an excess and a deficient type. The excess type arises because the amount of food the child eats is simply too much for even a relatively strong digestive system to cope with. The deficient type arises because the child's digestive system is so weak that it cannot cope with even a small amount of food. Figure 27.1 illustrates how Accumulation Disorder may arise.

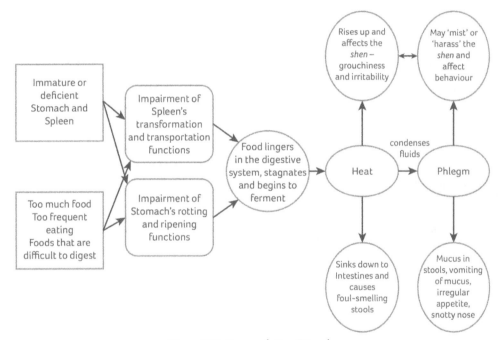

Figure 27.1 Accumulation Disorder

Excess (*shi*)-type Accumulation Disorder
Symptoms

- irregular bowel movements with foul-smelling stools

- stools may be green

- vomiting (of food or milk)

- swollen (and sometimes hard) tummy

- red cheeks

- green around the mouth

- worse when teething

- grouchy and bad tempered

- often temporarily better after a bowel movement

- disturbed sleep

- generally strong and robust child

- big appetite

- tendency to green mucus

Pulse: full, slippery, wiry

Tongue: thick, greasy coat

SUGGESTED TREATMENT
Points

M-UE-9 *sifeng*

Method: In children up to the age of three: prick the *sifeng* points of one hand (for a description of how to needle *sifeng*, please see Chapter 32)

In older children:

St 36 *zusanli*
St 25 *tianshu*
Ren 12 *zhongwan*

Method: sedation needle technique

Paediatric *tui na*
Routine to disperse accumulation of food:

Thick Gate *banmen* (straight pushing)
Eight Trigrams *bagua* (circular pushing anti-clockwise)
Four Wind Creases *sifengwen* (pinching)
Knead Ren 12 *zhongwan* (kneading clockwise)
Abdomen Stimulation *fuyinyang* (pushing apart)
Belly Corner *dujiao* (pinching)

It is vital to warn the parent that the child may have copious and urgent bowel movements in the twenty-four hours after the treatment.

Advice
With excess-type Accumulation Disorder it is essential to give the parent dietary suggestions, otherwise the condition will keep returning. The key points are:

- to allow intervals between feeds or meals

- to avoid whole foods, rich foods and too many different food types at one meal

- to avoid the baby or infant overeating.

CASE HISTORY: EXCESS-TYPE ACCUMULATION DISORDER

Main complaint: One-year-old girl with bouts of explosive diarrhoea every few days.

Other symptoms: Often fractious, sleep disturbed throughout the night, red and angry eczema.

Signs: Red cheeks, green colour around the mouth,* green nasal mucus, swollen tummy.

Diagnosis: Excess-type Accumulation Disorder (from diet consisting mainly of whole and raw foods or overeating).

Treatment: *Sifeng* points on one hand. Advice to mother to reduce raw foods and exchange brown bread, rice and pasta for good-quality white.

Outcome: The girl came back three times over a period of six months, whenever the symptoms returned. I repeated *sifeng* and reiterated the dietary advice to her mother.

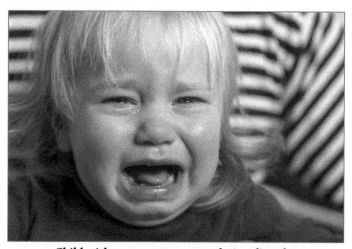

Child with excess-type accumulation disorder

Deficient (*xu*)-type Accumulation Disorder

The deficient (*xu*) pattern arises either from the long-term presence of the excess (*shi*) pattern, or in a child who is constitutionally deficient. The Spleen becomes too weak to effectively deal with even relatively small amounts of food.

Symptoms

- irregular bowel movements
- long periods of constipation
- stools not usually foul-smelling but may not be well formed
- pale or yellow complexion
- poor appetite
- weak cry
- may wake up frequently for short periods at night and sleep a lot during the day

---

* The green colour around the mouth reflects stagnation in the Liver channel as the deep pathway of the Liver runs around the mouth.

Pulse: deficient

Tongue: pale

Treatment principles: tonify Stomach and Spleen *qi*

SUGGESTED TREATMENT

Approximately two of the following points per treatment is usually sufficient.

Points

St 36 *zusanli*
Sp 3 *taibai*
Ren 12 *zhongwan*
Bl 20 *pishu*
Bl 21 *weishu*

Method: tonification

Other techniques: moxa

Paediatric *tui na*

Spleen *pijing* (straight pushing)
Thick Gate *banmen* (straight pushing)
Eight Trigrams *bagua* (circular pushing anti-clockwise)
Three Passes *sanguan* (straight pushing)
Knead the Navel *rou qi* (kneading anti-clockwise)
Knead Ren 6 *qihai* (kneading anti-clockwise)
Spinal Column *jizhu* (pinching from the bottom to the top of the back)
St 36 *zusanli* (kneading)

Note: It is important not to treat deficient-type Accumulation Disorder with the *sifeng* points as the child does not have enough *qi* to expel the food.

CASE HISTORY: DEFICIENT-TYPE ACCUMULATION DISORDER

Main complaint: Two-year-old boy with alternating constipation with bouts of unformed stools.

Other symptoms: Only wants to eat pasta and toast, very clingy.

Signs: Pale face, thin body with big tummy, weak limbs (did not react at all to my holding his legs).

Diagnosis: Deficient-type Accumulation Disorder from Spleen *qi* deficiency.

Treatment: Acupuncture to tonify Spleen *qi*, using points such as Ren 12 *zhongwan*, St 36 *zusanli* and Sp 3 *taibai*. I taught the mother a daily paediatric *tui na* routine to tonify Spleen *qi* and move Food Accumulation.

Outcome: After four weekly treatments, the boy's bowels were regular.

Lingering Pathogenic Factor

The concept of a Lingering Pathogenic Factor (LPF) (*xie yu*) is central to the treatment of children. Some of the most common childhood symptoms can be caused, at least in part, by an LPF. For example:

- recurrent ear infections

- recurrent tonsillitis

- recurrent bladder infections

- recurrent gastro-intestinal infections

- asthma

- cough

- headaches.

How does an LPF arise?

The most common cause of an LPF in a child is that he has not been able to entirely 'throw off' an illness. This may happen for the following reasons:

- an infection has been treated with antibiotics

- the child does not have sufficient and appropriate rest and care during and/or after an illness.

There are two other reasons an LPF may arise:

- it is transmitted to the child during pregnancy

- as a result of a vaccination.

An LPF strains the *qi* of the child. It is as if the child has to go about life carrying a heavy rucksack on his back. Everything consumes more *qi* than it should.

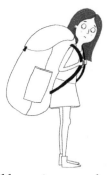

A child carrying around an LPF

What is the nature of the LPF?

There are various different ways in which an LPF may manifest in the body:

- **Thick Phlegm:**[*] This usually comes about because there has been an element of Heat to the illness which condenses the fluids. Thick Phlegm is generally too thick to 'flow', so the child will not appear full of mucus. It is most reliably felt as hard lumps in the glands in the neck (see Chapter 12 for a description of how to palpate lymph glands).[**]

- **Phlegm and Damp:** After an illness, a child may be left with abundant mucus in his nose and chest. There may also be mucus in the digestive system, which means his appetite may be irregular and he may be more picky about food than he was beforehand.

---

[*]   Scott and Barlow (in Chapter 3 of *Acupuncture in the Treatment of Children*) explain that the terms Lingering Pathogenic Factor and Thick Phlegm are considered synonymous in the Chinese literature. This is because the LPF blocks the flow of *qi* and fluids and Thick Phlegm arises as a result. However, in my experience, many children have an LPF that does not take the form of Thick Phlegm.

[**] The reason these hard lumps are often found in the neck is because the Gallbladder channel and the deep pathway of the Liver channel pass through the neck.

- **Heat:** An LPF may be Hot in nature. This is particularly likely after a 'Hot' illness such as a fever. The child may be left with symptoms that were not present beforehand, such as poor sleep, hyperactivity or emotional lability.

- **Cold:** An LPF may be Cold in nature. This is particularly likely after a 'Cold' illness such as an attack of Wind-Cold, or when the child has an underlying *qi* or *yang* deficiency. The child may be left with symptoms that were not present beforehand, such as cramping abdominal pain.

- **Qi deficiency:** Although it cannot really be called an 'LPF', *qi* deficiency is very often a part of the picture when an LPF is present. This is because the original illness itself has weakened the child's *qi*. However, the ongoing presence of the dormant pathogen also further weakens the child's *qi*.

What are the symptoms of an LPF?

There are two distinct phases in the manifestation of an LPF.

The dormant phase: There may be long periods of time when an LPF is present but does not cause the child to be 'ill' as such. However, the parent may report the following signs and symptoms:

0–3-year-olds

- child 'hasn't been himself' since an illness
- sudden and unexplainable energy crashes or mood changes
- swollen lymph nodes in neck and/or groin

School-age children

- child 'hasn't been himself' since an illness
- sudden and unexplainable energy crashes
- symptoms appear that were not there before an acute illness
- extreme emotional reactions
- seldom seems happy and contented
- swollen lymph nodes in neck and/or groin

Teenagers

- moody, emotionally complex
- makes decisions that do not seem to 'fit' personality*
- changes that go on around puberty are not smooth
- swollen lymph nodes in neck and/or groin

---

* For example, a fifteen-year-old girl with severe asthma had an LPF of Heat in the Lungs, which most likely stemmed from a bad bout of pneumonia when she was eight. The key trigger for an asthma attack was having to speak or perform in front of an audience, yet she had just decided to pursue drama at school with a view to studying performing arts at university. She had many other talents and therefore lots of other options were open to her!

The symptom of the child 'not being himself' is an important one. The reason for it is that the burden of carrying around the LPF distorts the child's personality. It is similar to an adult who may become more irritable, self-absorbed or needy if he is under a lot of stress, hormonally imbalanced or hungover. However, the effect is more significant in a child because his personality is still evolving and he is under strain anyway because he is growing and developing.

The flare-up phase: During a flare-up of an LPF, the child will suffer from a recurrence of a particular symptom, for example tonsillitis or a bladder infection. The LPF has 'woken up' and is making itself known. There are several reasons that a flare-up may occur:

- the child is especially tired or run down

- the child is stressed or there is an increased amount of stress in his family and he picks up on this (either consciously or unconsciously)

- the child has a shock

- the child is going through a phase of rapid growth or development and is not resting or eating properly throughout it.

Any of these factors depletes the child's *qi* and the LPF gains the upper hand. During easy times, the child's *qi* is strong enough to keep the LPF down and out of sight. The analogy of a see-saw, with *qi* on one end and the LPF at the other end, illustrates this ongoing 'contest' between them.

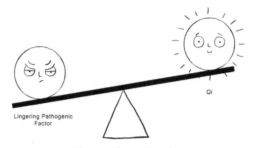

Qi keeps the LPF at bay

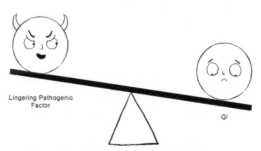

LPF gains the upper hand

In the dormant phase, a child may not be 'unwell' but may manifest some of the symptoms and/or signs listed. During the flare-up of an LPF, the child is likely to suffer from a bout of more severe symptoms that recurs periodically, such as an ear infection or sore throat.

How will the LPF manifest on the pulse and tongue?

There is no simple answer to this question. The manifestations of the LPF on the pulse and tongue will depend on the nature of the LPF and the degree of underlying *qi* deficiency in the child. However, very often there will be the following:

- A full quality somewhere on the child's pulses. This may be a wiry quality on the Wood pulse or a slippery quality on the Earth pulse, for example. Apart from this full quality, the pulses are otherwise often deficient.

- There may be red points on the tongue, either in the Lung or Liver area. There may also be a thick, and possibly coloured, tongue coating.

How long can an LPF stay?

An LPF may stay in the child for a few days, weeks, months or years. A child may be born with an LPF and it may stay with him his entire life. There are various windows of opportunity when the LPF may be more easily expelled from the child's body. These are:

- in the few weeks after it has become lodged in the child

- during a recurrence of the original illness

- during an acute infection that affects the same part of the body

- during the time that the child is transitioning between the seven- or eight-year cycles.

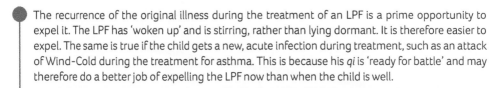

The recurrence of the original illness during the treatment of an LPF is a prime opportunity to expel it. The LPF has 'woken up' and is stirring, rather than lying dormant. It is therefore easier to expel. The same is true if the child gets a new, acute infection during treatment, such as an attack of Wind-Cold during the treatment for asthma. This is because his *qi* is 'ready for battle' and may therefore do a better job of expelling the LPF now than when the child is well.

How should an LPF be treated?

The practitioner needs to answer the following questions in order to effectively treat an LPF:

- Does the child have enough *qi* to throw off the LPF? If the child is *qi* deficient, then it is no use focusing treatment solely on clearing the pathogen. It is similar to trying to start a car with no fuel in it. It is necessary to strengthen the child's *qi* first as he will not be able to finally throw off the pathogen until his *qi* is strong enough to do so.

- What is the nature of the LPF? The practitioner must decide whether the LPF is Hot, Cold, Damp or a combination and choose points accordingly. The symptoms, pulse and tongue should reveal this information. Figure 27.2 illustrates the process of treating an LPF.

How is it possible to expel Thick Phlegm from the body with acupuncture?

Simply using points such as St 40 *fenglong* in order to clear Thick Phlegm is not usually effective. Before resolving the Phlegm, another treatment principle needs to be addressed, which is to loosen the Thick Phlegm. There are various points which are adept at doing this. Some of them loosen Thick Phlegm systemically, and some of them loosen Thick Phlegm in the local area.*

---

* Scott and Barlow use a combination of *bailao*, Bl 13, Bl 18 and Bl 20, needled with a moving technique, to loosen Thick Phlegm. Please see *Acupuncture in the Treatment of Children* (1999, p.52) for a description of this.

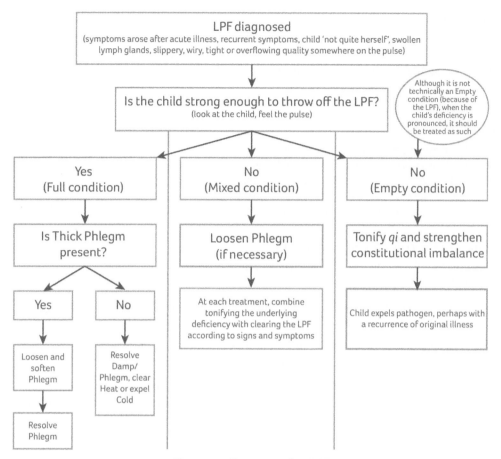

Figure 27.2 Treatment of an LPF

SOME POINTS WHICH ARE USEFUL WHEN CLEARING AN LPF
Thick Phlegm LPF

TB 17 *yifeng* loosens Thick Phlegm in the cervical lymph glands. Especially useful when treating chronic or recurrent ear conditions.

LI 18 *futu* loosens Thick Phlegm in the channels of the neck. Especially useful when treating chronic or recurrent tonsillitis and sore throats.

M-HN-30 *bailao* (2 cun superior to Du 14, 1 cun lateral to the midline) loosens Thick Phlegm in the upper part of the body.

TB 10 *tianjing* loosens Thick Phlegm in the upper part of the body.

GB 34 *yanglingquan* loosens systemic Thick Phlegm.

Liv 3 *taichong* does not loosen Thick Phlegm directly, but its ability to move *qi* aids the process of loosening Thick Phlegm. If the *qi* is flowing smoothly, it will help to break up the Phlegm and move it out of the body.

Extra point *pigen* is used to loosen Thick Phlegm in the abdomen or Lower Burner.

Hot LPF

Du 14 *dazhui* clears Heat that has been lurking in the body for a long time.

TB 5 *waiguan* clears Heat affecting all three Burners.

LI 11 *quchi* clears Heat from anywhere in the body.

Lu 10 *yuji* clears residual Heat from the Lungs.

He 8 *shaofu* clears residual Heat from the Heart.

Liv 2 *xingjian* clears residual Heat from the Liver.

Damp LPF

> Sp 6 *sanyinjiao* and Sp 9 *yinlingquan* resolve Damp, especially from the Lower and Middle Burners.
> Sp 3 *taibai* resolves Damp affecting the head and the Brain.
> St 8 *touwei* resolves Damp from the head.
> Ren 12 *zhongwan* resolves Damp in the Middle Burner.

Cold LPF

> Ren 6 *qihai* expels Cold in the Lower Burner.
> Du 4 *mingmen* expels Cold in the Lower Burner.
> St 36 *zusanli* expels Cold in the digestive system.
> Ren 12 *zhongwan* expels Cold in the digestive system.
> St 28 *shuidao* expels Cold in the Uterus or Bladder.

What are the consequences of an LPF?

There are both short-term and long-term consequences of an LPF being present.

The short-term consequences are the following:

- The child is carrying around the weakened pathogen. This in itself takes its toll on his *qi*. Everything he does consumes a little more *qi* than it otherwise would.

- The presence of the pathogen also disrupts the flow of *qi* and fluids in the child's body. This means that fluids often accumulate in the form of Damp or Phlegm.

- The *qi* in the local area becomes weakened by the long-term presence of the LPF. For example, in the case of recurrent ear infections, the *qi* of the ear becomes weakened. This obviously predisposes the child to further infections (see Figure 27.3).

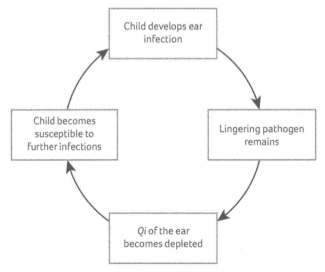

Figure 27.3 Interaction between an LPF and the qi of the local area

The long-term consequence is that if an LPF remains in the child past the age of seven or eight, and especially through adolescence, it begins to become a part of who he is. As the child's *qi* 'sets', it is, in part, moulded by the presence of the LPF. For example, if the LPF is in the Liver channel, it may predispose the child to an imbalanced expression of anger which may have a significant impact on both how he experiences the world and his relationships. It may also cause different Liver-related symptoms at different stages of his life.

One adult patient was a good example of how an LPF may manifest differently throughout a person's life. This woman had suffered from chronic and recurrent conjunctivitis (often Damp-Heat in the Liver channel) for the first eight years of her life. At the age of fourteen, when she began menstruating, she developed a strong propensity to an itchy and uncomfortable vaginal discharge (also Damp-Heat in the Liver channel). During the menopause, she suffered from severe irritability and hot flushes (both possible signs of Liver Heat). Who knows how her physical health may have been different if she had been able to expel the LPF in childhood?

What is the difference between an LPF and other chronic Pathogenic Factors?

The key difference between an LPF and other chronic Pathogenic Factors is in the pathogenesis. An LPF is usually the residue of an illness or vaccination. Therefore, it contains within it the resonance of the original illness. It does not build up over time as Damp often does if the child lives in a damp environment. Generalised Damp in the body may be worse on damp days but will generally cause chronic and ongoing symptoms such as heavy limbs and brain fog. An LPF may be 'silent' until such time as the child becomes run down or has a phase of stress. It then rears its head and causes symptoms that are similar to those of the original illness.

CASE HISTORY: LINGERING PATHOGENIC FACTOR – FULL CONDITION

Main complaint: Six-year-old girl with recurrent tonsillitis (came every six weeks or so – red, hot, swollen tonsils with a lot of pain).

Other symptoms: Extremely fiery temper.

Other signs: Constitutionally strong; physically robust; strong voice; confident; red face; strong, slightly rapid pulse; red tongue.

Diagnosis: Hot LPF.

Treatment: Clear Heat with LI 18 *futu*, LI 11 *quchi*, St 44 *neiting*, Liv 2 *xingjian* (sedation needle technique). I selected two of these points at each treatment.

Outcome: After six treatments, the pulse was no longer rapid and the girl's temper had calmed. I told the mother to come back if there was a recurrence of symptoms. She came back for two treatments after six months, having been free of symptoms until then. I never saw her again.

CASE HISTORY: LINGERING PATHOGENIC FACTOR – MIXED CONDITION

Main complaint: Ten-year-old boy with allergic asthma. Triggered by change in seasons, the wind and cats.

Other symptoms: Otherwise, relatively healthy, although needed more sleep than his peers; played a lot of football and had lots of energy for it; good sleep apart from occasionally waking up at night wheezing; good appetite.

Other signs: Hunched shoulders, thin body; thin pulse with an overflowing quality on the Wood pulses; Pc/TB pulses were the lowest; pale tongue with some red spots on the sides.

Diagnosis: Hot LPF in the Liver, Lung *qi* deficiency, Fire constitutional imbalance.

Treatment: At each treatment, I used points to clear the Hot LPF from the Liver (e.g. Liv 2 *xingjian*, Liv 3 *taichong*) and strengthen the Fire Element (e.g. *yuan* source points TB 4 *yangchi*, Pc 7 *daling*; or tonification points TB 3 *zhongzhu*, Pc 9 *zhongchong*). When I treated points on the Fire channels, the Lung pulse became much stronger, so I did not treat the Lungs directly.

Outcome: After three months of treatment, the boy had stopped using his inhaler which he had relied upon for years. The only time he needed it was if he was around cats for a long period of time.

> **CASE HISTORY: LINGERING PATHOGENIC FACTOR – DEFICIENT CONDITION**
>
> **Main complaint:** Two-year-old boy with chronic cough characterised by abundant mucus. Began after an invasion of Wind-Cold in the Lungs at three months old, treated with antibiotics.
>
> **Other symptoms:** Always tired, poor appetite, loose stools, unusually cold.
>
> **Signs:** Very pale, quiet, sat still on mother's lap for whole treatment, deficient pulses, normal tongue.
>
> **Diagnosis:** LPF of Damp/Phlegm in the Lungs with underlying Spleen *yang* deficiency.
>
> **Treatment:** Acupuncture and moxa to strengthen Spleen *yang* deficiency, including points such as St 36 *zusanli*, Bl 20 *pishu* and Ren 12 *zhongwan*. I taught the mother a paediatric *tui na* routine to descend Lung *qi*.
>
> **Outcome:** After the seventh treatment, the boy had what appeared to be an acute cough. He came to the clinic on the second day of the cough and I treated him to clear Phlegm in the Lungs and descend Lung *qi* (using Lu 5 *chize*, Bl 13 *feishu* and Ren 22 *tianshu*). After this illness, the original chronic cough was significantly improved. I treated him three more times (tonifying and warming Spleen *yang*) and by that time the cough had completely gone.

Phlegm and Damp

Some babies are born with substantial amounts of Phlegm and Damp. The pathogen may not affect just one particular Organ but the child is born with a Phlegm-type constitution (see Chapter 13). If circumstances in her early life are conducive to health, the child may, of her own accord, resolve the Phlegm and it need not necessarily lead to ill health. However, if, for example, the child has a poor diet, is perpetually overtired or is surrounded by family members who are depressed, the Phlegm and Damp may linger and cause symptoms. The symptoms described here most commonly arise in a child with a Phlegm-type constitution but describe a picture of pathology, rather than one of a constitutional type.

Symptoms

0–3-year-olds

- sleeps for long periods of time
- irregular appetite (sometimes eats a lot, sometimes not hungry)
- may generate a lot of mucus when ill
- frequent chesty coughs and snotty nose
- tendency to glue ear
- illnesses linger for a long time
- sticky stools
- may have lots of 'baby fat'

School-age children

- sleeps for long periods of time
- struggles to get going in the morning

- irregular appetite (sometimes eats a lot, sometimes not hungry)

- may generate a lot of mucus when ill

- frequent chesty coughs and snotty nose

- prone to glue ear

- illnesses linger for a long time

- sticky stools

- resists going out and getting moving but better for it once he gets going

- may be disconnected and in a world of his own

Teenagers

- struggles to wake up and get going in the morning

- bloating

- acne

- muzzy headed

- sluggish and lethargic

- may be disconnected and withdrawn

- depressed

Treatment principles: resolve Phlegm and Damp; tonify underlying deficiencies

SUGGESTED TREATMENT

The points chosen in each particular case should depend on the nature and location of the symptoms. Two points per treatment is usually sufficient.

Points

Sp 6 *sanyinjiao*
Sp 9 *yinlingquan*
Ren 12 *zhongwan*
St 40 *fenglong*
Lu 5 *chize*
GB 41 *zulinqi*
Ren 14 *juque*
Pc 5 *jianshi*

Points should also be chosen to treat the underlying deficiency according to which Organ or Organs are involved.

Method: sedation needle technique

Paediatric *tui na*

Heaven Gate *tianmen* (straight pushing)
Water Palace *kangong* (straight pushing)
Heart Gate *xinmen* (straight pushing)
Small Palmar Crease *zhangxiaowen* (straight pushing)

Hand *yin yang shaoyinyang* (pushing apart)
Eight Trigrams *bagua* (circular pushing)
Knead Ren 12 *zhongwan* (kneading)

In the clinic

- Phlegm and Damp in children is nearly always the result of an underlying deficiency of the Spleen. The amount of Phlegm and Damp present should be compared to the degree of the underlying deficiency. When the degree of deficiency is greater, the most effective way to resolve the Phlegm and Damp may be to strengthen the Spleen. The pulse is usually the most accurate guide as to which treatment principle should predominate.

- The Triple Burner plays an important role in the distribution of fluids. If the pulse indicates that the Triple Burner is deficient, consider whether this Organ also needs tonifying in order to get the fluids moving.

- Phlegm and Damp may combine with Heat, in which case there will be additional signs and symptoms such as:

  - coloured mucus

  - low-grade fever

  - fractiousness or irritability

  - thirst

  - poor sleep

  - red cheeks

  - rapid pulse.

A THREE-YEAR-OLD WITH PHLEGM AND DAMP

Owen had suffered from one thing after another since he was six months old. First, he had a chronic cough which got worse at night and disrupted his sleep. Then, his hearing deteriorated and he was diagnosed with glue ear. At the age of two, he developed eczema, which was oozing and particularly bad in his elbow and knee creases. He had a puffy face and sat on his mother's knee, seemingly uninterested in playing with any toys. I gave him acupuncture to resolve Phlegm and Damp (using the sedation method on points such as St 40 *fenglong*, Ren 12 *zhongwan* and Sp 9 *yinlingquan*). I taught his mother a paediatric *tui na* routine to tonify Spleen *qi*. It took several months of treatment but Owen's Phlegm and Damp gradually resolved. As this happened, his sparky character came more to the fore. Less weighed down by the Phlegm and Damp, he became brighter and more energetic and outgoing.

Heat

Some babies are born with Heat that they acquired whilst in the womb. Fevers, and, in particular, fevers with rashes, are an opportunity for a child to expel Heat that has accumulated in the womb. If a child does not find a way of expelling Heat,* it may remain and manifest with myriad symptoms.

---

* A child may not be able to expel Heat because he also has a 'layer' of Phlegm/Damp that traps Heat in his body. If he does get fevers but they are heavily suppressed with medication, that may also prevent the Heat from being expelled. Please see Chapter 3 on transformations and steamings for a discussion on the necessity of fevers in children.

Symptoms

At any age

- poor sleep (restless, throws off the bed clothes, needs help to settle)
- foul-smelling stools or constipation
- red face

0–3-year-olds

- finds it hard to settle
- clingy during the day
- hot temper
- strong emotional reactions
- tendency to high fevers

School-age children

- always on the go
- finds it hard to settle and be still
- strong emotional reactions
- difficulty concentrating
- impulsive
- seems to be able to survive on little sleep
- hot temper
- tendency to high fevers

Teenagers

- agitation
- restlessness
- panic attacks
- quick to anger
- tendency to red, angry-looking acne
- heavy periods in girls

Treatment principles: clear Heat; tonify underlying deficiencies

SUGGESTED TREATMENT

The choice of points used to clear Heat should be dictated by where the Heat is in the body. One or two points per treatment is usually sufficient.

Points

> Lu 5 *chize* – clears Heat in the Lungs
> St 44 *neiting* – clears Heat in the Stomach
> Liv 2 *xingjian* – clears Heat in the Liver
> TB 5 *waiguan* – clears Heat in the head, face and ears
> He 8 *shaofu* – clears Heat in the Heart
> GB 43 *xiaxi* – clears Heat in the GB channel affecting the head
> LI 11 *quchi* – clears Heat to reduce fever, and cools Blood
> Du 14 *dazhui* – clears Hot, retained Pathogenic Factors

Points should be chosen to tonify the underlying deficiency depending on which Organ or Organs are involved.

Method: sedation needle technique

Other modalities: *gua sha*

Paediatric *tui na*

> Palace of Toil *laogong* (kneading)
> Small Heavenly Heart *xiaotianxin* (kneading)
> Milky Way *tianheshui* (straight pushing)
> Six *Yang* Organs *liufu* (straight pushing)

In the clinic

- A common scenario is for a child to have a mixed condition of Heat with underlying deficiency. Sometimes it is necessary to clear Heat before strengthening the deficiency. In other cases, the deficiency is so great that the child needs to be strengthened before the Heat can be cleared. This decision should be made based upon signs and symptoms.

- A child may have pathogenic Heat at the same time as an underlying *qi* or *yang* deficiency. Or she may have Heat in one part of the body and Cold in another. For example, there may be Heat in the Lungs causing asthma and Cold in the Intestines causing tummy aches or diarrhoea.

> **A TWO-YEAR-OLD GIRL WITH HEAT**
> Maya walked into the clinic with bright red cheeks and an exhausted mother trailing behind her. Maya was a bundle of energy (or, more honestly, of hyperactivity) who had been awake for hours every night since she was born. She had been fully vaccinated and never had a fever. She had a red tongue, rapid pulse and a very loud voice. I taught the mother a paediatric *tui na* routine to clear Heat. After two weeks of diligently massaging her daughter twice a day, the mother rang despondently saying there had been no change. I urged her to continue for longer. Within a few days, the mother rang again to say that Maya had a high fever. I gave her some suggestions of how to help her daughter through the fever (see Chapter 70). After three days, the fever subsided. Maya came to the clinic the following week with her mother beside her with a broad grin. Maya had slept solidly through the night since the fever had subsided and was also far calmer during the day.

Cold
Symptoms
0–3-year-olds

- colic-type, strong tummy pain (full Cold)
- chronic, dull abdominal pain (empty Cold)
- vomiting of clear fluids
- diarrhoea
- easily feels cold
- white or clear mucus
- white complexion

School-age children

- strong, cramping tummy pains
- chronic, dull abdominal pain (empty Cold)
- dull pain over the bladder
- strong pain anywhere in the body
- painful and stiff muscles
- easily feels cold
- white complexion

Teenagers

- severe period pain in girls
- painful and stiff muscles
- easily feels cold

Pulse: slow or tight

Tongue: pale, thick-white coating

> **SUGGESTED TREATMENT**
> Points should be chosen according to where in the body the Cold is manifesting.
>
> **Points**
> Ren 6 *qihai* expels Cold in the Lower Burner
> Du 4 *mingmen* expels Cold in the Lower Burner
> St 36 *zusanli* expels Cold in the digestive system
> Ren 12 *zhongwan* expels Cold in the digestive system
> St 25 *tianshu* expels Cold in the digestive system
> St 28 *shuidao* expels Cold in the Uterus or Bladder

Method: needle technique will depend on whether the Cold is full or empty

Other techniques: moxibustion is essential

Paediatric *tui na*

> Two Men Upon a Horse *erma* (kneading)
> Lower Back Bl 23 *shenshu* (strong rubbing)
> Knead the Navel *rou qi* (kneading)
> Spinal Column *jizhu* (pinching from base to top)
> Outer Palace of Toil *wailaogong* (kneading)
> Wind Nest *yiwofeng* (kneading)
> Three Passes *sanguan* (straight pushing)

A ONE-YEAR-OLD WITH COLD

After Islay was born, she had terrible colic. Her parents assumed that, as with most babies, the colic would clear up after a few months. However, it did not. Every evening, she would scream in pain and pull up her knees until she was so tired she would eventually drop off to sleep. She had recently begun having similar bouts of colic-type pain in the afternoon too. Islay was a relatively strong and robust child, but her face was bright white and she had a blue colour around her mouth. I used acupuncture and moxibustion on points such as St 36 *zusanli*, Sp 4 *gongsun* and St 25 *tianshu*. I taught Islay's mother a paediatric *tui na* routine to warm *yang*. After approximately six weeks, Islay's bouts of colic-type pain had stopped.

SUMMARY

Accumulation Disorder

» Accumulation Disorder is generally seen in children up to the age of about three. It arises when the child is not able to process the quantity of food in his digestive system.

» This may be either because he has an underlying deficiency of Stomach and/or Spleen *qi*, or that his digestive system is under so much strain because of his diet and eating habits.

» The key symptom is irregular bowel movements. Other symptoms depend on whether it is an excess or deficient type of Accumulation Disorder.

» Full-type Accumulation Disorder is most effectively treated by using the *sifeng* points of one hand.

» Deficient-type Accumulation Disorder should be treated by strengthening the Stomach and Spleen.

Lingering Pathogenic Factor

» Lingering Pathogenic Factors (LPFs) are commonly seen in the treatment of children.

» They arise because a child is not able to completely recover from an infection, an infection is treated with antibiotics, or after vaccination.

» Having diagnosed an LPF and the nature of it, the practitioner needs to decide whether to treat the child as having a full, mixed or empty condition.

» Some LPFs are in the form of Thick Phlegm. Thick Phlegm needs to be 'loosened' before it can be resolved.

» An LPF of long-standing may be 'awakened' during the recurrence of an illness or during a new infection. This is a particularly opportune time to expel the LPF.

» The key to successful treatment of an LPF is to decide whether to (1) just do clearing treatments, (2) do a mix of both clearing and tonifying, or (3) just tonify.

Phlegm and Damp

» Phlegm and Damp are extremely common Pathogenic Factors in children.

» They most often (but not exclusively) occur in a child with a Phlegm-type constitution.

» They may cause physical and/or mental/emotional symptoms.

» They may be a part of many common childhood conditions such as glue ear, chronic cough and eczema.

» Treatment should not focus only on resolving the Phlegm and Damp, but should also include tonifying the underlying deficiencies.

» Relevant dietary advice is particularly important.

Heat

» Heat is also a commonly seen Pathogenic Factor in childhood conditions.

» Heat may cause physical symptoms but is especially likely to rise up and affect the *shen*.

» Heat is often present with a co-existing deficiency. Treatment needs to address both aspects of the condition.

Cold

» Cold most commonly affects either the digestive system (in young children) or the gynaecological system (in teenagers).

» It may cause either mild or strong pain, depending on whether it is full or empty.

» A combination of moxibustion and needles is the most effective way to scatter Cold and warm any underlying deficiency of *qi* and/or *yang*.

• Part 3 •

TREATMENT OF
CHILDREN

• Chapter 28 •

INTRODUCTION TO THE TREATMENT OF CHILDREN

Chinese medicine theory and diagnosis is enormously well suited to the kinds of problems for which children come for treatment. In nearly all cases, the practitioner, having heard the child's story and employed the relevant diagnostic methods, will feel that the picture makes sense to her and that Chinese medicine could help the child.

The stumbling block for both parents and practitioners is the delivery of the treatment. There is a widely held perception that most children in the West will simply not tolerate needles. Some people even believe it would be tantamount to cruelty to 'subject' a child to acupuncture needles. Practitioners sometimes struggle to find a way of delivering the treatment that is acceptable to the child. For these reasons, many children who would benefit hugely from treatment do not even make it to our doors. For those that do, the use of needles may mean the session does not go well and they do not last the course of treatment.

However, the reality is rather different to the perception. First, the vast majority of children accept being needled. They may not relish it (although some do), but most tolerate it when it is approached in the right way. Second, there are many other modalities available to the practitioner. If more parents were aware of this, it would mean more children coming to the clinic. Once there, these alternative modalities may be used either instead of or in conjunction with needles for the minority of children for whom this is necessary. For the practitioner, just the knowledge that she has other ways of administering the treatment can give her confidence that she can find a way to do what she needs to do. She will therefore be more relaxed and the child will pick up on this.

This part of the book will cover the three most important aspects of treating children:

- child-friendly needling
- alternatives to needling
- other Chinese medicine modalities that may be used on children.

Choosing the right treatment modality

Not all the modalities described will be available to every practitioner who works with children. Everybody comes to treat children with well-established preferences for how they like to carry out their treatment. Many practitioners will not own a laser machine, and some will not be familiar with paediatric *tui na* or *shonishin*.

However, when treating children, it is desirable to have available as many different methods as possible. Most children are coming because their parents have not been able to get sufficient help from anywhere else. Their child is suffering and they do not know what to do about it. In short, they are desperate. If we think that acupuncture can help, then it is beholden upon us to find a suitable method of carrying out the treatment the child needs.

The factors that influence which modality a practitioner will use with a particular child include:

- **The age of the child:** Paediatric *tui na* and *shonishin* are unlikely to be sufficient on their own with children beyond the age of around eight.

- **The nature of the child:** Lots of children are really happy to try needles. Some are petrified by the idea. It would be unwise (as well as, arguably, unethical) to force a child to try needles if it has the potential of destroying rapport.

- **Frequency of appointments:** If, due to geographical, financial or time restrictions, the child is not able to come for treatment as frequently as necessary, treatment modalities that the parent can use at home become more important.

- **Preferences of the practitioner:** A practitioner who feels especially confident using her hands may lean towards paediatric *tui na* or *shonishin*. A practitioner who is technologically confident may choose to rely on a laser machine.

Combining different treatment modalities

All the treatment modalities discussed in this book may be combined. For example, the practitioner may needle points on a child's limbs but use a laser pen on his back because he does not like being needled where he cannot see. The practitioner may use needles on a three-year-old and teach the parent a paediatric *tui na* routine to do daily at home between treatments. She may use *shonishin* at the start of the treatment and then move on to needles. She may use only moxibustion on one child, or *gua sha* and acupressure on another. Almost anything is possible, as long as it fulfils the relevant treatment principles. Children are constantly developing, and this is heightened if they are having acupuncture treatment. A child may not be ready for needles one week but ask for them the next week.* At each appointment, the practitioner should assess the situation as it is at that moment and choose her treatment modalities accordingly.

Becoming adept at a variety of treatment modalities

For any practitioner who would like to make paediatrics a central part of her practice, I encourage her to find courses where she can learn treatment modalities suitable for children. There is only so much that may be learned from a book about a practical method. I then encourage her to start using these modalities. She will then experience first-hand their effectiveness, and will find the ones with which she particularly resonates.

A word about 'trying to make it all better'

Those of us who are drawn to the healing professions usually have a strong desire to make people better. Practitioners who are drawn to working with children are likely to have a particularly strong desire to 'make it all better' for children. This is, of course, a valid incentive and often means a practitioner is conscientious and committed in her work.

However, the suffering of children and the profound effect that may have on the family can be hard to witness. The usual desire to help can go into overdrive and become a need to rescue. When this happens, the practitioner usually becomes less effective in her work. It is as if the depth of the desire gets in the way of her being able to see and work clearly. The practitioner's need permeates the atmosphere in the treatment room. Ironically, this means there is less 'space' available for the child and treatment does not usually go so well.

---

* A mother told me at the start of an appointment that her five-year-old son had been very upset after his last treatment. When I enquired why, she said it was because he had *really* wanted to have needles and I had not used them! Another child felt hard done by if I did not use as many needles on him as I did on his older brother.

I therefore strongly encourage a practitioner working with children to reflect on how she feels in relation to a particular child or family. If she catches herself thinking about them a lot outside of treatment time and with a desperate desire to take away all their suffering, it may be necessary to reflect on this and to take a step backwards. It is not always possible to take away the suffering of a child and family. This does not mean, however, that our treatment is of no value.

• Chapter 29 •

TREATING THE WHOLE CHILD

The topics discussed in this chapter are:

* Boosting resilience in the face of illness
* Boosting resilience in the face of life's challenges and stresses
* Easing the process of treatment
* Encouraging deeper healing

Introduction

The concept of treating the whole person, rather than just the illness, has always been a core principle of Chinese medicine. It is a system of medicine that lends itself beautifully to doing this. However, the extent to which the child is treated, as opposed to his physical symptom, has less to do with the particular medical system employed and more to do with the way it is practised.

In order to be an effective paediatric acupuncturist, the practitioner must often place her focus primarily on the child, and secondarily on the child's illness. The benefits of this are described below.

Boosting resilience in the face of illness

The same illnesses have very different effects on different children. One child who succumbs to a cold is able to carry on life much as normal. He may remain energetic throughout, and be right as rain within a couple of days. Another child who catches a cold may need time off school and be capable of nothing more than lying around on the sofa for a few days. It may take him a week or two to return to his previous, healthy state. The eighteenth-century medic Xu Dachun wrote, 'Illnesses may be identical but the persons suffering from them are different.'[1]

This difference in response to the same illness is based on several factors. First, the strength of the child's *jing* and upright (*zheng*) *qi* plays a part in determining how deeply a child succumbs to an illness and how long it lasts.

Second, and just as important, is the way in which a child responds emotionally to an illness. This is determined by her emotional constitution and the state of her spirit at the time. The stronger the child's spirit, the smaller the psychological impact of an illness.

There are many quotes in the Chinese classics that support this view and stress the importance of keeping the spirit strong. For example, *Su Wen* Chapter 25 says, 'In order to make all acupuncture thorough and effective one must first cure the spirit.'[2]

Zhang Jiebin made a similar point: 'When the Spirits are overwhelmed, they leave; when left in peace they remain. Thus the most important thing in the conduct and treatment of a being is maintenance of the Spirits, and then comes maintenance of the body.'[3] For this reason, when treating a child, it is vital to focus not only on the illness from which he is suffering, but also on the child himself and the state of the child's spirit. There are times when the physical illness is acute and severe and the practitioner's focus needs to be on that alone. However, in most chronic illnesses, focusing treatment at least in part on the child and his spirit is likely to bring about a faster and more long-lasting cure than merely treating the illness.

Boosting resilience in the face of life's challenges and stresses

There are many circumstances in children's lives that take their toll on the spirit (as discussed in Part 1). These stresses are a part of life and often cannot be avoided. However, treatment of a child's spirit will help to mitigate some of the negative effects these various stresses and strains would otherwise have.

Many Western medically trained paediatricians have long thought that the focus of the physician should be on the whole child, rather than just the illness or the part of the body that the illness is affecting. John Apley, for example, a renowned British paediatrician of the 1950s, wrote, 'The proper study for every doctor is not merely a symptom, organ, region or disease, but the whole patient, in the background of the family and the environment.'[4] He went on to say, 'There are no separate minds and bodies – only human beings. As children themselves might do, let me put this in a simple phrase: *the ill child is ill all over*.'[5]

Easing the process of treatment

Knowing the child helps the treatment to go more smoothly as the practitioner will have a sense of the best approach to take. It is necessary for the paediatric acupuncturist to be highly flexible in the way she approaches the treatment of each child. Of course, the practitioner must build rapport with adult and child patient alike. However, failure to do this well with a child may lead to poor outcomes. The child is less likely to allow the practitioner to administer the necessary treatment. Furthermore, she will not be sensitive enough to the changes in the child's *qi* to know whether her treatment is the right one and, crucially, when she has done enough.

Encouraging deeper healing

A failure to understand anything of the character of the child means the changes a practitioner is able to bring about are much narrower. The practitioner can only treat the *whole* child if she senses who that child is. Holding an awareness of the whole child as she goes about administering treatment will produce very different results compared with simply holding an awareness of the physical symptoms.

A child will sense and respond well to the fact that it is the whole of her that is being taken into account rather than simply her stomach that hurts or the fact that she finds it hard to concentrate at school. Sadly, many adults have lost the expectation that the whole of their being will be taken into account when they interact with the medical profession. A young child has rarely reached this point and she therefore has an innate assumption that the entirety of her is important.

Parents often notice that treatment has brought about changes in their child, as well as their child's symptoms. They may comment that their child 'seems more mature', 'has been kinder to her siblings', 'has been happier going to school' or 'is more relaxed'. Of course, acupuncture treatment will not take away the quirks and foibles that are part of normal childhood development, but these benefits that occur so often should not be underrated.

Conclusion

Focusing on the whole child, as well as her illness, brings about wider benefits than merely an eradication of symptoms. When the practitioner focuses her intention and her *qi* on the little human being in front of her, rather than a collection of symptoms, the influence of her treatment may include the mental–emotional well-being, growth and development of the child.

SUMMARY

» Treating the whole child has more to do with the approach of the practitioner than the system of medicine she practises.

» Treating the whole child has many benefits:

  − It helps a child to be more resilient when ill.

  − It helps a child to withstand the stresses in her life.

  − It helps the process of treatment to go smoothly.

  − It encourages healing of the whole child, rather than just eradicating her symptoms.

• Chapter 30 •

TREATMENT OF THE CHILD'S CONSTITUTIONAL IMBALANCE

The topics discussed in this chapter are:

- When to treat the Five Element constitutional imbalance
- Combining treatment of the Five Element constitutional imbalance with treatment of the Organ/Pathogen patterns
- Treatment techniques
- Use of points
- Intention
- Spirit points
- Five Element blocks to treatment

When to treat the Five Element constitutional imbalance

Treatment of the constitutional imbalance in a child can be of benefit in all situations, but there are various instances when this is particularly the case:

- when the child presents with a wide range of conflicting symptoms and signs
- when the child's spirit has been affected by her illness or by other circumstances in her life
- when the child's main complaint is mental–emotional
- when the child's physical complaint is predominantly caused by an internal cause of disease
- when the child has been ill for a long time and is not recovering as expected.

Treatment of the constitutional imbalance can be integrated with treatment of the Organ/Pathogen patterns.

CASE HISTORY: WHEN TREATMENT OF THE CONSTITUTIONAL IMBALANCE ALONE WAS ENOUGH

This case history illustrates how, sometimes, treatment on the Element of the constitutional imbalance is effective, even when the pathology lies in a different Element and Organs.

Sophie, who was thirteen years old, came for treatment because of her severe pre-menstrual syndrome. For at least a week before her period, she became aggressive and extremely moody.

Diagnosis: I diagnosed Liver *qi* stagnation and a constitutional imbalance in the Metal Element. Sophie's Wood pulse was wiry. Her voice was weeping, her colour was white and her Metal pulses were deficient.

Treatment: I decided to begin treatment by strengthening the Metal Element. I suspected that if Sophie's Metal Element were stronger, it would control Wood (via the controlling (*ke*) cycle) and that would reduce the Liver *qi* stagnation.

In the first treatment I used the *yuan* source points of the Organs related to Metal, LI 4 *hegu* and Lu 9 *taiyuan*. I noticed afterwards that the wiry quality on Sophie's Wood pulse had lessened. I continued using a variety of points on these channels at each treatment. Sophie's pre-menstrual syndrome was markedly improved after two months of weekly treatments. I never treated her Liver directly.

Combining treatment of the Five Element constitutional imbalance with treatment of the Organ/Pathogen patterns

There are certain instances when it is more likely the practitioner will need to combine these two styles of treatment, such as:

- when the child has a strong pathogen that has *not* originated in the Organs of the constitutional imbalance

- when there is a strong aetiological factor that particularly affects an Organ or Organs that are *not* related to the Element of the constitutional imbalance

- when the child was born with an inherited weakness in an Organ or Organs that are *not* related to the constitutional imbalance.

The following case histories illustrate when and how treatment of both the constitutional imbalance and the Organ/Pathogen patterns may be combined.

CASE HISTORY: WHEN TREATMENT OF THE ORGAN/ PATHOGEN PATTERNS ALONE WAS NOT ENOUGH

Treatment of the constitutional imbalance was used in this case because:

- treatment of the Organ/Pathogen pattern alone did not bring about a complete cure of the symptoms

- the main aetiology of the physical complaint was an internal cause of disease (i.e. intense emotions brought on by a break-up in the family)

- treatment of the Organ/Pathogen pattern did not bring about a change in the child's spirit.

Luke was nine years old and had suffered from headaches for the past two years. He rarely had more than a day at a time without a headache. The headaches had started when his father had, without warning, left when Luke was six. Luke came across as an unhappy boy, who rarely smiled or laughed.

Diagnosis and treatment: Luke's headaches were clearly due to Liver *qi* stagnation. His Wood pulses were wiry. My first treatment principle was to smooth Liver *qi*.

Luke's headaches showed some improvement immediately. They came less often, lasted less long and were less severe. However, they did not disappear completely. Moreover, Luke did not seem to change in himself at all. Despite my best efforts, I was never able to get him to spark up. I belatedly came to realise, based on Luke's predominant emotion, which was 'lack of joy', that his constitutional imbalance was in the Fire Element.

At Luke's fourth treatment, after smoothing his Liver *qi*, I then tonified his Pericardium and Triple Burner using the *yuan* source points Pc 7 *daling* and TB 4 *yangchi*.

After that treatment, Luke had a whole week without a headache. When he came back the following week, he told me quite enthusiastically about his fishing trip with his uncle. This was the first time I had seen him light up.

I continued smoothing Liver *qi* and using a variety of points to strengthen Luke's Fire Element. Luke went from strength to strength.

CASE HISTORY: WHEN TREATMENT OF THE CONSTITUTIONAL IMBALANCE ALONE WAS NOT ENOUGH

Treatment of the constitutional imbalance was used in this case because:

- the constitutional imbalance was in the Element related to the Organ patterns causing the main complaint
- there was a strong emotional component to the condition
- the child had not recovered from a prior acute illness in the expected way.

Lara (eight years old) had had a lot of time off school over the past year because of stomach aches. They had begun after an acute bout of gastroenteritis on a family holiday to Morocco when she was seven. The tummy aches were dull and came and went seemingly randomly. Her appetite was low.

Lara openly talked about hating school. She said that, if she could, she would happily stay at home with her mum all day. She had always been a 'Mummy's girl' and still often slept in her parents' bed at night.

Diagnosis and treatment: I diagnosed Lara as having an Earth constitutional imbalance. She had a yellow colour beside her eyes and a singing voice, and seemed to find it hard to accept sympathy. I thought that treating this would be enough to help her tummy aches, which I assumed were tied up in finding separation from her mum difficult and hating school.

I began by strengthening Lara's Earth Element with a variety of points on the Stomach and Spleen channels. I included several points which are known to affect the spirit. After four sessions Lara said that she felt more relaxed, found it easier going to school and had slept in her bed the whole night for the past two weeks. However, she was still getting the tummy aches.

I then added in points to clear a Lingering Pathogenic Factor of Damp, probably stemming from the gastroenteritis when she was seven. I continued strengthening her Earth Element. It was a combination of these two treatment principles that enabled both Lara and her stomach aches to get better.

Treatment techniques
Needles
Practitioners of Five Element constitutional acupuncture use two different needle techniques, 'tonification' and 'sedation'. Tonification is used far more frequently than sedation. That is because practitioners of this style are generally focused on strengthening the underlying constitutional imbalance. Deficiencies are far more common in the Element of the constitutional imbalance than excesses.[*]

See Chapter 31 for a fuller description of the child-friendly needle technique.

Tonification technique
Tonification is used to strengthen a child's *qi*. It involves inserting the needle to contact the child's *qi* and then immediately and quickly removing it. During the mere one to two seconds that the

---

[*] The exception to this is the treatment of a child with a Wood constitutional imbalance, when the practitioner is just as likely to use the sedation method as tonification.

needle is inserted, the practitioner should turn the needle 180 degrees in a clockwise direction. This style of needling is obviously particularly well suited to the treatment of young children, most of whom would find it difficult or impossible to lie still for any length of time.

Sedation technique

The sedation technique is used to clear an excess condition. When treating adults, practitioners of this style insert the needle and leave it in place for twenty to thirty minutes. This is obviously not possible when treating young children. Instead, the practitioner should insert the needle, turn it 360 degrees anti-clockwise and then withdraw it slowly.

When the child is old enough for the needles to be retained, the length of retention should be determined by the changes that take place on the pulse. Up until the teenage years, somewhere between three and ten minutes usually suffices.

Alternatives to needling

Any of the alternatives to needling discussed in Chapter 33 may be used to treat the constitutional imbalance. However, direct moxibustion deserves a special mention.

Moxibustion

Moxibustion is considered an important treatment technique in Five Element constitutional acupuncture. It is used to warm a patient who is cold, but also alongside or instead of needles as a method of tonification. Most commonly, the form of moxa used is that of small cones which are placed on the acupuncture points and lit.

For a discussion on the use of moxa generally in children, see Chapter 33.

Use of points

The points that are most commonly used in Five Element constitutional acupuncture are described later in this chapter and summarised in Table 30.1. The question remains as to how the practitioner goes about choosing which points to use in each treatment.

There are two main criteria which inform the point choice:

* **type of point:** whether the point is a *yuan* source point, back *shu* point, Element point, tonification point, etc.

* **name of point:** the name may inform the practitioner as to which level of the person the point is particularly suited to treating. For example, He 7 *shenmen* clearly treats the mind/ spirit of the person.

See Chapter 32 for other criteria used when choosing points in children.

Pairing points on the *yin* and the *yang* channels of the Element

When treating the Five Element constitutional imbalance, the practitioner will generally choose to needle one point on the channel of the *yang* Organ and one point on the channel of the *yin* Organ related to that Element. So, for example, if the constitutional imbalance is in Metal, she may choose to needle the *yuan* source points of the Lung and Large Intestine channels, Lu 9 *taiyuan* and LI 4 *hegu*. She will then take the pulse to ascertain whether the treatment has brought about the required change.

Before carrying out the treatment, the practitioner will have decided in what way she wants the pulses to change. It may be that all the pulses are deficient and the desired outcome is that they should all be stronger. Or it may be that one particular pulse position seems to be very different in quality or quantity to the rest and a key aim is for that position to become more like the others.

Variation of points

If treatment on a particular Element produces the desired changes in the child and to her pulse,* the practitioner will generally vary the points she uses each time she treats the child. For example, she may use the back *shu* points in one treatment, followed by the tonification points in the next and the *luo* junction point in the next. It is considered important in the practice of Five Element constitutional acupuncture to vary the point choice. Each point will have a subtly different impact on the *qi* of the child.

Table 30.1 Points commonly used in Five Element constitutional acupuncture

	Yuan source	Tonification	Sedation	Xi cleft	Luo junction	Horary	Back shu	Front mu
Liver	Liv 3	Liv 8	Liv 2	Liv 6	Liv 5	Liv 1	Bl 18	Liv 14
Gallbladder	GB 40	GB 43	GB 38	GB 36	GB 37	GB 41	Bl 19	GB 24
Heart	He 7	He 9	He 7	He 6	He 5	He 8	Bl 15	Ren 14
Small Intestine	SI 4	SI 3	SI 8	SI 6	SI 7	SI 5	Bl 27	Ren 4
Pericardium	Pc 7	Pc 9	Pc 7	Pc 4	Pc 6	Pc 8	Bl 14	Ren 17
Triple Burner	TB 4	TB 3	TB 10	TB 7	TB 5	TB 6	Bl 22	Ren 5
Spleen	Sp 3	Sp 2	Sp 5	Sp 8	Sp 4	Sp 3	Bl 20	Liv 13
Stomach	St 42	St 41	St 45	St 34	St 40	St 36	Bl 21	Ren 12
Lung	Lu 9	Lu 9	Lu 5	Lu 6	Lu 7	Lu 8	Bl 13	Lu 1
Large Intestine	LI 4	LI 11	LI 2	LI 7	LI 6	LI 1	Bl 25	St 25
Kidney	Ki 3	Ki 7	Ki 1	Ki 5	Ki 4	Ki 10	Bl 23	GB 25
Bladder	Bl 64	Bl 67	Bl 65	Bl 59	Bl 58	Bl 66	Bl 28	Ren 3

Intention

Simply needling a point that is thought to have a strong impact on the *shen* is, of course, not enough. Practitioners of all styles know that intention is important, but Five Element constitutional acupuncturists place a particularly high value on it. Sun Simiao wrote, 'Medicine is intention (*yi*). Those who are proficient at using intention are good doctors.'[6]

Many points have the ability to affect both the level of the body and *shen*. The intention of the practitioner is, to a large degree, what determines which aspect of the person will be affected. A practitioner may, for example, needle Liv 14 *qimen* (Gate of Hope) with the intention of moving *qi* to aid digestion. Or she may needle it on a depressed teenager with the intention of helping her to regain a sense of hope in the future. The clarity and focus of the practitioner is paramount. She must at all times hold an awareness of what she is trying to achieve in needling a particular point.

If the practitioner has employed great sensory acuity, intuition, clarity and focus whilst diagnosing the nature of the child's imbalance, she will have gained a sense of who the child is and of the nature of the imbalance in her spirit. A child, and even a young baby, will sense that this has taken place. They are hard to fool. The practitioner must hold an awareness of all these aspects of the child when she needles her in order to bring about the desired change in her spirit.**

---

* These may include a change in colour, sound, emotion or odour and a 'harmonisation' of the pulse. The child may have an increased sense of well-being and symptoms may improve.

** I refer the reader who is interested in ways of honing this skill to Chapter 6 of *Five Element Constitutional Acupuncture* by Hicks et al. (2011).

Spirit points

If the practitioner perceives that the problem resides at the level of the child's spirit, points that are known to be adept at treating this level of a person may need to be considered. Whilst any point on the body has the potential to bring about change in the child's mind and spirit, there are some points that have a heightened ability to achieve this.

Points that primarily affect the spirit are most often used on the channels of the Organs related to the Element of the child's constitutional imbalance.

Whichever points are chosen, the child's spirit will only respond if there is rapport between practitioner and child, and if the practitioner has focused intention whilst needling. For a further discussion of these issues, please see the sections on building rapport at the end of Chapters 16 to 20.

Broad categories of spirit points

- Spirit points on the head, face and neck may be used when the child needs to reconnect with 'the *qi* of the heavens'. This connection may be blocked because of a pathogen, such as Phlegm or Heat, or because there is not enough clear *yang* in the upper part of the body. Symptoms may include depression, lack of inspiration, feelings of hopelessness, loss of purpose or agitation.

- Spirit points on the chest or upper back may be used when the child is struggling in his relationships with other people. Points in this region tend to strengthen the Organs of the Fire Element, which must be strong if a child is going to thrive in his relationships. Symptoms may include vulnerability, lack of emotional robustness, shyness, inappropriate openness, avoiding contact with friends and family, and difficulty coping with social situations.

- Spirit points in the Lower and Middle Burners may be used when the child is not rooted to the earth. Symptoms may include anxiety, insecurity or hyperactivity.

Table 30.2 shows some points that are known to particularly affect the spirit.

Table 30.2 Points whose names contain reference to the spirit

Tian (heavenly)	*Shen*	*Ling* (spirit)
LI 17 *tianding* Heavenly Vessel	GB 13 *benshen* Root of the Spirit	GB 18 *chengling* Receiving Spirit
Sp 18 *tianxi* Heavenly Stream	He 7 *shenmen* Spirit Gate	Ht 2 *qingling* Blue-Green Spirit
SI 11 *tianzong* Heavenly Ancestor	Bl 44 *shentang* Spirit Hall	Ht 4 *lingdao* Spirit Path
Bl 7 *tongtian* Heavenly Connection	Ki 23 *shenfeng* Spirit Seal	Ki 24 *lingxu* Spirit Burial Ground
Pc 2 *tianquan* Heavenly Spring	Ki 25 *shencang* Spirit Storehouse	Du 10 *lingtai* Spirit Tower
TB 10 *tianjing* Heavenly Well	Ren 8 *shenque* Spirit Gate	
TB 15 *tianliao* Heavenly Foramen	Du 11 *shendao* Spirit Path	
	Du 24 *shenting* Spirit Hall	

Outer back *shu* points

The outer back *shu* points have a particular effect on the spirit of each Organ. The names of the points contain words which refer to a part of a building, such as 'dwelling' or 'abode' (see Table 30.3). This suggests that these points help to give each spirit a 'residence' if it is agitated or depleted.

Table 30.3 Outer back *shu* points

Name	Number
Door of *Po pohu*	Bl 42
Shen Hall *shentang*	Bl 44
Hun Gate *hunmen*	Bl 47
Yi Dwelling *yishe*	Bl 49
Zhi Room *zhishi*	Bl 52

Kidney chest points

The points on the chest from Ki 22 to Ki 27 are often referred to as the 'Kidney chest points' (see Table 30.4). Although on the Kidney channel, these points come after the Exit point (Ki 22 *bulang*) and have as strong a connection with the Organs of the Upper Burner as they do the Kidneys. Chapter 16 of the *Ling Shu* alludes to this fact when it describes how 'the *qi* entering the Kidneys and flowing into the pericardium, it scatters in the chest...'[7]

Three of the Kidney chest points have the word *shen* or *ling* (terms which refer to the spirit of the Heart) in their name. These points are particularly helpful to assist a child who is struggling with her ability to relate to other people in some way.

Table 30.4 Kidney chest points

Ki 22 *bulang* Walking on the Verandah
Ki 23 *shenfeng* Shen Seal
Ki 24 *lingxu* Spirit Burial Ground
Ki 25 *shencang* Spirit Storehouse
Ki 26 *yuzhong* Elegant Centre
Ki 27 *shu fu* Central Treasury

Window of Heaven points

This group of points, listed in Table 30.5, is given in Chapters 2, 5 and 21 of the *Ling Shu*. Most of them contain in their name the word *tian*, which is usually translated as heaven. They are all positioned on the upper part of the body, which has always been regarded as being resonant with Heaven. These points are indicated when a child has become disconnected with the inherent beauty and meaning in life.

Table 30.5 Window of Heaven points

Fire	SI 16 *tian chuang* Heavenly Window
	SI 17 *tian rong* Heavenly Appearance
	Pc 1 *tian chi* Heavenly Pond
	TB 16 *tian you* Heavenly Window
Earth	St 9 *renying* People Welcome
Metal	Lu 3 tian fu Heavenly Treasury
	LI 18 *futu* Support the Prominence
Water	Bl 10 *tian zhu* Heavenly Pillar
Ren mai	Ren 22 *tian tu* Heavenly Chimney
Du mai	Du 16 *fengfu* Wind Treasury

These are by no means the only points which may be used to treat the spirit. However, they are some of the most commonly used. The reader is encouraged to read other texts on point interpretations and to gain as much experience as possible through using a wide variety of points.

Five Element blocks to treatment

Five Element constitutional acupuncturists recognise certain 'blocks' that may present in a patient. These blocks often cause significant physical or psychological problems and may prevent treatment on the constitutional imbalance being effective.

The four blocks are:

- Aggressive Energy

- Possession

- Husband–Wife imbalance

- Entry–Exit blocks.

It is not within the scope of this book to discuss each block in detail, and this has been explained excellently in Chapter 30 of *Five Element Constitutional Acupuncture* by Hicks et al. (2011). However, I will briefly discuss here the presence of Aggressive Energy and Possession, which, in my experience, are the blocks most commonly found in children. I have rarely found a Husband–Wife imbalance in a child.*

Entry–Exit blocks are relatively common in children, but their manifestation and treatment does not differ from that of adults, so I refer the reader to the text *Five Element Constitutional Acupuncture*, as mentioned above, for further information on them.

Aggressive Energy

Aggressive Energy is understood as evil or unhealthy (*xie*) *qi*. It may be present in one or more of the *yin* Organs and it travels between the *yin* Organs along the *ke* cycle (as opposed to upright (*zheng*) *qi* which travels along the *sheng* cycle).

Causes of Aggressive Energy in children

Aggressive Energy may arise either from an emotional trauma or from an External Pathogenic Factor which invades the body, which may be climatic or may come in the form of medication or recreational drugs. In children, it most commonly arises:

- in the womb or during labour if the mother requires strong medication or suffers a shock

- after a vaccination

- after a strong, sudden trauma or an ongoing, severely stressful emotional situation

- in serious illness.

Diagnosing Aggressive Energy in children

The practitioner may suspect the presence of Aggressive Energy in a child if:

- there are unexpected or unusual reactions to treatment

- there is a serious physical or psychological condition.

---

* The only time I have come across a Husband–Wife imbalance in a child was in an eight-year-old who had a terminal illness.

I also look for Aggressive Energy by performing the paediatric *tui na* technique *jizhu* (see Chapter 34) along the Bladder channel on the back. If the area around the back *shu* points related to a particular *yin* Organ 'pink up' more strongly or quickly than others, this suggests there may be Aggressive Energy in that Organ.

Treatment of Aggressive Energy in children

The usual treatment of Aggressive Energy in adults is to shallowly insert needles in the back *shu* points related to each of the *yin* Organs and to leave them in place for as long as it takes the erythema to clear. However, this is not practical in most young children for obvious reasons. Instead, I have found the following methods effective for clearing Aggressive Energy:

- With a smooth shell or the back of a spoon, rub the area around the back *shu* point in a lateral direction (i.e. away from the spine towards the flanks) until the colour that comes up no longer intensifies.

- Leave a retained needle (see Chapter 33) on the point for the duration of the treatment.

Outcome of treatment

The practitioner may find that, after clearing Aggressive Energy, long-standing physical or emotional symptoms clear up. The child may feel much better in herself and the parent may report a 'positive' change in the child's behaviour or moods.

CASE HISTORY: AGGRESSIVE ENERGY

A nine-year-old girl with chronic fatigue syndrome who had a Metal constitutional imbalance used to become hyperactive for a couple of days after treatment. After clearing Aggressive Energy from the Lung, this abnormal reaction to treatment stopped. It also marked a turning point in her health, and she began to regain her energy.

Possession

To a Five Element acupuncturist, the term 'Possession' denotes a person having lost control of their mind or spirit in some way. This may manifest as obsessive or ungrounded thinking, or unusual, reckless behaviour.

Causes of Possession in children

In children, the most common causes of Possession are:

- shocks or prolonged emotional instability

- physical trauma

- drugs or alcohol (in teenagers).

Of course, not everybody becomes possessed after experiencing one of these factors. Possession usually occurs in a child whose *shen* is not robust. Hsu Ling-t'ai said, 'If a person's essence and spirit are firmly established, no evil outside of the body will venture an assault. But whenever that which protects the essence and spirit fails, the harmful agents will collect in its place.'[8]

Diagnosing Possession

As Hicks et al.[9] note, each patient is possessed in her own unique way. The practitioner is often struck that there is something 'unusual' or 'other' about a child who is possessed. Some common manifestations of Possession are:

- the practitioner feels the child cannot be reached or that she is disconnected in some way

- the child appears to have 'veiled' eyes
- the child has obsessive thoughts or behaviours
- the child has repeated, terrifying dreams.

Treatment of Possession

The treatment of Possession is to use one of two possible formulae of particular points. The first is called the Internal Dragons, and should be used when the cause of the Possession is internal. The seven Internal Dragon points are:

- Extra point 0.25 cun below Ren 15 *jiuwei*
- St 25 *tianshu*
- St 32 *futu*
- St 41 *jiexi.*

Less commonly used in children are the seven External Dragon points, which are indicated when the cause of the Possession was something that came from outside, such as a physical trauma or drugs. The seven External Dragon points are:

- Du 20 *baihui*
- Bl 11 *dazhu*
- Bl 23 *shenshu*
- Bl 61 *pucan.*

In both cases, the needles are left in for approximately fifteen to twenty minutes.

In a young child, this of course may not be possible. In this case, the best alternative is to use press-spheres or retained needles for a similar length of time or a little longer (see Chapter 33 for a discussion on the use of press-spheres and retained needles).

Outcome of Possession treatment

A child often experiences a profound change in his spirit after having a Possession treatment. He may feel 'more himself', find he can relax in his class at school where before he could not, or be able to relate to his siblings in an easier way. Both parent and child are often astounded by the change that has taken place.

CASE HISTORY: POSSESSION

The mother of Lenny, a four-year-old boy, told me tearfully on the telephone that she felt she had 'lost' her son. In the past six months he seemed to be in a world of his own, had cut off from the rest of the family, endlessly chatted to himself and had stopped responding when he was spoken to. She said this did not seem out of defiance, but simply that he was 'in another world' and really did not hear. I asked her what was going on when this happened and she said that her mother, who lived with the family, had died suddenly of a heart attack in front of Lenny.

When Lenny came for his first appointment, I immediately recognised how his mother had described him. He did not seem present at all and I struggled to have a conversation with him. I used the seven Internal Dragon points to treat Lenny, placing a retained needle on each one for twenty minutes.

Lenny went home and, unusually, slept for fourteen hours that night. His mother said that it was 'as if a miracle had happened'. The family sat at breakfast the following morning and Lenny chatted away to the family as he used to before his grandmother's death. As his mum said, 'He came back to us!'

SUMMARY

» Sometimes a practitioner will treat only the Five Element constitutional imbalance, and sometimes it will be combined with treatment of the relevant Organ/Pathogen patterns.

» The tonification needle technique is used more commonly than the sedation needle technique by Five Element constitutional acupuncturists.

» Moxibustion is often used to tonify, as well as to treat Cold.

» Points are often chosen according to type and name.

» When treating the Five Element constitutional imbalance, a point from the *yin* and the *yang* channels of the related Organs are often combined.

» It is considered important to vary the points used when treating the Five Element constitutional imbalance.

» It is usual to incorporate only one or two spirit points into each treatment. Very often, the practitioner will use one spirit point on each channel in an Element.

» Spirit points on the channels related to the child's constitutional imbalance are most commonly chosen, as well as points that are known to affect the Organs related to the Element of the constitutional imbalance, such as Ren 14 *juque* for a child with a Fire constitutional imbalance.

» The blocks to treatment most commonly seen in children are Aggressive Energy, Possession and Entry–Exit blocks.

• Chapter 31 •

CHILD-FRIENDLY NEEDLING

The topics discussed in this chapter are:

- The thorny issue of needles and children
- Length and gauge of needles
- Type of needle
- Preparing for needling
- Insertion technique
- The child's response to the needle insertion
- Obtaining *deqi*
- Manipulation of the needle
- Retaining the needles
- Number of needles

The thorny issue of needles and children

The widely held perception that needles hurt and would be traumatic for a baby or young child is probably the biggest barrier to more children having acupuncture treatment in the West. The reality is that, when practised in the right way, acupuncture can be almost painless and is accepted by the vast majority of children.

However, there is a small percentage of children for whom being needled is genuinely terrifying. There are several reasons to avoid pushing a child to be needled when it is distressing for him:

- The child may spend the time between treatments worrying about the needles at the next treatment. This is not conducive to improving his health.

- If the child does not enjoy the treatment, he may persistently moan to his parents about the fact he has to come. Over time, busy and overstretched parents may be worn down by this and stop treatment prematurely. The family are then back in the position they started from and the end result is that we have not helped the child.

- Distress and upset cause strong movements of *qi* which are bound to negatively impact the efficacy of the treatment.

Having said this, there are odd occasions when the possible benefits of needling a child are so great, and the outcome of not needling them so dire, that it is necessary to do it even when the child shows some resistance. For example, acupuncture during an acute asthma attack can be nothing short of miraculous. If this prevents the child having to go into hospital and be given a nebuliser then it is nearly always worth doing. Even on these occasions, however, there will be times when the child's resistance is so strong that the practitioner feels the child has plainly not given his consent to be treated and this should always be respected. The practitioner should also be guided by what the parent wants, especially with younger children.

Length and gauge of needles

Very fine needles are best used when treating children and are sufficient to bring about the required change. The length and gauge of needles used is partly a matter of personal preference for the practitioner. However, Table 31.1 gives a useful guide.

Table 31.1 Length and gauge of needles according to age

Age	Length	Diameter (mm)
0–3 years old	15 mm	0.14 to 0.16
3–8 years old	15 mm or 30 mm	0.16 to 0.18
8–12 years old	30 mm	0.16 to 0.18
12 years old plus	30 mm	0.18

Type of needle

Japanese needles have particularly good insertion characteristics and, whilst the technique of the practitioner is the most important factor, these very fine needles also help to reduce any pain on insertion.

Preparing for needling

It can be helpful to remember 'the four Ps' before needling a child for the first time.[10]

- **Prepare the practitioner (i.e. yourself!):** A child will sense if the practitioner is rushed, cross about something or preoccupied.

- **Prepare the parent:** If the parent is concerned and anxious about their child being needled, the child will be anxious. It can be helpful to needle the parent in a 'non-point' so that they can then reassure the child that it feels all right.

- **Prepare the patient:** When a child is old enough to understand, the practitioner needs to explain clearly what she would like to do and to gain her consent.* A young child cannot usually take in lots of information all at once, so it helps to break things down into bite-sized chunks. Explaining that you will start with one point and then see how it goes reassures the child that she has a get-out clause if she needs it.

- **Prepare the point:** Rubbing a point before needling reduces the chances of a strong needle sensation.

Insertion technique

There is no one way of inserting a needle that is right for all children, or indeed for all practitioners. The best method of needling a child is usually for the practitioner to adapt the method that she uses on adults. This is because one of the most important criteria is for the practitioner to be

---

* Gaining the child's consent must be done without the practitioner being hesitant. At the same time as explaining what she would like to do, the practitioner should have a firm intention that this *is* what is going to happen. If the child senses the practitioner is unsure about needling her, she will feel unsure about it herself.

comfortable, relaxed and adept when needling a child. To learn a new insertion technique may reduce confidence levels in the practitioner, and this will be detrimental.

Having said that, needle technique is even more important when treating children than when treating adults, and therefore it is an area that the practitioner may need to focus on. There is no substitute for practice and there are no shortcuts to developing the skill of painless needle insertion. The practitioner should practise on herself or on a friend or family member using a 'non-point' until she can reliably insert the needle painlessly.

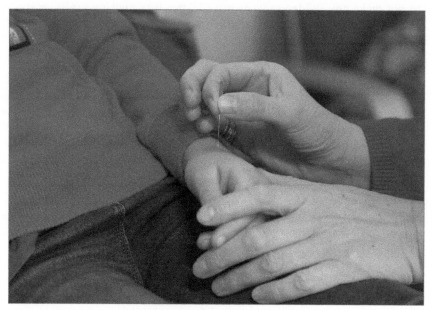

Child being needled without a guide tube

Guide tube insertion versus non-guide tube insertion

Every paediatric acupuncturist will have his own view on whether or not it is best to needle a child using a guide tube or not. For example, Scott[11] does not use a guide tube whereas Birch[12] does. As with most things, there are pros and cons of each technique (see Table 31.2).

Table 31.2 Guide tube versus non-guide tube needle insertion

	Pros	Cons
Guide tube insertion	Insertion can be made less 'sudden' by tapping the needle in Pressure of guide tube on skin can distract child from the sensation of the needle	Guide tube may be one too many things to contend with along with needle, wriggly baby, etc. Hard to get accuracy of location on small points
Non-guide tube insertion	A well-executed insertion can be quick and painless Practitioner does not have to manage guide tube (as well as needle and child)	Can be painful when executed badly

Whilst every practitioner needs to find their own way, there are a few guidelines that may be useful:

- **Be open with the child about what you are doing:** Whilst it is true that, with good distraction techniques, it may be possible to needle a child without him having any idea what you are doing, if this approach backfires then the child will lose all trust in the practitioner. Even if the needling is painless, a child frequently has a strong emotional response to a particular point being needled. This means the child will know something has happened about which he was not forewarned. The exception to this is obviously a baby, when it is not possible to explain to him what you are about to do.

- **Do not make any sudden movements:** Children hate anything sudden or shocking. Therefore, the moment of needle insertion should never feel to her that it comes out of the blue. It should be seamlessly woven into the practitioner's interaction with the child. The interaction should include a level of rapport, conversation and touch.

- **Do not make the needling the 'main event':** The moment of needling should not define the child's experience of being in the treatment room. It should be a relatively small part of what takes place. The practitioner should avoid creating any sense of a build-up to the needle insertion. The more focus that is put on this unknown and potentially frightening event, the more the child will feel it as 'a big thing'. The aim is to walk a middle ground between preparing the child and seamlessly integrating the needling into the whole experience.

- **Do not minimise the child's experience of pain:** If a child says that the needle hurt him, it is never a good idea to tell him that it did not hurt! Pain is a very complex phenomenon and, even if the practitioner is convinced that her needle insertion technique is absolutely painless, the child may still have experienced the moment as painful.

  A better approach is to acknowledge to the child that he felt some pain, and then to point out to him that, despite this, he was able to manage it. If the child is old enough, it is also useful to help him distinguish between pain and discomfort. The vocabulary of extremes (I 'hate' sausages, I had the 'worst' day ever, this is 'impossible') may come more easily to a child than that of the grey area in the middle (Sausages are not my favourite food, I had some tricky moments today, I am finding this challenging). By offering a child some words to describe something that was bearable even though it was not wholly pleasant may help him to feel he can tolerate it.

A FEW OTHER TIPS THAT MAY BE USEFUL WHEN NEEDLING A CHILD

» A child who is verbal will usually enjoy being involved in the treatment. Explain to the child that you need her help for the magic to work. When you have tapped the needle in, you are going to say the magic words 'bippety, bippety bop' together. This makes things fun, distracts the child from being needled and helps her to feel that she is not having something done 'to her' but that you and she are doing something together.

» Sound effects work wonders. When using a guide tube insertion, it can be helpful for the practitioner to start saying 'tap, tap, tap' when the guide tube is resting on the skin but before she taps the needle in. The child is then focused on the sound rather than the sensation on her skin.

» Keeping eye contact with the child (when working on the front torso and limbs) helps to gain trust and keep her involved in the process.

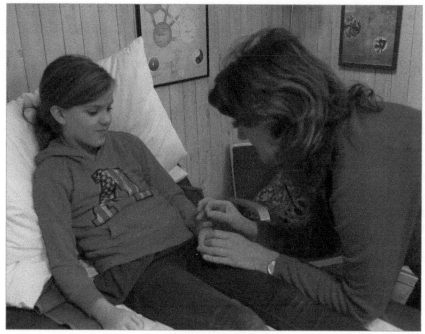

Child being needled

The child's response to the needle insertion

Children with different patterns of imbalance show tendencies towards certain reactions to the needle insertion. Therefore, a knowledge of which patterns of imbalance a child has can help a practitioner to adapt her needle technique accordingly.

The main tendencies are:

- **Phlegm/Damp:** A child with a lot of Phlegm tends not to feel the needle strongly, if at all. His sensations are dulled. It is a sign of progress when he starts to be more aware of the needles.

- **Deficient:** A child with *qi* deficiency may also not feel the needle insertion strongly, or at least not have sufficient *qi* to react strongly to it. Again, it is a sign of progress when he starts to protest more strongly to the needles.

- **Kidney deficiency:** A child with Kidney deficiency may be genuinely fearful of needles and become truly upset. It is usually best to avoid using needles at all on this child. Again, as treatment progresses, he may become more willing to try a needle and to tolerate being needled.

- **Weak *shen*:** A child with a weak *shen*, whether inherited or due to Blood deficiency, may feel easily startled by a sudden needle insertion. With this child, it is often better to do a series of gentle taps with a guide tube in order to insert the needle.

- **Qi stagnation:** A child with *qi* stagnation may have a sudden and strong outpouring of emotion on being needled. The needle has the effect of stirring up an emotion that has been 'stuck'. Ideally, the practitioner should calm and reassure the child whilst the needle is left in and let the child settle. However, in some cases it may be necessary to take the needle out.

Obtaining *deqi*

It is obviously not possible to rely on feedback from a baby or young child as to what he is feeling. Not only may he be pre-verbal but asking him what he is feeling draws his attention to the needle. This is often counter-productive, at least in young children. With experience, the practitioner will often sense that the needle is being 'grabbed' and this will indicate that *deqi* has been found. However, there are other signs to look out for too.

When *deqi* is obtained on a baby, his response is often to stop wriggling and to become inwardly and outwardly still for a second or two. It is almost as if the baby momentarily goes into a different 'zone'. He may also break out into a smile. If the process is approached in the right way, and the baby is neither hungry nor tired at the time, he rarely cries as a response to being needled.

When treating an older child, he may feel empowered by being involved in the process and enjoy describing the different sensations he feels as he is needled.* The practitioner must decide with each child whether it works better to involve the child in the process or trust herself enough to decide whether *deqi* has been obtained.

When treating teenagers, the vast majority are able to fully engage with the process of being needled and are able to differentiate between the feeling of the needle and the feeling of *deqi*.

Manipulation of the needle

The practitioner must be very clear before he inserts the needle whether he wants to tonify the *qi* or reduce an excess. The needle should then be manipulated, as with adults, in the appropriate way. Most children respond quickly and strongly to any intervention and therefore it usually suffices to manipulate the needle very mildly. If the condition is severe and the child is robust, stronger manipulation can be used.

Retaining the needles

Babies and toddlers

It is not necessary (let alone possible) to retain needles on a child up to the age of four years old, purely because he will wriggle and move. The needle should be withdrawn as soon as the required manipulation has been performed.

School-age children and teenagers

It is possible to successfully treat children up to their teenage years without retaining any needles. However, some children, even as young as four or five years old, can tolerate needles being retained for a few minutes. If the child is of an age where he cannot be relied upon to keep still, the parent can be asked to place her hand on the limb that is being needled. If there is a needle retained in more than one limb, the practitioner can watch over the second limb.

The advantage of being able to retain a needle is that it means less manipulation of the needle is necessary. Some children prefer to have the needle left in for a few minutes rather than have a few seconds of manipulation. Other children prefer the opposite. The practitioner should use whichever method is best suited to the child.

If the needle is retained, it is usually only necessary to retain it for a short period of time. For a child who is five years old, three or four minutes is usually sufficient. The length of time the

---

* Children often come up with the most wonderful descriptions of *deqi*. Amongst my favourite are 'That felt like the gooey bit in the middle of a chocolate cookie' and 'That gave me a buzzy feeling under my skin'. Even when the sensation is not pleasant, naming it can help the child to tolerate it. One good example given by a ten-year-old boy was 'That was a bit like finding a green vegetable in the middle of a gooey cheese pie'.

needle is retained can be slowly increased with age. With teenagers, needles may be retained for up to fifteen or twenty minutes.

The criteria which should be used to decide on the length of time of retention are:

- the age of the child
- the maturity of the child
- the stature of the child (the bigger and more developed the child, the longer the needle can be retained)
- the strength of *qi* of the child (the stronger the *qi*, the longer the needle can be retained)
- the nature of the condition (the fuller the condition, the longer the needle should be retained).

Table 31.3 gives a rough guide to needle retention times.

Table 31.3 Needle retention time according to age

Age	Suggested time of needle retention
0–4 years old	No retention
4–8 years old	No retention or retention for three or four minutes
8–12 years old	Retention for up to ten minutes if necessary
13 years plus	Retention for up to fifteen to twenty minutes if necessary

 Some children become upset or agitated by looking at the needle when it is retained, even though they cannot feel it. When this is the case, the best thing is to distract their attention from it by reading a story or chatting.

Number of needles

A child, especially below the age of seven, usually needs minimum intervention. Therefore, only a few points need to be used. Two points per treatment is often sufficient. Furthermore, using too many points in a treatment may produce an adverse reaction.[*]

Needling unilaterally (in nearly all cases) is just as effective as needling bilaterally. This is particularly useful in the treatment of children, where the fewer needles used the better.

The criteria that influence the number of needles used per treatment are shown in Figure 31.1.

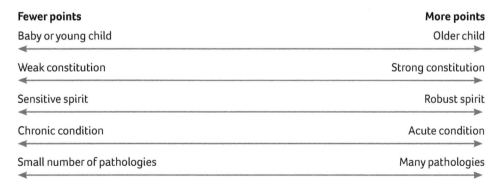

Fewer points	More points
Baby or young child	Older child
Weak constitution	Strong constitution
Sensitive spirit	Robust spirit
Chronic condition	Acute condition
Small number of pathologies	Many pathologies

Figure 31.1 Number of needles used per treatment

---

[*] Birch writes at length on the 'dosage' of treatment in Chapter 4 of *Shonishin: Japanese Pediatric Acupuncture* (2011).

SUMMARY

» The vast majority of children accept being needled.

» For those who do not, the practitioner needs to find other ways of delivering the treatment.

» The practitioner should prepare herself, the parent, the patient and the point before needling.

» The practitioner needs to find a way of needling children that she feels confident about, and which is as close to painless as possible.

» Needles are rarely retained on children below the age of approximately seven or eight.

» It is easy to over-treat a child. Very few points should be used during each treatment.

Chapter 32

POINTS COMMONLY USED TO TREAT CHILDREN

The topics discussed in this chapter are:

- Choosing points
- Points commonly used to treat children

Choosing points

The practitioner's approach to choosing points when treating children should be based on somewhat different criteria than when treating adults:

- The treatment of children has to be approached in a very practical way. Points that are accessible should be used over ones which are not. For example, if a baby is happily lying on his back, then it would make sense to choose a point on one of his limbs or front torso, rather than moving him onto his front to access a point on the back, as the process of doing this may make him unhappy or cross. There are times when only one point will do. Usually, however, there is more than one point that the practitioner may use to achieve her desired treatment outcome.

- As discussed in Chapter 2, the channel system and points are not fully developed until approximately the age of seven or eight. There may be little discernible difference in impact, therefore, between one point on a channel and the next. Consequently, the practitioner may be guided in her point choice by the degree of discomfort that a point may induce in the child, and the location of the point, as much as the action of the point.

- The paediatric acupuncturist is likely to turn to more commonly used points and fewer rarely used points than when treating adults. In the still-maturing channel system, there may be more *qi* available at points such as the *yuan* source points and points which are known to have a widespread and particularly potent effect, such as St 36 *zusanli*.

Points commonly used to treat children

This section includes a description of points which are relied upon more heavily in paediatric acupuncture than in adult acupuncture and of which some readers may therefore be unfamiliar. It also includes some points that are especially important for the paediatric acupuncturist because they are used in conditions to which children are especially prone. Of course, the full repertoire of acupuncture points may be used on a child. The reader is referred to a text on the locations and uses of points such as *A Manual of Acupuncture* by Deadman et al. (1998).

For further discussion of particular points used in the treatment of children see Chapter 30.

Sifeng (M-UE-9)

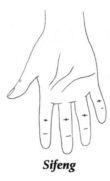

Sifeng

Location: The *sifeng* points are a group of extra points located on the palmar surface of the hand, at the midpoints of the transverse creases of the proximal interphalangeal joints of the four fingers.

Action: The action of the *sifeng* points is to dissipate accumulation in the digestive system. The result of this is that the baby or infant will often have a succession of foul-smelling and sometimes explosive bowel movements during the twenty-four hours after the treatment. Less frequently, he may also vomit too. Of course, both of these outcomes are a sign that the accumulation has been successfully dispelled. However, it may alarm the parent, who should be warned beforehand that this may happen.

Indications: Accumulation in the digestive system may manifest in a child as Accumulation Disorder, which may lead to common symptoms such as irregular bowel movements, abdominal pain, vomiting, cranky mood and poor sleep (see Chapter 27 for further discussion of Accumulation Disorder).

Method of use: All four points should be needled, one after the other. Needling each of these four points once on one hand constitutes a treatment. The hand of the baby or infant should be firmly held, palm facing upwards. The practitioner should prick each of the four points, in quick succession.

It is preferable to needle these points without using a guide tube. This is because speed is of the essence. With some skill and practice, it is possible for the practitioner to have needled all four points before the baby or infant has had the time to realise that he does not like the feel of it. Sound effects and funny faces also help the process.

If the treatment needs to be repeated at a further session, then the alternative hand should be used.

Contraindications: Due to the fact that *sifeng* has a strong dispersing action, it should not be used in cases of pure deficiency.

Frequency of use: Although it may be necessary to use the *sifeng* points repeatedly during an acute condition, in general they should be used sparingly. There are two reasons for this. First, if overused, they may begin to deplete the *qi* of the child because of their dispersing action. Second, if the child is developing Accumulation Disorder, then it is likely that his diet needs changing.

Dingchuan (M-BW-1)

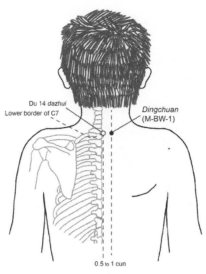

Du 14 dazhui
Lower border of C7

Dingchuan
(M-BW-1)

0.5 to 1 cun

Dingchuan

Location: *Dingchuan* is located 0.5 to 1.0 cun lateral to Du 14 *dazhui*, below the spinous process of the seventh cervical vertebra.

Action: *Dingchuan* is used in the treatment of acute asthma, in order to calm wheezing. It is a valuable point when treating a child during an asthma attack.

Method of use: The point should be needled bilaterally with the child sitting up on the couch. The practitioner should intermittently perform a reduction technique on the needles. In some cases, it is enough just for the needles to be left in and no reduction done.

Once the needles have been inserted into *dingchuan*, the practitioner should then needle whichever other points are indicated, for example Lu 6 *kongzui*, Bl 13 *feishu* and Ren 17 *shanzhong*. If the child is too young to sit still, the practitioner may need to needle *dingchuan* with the reduction technique for as long as is possible and then take the needles out. In a slightly older child, the needles may be able to be left in if the parent sits right beside the child to make sure that he does not try to lie down.

In nearly all cases, the child's acute asthma will start to calm within a few minutes of *dingchuan* being needled. At the end of the treatment, the practitioner may place a press-sphere or retained needle on the point, having given instructions to the parent to remove it and safely dispose of it later (see Chapter 33).

RED FLAGS: ASTHMA

It should be remembered that an asthma attack is a potentially life-threatening situation. In some cases, the most appropriate course of action is for the child to be taken to hospital immediately. When practical, **dingchuan** may be needled whilst the child is waiting for medical intervention.

Bailao (M-HN-30)

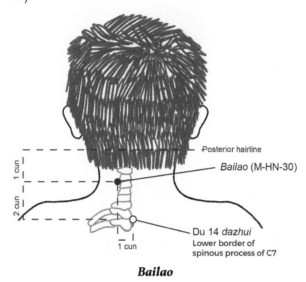

Bailao

Location: *Bailao* is located on the back of the neck, 2 cun superior to Du 14 *dazhui* and 1 cun lateral to the midline.

Action: *Bailao* has the effect of softening Thick Phlegm, particularly in the upper part of the body.

Indications: Thick Phlegm in children is often related to the presence of a Lingering Pathogenic Factor and may cause a wide range of symptoms (see Chapter 27). When located in the upper part of the body, it may be involved in chronic or recurrent ear problems or tonsillitis, blocked sinuses, chronic cough, asthma or headaches.

Method of use: The point should be needled with a sedation or reduction needle technique. The needle may or may not be retained depending on the age of the child. *Bailao* should be treated in conjunction with other indicated points depending on the patterns involved.

Pigen

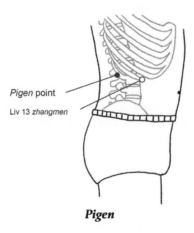

Pigen

Location: *Pigen* is found 3.5 cun lateral to the spinous process of the lumbar vertebra, in a depression below the margin of the twelfth rib, not quite as far as GB 25 *jingmen*.[13]

Action: *Pigen* has the effect of softening Thick Phlegm and dispelling accumulation. It is especially effective at softening Thick Phlegm in the digestive system or the lower part of the body.

Indications: Thick Phlegm in children is often related to the presence of a Lingering Pathogenic Factor and may cause a wide range of symptoms (see Chapter 27). When located in the Middle or Lower Burner, it may be involved in chronic or recurrent abdominal pain, food allergies or bowel symptoms.

Uranaetei

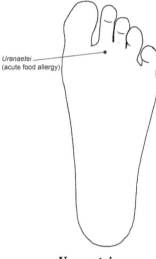

Uranaetei

Location: *Uranaetei* is found on the sole of the foot proximal to the second toe.

Action: This point may be used to treat acute symptoms of the gastro-intestinal system, including vomiting and diarrhoea, which may derive from a number of different sources, such as food poisoning or food allergy.

Method of use: Direct moxibustion only is used. Cones should be applied to the point bilaterally, and then directed to the foot that takes longer to feel the heat at that point. Moxa should continue to be applied until both feet have felt the heat three times.[14]

Du 12 *shenzhu*

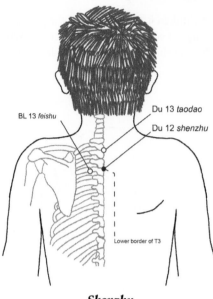

Shenzhu

Location: Du 12 *shenzhu* is located on the midline of the upper back, between the spinous processes of the third and fourth vertebrae.

Action: In the Japanese acupuncture tradition, Du 12 *shenzhu* is used in the treatment of nearly all paediatric conditions. Birch[15] explains that historically the point was treated with moxa to help prevent illness and to help children recover from illness. This point often has a strong calming effect on children, which ties in with the TCM view of the actions of this point, one of which is that it calms the spirit.[16]

SUMMARY

» The practitioner should employ a flexible approach when choosing points to use on children, taking into account the practicalities of locating the point, the degree of discomfort it may cause and the preferences of the child.

» The four *sifeng* points on one hand constitute a treatment.

» *Sifeng* points should not be used on a deficient child.

» *Bailao* softens Phlegm affecting the upper part of the body.

» *Pigen* softens Phlegm in the lower part of the body.

» Du 12 *shenzhu* has a strong action on calming the *shen* of the child.

• Chapter 33 •

ALTERNATIVES TO NEEDLING
· ·

The techniques discussed in this chapter are:

- Moxibustion

- Laser pens

- Microcurrent stimulation

- *Gua sha*

- Cupping

- Acupressure

- Press-spheres

- Retained (semi-permanent) needles

- Auricular acupuncture

Moxibustion

The use of moxibustion is invaluable in the treatment of children. This is because so many children suffer from Cold and/or deficient pathologies.

Reasons to use moxibustion

There are four main uses of moxa in the treatment of children:

- **Expel Cold:** Moxa may be used to expel full Cold in both acute conditions, such as Wind-Cold in the Lungs, and chronic conditions, such as Cold in the digestive system.

- **Warm *qi* and *yang*:** Moxa may be used to warm *qi* and *yang*. It may be used instead of or alongside needles for this purpose. In young children, moxa alone is often enough and can be a convenient alternative for a child for whom the thought of needles creates anxiety. The *qi* of a particular Organ may be warmed by using moxa on a point on the related channel. An area of the body, such as the stomach or the lower back, may also be targeted.*

- **Stimulate an acupuncture point:** Moxa may be used to stimulate an acupuncture point, even when the *qi* of that channel and Organ are not particularly Cold, but as long as they are not particularly Hot.

- **Draw Heat downwards:** Moxa may also be used to draw deficient Heat downwards in the child's body. For example, the child may be Kidney deficient with Empty Heat rising up to the Heart and agitating the *shen*. It can be beneficial to use moxa on a point such as Ki 1 *yongquan* to draw Heat down from the Heart and strengthen the Kidneys in the process.

---

* Scott (personal conversation) has the simple yet clear rule of thumb that moxa may be used on any part of the body that feels cold and may not be used on any part that feels warm or hot.

Suitable methods of moxibustion

The method of moxa used with children will be partly determined by the practitioner's personal preference but should always be guided by what is practical considering the age and nature of the child.

Moxa stick

A moxa stick may be held over a point or an area of the body. In a child who is too young to verbalise when it feels too hot, a finger should be placed either side of the point so that the practitioner can easily keep a check on the pace at which it is warming up. If an area such as the abdomen is being warmed, then the practitioner should place the palm of her hand on the area every five to ten seconds to feel the degree of warmth.

The application of moxa in this way should be stopped either when the child indicates that it feels too warm or the practitioner feels it is getting close to that point. It is useful to return to the point or area after a few minutes. If it does not still feel warm, then more moxa should be applied. Another indication that the moxibustion may be stopped is that the child becomes extremely relaxed. Warmth helps the *qi* to become less constricted and to flow more easily. Signs that this is happening may be that the child starts breathing more deeply, her body becomes more floppy or she becomes more still.

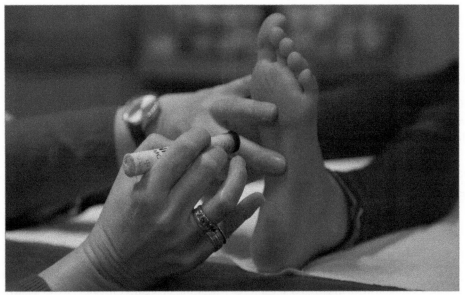

Using a moxa stick to treat Ki 1 *yongquan*

Direct moxa cones

Some practitioners prefer not to use moxa cones on young children at all, because of the risk of the child moving when the cone is burning down or because they perceive that the heat sensation may be too strong. However, using the Japanese *okyu* method of direct moxa as described by Birch[17] is tolerated by most babies and infants and can be performed safely by a practitioner who has some experience of it. The end of the moxa cone that comes into contact with the child's skin is incredibly fine, and the cone may be removed once it has burned down approximately 50–60 per cent of the way, at which point the child will feel no more than a very short-lived pinch of heat. Usually, between three and seven moxa cones are sufficient to bring about the desired effect, which can be monitored by changes in the child and on her pulse. Direct moxa is, of course, a well-tolerated and useful treatment method on older children.

Particular cautions when using moxa in the treatment of children

It goes without saying that fire and young children should only be put in the same vicinity when extreme caution and care is used. Many young children have a propensity to grab things that look interesting, such as a lit moxa stick. Therefore, the practitioner should at all times keep firm hold of the moxa stick and make sure that the child, or a sibling who happens to be in the room, cannot grab it. Young children also have a propensity to move their limbs around, sometimes out of the blue. Therefore, the practitioner should gently place his non-dominant hand on the limb where he is using the moxa to keep it still.

Parents may have some concerns about the use of moxa. It is always prudent, therefore, to explain to them what you are going to do and why you are doing it before beginning the process. Once the child is old enough, a simple explanation of what you are about to do is also vital. When using a moxa stick, it is especially important to explain to the child that the lit end of the stick is not going to touch her skin. It can be helpful for the practitioner to demonstrate what he is going to do on his own hand before beginning the process on the child.

Apart from the extra care that should be taken with fire around children, all the normal contraindications of using moxibustion also apply. On top of this, it is also important to note that some asthmatic children, or those with respiratory allergies, may have an adverse reaction to moxa smoke. In this case, either smokeless moxa or a heat lamp should be used instead.

Laser pens

Laser acupuncture includes the treatment of acupuncture points and areas of the body with laser pens, laser needles and laser showers. The following is a discussion of the use of laser pens in the treatment of acupuncture points, as this is the method I use.

What are laser pens?

A laser pen applies a quantity of therapeutic light to the acupuncture point over which it is held. A laser pen can be used on any point on the body. The process is totally painless for the child, and this is the most important factor. Laser pens mean that a child who cannot face the thought of needles, or deal with the experience of them, can still receive treatment.

There are many laser pens of different strengths on the market. Generally speaking, the more powerful the laser pen, the more expensive it is. A higher-performance pen means that the correct dose can be delivered in a shorter time, which has obvious advantages especially in the treatment of very young children who find it hard to stay still. At the time of writing, the most powerful pen on the market is 500mW, which means that it rarely needs to be held over a point for more than ten seconds.

How are laser pens used?

Before using the laser pen, the practitioner must set the dose that is required. This may be anywhere between 0.5 joules and 4 joules. The younger, or more sensitive, the child, the lower the dose needed. The laser pen is held at a perpendicular angle over an acupuncture point and a button is then pressed on the pen so that it begins the treatment. The pen will then beep when the treatment of that point is finished. The time it takes will depend on the power of the laser pen, but with a 200mW pen, it will take between 2.5 and 20 seconds to deliver a dose of between 0.5 and 4 joules.

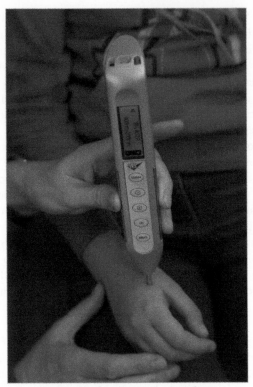

Using a laser pen to treat LI 4 *hegu*

How does using a laser pen differ from using a needle?

In an ideal world, there would be no need for an acupuncturist to use a laser pen. However, the world is far from ideal, and the invention of laser pens has meant that more children receive acupuncture treatment than otherwise would.

There are some differences to the planning and carrying out of the treatment when using a laser pen instead of a needle:

- The laser pen should be used bilaterally, whereas it is often sufficient to needle a point unilaterally. This is because it takes a little more to achieve the same effect with a laser pen than with a needle.

- More points need to be used to bring about the desired effect with a laser pen than with a needle. For example, if the treatment principle is to tonify Spleen *qi*, it may be sufficient purely to needle St 36 *zusanli* with a needle, but the practitioner may need to stimulate St 36 *zusanli* and Ren 12 *zhongwan* or Bl 20 *pishu* with a laser pen to bring about the same change.

- It is a little more difficult to differentiate between tonification and reduction with a laser pen than it is with a needle. Various authors disagree on this issue. Scott believes that laser pens are only really effective at tonification.[18] Kreisel and Weber, on the other hand, believe that it is possible to clearly determine the desired needle technique in the following way: 'Tonification effects can often be achieved with a short irradiation time and high-power output and sedation effects with a longer irradiation time and low power output.'[19]

In my experience, it is possible to use the laser pen both to tonify and/or to reduce a point, by changing the settings on the laser pen accordingly. However, when the intention is to reduce, it is helpful to do some strong acupressure on the point before and after using the laser in order to encourage the *qi* to disperse.

Are laser pens safe?

If used properly, laser pens are completely safe. Even the most state-of-the-art laser pen delivers a very low-level laser which does not have the power to damage tissue. The most important safety measure is to make sure that the laser is not beamed at the child's eyes. Laser pens are sold with protective glasses that the child may wear during the treatment. The practitioner should always be conscious of the fact that many children are attracted to shiny machines with buttons to press, so should never leave it placed where the child might be able to grab it.

Kreisel and Weber also list some contraindications that are relevant to the use of laser acupuncture with children. The following areas should not be stimulated with a laser pen:

- open fontanelles
- the eye
- the testicles
- cancerous or pre-cancerous tumours
- skin which is damaged due to UV light or radiation.

Microcurrent stimulation

Another way of treating a child is with a handheld microcurrent device. These small, pen-sized machines place controlled voltage at the acupuncture point to stimulate it by passing a microcurrent through it. They are totally painless and a relatively quick method of treatment. Depending on the machine, it usually needs to be held over a point for anywhere between five and twenty seconds.

Children are generally very happy to receive treatment in this way. The machines usually make beeping noises, which are always popular. A microcurrent device may be used on either body or ear points.

As with the laser pen, it can be harder to differentiate between tonification and sedation using a microcurrent device.

Gua sha

Gua sha is a very useful and widely used method of treatment for children. Traditionally a blade that is roughly rectangular but with curved edges, known as a *gua sha ban*, was used. However, to guard against the theoretical risk of cross-infection, practitioners should use a disposable implement. Honey pot lids, which have a smooth round lip, are ideal for this purpose. They can be bought in bulk and disposed of after use.

Indications for *gua sha*

- **Release the exterior:** *Gua sha* is one of the most effective and well-tolerated ways of releasing the exterior on a child. Ideally, the child will be brought to the clinic at the first signs of invasion from an External Pathogenic Factor. Timely *gua sha* can stop the pathogen from penetrating into the interior and thus prevent a more serious and prolonged illness.

- **Clear excess Heat:** *Gua sha* can be used to 'vent' Heat from the body, whatever the cause. A common clinical situation in children is Heat trapped in the interior because of an outer layer of Damp or Phlegm. Treating the surface of the body with *gua sha* helps to disseminate fluids. Once the fluids are dispersed, the Heat trapped beneath is more able to find a way out of the body.

- **Moving *qi* and Blood:** The most common reason for *qi* and Blood stagnation in young children is an invasion of Cold. Older children who play an excessive amount of sports are also prone to *qi* and Blood stagnation because of overuse of the limbs or injury. *Gua sha* is useful in all cases where there is pain but is especially beneficial when the pain is Full (*shi*) in nature.

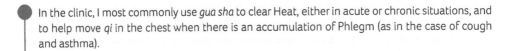

In the clinic, I most commonly use *gua sha* to clear Heat, either in acute or chronic situations, and to help move *qi* in the chest when there is an accumulation of Phlegm (as in the case of cough and asthma).

Preparation of the parent and child

Before undertaking *gua sha* on a child, it is imperative to explain clearly to the parent, and depending on her age the child, what you would like to do and why you would like to do it. It can be helpful for the practitioner to use his own arm in order to demonstrate to the child what will happen. A part of the explanation must be to explain that the child will be left with red marks over the area the *gua sha* is performed on and that they may take a day or two to fade.[20]

Before embarking on *gua sha*, the practitioner should make it clear to the child that if at any point she would like the practitioner to stop, she should clearly say so. The practitioner should also check in with the child as the treatment is being carried out, to make sure that she is comfortable with it.

Preparation of the area to be treated

The area to be treated must be lubricated with a balm or an oil (balms have the advantage of being less runny). Before applying any balm to the child's skin, the practitioner should check with the parent that the child has no known allergies to any of the ingredients. There are many balms that can be used, some of which have particular warming or cooling properties, as well as neutral ones. The practitioner should choose one which is best suited to the child's condition.*

Method

The force with which *gua sha* is performed should largely be determined by what is acceptable to the child. Older and more robust children often enjoy quite strong *gua sha*, whereas younger and more deficient children will only tolerate it when done lightly. *Gua sha* should be performed on the appropriate part of the body until the skin becomes red. It is not always necessary to make petechiae appear on the skin, as is the case when treating adults.

---

* Balms can be purchased from most acupuncture supply companies.

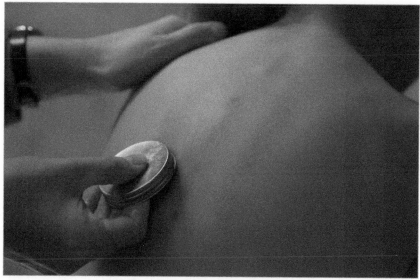

Gua sha **on the back using a honeypot lid**

Cupping

Cupping is a useful adjunctive therapy in the treatment of children. With the right preparation, the vast majority of children enjoy the experience of being cupped. It is most commonly used in the following circumstances:

- to help expel an external pathogen, especially an invasion of Wind in the Lungs

- to loosen Thick Phlegm, as in the case of a Lingering Pathogenic Factor

- to help in the treatment of asthma or chronic cough by moving Lung *qi* that is constrained by Phlegm, Heat or *qi* stagnation

- in older children, to move *qi* and Blood in painful conditions.

Types of cups

The most commonly used methods of cupping are fire cupping, where a flame is used to create suction, and suction cups. Cups are usually made out of glass, bamboo or plastic. The type of cup used, and the method employed in order to create suction, will largely depend on the practitioner's personal preference and experience.

However, it is not advisable for a practitioner who lacks extensive experience of fire cupping to use this method around children. It only takes a momentary lapse in concentration for something to go horribly wrong. When working with young children, there is always the chance that the child will make a sudden, unexpected movement, or that she cannot resist suddenly trying to grab the lighter or the alcohol used to soak the cotton wool. There may be several siblings present too who are bored and think it might be fun to take a closer look at what you are doing. It may not be possible for one practitioner, with only one pair of hands, to manage this situation in a way which is entirely safe.

Consequently, I normally do not use fire cupping when working with children, especially young ones. Suction cups, as well as being safer, have the added advantage of allowing for a little more control over the degree of suction created. It is now possible to buy cups made out of biocompatible silicone, with varying degrees of hardness, which are ideal for using with children. Their application feels much gentler and less sudden than that of glass or bamboo cups.

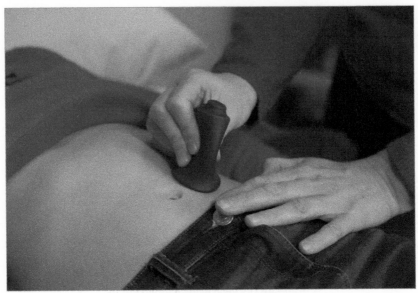

Using a silicone cup on the abdomen

Preparation of the parent and child

Before cupping a child, the practitioner must take great care to explain to both parent and child exactly what she is going to do. It can be helpful for the practitioner to use her own arm in order to demonstrate to the child what will happen. The explanation should include the fact that the child may be left with red marks that may take a day or two to fade.

Cupping methods

Several different cupping methods may be used when treating children:

- **Static cupping:** When a particular acupuncture point is being targeted, such as Bl 13 *feishu* in the treatment of an external Lung condition, the cup may be applied over the point and left in position for the duration of the treatment. On young children, just two or three minutes is usually long enough. As a child gets older, the cups may be left in place for a slightly longer period of time. It is rarely necessary to leave a cup in position for more than ten minutes with a child under the age of fourteen.

- **Sliding cupping:** When treating an area or a channel, rather than a point, sliding cupping may be used. The skin must be lubricated with balm beforehand. Sliding cupping may be used over the upper back, for example if the child's Lungs are congested with Phlegm. It may be used along a channel, for example the Gallbladder channel when there is pain from *qi* and/or Blood stagnation. Sliding cupping may be used on the abdomen to clear a condition of full Cold.

- **Flash cupping:** Traditionally, flash cupping is done using fire cups. However, it is possible to use silicone cups to perform flash cupping on a child. It can be effective at loosening Thick Phlegm, a common pathology in children especially when there is a Lingering Pathogenic Factor present. Flash cupping can be done on the back or over the abdomen.

Contraindications

Cupping should be used sparingly in deficient conditions. It should not be performed over skin which is broken or eczematous.

Acupressure

Acupressure can be used in place of needles. It therefore may be used with children for whom the thought of a needle or the reality of being needled is too upsetting. However, it is far more time-consuming than acupuncture and is considerably less effective in most conditions.

Acupressure of certain points may be taught to the parent so that they can use it on their child at home. It is effective in chronic conditions, where daily treatment may be beneficial. It may also be useful during the flare-up of a recurrent condition, if the child is not able to get to the clinic.

There are many ways of performing acupressure. The practitioner should feel her way into it and adapt her method according to the individual needs of the child. Strong, robust children need acupressure to be done with a quite forcible touch, whereas a more deficient child needs it to be performed more gently. Generally speaking, slow, clockwise movements on a point will tonify, and rapid, anti-clockwise movements will disperse.

Press-spheres

Press-spheres are tiny balls in the middle of a small, round, hypoallergenic sticker which can be placed directly on the skin. Press-spheres may be used both on body points and ear points.

Uses

Press-spheres have the effect of giving a continual, very low-dose stimulation to a point. Gold-coloured press-spheres are used to tonify a point, and silver-coloured ones are used to disperse.

Method

The practitioner may place press-spheres on a relevant point or points at the end of the treatment and the child may be sent home with them in place. It is much easier to apply them with a small pair of tweezers than with the hands, to which they have a habit of sticking. The parent may be given spare press-spheres. It is useful to advise parents to check the press-spheres each evening. If they look like they are beginning to become unstuck, the old one can be removed and a new one put in its place. The original one will leave a mark which makes the correct positioning of the new one straightforward.

Precautions

Press-spheres should only be used on children who are old enough not to peel them off and put them in their mouths.

Occasionally, a press-sphere, or even the tape which is used to stick it to the skin, may cause irritation on the child's skin. This is another reason for the parent to check them every evening. When there is irritation, their use should be stopped on that point until the irritation has disappeared. This should not preclude the practitioner from trying again in the future as, especially after further treatment, the child may not react in the same way.

Press-spheres should not be placed on points where they may cause discomfort, such as Ki 1 *yongquan* on the sole of the foot or any point on the buttocks or the backs of the thighs.

Occasionally, a child is resistant to press-spheres for aesthetic reasons or purely because she does not like anything that may draw attention to her. It is rarely worth insisting upon their use if this creates upset in the child. It should also be said that a child may ask for them to be placed in specific places, particularly on the ears, because she likes the look of them!

Retained (semi-permanent) needles

There are various different types of retained needles. Those most suited to the treatment of children are extremely short, thin-gauge needles embedded into a plastic base with a surrounding piece of hypoallergenic tape used to stick the needle onto the skin. The shortest ones are 0.3 millimetres in length, and the longest are 0.9 millimetres in length. They are 0.2mm gauge.* They are easily removed and cannot become embedded under the skin.

Uses

As with press-spheres, retained needles give a continual, low-dose stimulation to the point on which they are placed. Their effect is slightly stronger than that of a press-sphere. The longer the retained needle is, the stronger the effect on the *qi*. Therefore, the shortest ones tend to be used on babies and young children, or particularly deficient or sensitive older children. The longer ones may be used on older children.

Method

The method of using retained needles is the same as that of press-spheres (see the section 'Press-spheres' above). If a child is being sent away with retained needles in place, the parent should be given a small sharps box to take home in which to dispose of the retained needles.

Contraindications and precautions

Retained needles should not be used on a child who has an artificial or damaged heart valve. They are also contraindicated if the child has a prosthetic joint. Otherwise, precautions are the same as for press-spheres. Practitioners should also check the current guidelines of their professional body concerning the use of retained needles.

Auricular acupuncture

Auricular acupuncture is a useful addition in the treatment of children. I tend to use it on children from about the age of four upwards. The ears of babies and infants are so small that it is extremely difficult to locate the point and accurately stick a press-sphere on it – all of which would need to be done whilst she is most likely wriggling or moving.

Uses

Auricular acupuncture may be used to enhance the child's treatment. Some points on the ear may be used to address specific symptoms, whilst body acupuncture is used to treat the underlying imbalance. For example, ear *shenmen* may be used on a child who is hyperactive because of its calming effect, whilst body acupuncture is used to clear Heat that is causing the hyperactivity. Auricular acupuncture should not be used in place of a sound, differential diagnosis however, but as an auxiliary to treatment of the underlying Organ and Pathogen patterns.

Some of the most commonly used ear points in children are as follows:

- **Shenmen:** for any sleep disorders, hyperactivity, difficulty with attention, anxiety, depression and all other emotional problems.

- **Lung:** for coughs, both acute and chronic, asthma and respiratory allergies.

- **Kidney:** for developmental disorders, bedwetting or any other disorder involving a Kidney deficiency.

---

* These are called Pyonex and are made by Seirin.

- **Spleen:** for all digestive disorders, overthinking, worrying and anxiety (especially around exam time).

- **Liver:** for hyperactivity, problems with expression of anger, some sleep problems and digestive problems.

- *Fengxi* **and the allergy point:** for allergies.

Method

Whilst of course points on the ear may be needled, in order to be effective, they should be left in for at least twenty minutes. Ear points may also be more painful than body points. Therefore, with a child, the most common method is to place press-spheres on the points instead. In order to find the point, it can be helpful to use a handheld electrical stimulation machine, such as the Stimplus Pro. This indicates with a light or a beeping sound when a point has been found. It can then be used to leave a tiny indent, indicating where the sticker can then be placed.

Either vaccaria seeds or gold- or silver-coloured seeds may be used. These can be left in place and the child sent home with them. It is not uncommon to find that they are still in place a week later when the child next comes for a treatment, despite the child having had baths and showers. However, parents may be given spare seeds and asked to check each evening whether the original ones are still firmly in place. If they are not, or if they look as if they may be beginning to lose their stick, then a new seed can be put in place. Even if the original one has fallen off, there will usually be a small indentation which will show the parent where the new sticker should be placed.

Most children love having press-spheres in place. Some younger children who aspire to have their ears pierced even ask for them. However, older children and teenagers may object on aesthetic grounds to being given press-spheres. In such cases the tacks can be placed on the back of the ear corresponding to the point on the front of the ear to be treated, but out of sight, and the child shown how to press the tack which will activate the reflex point. Parents and children should be told that, if the ear tacks begin to become uncomfortable or unwanted, they can always be removed.

Precautions

The practitioner should ask the parent to check the child's press-spheres regularly, particularly the first time. This is to ensure that no skin irritation has developed and the child does not have an allergy to the seed or the sticker holding it in place.

Table 33.1 summarises the advantages and disadvantages of the alternatives to needling that have been discussed in this chapter.

Table 33.1 Advantages and disadvantages of alternatives to needling

	Key advantages	Key disadvantages
Needles	Can treat any pathology	May be resisted by child
	Most powerful way of contacting *qi*	May be uncomfortable
Moxibustion	Painless method of tonifying *qi, yang* and Blood	Risk of burning
		Contraindicated in Hot or excess conditions
		Moxa smoke may irritate allergies in some children
Laser pen	Entirely painless	More time-consuming
		Less effective in excess conditions

	Key advantages	Key disadvantages
Microcurrent stimulation	Entirely painless	More time-consuming Less easy to differentiate between tonifying and sedating
Gua sha	Effective way of clearing Heat, full and pain conditions	Limited scope Sha may cause alarm in others Older children may be self-conscious about sha
Cupping	Effective and comfortable way of releasing the exterior	Limited scope Some children find it uncomfortable
Acupressure	Painless No tools needed Parents may use it at home	Less powerful way of contacting qi
Press-spheres	Useful home treatment Can be used on ear or body points	Some children may be allergic Older children may be self-conscious May be fiddled with
Retained needles	Useful home treatment	Some governing bodies have disallowed use outside treatment room Some children may be allergic Badly tolerated by some May be fiddled with
Auricular acupuncture	Avoids need to undress Painless press-spheres may be used Useful for symptomatic treatment	Needles in the ear may be painful Older children may be self-conscious Can be hard to locate a point accurately on the ear of a small child

Chapter 34

PAEDIATRIC *TUI NA*

The topics discussed in this chapter are:

* Age of child

* Paediatric *tui na* in the clinic and at home

* Types of manipulations used in paediatric *tui na*

* Points, lines and areas used in paediatric *tui na*

* Teaching parents paediatric *tui na*

* Using *tui na* in the treatment of specific disorders

Introduction

Paediatric *tui na* (*xiao er tui na*) is a wonderfully effective system of massage. Whilst being a systematic, medical treatment, it developed out of a mother's innate instinct to stroke, touch and caress her baby or young child. Therefore, it is practical, intuitive and easy to deliver. Babies and children in the main love it.

Paediatric *tui na* involves using a variety of different movements, ranging from stroking to tapping, on different parts of the child's body. Some of the areas it uses are acupuncture points on the main channels or extra points. However, most are areas which are specific to children and not connected to the main channel system. These areas are 'open' in children and are understood to be of therapeutic use. This is one of the ways in which paediatric *tui na* is so practical. The areas that are used are ones that are easily accessible on babies and young children. Furthermore, because it is mostly focused on areas rather than points, it avoids the need for accuracy that can be so difficult on a wriggling baby or infant. Massage is done:

* along lines of the body, for example between the wrist and elbow, or along the edge of a finger

* in circular areas, for example around the palm of the hand

* on specific non-acupuncture points, such as between the bases of the two thenar eminences of the hand

* on acupuncture points, for example St 36 *zusanli*

* on large areas, such as the lumbar area of the back.

Paediatric *tui na* can be taught to parents to enable them to give 'home treatment'.

Age of child

There are differences of opinion as to what the age limit is for paediatric *tui na* to be effective. Flaws writes that, beyond the age of six, adult *tui na* should be used instead.[21] Fan Ya-li, on the other hand, suggests that paediatric *tui na* may be used on children up to the age of twelve. The younger the child, the more effective it is.[22] So much of paediatric practice is driven by what is practical and possible with each individual child at any given moment. It is certainly true that paediatric *tui na* alone is capable of transforming the health of babies and young children. With children above the age of approximately six or seven, it is often more effective to combine paediatric *tui na* with acupuncture.

Paediatric *tui na* in the clinic and at home

A sequence of paediatric *tui na* movements may be performed by the practitioner in the clinic. A sequence or routine may be made up of between five and fifteen moves. It may be that this is all the practitioner does in one treatment, or that it is combined with other modalities such as needles or moxibustion.

One of the greatest benefits of paediatric *tui na*, however, is that it can be taught to the parent and then done every day at home. There are many benefits to this. It means that improvement is quicker and the child need not come to the clinic so often. It also often means that some magic may happen in the relationship between parent and child, which may have become strained by the child's illness. The child benefits from being the sole focus of the parent's attention for a few minutes each day, and the parent feels empowered that she is doing something to help her child.

Types of manipulations used in paediatric *tui na*
Straight pushing (*zhi tui fa*)

Straight pushing is the most commonly used stroke and is used on all the linear points.

Method: Pushing in a straight line over an area of the body with either the pad of the thumb or the pads of the index and middle fingers held together. This should be done quite rapidly (approximately 100–200 times per minute). The thumb or fingers should remain in contact with the skin. Whilst strong force is not necessary, firm contact should be made. It should be more than just a tickle. The force of contact and rhythm of stroking should be consistent.

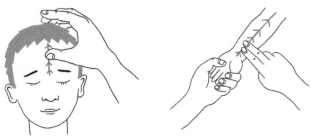

Straight pushing

Pushing apart (*fen tui fa*)

Pushing apart is a variant of straight pushing. It is also used on linear points, when it is necessary to push from the middle outwards. It is sometimes translated as 'separating pushing' or 'opening up'.

Method: Pushing in a straight line from the middle of a linear point to both ends, using the radial corner of the pads of the thumbs (or, less commonly, the pads of the index and middle fingers held together). This should be done quite rapidly (approximately 100–200 times per minute).

The thumb or fingers should remain in contact with the skin. Whilst strong force is not necessary, firm contact should be made. The force of contact and rhythm of stroking should be consistent.

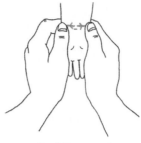

Pushing apart

Circular pushing (*yun fa*)

Circular pushing involves pushing in a circle, rather than along a straight line.

Method: Circular pushing should be done using the top part of the thumb pad or the tops of the pads of the second and third fingers. The pads of the fingers or thumb should maintain contact with the skin. The contact should be firm but not forceful. The speed should be slow relative to the other movements described (approximately 80–100 times per minute).

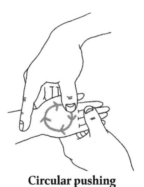

Circular pushing

Kneading (*rou fa*)

Kneading involves manipulating a point or area by massaging in either a clockwise or anti-clockwise circular motion. A clockwise movement is used to sedate, and an anti-clockwise movement to tonify.

Method: This method is most commonly done with the tip of a finger or the tip of the thumb. On the stomach, the palm of the hand or the palmar surface of the four fingers held together may be used. In all cases, whichever part of the hand the practitioner is using should remain fixed on the point, whilst moving in either a clockwise or anti-clockwise direction. A firm but soft touch should be used. The movements should be rhythmic and done at a moderate pace (approximately 100–160 times per minute).

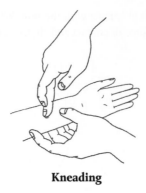

Kneading

Circular rubbing (*mo fa*)

Circular rubbing involves rubbing in either a clockwise or anti-clockwise direction.

Method: This method involves placing either the palm of the hand or the palmar surface of the four fingers on the child's body and rubbing either in a clockwise or anti-clockwise direction. The hand should keep contact with the skin, and the force used should be that which is naturally derived from the weight of the hand. The movements should be done at a moderate speed (approximately 100–120 times per minute) and in a rhythmic fashion.

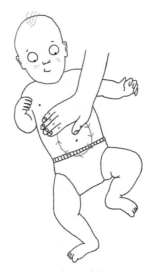

Circular rubbing

 When kneading, the hand or fingers stay in the same position on the child's skin whilst rotating in the appropriate direction. When circular rubbing, the hand moves over the skin.

Pinching (*nie fa*)

Pinching involves holding the skin between the pads of the thumbs, and the index, middle and ring finger of each hand. When used on the hands, the skin is simply pinched and then released. When used on the back, the skin is pinched upwards and the practitioner, whilst maintaining contact with the skin, moves her fingers and thumbs forward. Therefore, a kind of rolling effect is created. The hands are moved at a steady pace and in a straight line.

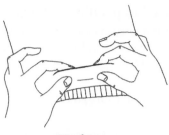

Pinching

Strong rubbing (*ca fa*)

Strong rubbing involves placing the entire hand, palmar surface down, on the desired area of the body. The hand is then quickly and quite forcefully rubbed back and forth over the skin. It is not necessary to press downwards strongly, but the movement should be performed vigorously. This should be done for one to two minutes.

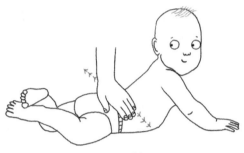

Strong rubbing

Tapping (*kou fa*)

Tapping involves using the tip of a finger to tap a point rapidly and rhythmically. The wrist should remain loose whilst tapping. This should be done for between one and two minutes.

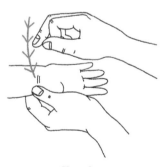

Tapping

> When performing *tui na*, the above guidelines should be followed. However, they are only guidelines. Rather than slavishly counting the number of taps or the amount of time spent on each move, the practitioner should adapt her approach to treat the individual child.

Points, lines and areas used in paediatric *tui na*

As mentioned above, some of the areas used in paediatric *tui na* correspond to regular acupuncture points. Most, however, are areas that are considered to be 'open' in children but not of any particular therapeutic significance in adults.

Areas that correspond to particular Organs

The seven finger points

These are areas on the fingers that correspond to each of the five *yin* Organs and to the Small and Large Intestines. These areas are particularly used on babies and toddlers. They are easy to access on a baby when she is being held or when feeding, without the need for her to lie in a certain position or take any clothes off. They may also be used on older children but in this case would need to be combined with other areas on the torso.

When working on these areas, the straight pushing technique is always used. However, it is important to distinguish between the two different ways of using this technique:

- straight pushing from the tip of the finger to the base has a **tonifying** action
- straight pushing from the base of the finger to the tip has a **sedating** action.

It is essential that contact is made all the way down the finger, with a particular focus on the pads of the fingers.

SPLEEN (*PIJING*)

Location: along the radial surface of the thumb

Technique: straight pushing

Indications: Spleen *qi* deficiency

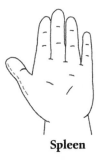

Spleen

LARGE INTESTINE (*DACHANGJING*)

Location: along the radial surface of the index finger

Technique: straight pushing

Indications:

- *qi* deficiency affecting the Large Intestine with the tonification technique
- Full Heat or Damp-Heat in the Intestines with the sedation technique

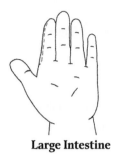

Large Intestine

LIVER (*GANJING*)
Location: along the palmar surface of the index finger

Technique: straight pushing

Indications:

- stagnation, Heat or Wind in the Liver with the sedation technique
- Liver Blood or *yin* deficiency with the tonification technique

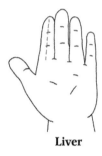

Liver

HEART (*XINJING*)
Location: along the palmar surface of the middle finger

Technique: straight pushing

Indications:

- Heart *qi* or Blood deficiency with the tonification technique
- Heat in the Heart with the sedation technique

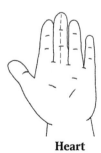

Heart

LUNG (*FEIJING*)

Location: along the palmar surface of the ring finger

Technique: straight pushing

Indications:

- Lung *qi* deficiency with the tonification technique
- expels Wind-Heat, Wind-Cold, Heat and Phlegm from the Lungs with the sedation technique

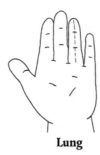

Lung

KIDNEY (*SHENJING*)

Location: along the palmar surface of the little finger

Technique: straight pushing

Indications: Kidney deficiency with the tonification technique

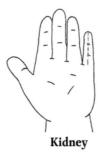

Kidney

SMALL INTESTINE (*XIAOCHANGJING*)

Location: Ulnar surface of the little finger

Technique: straight pushing

Indications:

- Heat, stagnation and pain in the Small Intestine with the sedation technique
- deficiency of the Small Intestine with the tonification technique

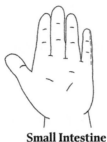

Small Intestine

Areas that strengthen and tonify the body

Kidneys

Two Men Upon a Horse (*ERMA*)

Location: on the dorsal surface of the hand, just proximal to the metacarpal-phalangeal joint, between the fourth and fifth metacarpal bones

Technique: kneading

Indications: Deficiency of Kidney *qi*, *yin*, *yang* or *jing*

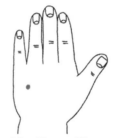

Two Men Upon a Horse

> Two Men Upon a Horse (*erma*) lies on the Triple Burner channel. Kidney *yang* and the Triple Burner are closely inter-related, which might explain the use of this point to strengthen the Kidneys.

Lower back (area around Bl 23 *shenshu*)

Location: the area from one side of the back to the other, at the level of the lumbar vertebrae

Technique: strong rubbing

Indications: Kidney deficiency, especially Kidney *yang* deficiency

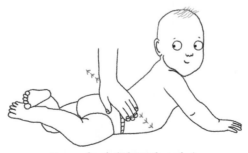

Lower back (Bl 23 *shenshu*)

Spleen and Stomach

STOMACH (*WEIJING*)

Location: along the radial edge of the thenar eminence of the thumb

Technique: straight pushing

Indications:

- Stomach *qi* or *yin* deficiency with the tonification technique
- Accumulation Disorder, Cold in the Stomach, Heat in the Stomach, Rebellious Stomach *qi* with the sedation technique

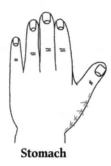

Stomach

KNEAD *ZHONGWAN* (*ROU ZHONGWAN*)

Location: the area of Ren 12 *zhongwan*

Technique: kneading

Indications: Spleen and Stomach *qi* deficiency manifesting with digestive symptoms, especially nausea, vomiting and reflux

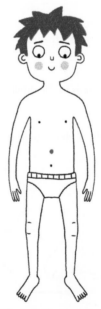

Knead *zhongwan*

KNEAD THE NAVEL (*ROU QI*)
Location: the area of Ren 8 *shenque*

Technique: kneading

Indications: either fullness in the digestive system, or deficiency of the Spleen manifesting with digestive symptoms, especially loose stools, poor appetite and weakness

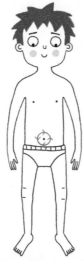

Knead the Navel

KNEAD THE LOWER ABDOMEN (*ROU QIHAI*)
Location: the area of Ren 6 *qihai*

Technique: kneading

Indications: either fullness in the digestive system, or deficiency of the Spleen manifesting with digestive symptoms, especially loose stools and abdominal pain

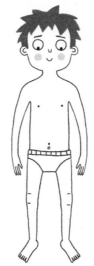

Knead the Lower Abdomen

The three manipulations described above, all of which treat the Stomach and Spleen, may be combined or done separately. On a young baby, they can all be done simultaneously as the hand of an adult will cover all three areas. Kneading any of them in a clockwise direction is sedating, and in an anti-clockwise direction is tonifying.

All the zangfu
SPINAL COLUMN (A) (*JIZHU*)

Location: all along the back, from the sacrum to the top of the thoracic area, either side of the spine

Technique: pinching, from the bottom to the top of the spine

Indications: generalised deficiency of *qi*

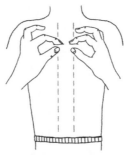

Spinal Column (a)

SPINAL COLUMN (B) (*JIZHU*)

Location: all along the back from the top of the thoracic area to the sacrum, either side of the spine

Technique: straight pushing

Indications: excess Heat in any Organ[*]

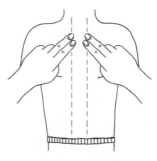

Spinal Column (b)

Note: Both the above methods of treating the Spinal Column may be used over the entirety of the back to affect every Organ. Alternatively, they can be focused on one area of the back, for example the top of the back for respiratory problems or the middle of the back for digestive problems.

---

[*] I also use *jizhu* diagnostically. An area on the back that becomes red more quickly or strongly than another area may indicate Heat or fullness in the Organ related to that back *shu* point.

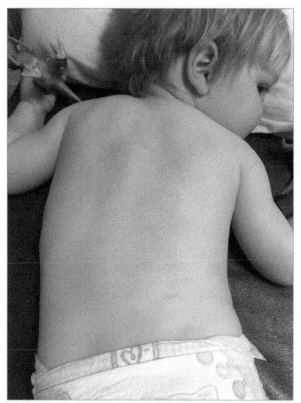

Redness on the back after using Spinal Column (*jizhu*) treatment

Any acupuncture point on the body can be kneaded (*rou*) in order to strengthen the *qi* of any Organ, as part of a complete *tui na* routine. Points that are commonly kneaded are the back *shu* points, St 36 *zusanli*, TB 5 *waiguan*, LI 4 *hegu*, Sp 6 *sanyinjiao* and Ki 1 *yongquan*.

Intestines
SEVEN BOUND BONES (*QIJIEGU*)

Location: along the lumbar and sacral spine, between the fourth lumbar vertebra and the coccyx

Technique: straight pushing, downwards to disperse and upwards to tonify

Indications: either fullness or deficiency in the Intestines

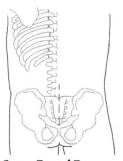

Seven Bound Bones

TURTLE'S TAIL (*GUIWEI*)
Location: at the tip of the coccyx

Technique: kneading anti-clockwise

Indications: deficiency in the Intestines manifesting in loose stools or diarrhoea

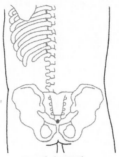

Turtle's Tail

Bladder
WINNOWER GATE (*JIMEN*)
Location: along the medial aspect of the thigh

Technique: straight pushing

Indications:

* Damp-Heat in the Bladder causing urinary symptoms (from groin to knee)

* Bladder deficient and Cold (from knee to groin)

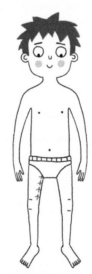

Winnower Gate

Areas that clear Heat and calm the *shen*

PALACE OF TOIL (*LAOGONG*)
Location: this point corresponds to Pc 8 *laogong*

Technique: kneading

Indications: Full Heat affecting the *shen*

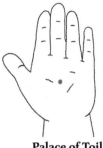

Palace of Toil

SMALL HEAVENLY HEART (*XIAOTIANXIN*)

Location: at the central point at the base of the palm, between the thenar and hypothenar eminences

Technique: kneading

Indications: Full Heat affecting the *shen*

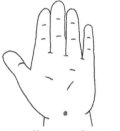

Small Heavenly Heart

MILKY WAY (*TIANHESHUI*)

Location: along the central line of the ventral surface of the forearm, between the wrist and elbow

Technique: straight pushing from the wrist to the elbow

Indications: any type of Heat, but particularly Heat from deficiency

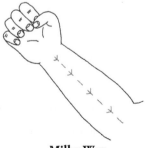

Milky Way

Milky Way (*tianheshui*) follows the line of the Pericardium channel, a Fire Organ which is susceptible to being affected by Heat. It also involves pushing towards the elbow, where three Water points are located (Lu 5 *chize*, He 3 *shaohai* and Pc 3 *quze*). Both of these facts might help to explain why this *tui na* move is so adept at cooling a child.

Six Yang Organs (*LIUFU*)

Location: on the ulnar side of the ventral surface of the forearm, on a line between the elbow crease and the wrist crease

Technique: straight pushing from the elbow to the wrist

Indications: Full Heat, especially when it affects the Intestines

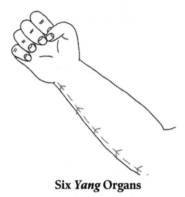

Six *Yang* Organs

 Six *Yang* Organs (*liufu*) roughly follows the path of the Small Intestine channel along the forearm, which may help to explain its ability to clear Heat from the Intestines.

Heaven Gate (*TIANMEN*)

Location: on a line on the forehead, from *yintang* (M-HN-3) to the anterior hairline

Technique: straight pushing upwards towards the hairline

Indications: disturbed *shen*; also used in invasions of External Pathogenic Factors causing symptoms in the head

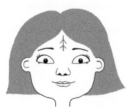

Heaven Gate

Water Palace (*KANGONG*)

Location: along a line on the forehead, 1 cun above the eyebrows

Technique: pushing apart from the midline outwards to a point roughly level with the lateral end of the eyebrows

Indications: disturbed *shen*; also used for invasions of External Pathogenic Factors causing symptoms in the head

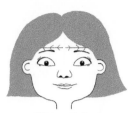

Water Palace

HEART GATE (*XINMEN*)

Location: on a line backwards from approximately Du 24 *shenting*

Technique: straight pushing

Indications: disturbed *shen*

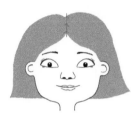

Heart Gate

Heaven Gate *tianmen*, Water Palace *kangong* and Heart Gate *xinmen* pass over two points which are particularly adept at calming the spirit, M-HN-3 *yintang* and Du 24 *shenting*. These three paediatric *tui na* moves have such a strong ability to calm a child's *shen* that it is not uncommon for a baby or toddler to fall asleep whilst she is being treated.

Areas that warm *yang* and expel Cold

OUTER PALACE OF TOIL (*WAILAOGONG*)

Location: on the dorsal surface of the hand, between the third and fourth metacarpal bones

Technique: kneading

Indications: *yang* deficiency of any Organ

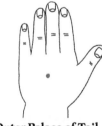

Outer Palace of Toil

WIND NEST (*YIWOFENG*)

Location: on the dorsal surface of the wrist, at the centre of the wrist crease

Technique: kneading

Indications: *yang* deficiency and internal Cold

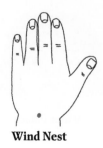

Wind Nest

THREE PASSES (*SANGUAN*)

Location: on the radial side of the ventral surface of the forearm, on a line between the wrist crease and the elbow crease

Technique: straight pushing from distal to proximal

Indications: *qi* and *yang* deficiency of any Organ

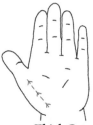

Three Passes

 Three Passes *sanguan* roughly follows the Large Intestine channel on the forearm. This may explain its ability to ease the symptoms of colic in a baby, when it stems from a deficiency of *qi* and *yang*.

Areas that move Food Accumulation

THICK GATE (*BANMEN*)

Location: along the thenar eminence, from the wrist crease to the base of the thumb

Technique: straight pushing

Indications: Food Accumulation

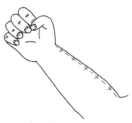

Thick Gate

EIGHT TRIGRAMS (*BAGUA*)

Location: a circle on the palm of the hand, which runs through Pc 8 *laogong* and He 8 *shaofu*

Technique: circular pushing, either clockwise or anti-clockwise

Indications: Food Accumulation, accumulation of Phlegm

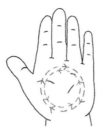

Eight Trigrams

> Eight Trigrams has the ability to raise *qi* when pushed in a clockwise direction, and to descend *qi* when pushed in an anti-clockwise direction. As so many children's conditions involve counterflow *qi*, this move, performed in an anti-clockwise direction, is therefore included in routines to address multiple, common conditions (such as cough, hyperactivity, insomnia, headaches and mouth ulcers, to name but a few).

FOUR WIND CREASES (*SIFENGWEN*)

Location: on the palmar surface of the hand, at the midpoints of the transverse creases of the proximal interphalangeal joints of the four fingers

Technique: pinching

Indications: Food Accumulation

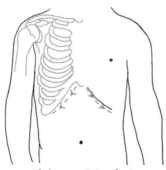

Four Wind Creases

ABDOMEN STIMULATION (*FUYINYANG*)

Location: from the midline outwards, following the line just below the ribs on either side of the abdomen

Technique: pushing apart

Indications: Food Accumulation

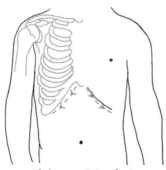

Abdomen Stimulation

Belly Corner (*dujiao*)

Location: a point on either side of the navel, below the tip of the eleventh rib

Technique: pinching, two or three times

Indications: Food Accumulation

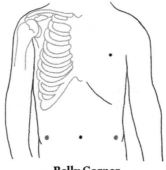

Belly Corner

 Abdomen Stimulation *fuyinyang* and Belly Corner *dujiao* both coincide approximately with the line of the Liver channel and, in the case of Belly Corner, Liv 13 *zhangmen*. This helps to explain why these moves are effective in excess digestive complaints in a child.

Areas that resolve Phlegm

Small Palmar Crease (*zhangxiaowen*)

Location: on the palm of the hand, just proximal to the base of the little finger

Technique: straight pushing

Indications: accumulation of Phlegm in the chest

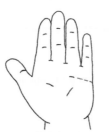

Small Palmar Crease

Hand *yin yang* (*shouyinyang*)

Location: along the central crease at the palmar surface of the wrist, from the midpoint to both sides

Technique: pushing apart

Indications: Thick Phlegm in the chest

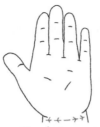

Hand *ying yang*

Hand *yin yang* passes over He 7 *shenmen*, Lu 9 *taiyuan* and Pc 7 *daling*, all of which are Earth points. This may help to explain the ability of this move to transform Phlegm in a child, which usually stems from a deficiency of the Spleen.

Areas that release the exterior and expel invasions of External Pathogenic Factors

Two Panels Gate (ERSHANMEN)

Location: two points on the dorsal surface of the hand, both just proximal to the metacarpal phalangeal joint; one is between the second and third metacarpal bones, and the other between the third and fourth

Technique: pinching and kneading

Indications: invasions of Wind in the Lungs

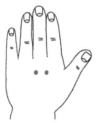

Two Panels Gate

Taiyang (M-HN-9)

Location: in a depression posterior to the lateral orbital ridge of the eyes

Technique: kneading

Indications: invasion of External Pathogenic Factor causing headache

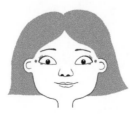

Taiyang

BEES ENTERING THE CAVE (*HUANGFENG RUDONG*)
Location: two points just below the opening of each nostril

Technique: kneading

Indications: invasion of External Pathogenic Factor with blocked nose

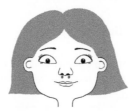

Bees Entering the Cave

WIND POND (*FENGCHI*)
Location: in the dip posterior to the mastoid process and inferior to the occiput, on each side of the neck (GB 20 *fengchi*)

Technique: kneading

Indications: invasion of External Pathogenic Factor

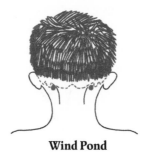

Wind Pond

BIG BONE BEHIND THE EAR (*ERHOU GAOGU*)
Location: behind the earlobe at the apex of the mastoid process

Technique: kneading

Indications: invasion of External Pathogenic Factor, especially causing pain in the ears

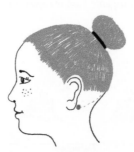

Big Bone Behind the Ear

Areas that move *qi* and send *qi* downwards

CELESTIAL PILLAR BONE (*TIANZHUGU*)

Location: a line on the midline of the back of the neck, from the posterior hairline to the base of the neck

Technique: straight pushing

Indications: counterflow *qi* rebelling upwards, causing vomiting or fever

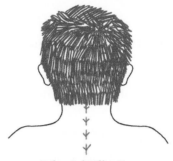

Celestial Pillar Bone

CENTRAL ALTAR (*SHANZHONG*)

Location: two lines, one level with the nipples on the midline of the chest and one downwards on the midline from Ren 22 *tiantu* to approximately the level of Ren 15 *jiuwei*

Technique: pushing apart and straight pushing

Indications: counterflow *qi* rebelling upwards causing cough; Phlegm in the chest

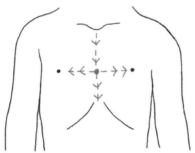

Central Altar

BREAST SIDES AND BREAST ROOT (*RUPANG* AND *RUGEN*)

Location: two points on the chest, just lateral and just inferior to each nipple

Technique: kneading

Indications: stagnation of *qi* in the chest and Phlegm, causing cough

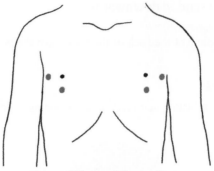

Breast Sides and Breast Root

FLANKS AND RIBS (*XIELEI*)

Location: on the lateral costal region at the sides of the torso (the flanks) from the armpit to a point approximately level with the navel

Technique: straight pushing with the palms of the hands

Indications: counterflow *qi* rebelling upwards and stagnation of *qi*, causing cough

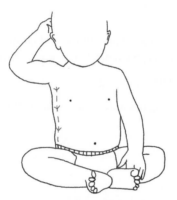

Flanks and Ribs

LUNG TRANSPORT (*JIANJIAGU*)

Location: a curved line just medial to the inner border of the scapula, on both sides

Technique: pushing apart, from above to below

Indications: stagnation of *qi* in the chest, manifesting with cough or difficulty breathing

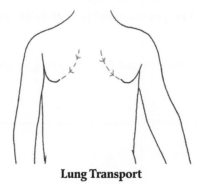

Lung Transport

Areas to reduce a fever

FISHING FOR THE MOON IN THE WATER (*SHUIDI LAOYUE*)

Location: on the palm of the hand, from the base of the little finger towards the base of the hand, and then upward towards the centre of the palm

Technique: pushing

Indications: fever, either acute or chronic and low grade

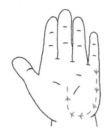

Fishing for the Moon in the Water

Fishing for the Moon in the Water *shuidi laoyue* ends around the point Pc 8 *laogong*. This helps to explain the efficacy of this move to reduce a fever in a child.

FIVE CHANNELS (*WUJING*)

Location: on the palmar surface of the hand, from the base of the palm upwards towards the tip of each finger and thumb

Technique: straight pushing

Indications: fever

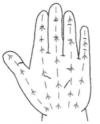

Five Channels

Teaching parents paediatric *tui na*

As mentioned above, one of the many benefits of paediatric *tui na* is that it can be taught to parents to perform daily on their child at home. The following is a helpful protocol to follow to ensure that parents perform it as well as possible on their child, and that they feel supported in doing so:

- **Demonstrate:** The complete *tui na* routine should be demonstrated to the parent on her child in the clinic.

- **Give feedback:** During the same session, the parent should be given the chance to try out each of the moves and the practitioner should give her feedback and correct anything that is not right.

- **Video:** The parent should be offered the opportunity to video the practitioner doing the *tui na* routine on a mobile device, providing she has one.

- **Written record:** A sheet with diagrams and clear instructions can be given to the parent to take home with them.

- **Ongoing support:** The practitioner should make it clear to the parent that she may contact him if she is unsure about what she is doing or if her child's condition changes.

- **Checking in:** The practitioner should ask the parent to show him how she has been doing the *tui na* routine at the next appointment so that the method can be checked and corrected if necessary.

Using *tui na* in the treatment of specific disorders

Part 5, Treatment of Physical Conditions, includes suggested *tui na* routines where applicable. They are only included in the sections describing the treatment of babies and toddlers, and sometimes school-age children. However, this is not to say that paediatric *tui na* cannot be used on older children.

I have found paediatric *tui na* especially helpful when treating older children who are developmentally younger than their age. For example, it was the only treatment that one fourteen-year-old girl who was on the autistic spectrum would tolerate and it had a remarkably beneficial effect on her. It is far better to try using *tui na* if it is the only treatment option available than to turn the child away without having tried to help.

SUMMARY

» Paediatric *tui na* is a system of medical massage that may be used on babies, infants and school-age children.

» A routine or sequence usually consists of anywhere between six and fifteen moves.

» A routine should be put together for each child, based on her constitution, signs and symptoms.

» Paediatric *tui na* routines may be performed in the clinic and taught to parents to be used daily at home.

• Chapter 35 •

SHONISHIN

· · · · · · · · · · · · · · · · · · · ·

The topics discussed in this chapter are:

- Method of application

- When might *shonishin* be useful in clinical practice?

- What is the clinical effect of *shonishin*?

- Core non-pattern-based root treatment

- Home treatment

- Using *shonishin* in the treatment of specific disorders

Introduction

The Japanese term *shonishin*, meaning 'children's needle' or 'children's needling', refers to a method of treating children that dates back to the 17th century.[23] However, it is a method that does not actually use needles. Instead, the practitioner uses various tools to stroke or tap areas on the child's body. There are many benefits of using *shonishin* treatment for children. Some of the key ones are outlined below:

- The basic treatment can be applied without having to first make a differential diagnosis based on Organ/Pathogen patterns.

- Treatment can be applied without using needles.

- In most cases, children enjoy the treatment.

- The treatment time is short.

- *Shonishin* can be combined with whichever style of acupuncture the practitioner practises.

- Parents can be taught to apply the treatment daily at home (this innovation was introduced by Birch in the 1980s).[24]

Shonishin is a pragmatic and flexible way of treating a child that can be adapted, not only to the needs of the child being treated, but also to the preferences of the practitioner giving the treatment. Most importantly, however, *shonishin* can be a very powerful treatment. It is a light and non-invasive method of treatment which can bring about profound changes in a baby or child.

> As with all techniques, the best way of learning the subtleties of their application is to attend a course. The reader is advised to find a *shonishin* course in order to hone the skills described in this chapter.

Method of application

When treating babies or children up to the age of approximately five years old, *shonishin* is applied using a range of tools. The practitioner strokes and taps various parts of the body with these tools. In older children, this non-invasive treatment may be combined with regular acupuncture needles too. There is a plethora of tools to choose from. Most practitioners will find they lean towards using one or two.* Some examples of the tools used are shown below.

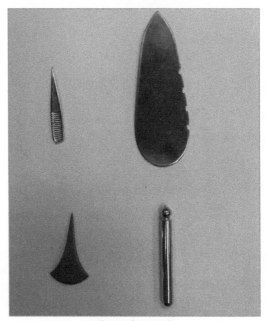

***Shonishin* tools**

However, it is not necessary to buy any specially designed tools. It is possible to apply the treatment using natural objects such as shells, and household objects such as hair grips (for tapping) or spoons (for stroking).

When might *shonishin* be useful in clinical practice?

Non-pattern-based root treatment *shonishin* may be applied, and is beneficial, in almost all cases. However, there are particular instances where it may be the treatment of choice. Some of these are listed below:

- In pre-term babies who are not 'ill' as such, but who may be prone to developmental problems because they were not able to complete the usual developments that take place in the womb.

- In very small babies.

- In babies who do not necessarily have a particular Organ/Pathogen pathology but who are unsettled, unhappy or not feeding properly.

- At the beginning of a treatment with a child of any age as a way of helping him to relax before needling. Starting treatment with the non-pattern-based root treatment also helps to build rapport between practitioner and child.

---

* Readers are advised to see the range of tools available from Japanese acupuncture supply companies.

- In any child, whether neurotypical or on the autistic spectrum, who has sensory processing issues, particularly ones related to tactility. *Shonishin* may help balance and normalise the sensations these children feel coming from their environment and in their bodies.

- Perhaps surprisingly, *shonishin* seems to be particularly well tolerated by children, many of them on the autistic spectrum, who usually cannot tolerate touch.

- In any child who has a pathology related to counterflow *qi* rising up to the head. The stroking action of the non-pattern-based root treatment helps to 'train' the *qi* to prevent it rising up so readily.

Age of child

There are differing opinions as to the effectiveness of *shonishin* on children of different ages. Birch recommends using a non-pattern-based root treatment on all children up to the age of five, most children between the ages of five and ten, and on some teenagers.[25] Wernicke, on the other hand, suggests *shonishin* can be effective on children of any age and adults too.[26] My experience is that *shonishin* is especially beneficial for children up to the age of approximately seven or eight but may also be effective in some older children and teenagers.

What is the clinical effect of *shonishin*?

There are different ways of understanding the effect of *shonishin*. Birch describes the non-pattern-based root treatment outlined below as having the ability to 'restore and stimulate the body's natural healing mechanisms'.[27] In this sense, it can be understood as a gentle method of supporting a child's maturing health and general development, or as a way of tenderly encouraging a child's body back to a place of health. Wernicke,[28] choosing a more scientific explanation, describes *shonishin* treatment as a way of regulating the autonomic nervous system of the child. Research in Sweden has shown that stroking may also lead to the release of oxytocin in the body.[29] Oxytocin is known to have a strong calming effect. It is also sometimes described as 'the happy hormone', as it tends to increase a sense of well-being.

On a very simple and intuitive level, *shonishin* can be understood as a way of helping to counteract the tendency of *qi* in a young child to rise up to the head. The downward-stroking action involved in the non-pattern-based root treatment (described later in this chapter), in particular, has this effect. Counterflow *qi* is a part of so many of the conditions for which children most commonly seek treatment, for example asthma, insomnia, hyperactivity, vomiting and headaches, to name but a few. A downward-stroking movement encourages *qi* in the same direction. The application of this in paediatric practice is extremely widespread.

As well as stroking, a tapping action is also used in the non-pattern-based root treatment. My experience of tapping is that it helps to stimulate the *qi* of the point or the area that is tapped. This is useful in deficient conditions.[*] It is also useful when trying to bring *qi* to a particular area. For example, when treating a child with chronic or recurrent ear or throat symptoms, *qi* may be brought to that part of the body in order for subsequent treatment of the Organ/Pathogen patterns to be effective.

Core non-pattern-based root treatment

The core of *shonishin* treatment is a non-pattern-based root treatment that can be used on all children at all times (with one or two notable exceptions which are listed below under 'Contraindications and precautions for the non-pattern-based root treatment'). In particular, it can be used:

---

[*] However, tapping should be used cautiously on a child who is easily overstimulated.

- when a child has an acute or chronic illness, in order to help him recover

- when a child needs support through a stressful time, such as starting school, in order to help maintain his health

- to help a child through a particular developmental stage, such as learning to walk or becoming dry at night

- as a preventive treatment and to enhance well-being.

There are various methods of delivering this core treatment. The method described here involves tapping and stroking certain areas of the body.

- **Stroking:** Stroking here refers to a gentle movement over the body's surface, applied with a smooth instrument, and going in one direction only. Birch suggests stroking at a rate of between 70 and 100 times per minute.[30] With a little experience, the practitioner will find a rate and method of stroking which she can adapt according to the child she is treating.

- **Tapping:** Tapping involves a rapid movement to a point or an area. In young children, it is more effective to tap the area around a point, rather than merely the point itself. This is because points are not fully formed until approximately the age of seven or eight. Birch suggests 100–200 taps per minute.[31] Rather than counting the number of taps, the practitioner should find a fast pace at which she can tap whilst maintaining a relaxed hand.

Stroking

The areas that are stroked are illustrated below. The stroking should always be done in a downward direction, from above to below. It should be performed only on the surfaces of the body where the *yang* channels run. My preferred method is to begin the treatment with the baby or child lying on his back and to stroke down the arms, torso and then legs. Afterwards, the baby or child is turned onto his front and the stroking is done down the backs of the arms, down the back and down the backs of the legs. However, this is all well and good if the child is happy to go along with this. It may, however, be necessary to employ a more flexible approach if the child is resistant to having the treatment done in this way.

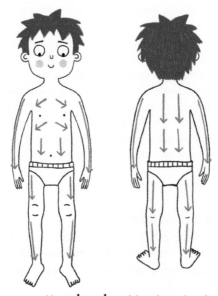

Core non-pattern-based root treatment – stroking

Number of strokes

The number of strokes depends on the age, constitution and health of the child being treated. The lowest dose of treatment would be two strokes in each area, and the most would be approximately six strokes in each area. Some general guidelines to help the practitioner decide on the number of strokes a child needs are the following:

- The younger the child, the fewer strokes needed.

- The weaker the child's physical constitution, the fewer strokes needed.

- The more emotionally sensitive the child, the fewer strokes needed.

- The more acutely ill, the fewer strokes needed.

The strokes are performed with a tool in the dominant hand, such as the *yoneyama* (see the picture of *shonishin* tools on page 344). The non-dominant hand should immediately follow the path of the dominant hand. This is so that the practitioner may assess changes that occur on the skin as the treatment is carried out. If the skin becomes warmer, looser or softer, then the practitioner should move on to the next area of the body to be stroked.

Tapping

The non-pattern-based root treatment includes tapping around the area of Du 12 *shenzhu*. This point has been used historically with moxa to prevent illness in children, but it also has a very important calming action.[32] This somewhat concurs with the TCM view of the actions of this point. Deadman et al.'s[33] list of actions for this point includes calming the spirit, and it is also included as a point which is used to treat childhood fright epilepsy. Tapping is carried out with the pointed end of a *shonishin* instrument, such as a *yoneyama*.

Tapping can also be performed on other areas which are indicated for each particular child. For example, the practitioner may decide to tap the area around Bl 23 *shenshu* at the end of the non-pattern-based root treatment on a child with Kidney deficiency. The occiput and interscapular areas are also common areas for tapping, as they have a calming effect.

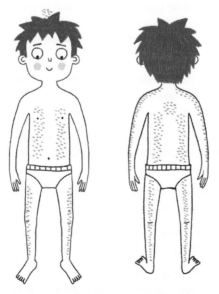

Core non-pattern-based root treatment – tapping

Number of taps

The criteria for deciding on the number of taps are the same as those listed above for deciding on the number of strokes. The smallest number of taps may be just eight or ten, and the highest number of taps may be up to approximately twenty or twenty-five.

 OVER-TREATMENT

The practitioner should always be mindful of 'over-treating' when giving acupuncture to a child. This applies equally when using *shonishin*. It can be tempting because the treatment takes such a short time and does not visually amount to much. The practitioner may feel she 'should' do more because the parent has an expectation of this and the family have come a long way for the treatment.

Contraindications and precautions for the non-pattern-based root treatment

As mentioned above, the non-pattern-based root treatment is beneficial in nearly all children nearly all the time. However, the following exceptions should be noted:

- It should not be carried out in a child who is feverish, as it can temporarily slightly raise the child's body temperature.

- It should not be carried out over broken skin or skin lesions. In children with skin conditions such as eczema, it is possible to tap around the eczematous areas but not over them.

For the reader who has no other knowledge of or training in *shonishin*, it is recommended to combine the core treatment using stroking and/or tapping with symptomatic treatment involving tapping of the relevant area of the body (e.g. the upper back in asthma or the lower back in bedwetting).

Home treatment

Birch developed the idea of teaching parents to do *shonishin* treatment on their children at home.[34] In the West, many of the children we treat travel a long way to get to us. Home treatment means visits can be less frequent than they would otherwise need to be. The following is a helpful protocol to ensure that parents perform it as well as possible on their child, and that they feel supported in doing so:

- **Demonstrate:** The complete *shonishin* routine should be demonstrated to the parent on his child in the clinic. It is also useful to do a 'sample' stroke and tap on the parent so he can feel how light the touch is.

- **Give feedback:** During the same session, the parent should be given the chance to try out the routine and the practitioner should give him feedback and make any necessary corrections.

- **Video:** The parent should be offered the opportunity to video the practitioner doing the *shonishin* routine on a mobile device, providing he has one.

- **Written record:** A sheet with diagrams and clear instructions should be given to the parent to take home with him.

- **Ongoing support:** The practitioner should make it clear to the parent that he may contact her if at any time he is unsure about what he is doing or if his child's condition changes.

- **Checking in:** The practitioner should ask the parent to show her how he has been doing the *shonishin* routine at the next appointment so that the method can be checked and corrected if necessary.

Using *shonishin* in the treatment of specific disorders

Part 5, Treatment of Physical Conditions, includes suggested *shonishin* treatments where applicable. They are only included in the sections describing the treatment of babies and toddlers, and sometimes school-age children. However, this is not to say that *shonishin* cannot be used on older children.

I have found *shonishin* especially helpful when treating older children who are developmentally younger than their age or who need help to relax at the start of a treatment. Even if the therapeutic effect is stronger on a younger child, using *shonishin* on an older child seems to have the effect of preparing the *qi* of the child so that the treatment that follows is especially well assimilated.

With *shonishin* probably more than any other treatment modality, the practitioner may be flexible in its application. For example, some practitioners may only use the stroking technique, whilst others may only use the tapping technique. As her experience deepens, the practitioner should apply *shonishin* techniques to her practice in the way that most benefits the children she treats.

SUMMARY

» *Shonishin* is a Japanese method of treating children which uses various instruments to stroke and tap the skin.

» The core non-pattern-based root treatment may be combined with any style of acupuncture and used without having first made a diagnosis of Organ/Pathogen patterns.

» This root treatment involves both stroking down the *yang* channel surfaces and tapping around particular points or areas.

» *Shonishin* may be taught to parents to perform daily at home.

• Chapter 36 •

ADVICE

· · · · · · · · · · · ·

The topics discussed in this chapter are:

- Finding a balance and rhythm to life

- Diet

- Protection from Pathogenic Factors

- Sleep

- Exercise

- Over-scheduling and overstimulation

- Pressure and expectation

- Studying

- Screen time

- Care during illness

- Emotions

- Support for the primary caregiver

Introduction

When giving any advice to parents, the practitioner should bear in mind two things. The first is that a parent is often very prone to feelings of guilt. The second is that a parent is often sensitive to feeling that she is being criticised. The practitioner must choose her words very carefully. Even more importantly, she should speak to parents from a place of compassion and understanding, and ideally with some degree of rapport having been made. This will mean that advice will generally be better accepted.

There are a few other points to bear in mind when giving advice:

- Advice should be given in bite-sized chunks. A long list of suggestions often feels overwhelming and is less likely to be followed.

- The practitioner should only give advice that she thinks is really pertinent to that individual child. There are many different reasons for a child to be Spleen *qi* deficient, for example. In most cases, only one or two will apply to each child.

- Ideally, advice is best given to parents in written form. Sleep deprivation, or merely the fact that parents generally have to keep so many things in their minds, means that it is more likely to be remembered correctly if written down.*

---

* Obviously, writing down advice is only really applicable when the advice is specific, such as foods to include and foods to avoid. More general advice, such as aiming to make bedtime a little earlier, does not generally need to be written down.

Finding a balance and rhythm to life

Babies and toddlers

A cactus will only thrive in the hot, arid desert. A young maple tree needs protection from the wind. Some shrubs and plants grow only in damp, waterlogged soil. Equally, every baby needs a different environment in which to thrive. One baby will be happier if she has lots of time at home. Another will love being out and about and watching the world go by. One baby may become easily unsettled by loud noises and lots of people, whilst another may be unperturbed.

It may be useful for the practitioner to chat with the parent and to get a sense of whether there is an obvious misfit between the nature of the baby and her routine. For example, it may be apparent that the baby is an excess type, who gets easily bored and restless but who spends virtually all day at home. Conversely, it may be that the baby is rather vulnerable and sensitive but is being taken to lots of loud, busy toddler groups. A baby who has a lot of Heat and becomes easily agitated will probably feed better in a quiet room, whereas another baby will feed well when she is out and about.

It is not always possible to provide the 'perfect' environment. However, if the practitioner perceives that there is an aspect to the life and routine of the baby that is causing the condition for which she is being brought for treatment, then this needs to be discussed with the parent.

School-age children and teenagers

A child will tend to become gradually more adaptable as she grows. However, a child will still struggle to thrive with a routine that does not suit her constitution. This is usually in the area of how busy a child is and is discussed in the section 'Over-scheduling and overstimulation' below.

Diet

(See also Chapter 8, Miscellaneous Causes of Disease, and Chapter 45, Problems with Eating and Appetite.)

Babies and toddlers

A baby's digestion is a finely tuned system. It takes very little for it to go out of kilter. The following pieces of dietary advice are appropriate for nearly all babies. Different ones may be emphasised depending on the nature of the baby.

Spacing of feeds and meals

If a baby is feeding much of the time, her Spleen never gets a chance to rest. Most babies need at least a two-hour break between the end of one feed and the start of another. This applies to both bottle- and breastfed babies. When a baby starts solids, the same applies. Meals should be regular and well spaced. The Spleen likes regularity. The Stomach needs time to rot and ripen food, then to empty and then to rest, before starting the process again.

Breast or bottle

There is little doubt as to the benefits of breastfeeding over bottle feeding. From the Chinese medicine perspective, cow's milk formula places a larger strain on the Spleen and promotes the formation of Damp and Phlegm in the body. Various alternatives to regular cow's milk formula are available. These may, for example, be extensively hydrolysed formulae based on meat derivatives, amino acid-based formulae or soy-based formulae. Although they may be slightly less detrimental to the Spleen than cow's milk formula, they are still much harder for a baby to digest than breast milk. They are often energetically Cold and lacking in *qi*.

Introducing solids

Solids should be introduced when the baby shows an interest in them. However, a baby's taste for solid food may be further developed than his digestive system. Although it goes against a very deep maternal instinct, it may sometimes be necessary for a parent to restrict the food intake of her baby. A baby should be allowed to stop eating when she has had enough rather than coaxed into eating more.

> A one-year-old baby was brought to the clinic with a host of digestive problems stemming from Accumulation Disorder. When I asked the parent about what he ate, she replied that he liked eating *everything*. She said that the baby ate what was not far off an adult portion of the same food she and her husband ate every evening. After I talked to the mother about the delicate nature of a baby's digestion, she began to give him smaller portions of simpler foods. With some treatment too, his digestive problems were soon resolved.

New foods should be introduced one at a time, with about a week in between. Most babies benefit from their first foods being either energetically neutral or slightly warming. Good first foods are rice- or millet-based products.

Energetics of food

Those not versed in the theory of Chinese medicine tend to view foods purely based on their nutritional content. A parent with the best intentions may feed her baby raw vegetables and fruit knowing that the vitamin content is high. It is common in the West to eat foods straight from the refrigerator. Babies born into Asian families may be weaned on spicy foods.

The practitioner might advise on which foods are appropriate for the baby based on the nature of the baby's *qi*. Many babies need a diet that is energetically warmer than the one they are receiving. A few need one which is less heating. Some 'rules' which benefit almost every baby are the following:

- Limit the amount of whole foods in the diet (so white rice is better than brown rice, for example).

- Lightly steamed fruit and vegetables are easier for a child to digest than raw vegetables. This is especially true in the winter months.

- Food should be eaten at room temperature or warmer.

- Rich, fatty and greasy foods should be kept to a minimum.

- Refined sugar products should not be given to babies.

- Foods containing additives (e.g. preservatives, artificial flavours) should not be given to babies.

School-age children

From the age of approximately seven, the digestive system of a child becomes stronger. From this age, children are therefore usually able to handle more diverse foods, and not be thrown out of kilter by eating something occasionally that is energetically not suitable for them.

Different aspects of diet become a cause of ill health during the school years. The key points are the following:

- Meals should be regular.

- The child should not read, look at a screen or do her homework whilst she is eating.

- Meals should be eaten together with family or other members of the community whenever possible.

- Refined sugar should be kept to a minimum.

- Fresh, unprocessed food should be eaten whenever possible.

- Food appropriate to the season should be eaten; for example, no ice cream in winter.

- Artificial additives should be avoided.

- Children should be encouraged to eat a wide variety of food.

Beyond these key points, advice should be given based on the condition of the individual child.

Teenagers

The same key points listed for school-age children apply to teenagers. On top of this, there are a couple of other considerations:

- Teenagers often have phases of eating insatiably. At the same time, a parent usually has less control over what a teenager eats partly because she may be out with friends more of the time. Parents should do what they can to ensure that teenagers eat proper meals at mealtimes, and that they do not eat sugary and salty snacks throughout the day in lieu of this.

- It is important for teenage girls, in particular, to eat a good amount of Blood-nourishing foods.

Protection from Pathogenic Factors

(See also Chapter 9, External Causes of Disease.)

Babies

A baby is more vulnerable to invasion from an External Pathogenic Factor than an adult. Whilst fresh air is important for the baby's Lung *qi* to grow strong, he should be wrapped up appropriately when he goes outside. In cold weather, he should be wrapped up in warm clothes, especially his head, back of neck, tummy and lower back, hands and feet. In wet weather, he should be kept dry or taken out of damp clothes as soon as possible. In hot weather, he should be shaded from direct sun.

When a baby is invaded by an external pathogen, his *yin* being insubstantial, he is not able to keep the Heat in check and therefore may quickly develop a high fever. Therefore, when a baby has a fever, measures should be taken to avoid exacerbating the Heat. See Chapter 70 on the treatment of acute illnesses for suggestions of how to do this.

As well as causing possible digestive issues as discussed, another consequence of the baby's immature Spleen is that he will struggle to transform and transport fluids after an invasion of an External Pathogenic Factor. This means that his head, nose, chest and digestive system may easily become clogged with Phlegm and/or Damp. The best protection against this is to avoid the invasion of the External Pathogenic Factor in the first place. When this is not possible, then advice may be given to the parent about diet, avoiding damp places such as swimming pools, and giving him the opportunity to move as much as possible (when he is at an age when he can crawl or walk).

School-age children and teenagers

From the age of approximately seven, a child's defensive (*wei*) *qi* will have become more mature, her *yin* more substantial and her Spleen stronger. Therefore, she is better able to resist external invasions and to recover more quickly and more completely if she does succumb. However, depending on the nature of the child, there are still some key pieces of advice:

- Pre-pubescent and adolescent girls should keep their lower back and abdomen protected against the cold and damp to avoid these pathogens entering the gynaecological system.[*]

- All children should protect the lower back and abdomen against invasions of Cold and Damp, especially when going through intense periods of change and development (such as happens at the changeover of the seven- and eight-year cycles). These changes are fuelled by the Kidneys, which are particularly susceptible to imbalance when they are working so hard.

- A child should be encouraged to protect herself against the elements when she is exercising. Sweating opens the pores and makes her more vulnerable.

Sleep

(See also Chapter 8, Miscellaneous Causes of Disease, and Chapter 43, Sleep Problems.)

Few babies and infants remain healthy without the appropriate amount of sleep. Sleep, and the amount of sleep a child needs at each age, is discussed in Chapter 43. Some babies and children do not sleep because of an imbalance in the *qi*. It is very hard for the parent to do anything about this, and treating the imbalance is the best solution. However, there are many other reasons why babies and children do not sleep enough.

For a baby or child, going to sleep involves separating from a parent. This fact alone makes it a complex area that can arouse fear and anxiety in the child, and guilt, frustration and worry in the parent. Dynamics at bedtime often reveal a deeper dynamic in the family. As a consequence, they can be tricky to change. Explaining to the parent the importance of sleep, and the impact that not enough may be having on her child, is essential and a good place to start.

---

[*] An excellent way of doing this is by using a *haramaki*, a Japanese Kidney warmer. These are easy to buy on the internet. They come in a range of different fabrics and colours, which can make them appealing to teenage girls.

The most pertinent points of advice in regards to sleep are given below.

Babies and toddlers

The best sleep environment should be found for the baby. Some sleep quite well whilst out and about and being carried in a sling, others only sleep whilst in a quiet room at home. One baby may sleep better in the comfort of her parent's bed, whilst another may be overstimulated by the presence of a parent. The parent may have deeply held views about how a baby *should* sleep, and these may not fit with how her baby wants to sleep.

Some parents have a fear that a baby who sleeps a lot in the day will sleep less well at night. The opposite is usually true. The practitioner can explain to the parent that the *qi* of a baby has a strong tendency to rise upwards. The more tired she becomes, the more this is likely to happen. The more this happens, the harder it is for the baby to sleep.

> The sleep problems of one nine-month-old baby who came to the clinic were simply solved by suggesting to the parents that they put the baby to bed in the early evening rather than keeping her up with them. This meant the baby was no longer tired, fell asleep much more easily and slept more soundly.

School-age children

Separation from the parent at bedtime is a common problem for school-age children. This may be because the child does not see her parent in the day and therefore is not ready to separate from her when they have only just come together at bedtime. It may also be because the parent is struggling to separate from the child (especially if that means facing a partner with whom there are difficulties). The practitioner should stress to the parent the importance of sleep during the early evening, and work with her to come up with suggestions of how to make bedtime easier. This may be spending more time with the child during the day, reward charts, ensuring the household has a calm atmosphere at bedtime or involving another adult figure at bedtime who is better able to keep firm boundaries.

Teenagers

Sleep is as important in the teenage years as at any other time. The most common issue for a teenager is her reluctance to go to bed early enough, and difficulty getting up in time for school. Of course, a teenager may resist being told by her parent that she needs to go to bed early enough. However, if she is told by the practitioner, and the connection between lack of sleep and the condition for which she is being treated is explained, she is more likely to take the advice on board.

Suggestions for helping teenagers to sleep well are the following:

- Keep screens out of bedrooms.

- Come off all screens at least an hour before bedtime.

- Stop studying at least an hour before bedtime.

- Exercise during the day.

- Avoid eating a big meal just before bedtime.

Exercise

(See also Chapter 8, Miscellaneous Causes of Disease.)

Babies and toddlers

Once a baby starts crawling or walking, she should be given the opportunity to move about as much as possible throughout the day. This helps to counteract the tendency to stagnation in the digestive system that is such a problem in the early months.

School-age children

Children need ample opportunity to run around and move. A child has an abundance of *yang*, and if this does not get expression then it may lead to imbalance and illness.

However, at the same time, a child is growing and developing at an extraordinary rate. She should therefore not be expending too much of her *qi* on exercising. She should be able to stop running around or doing whatever sport she is doing when she gets tired. It is entirely inappropriate for a child of this age to be 'pushed' physically to the point where she has to dig into her reserves in order to keep going.

The key pieces of advice for school-age children regarding exercise, therefore, are the following:

- Provide ample opportunity for and encourage physical activity and movement.

- Reduce or exclude organised sport where the child is required to train for extended periods of time to the point of exhaustion, or to train on a daily basis.

- Avoid sports where one part of the body is overused in order to prevent injury.

- Intense aerobic exercise, such as running, is too depleting for almost all children until they are through the early teenage years.

Teenagers

Teenagers seem to be divided into those who eschew leaving the house under any circumstances and those who train excessively for a particular sport. Of course, a balance in the middle of those two things is the ideal. Excessive sport at a time of such rapid growth and development can be depleting. On the other hand, not moving around at a time when there is such a surge of *yang* can be equally detrimental.

The following tips may be useful:

- Girls should be encouraged to limit hard exercise during and after menstruation, when the body needs its resources to build up Blood.

- If a teenager is doing hard training for a particular sport that she is not willing to give up, encourage her to have whole days off exercise whenever possible and to cut out any peripheral physical activity that she cares less about. It should be stressed that, because she is training to that level, sleep and diet are even more important.*

---

*   The practitioner should remember that it is entirely contrary to the view of most people in the Western world that doing lots of exercise can be harmful. It is therefore vital to explain our thinking behind advising a teenager to do less.

- If a teenager is not doing enough exercise, it is again important to explain to her exactly why doing some more will help her condition.* Exploring with the teenager and parent what kind of exercise might be the most palatable to her may be helpful. It may even be possible to build exercise into the young person's daily life by cycling to school, for example.

Over-scheduling and overstimulation

(See also Chapter 7, The Challenges of Life.)

An overly busy schedule and a lack of downtime is at the root of a lot of depletion and *qi* stagnation in children. One of the most common reasons for a child to discontinue treatment is that the family cannot fit coming to the clinic into their busy schedule. A fast and full life has become so much the norm that it is often not recognised as being problematic. Children are growing and developing, and doing it fast. They need downtime in order to do this successfully and, more fundamentally, simply to be able to breathe.**

> I once received an email from the mother of a ten-year-old girl who was suffering from constant tension headaches. She wanted to book an appointment and said that they would be able to attend the clinic between 4.15 and 5.15pm on a Thursday. On all other days after school, and after 5.15pm on a Thursday, the girl had other activities which she could not miss. We eventually managed to make an appointment. A few days before, the mother cancelled it saying that her daughter had extra swimming training so would not be able to make it. No wonder she suffered from tension headaches!

Each child will have different needs in terms of how much downtime she needs and how full a schedule she can handle. Parents who thrive off a busy and full life may find it hard to recognise that their child is not able to handle such demands and such a pace.

The key pieces of advice related to downtime are the following:

- A child needs periods of time in her weekly schedule when she is at home, not being rushed to the next activity and not doing homework or other chores. Cutting down on extra-curricular activities is usually possible, although it may take a strong parent to resist the pressure for the child to be taking part in everything on offer.

- Most children need an absolute minimum of one day a week at home and with an opportunity to switch off and relax.

- The definition of downtime is time that induces a feeling of relaxation and unwinding. For most children, playing computer games and going on sleepovers is not downtime. Running around and exploring in the countryside would constitute downtime for most children, whereas playing a competitive sport would probably not.

- Time in nature is especially valuable downtime. This is not just because the child will breathe in fresh air and get exercise. Research has shown that being in a natural environment actually helps a child's senses to develop and work at a more refined level. Children relax when they are in nature and can express their wild sides – which get so little expression in everyday life.

- A child will go through periods of especially rapid growth and development. During these times, she will need more rest and downtime than usual. Ideally, a family's schedule will

---

* For example, 'In Chinese Medicine terms, your acne has arisen because of a build-up of too much heat in your body. Exercising will help to disperse this heat and that will mean it does not need to find its way out via your skin.'

** Downtime has many additional benefits. For example, family members can really get to know each other. Being bored stimulates creativity and imagination. If a child does not learn how to 'do' downtime, she is likely to become an adult who is unable to stop.

be able to accommodate this. It is especially important not to overstimulate a child during these times too. She needs to be allowed to go inwards and to conserve her *qi* for the process that is at work within her. Simple, quiet activities, rather than intense and frenetic ones which excite and stimulate, are always beneficial, but especially during these times.

- After an intense time, such as an exam period or a major sporting event, a child needs extra downtime in order to unwind and recuperate.

Pressure and expectation
(See also Chapter 7, The Challenges of Life.)

Too much pressure and expectation has a similar impact to being over-scheduled. It demands too much of a child whilst she already has her work cut out with growing and developing. It can lead to constraint of *qi* as well as depletion.

This is an area where it is hard to give advice. Parents are often unaware of the subtle ways in which they themselves may be putting added pressure on a child. However, the practitioner may be able to open up discussions that help to bring about a shift in the dynamic. Talking to a parent about his child's constitution from the Chinese medicine perspective may help him to understand the particular sensitivities their child may have.

The key points to bear in mind are the following:

- A child usually feels more than enough pressure at school, academically and socially. Home, as far as is possible, needs to be a place of refuge from pressure.

- The focus should be on long-term physical and mental health for a child. Pressure to achieve goals in the short term (e.g. being top of the class, excelling at a sport, being socially mature) may come at the expense of health and happiness in the future. If too much is asked of a child over a period of time, some aspect of her will usually crack.

- Breaks away from the habitual school and social environment often help a child to escape the pressure she feels to be a certain way and behave in a particular fashion.

Studying
(See also Chapter 7, The Challenges of Life.)

Studying cannot, of course, be avoided. The practitioner often needs to point out, however, that too much of it may be having a detrimental effect on the child.* The key points to consider are the following:

- Too much studying before the age of seven is particularly depleting for a child.

- A child should stop studying an hour before bedtime, in order to give her time to quieten her thoughts before attempting sleep.

---

* Explaining to a child and parent the role of the digestive system in taking in information as well as food often helps them to understand why studying may be depleting.

- Studying should be interspersed with movement.

- Studying should not be done whilst eating, watching television or communicating on social media. Creating the right environment to study in means work will be got through more quickly and be done better.

Screen time
(See also Chapter 7, The Challenges of Life.)

Screen time, and how to negotiate it with a child, is often the bane of a parent's life. When a child's relationship to the online world becomes a cause of imbalance, the practitioner may be able to help the parent to instil new 'rules' about the child's screen time.

The key points to bear in mind are the following:

- Parents should be in charge of how much time their child spends on a screen.

- The earlier in a child's life that she begins having screen time, the more potentially negative impact it may have.* Therefore a parent should hold out against her child using computers, mobile phones and tablets for as long as possible.**

- A child should not be given time on a device as a way of comforting her when she is upset.

- Short periods on a device are better than long ones. So, it is less detrimental for a child to have two half-hour slots a day than it is to have one hour-long slot.

- Screen time should not be allowed within an hour of bedtime.

- Devices should not be allowed in bedrooms.***

- Screen time should be interspersed with a mix of other activities.

- The child should be given opportunities to develop a range of interests so that being on a device is not the only way she knows of filling her time.

- The more a child protests when she is told to come off her device, the more it indicates that screen time has become too big a feature in her life.

- Parents who are too attached to their electronic devices will find it hard to instil sensible use of them in their children.

- Parents should monitor exactly what their child is doing online and make sure it is age appropriate.

---

* Some of the documented negative impacts include poor posture, eye strain, social difficulties and an increase in mental health disorders.

** In 2015, the Taiwanese government made it illegal for parents to allow a child under the age of two to use an electronic device such as a smartphone, tablet or television. The law also stated that parents must ensure that a child under the age of eighteen use electronic devices for a 'reasonable' length of time.

*** Devices in bedrooms are known to be a major cause of sleep deprivation in teenagers.

I once treated a three-year-old boy for insomnia. He would walk into the clinic staring at his tablet and continue staring at it throughout the treatment. I suggested to his mother that the treatment would have more effect if he was not on the tablet, and that in general the amount of time he spent on a screen was contributing to his sleep problem. His mother said he would be furious if she took it away from him and would not consent to the treatment. I suggested we try. As predicted, the boy had an enormous tantrum. However, once he had got through this and I had managed to engage him in chat, he started giggling and really enjoyed his treatments. This helped model to his mother that it was possible. It can be hard for parents, dealing with the many strains of parenthood, to change a dynamic that has become embedded between them and their child. As an outsider, we can sometimes show how this is possible.

Care during illness

There is a widely held view that a child should take some paracetamol and keep going through a minor illness. This belief, as well as practical concerns about childcare, also means a child will get back to school or childcare as soon as possible after a bigger illness. This is contrary to Chinese medical opinion. A child needs a quality of care during illness and time to recuperate afterwards. This hugely reduces the chance of a Lingering Pathogenic Factor forming.

The key points of advice are the following:

- When ill, a child should ideally stay at home, and be cared for by her primary caregiver or someone with whom she is deeply familiar.*

- During a febrile illness, the child should avoid being on a screen, which encourages *qi* and Heat to rise up to the brain.

- A child should, in an ideal world, have a day of recuperation after an illness for each day that the illness lasted. So, if the illness lasted three days, the child should stay at home for three more days when she is better. When she does return to school, she should avoid all extra-curricular activities for a while.

- If a child is not hungry when ill, she should be allowed not to eat. If she is hungry, she should be given simple foods, and avoid sugary, spicy, rich or fatty foods.

Suppression of fevers

Fevers used to kill children and, in the collective unconscious, there is still a deep fear of them. It goes without saying that a fever should be taken seriously, especially when it is accompanied by a rash.

However, there is a widespread tendency to suppress fevers with medication. Whilst this may be necessary, it is sometimes done in lieu of proper care. If the fever is mild, the child is coping with it well and she is otherwise healthy, it is probably advisable not to intervene. Suppressing a fever can mean that a child is unable to expel Heat, which may then remain in her body after the illness and cause chronic symptoms.

Parents often ask how high they should let a fever go before they medicate the child. Rather than looking at the thermometer, it is best to look at the child. A child may be very ill with a low fever or relatively well despite a high fever.

Please see Chapter 70, Treatment of Acute Conditions, for advice on how to support a child through a fever.

---

* Parents often notice they feel very tired after caring for a child through an illness. This is because the child feeds off the parent's *qi* in order to get better. So it is appropriate that the parent should feel that way.

Emotions
(See also Chapter 5, Emotions.)

It is very hard to give advice about emotions. Acupuncture is often the most effective way of helping to bring about greater emotional equilibrium in a child. Conversation with the parent and child can be helpful too. If the parent and/or child can be helped to see the connection between the physical imbalance and an emotion, it may pave the way for change to take place. Simply acknowledging an emotion may help it become unstuck. The practitioner should remember that the reason a child may be suppressing an emotion is because the parent feels uncomfortable with that emotion and it is taboo in the family.

The following points may be helpful:

- **Anger:** A child with an imbalance in her expression of anger, frustration or pressured feelings needs an outlet for these emotions. If she is generally a 'good girl' and overly compliant, exploring ways she can also express her defiant, assertive and independent side is important. Some examples may be beating a pillow against a bed, mucking around in nature, playing the drums or being given permission to argue a bit more.*

- **Worry:** A young child who has a tendency to worry may benefit from having a 'worry tree' where she can hang all her worries before bedtime. It is often useful to allow a child to talk about her worries rather than responding with a platitude of 'Don't worry, it will all be fine'. Expressing worries helps the *yi* to become unstuck. Having said this, it is sometimes advisable to tell a child who is worried and anxious before bedtime that you will talk about her worries in the morning when she is not so tired. A balance needs to be struck between allowing a child to express her worries but also encouragement not to dwell on them.

- **Fear:** Fear and anxiety come from the Kidneys which reside in the Lower Burner and are rarely alleviated by words which do not touch this primal part of a child. It is not always possible to banish from her life something that makes a child fearful, but giving her a space to talk about it in the treatment room can help to diminish its power. A child may be able to verbalise something in the treatment room she is not able to at home. Treatment often helps her to feel more empowered in the face of something she has previously found frightening.

- **Sadness:** Treatment of the Lungs, as well as the Organs related to the Fire Element, often helps a child to release sad feelings that have been somatised. A young child may find it easier to draw a picture of her sad feelings rather than talk about them. Letting a child cry rather than trying to cheer her up is often cathartic.

- **Joy:** A child needs laughter in her life. A family who are busy, rushed, strained and over-scheduled may forget to laugh. Most children have a wonderful ability to find humour everywhere. Talking to a child and her parent about what makes her light up, and reminding them to make time for this, is so simple yet can make such a difference.

---

* It may be that the parent or parents have low tolerance for an assertive child. Allowing siblings to argue a bit more, and not reprimanding teenagers for throwing strops, is sometimes advisable. Of course, certain behaviour is unacceptable, but parents need to pick their battles so as not to become too suppressive.

Support for the primary caregiver

Babies and toddlers

A baby feeds off the *qi* of the main caregiver. Apart from the basics of food and practical care, the aspect of life that has most influence on a baby is the relationship he has with his primary caregiver, usually his mother. This will be largely determined by the emotional state of this person. The more relaxed, happy, secure and loved the mother is, the better able she will be to meet her baby's needs.

Therefore, when a mother brings her baby for treatment, the most important advice we give may be for the mother to make some changes in her life. This may involve her being encouraged to access more practical support, receiving acupuncture treatment, reminding her of the importance of eating well or sleeping when her baby sleeps. In the fog of sleeplessness, and overwhelmed by being responsible for the needs of her baby, it is easy for a mother to entirely forget about her needs. The practitioner can play an important role in reminding her of them.

The reader will be familiar with the Five Elements concept of 'treating the mother to treat the child'. In many cases, unless the mother is well it is impossible for a baby to thrive and be healthy. A baby is drinking in the *qi* of the mother to such an extent that his health often depends to a large degree on that of the mother.

School-age children and teenagers

The primary objective for a parent and her baby or toddler is to bond as strongly as possible. After the age of seven or eight, the objective becomes to support a child gradually in taking steps towards independence. The happier a parent is in her own life, the easier it will be for her to do this.

So, support is still needed but to a different end. Parenting in isolation is difficult with a child of any age. Simply bringing her child for treatment may feel supportive to a parent. There may sometimes be an opportunity to encourage a parent to seek support in other areas, such as from other healthcare professionals, friends or family. Treating the child may mean she is less demanding of her parent, and this, in turn, helps the parent to feel less strained.

Tables 36.1, 36.2 and 36.3 summarise advice according to Organ pathology, Pathogenic Factors and Vital Substances/non-Organ pathologies respectively.

Table 36.1 Areas of advice according to Organ pathology

Spleen *qi/yang* deficiency	Lung *qi* deficiency	Kidney deficiency	Liver *qi* stagnation
Worry and overthinking	Expression of sad feelings	Insecurity and fear	Expression of anger and related emotions
Amount of study	Lack of fresh air	Over-scheduling	Lack of exercise and movement
Diet	Too much cardiovascular exercise	Excessive, intense exercise	
Amount and type of exercise	Protection from External Pathogenic Factors	Pressure and expectation	Pressure and expectation
Nurture and care		Long-term poor diet	Over-scheduling
Lack of sleep	Lack of sleep	Lack of sleep	Excessive screen time
		Computer games	Atmosphere at mealtimes

Table 36.2 Areas of advice according to Pathogenic Factors

Phlegm/Damp	Heat	Cold
Diet	Internalised emotions	Diet
Damp environment	Diet	Protection from energetically Cold medications (e.g. paracetamol, antibiotics)
Lack of movement/exercise	Excessive pressure and stress	
Any cause of Spleen deficiency	Any cause of Liver *qi* stagnation	Any cause of Spleen *qi/yang* deficiency

Table 36.3 Areas of advice according to Vital Substances and non-Organ patterns

Blood deficiency	Accumulation Disorder	Lingering Pathogenic Factor
Too much exercise	Too much whole and/or raw food	Rest
Worry		Care through illness
Excessive reliance on social media	Overeating	
Excessive studying	Lack of space between feeds	
Lack of Blood-nourishing foods	Stressed while eating or feeding	

Advice according to Constitutional Imbalance should address the following issues.

(See also Chapters 16 to 20.)

Fire

- Lots of love, warmth, communication and intimacy
- Emotional stability and constancy
- Fun, joy and laughter
- Permission to be low sometimes
- Balance between time alone and time with others
- Support in navigating friendships

Earth

- Consistent, responsive, nurturing
- Neither a 'lack' of mothering nor 'smothering'
- To feel heard and understood
- An emotionally and physically stable home environment
- Support to take notice of and respond to own needs
- Rhythm and routine

Metal

- Support in dealing with loss
- An appropriate and present father figure

- Meaningful acknowledgement and praise

- An orderly environment

- Permission to be less than perfect

- The right kind and amount of physical contact

- Support in learning to connect with others

Water

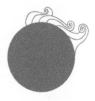

- A feeling of safety

- Reassurance

- Patience

- Allowed to develop at their own speed and in their own time

- Permission to 'go with the flow'

- Trustworthy, solid and reliable adults

- Support with assessing age-appropriate risk

- Support to know when to keep going and when to rest

Wood

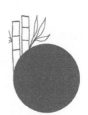

- The right balance between boundaries/rules/guidance versus freedom/ independence

- Support with the expression of emotions in the anger family

- Adventure and exploration

- Impartiality

- Peace and quiet

- Time to dream

- Permission to express individuality

Conclusion

Lifestyle advice is an essential part of treatment. As with the other aspects of treatment, less is often more. There is great value in pinpointing the key aspect of the child's life that is causing her to be ill, and addressing this with the child and/or parent. Lifestyle advice is not usually something that needs to be spoken about once and then forgotten. Just as with the other aspects of treatment, it needs to be returned to, sometimes again and again, and discussed from many different angles.

For example, the concept of 'deficiency' may be one to which a parent or older child simply does not relate. Unless she is not getting enough sleep or is conscious of feeling exhausted, it can be hard for a child or her parent to understand that she is depleted. Often, a deficient child is seemingly full of energy because she is 'running on empty'. Lifestyle advice, therefore, is sometimes not just about changing something on a practical level, such as not eating bananas. It can be about enabling a family to gain an entirely new perspective on what is health-giving and what is not. This can be as challenging as finding exactly the right treatment principles and point combination, but it can be equally miraculous and beneficial in its effect when done well.

A seven-year-old girl came to the clinic with alopecia. She was at school six days a week, played three musical instruments, swam and played netball for her school team. School holidays were filled with endless activities. She was very depleted indeed. Her parents, when I explained this, initially said this could not be right because none of her teachers or coaches had pointed out to them that she was tired, and she seemed to have lots of energy. I used the analogy of a battery to explain what I meant. Even when a battery only has 10 per cent charge, it still appears to work as well as one which has 100 per cent charge. Their daughter needed time resting to 'recharge'.

• Part 4 •

TREATMENT OF MENTAL– EMOTIONAL CONDITIONS

Chapter 37

INTRODUCTION TO THE TREATMENT OF MENTAL–EMOTIONAL CONDITIONS

The following chapters focus on the treatment of the mental–emotional conditions that are most commonly seen in my clinic. Whilst there is a sadness to the fact that these conditions are now so prevalent amongst young people, it is encouraging that there is a growing awareness that acupuncture can provide support.

Mental–emotional conditions often arise because a child is ill-equipped to deal with intense emotions and does not know how to express her pain in a 'healthy' way. She may become depressed or anxious, or turn to a self-destructive strategy such as starving herself or self-harming. Most children have little or no guidance in learning to identify and understand their emotions. It is no wonder that so many then end up overwhelmed and desperate.

How far can acupuncture help in the treatment of complex mental–emotional conditions?

It is my experience that acupuncture can be of great benefit to a child suffering from a mental–emotional condition. It is particularly beneficial because treatment of the child's *qi* will influence her relationship with her emotions, her expression of emotion and her felt experience of being in the world. It can do this without the child necessarily needing to talk in any great detail about how she feels. Therefore, acupuncture has an advantage over talking therapies for many children who find it hard to articulate the nuances of their emotional landscape or feel threatened by the requirement to do so. If acupuncture helps a child to feel better about herself and more comfortable in her own skin, then conditions such as eating disorders, self-harm, anxiety and depression may begin to have less hold.

Expectations

Having said this, it is prudent for a practitioner who sees a child with a complex, mental–emotional condition to be mindful of her expectations. Whilst it may be possible for treatment to 'cure' an eight-year-old with mild anxiety, it is less likely that acupuncture alone will 'cure' a fifteen-year-old who is in the grips of severe anorexia. In the latter case, the child will probably need treatment from a range of healthcare professionals who are trained in the particular complexities of eating disorders. In the case of a child on the autistic spectrum, the practitioner needs to remember that the child will most likely always struggle, to some degree and with some areas, in a largely neurotypical world. Treatment can help to lessen the child's struggle and make life a little easier for her. It cannot, of course, change the nature of any child.

Limits to competence

A practitioner may find she feels overwhelmed, upset or intimidated when treating a child with a mental–emotional condition. It is wise for her to reflect on the limits to her competence before agreeing to treat a child with, for example, severe depression. It is also important for the practitioner to communicate with the parent to ensure that the child is receiving the support she needs from other healthcare professionals, and to communicate with them when possible.

Unless the practitioner has additional training or skills, she may find it helpful to remind herself that, even when treating a child with a complex and deep-rooted mental–emotional condition, her role is to diagnose the imbalances she finds in the Elements and Organs and to treat them to the best of her ability.

How does treatment of a mental–emotional condition differ from that of a physical condition?

A physical symptom may, of course, often arise as a result of an imbalance in the emotions or the spirit. However, a mental–emotional problem always does. Therefore, the practitioner may need to include a range of points known to particularly affect the spirit, such as those listed in Chapter 30, in her point choice. Similarly, whilst treatment of the constitutional imbalance is frequently of benefit in the treatment of physical conditions, it is nearly always of benefit in the treatment of mental–emotional conditions.

A few other issues to bear in mind

- The reader will note that there are no paediatric *tui na* or *shonishin* treatments included in this part of the book. This is because the majority of children who come with these conditions are at an age when these treatments will be less effective. However, this is not to say that they should not be used, or that younger children will not sometimes come with these conditions too.

- The patterns listed are the ones I most often see. However, as always, the practitioner should treat what she finds (which may not be one of the patterns listed here).

- Similarly, the points listed are suggestions and the practitioner should choose points according to the child in front of her, as well as her own particular preferences.

• Chapter 38 •

HYPERACTIVITY, INATTENTIVENESS AND LEARNING DIFFICULTIES

· ·

The topics discussed in this chapter are:

- Organs

- Aetiology and pathology

- Patterns

- A Five Element view of hyperactivity, inattention and learning difficulties

- Other treatment modalities

Introduction

Most children are inattentive at times, and most are hyperactive at times too. Many children struggle with some aspects of learning but not with others. It can be hard to determine when the line is crossed between normal behaviour and a diagnosable condition that needs treatment. However, attention deficit disorder (ADD) and attention deficit hyperactivity disorder (ADHD) are two of the most commonly diagnosed mental disorders of childhood.

From the acupuncturist's perspective, it does not matter whether or not the child falls into the diagnostic category defined via the DSM-IV criteria.[1] The child will most likely have been brought to the clinic because her behaviour is causing problems at home and/or school. Hyperactivity or inattentiveness may not only be disrupting her ability to learn but may also be getting in the way of her making and sustaining friendships. Thankfully, acupuncture is usually a wonderfully effective way of helping this child.

Symptoms

Symptoms can be divided into two broad categories: those related to inattention and those related to hyperactivity. Some of the most common are shown in Table 38.1.

Table 38.1 Symptoms of inattention and hyperactivity

Symptoms of inattention	Symptoms of hyperactivity
Difficulty paying close attention to detail in school work, etc.	Unable to sit still
Difficulty sustaining attention either at school or when playing	Constantly fidgeting
Difficulty listening when spoken to	Needs to move all the time
Does not follow through on instructions or finish things	Excessive talking
Easily distracted	Unable to wait his turn
Avoids tasks that require sustained attention	Interrupts conversations
Difficulty organising himself, tasks or activities	Reckless behaviour
Forgetful and loses things	Impulsive behaviour

Learning difficulties

In the West, it is often assumed that thinking and feeling are two entirely separate processes. In Chinese medicine, however, the ability to learn and have clear thoughts is intimately related to the state of a child's *jingshen* and therefore to her emotions. For example, the character for *yi*, usually translated as intellect, also includes the radical for the Heart:

This character means 'the process of establishing meaning in the world with words that come from the Heart'.[2] Without the involvement of the Heart, a child's thoughts will be ungrounded and will not reflect who the child is.

The significance of this is that treatment of learning difficulties often needs to be focused, at least in part, on the *shen*. Furthermore, it conveys the fact that if a child is overwhelmed with a particular emotion, it is likely to affect her ability to learn.

When a parent reports that her child is struggling academically, the practitioner should not always assume a pathology is present, however. It should be remembered that some children's gifts do not lie in the area of the intellect. It may simply be that too much is being asked of a child, and that her parents and/or school have unrealistic expectations of her.

Organs

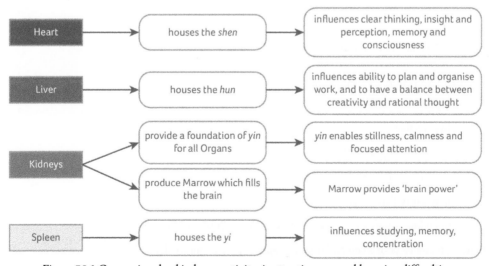

Figure 38.1 Organs involved in hyperactivity, inattentiveness and learning difficulties

Aetiology and pathology

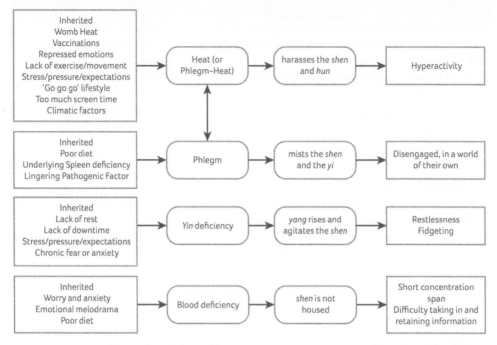

Figure 38.2 Aetiology and pathology of hyperactivity, inattentiveness and learning difficulties

Patterns

All these patterns are commonly seen in the clinic. In severe cases Heat and/or Phlegm are usually present, against a background of deficiency. In a child with milder difficulties, there may only be one of the deficient patterns present.

Below we consider:

- Heat in the Liver and/or Heart

- Phlegm misting the Mind

- Kidney and/or Liver *yin* deficiency

- Spleen *qi* and Heart Blood deficiency

Heat in the Liver and/or Heart

Key symptoms

- hyperactive

- physically fidgety and restless

- mentally active and very talkative

- may easily flare with anger

- unending supply of energy but may suddenly crash with exhaustion

Other symptoms: poor sleep and does not appear to need much sleep

Pulse: overflowing, rapid

Tongue: red, may have a yellow coat

Treatment principles: clear Heat; calm the *shen*

> **SUGGESTED TREATMENT**
> It is usually sufficient to use two points per treatment, one to clear Heat and one to resolve Phlegm.
>
> **Points**
> To clear Heat and calm the *shen*:
>
> > Liv 2 *xingjian*
> > Liv 3 *taichong*
> > He 7 *shenmen*
> > He 8 *shaofu*
> > M-HN-3 *yintang*
> > LI 11 *quchi*
>
> To resolve Phlegm:
>
> > Pc 5 *jianshi*
> > St 40 *fenglong*
>
> **Note:** If the Heat is also in the Stomach, add St 44 *neiting*.
>
> **Method:** sedation needle technique
>
> **Paediatric *tui na*** to clear Heat
>
> > Heart *xinjing* (straight pushing sedation)
> > Liver *ganjing* (straight pushing sedation)
> > Heaven Gate *tianmen* (straight pushing)
> > Heart Gate *xinmen* (straight pushing)
> > Water Palace *kangong* (pushing apart)
> > Inner Palace of Toil *neilaogong* (kneading)
> > Small Heavenly Heart *xiaotianxin* (tapping)
> > Milky Way *tianheshui* (straight pushing)

Phlegm misting the Mind

Symptoms

- difficulty concentrating

- unengaged

- disconnected

- hard to reach

- appears to not hear requests or instructions from parents or teachers

- confused thinking

Pulse: slippery or wiry

Tongue: thick, sticky coat

Treatment principles: resolve Phlegm

SUGGESTED TREATMENT

One or two points per treatment is usually sufficient.

Points

> Pc 5 *jianshi*
> St 40 *fenglong*
> GB 13 *benshen*
> GB 41 *zulinqi*
> Ren 14 *juque*
> Ren 15 *jiuwei*

Method: sedation needle technique

Paediatric *tui na*

> Heaven Gate *tianmen* (straight pushing)
> Heart Gate *xinmen* (straight pushing)
> Water Palace *kangong* (pushing apart)
> Inner Palace of Toil *neilaogong* (kneading)
> Small Heavenly Heart *xiaotianxin* (tapping)
> Small Palmar Crease *zhangxiaowen* (straight pushing)
> Hand *yin yang shouyinyang* (pushing apart)

Kidney and/or Liver *yin* deficiency

In children, a deficiency of the Liver and Kidneys means the propensity for *qi* and *yang* to rise up to the head becomes pronounced. In some cases, it could be described more accurately as a bad distribution of *qi* rather than a deficiency. There is too much *qi* in the head and not enough in the body.

Key symptoms

- hyperactivity which is worse when tired, as the day goes on and when overstimulated
- becomes worse as the term goes on
- easily distracted when tired
- a bit fidgety and restless

Other symptoms: finds it hard to go to sleep when overtired or overstimulated

Pulse: deficient, floating

Tongue: slightly red, may be peeled

Treatment principles: nourish Kidney and/or Liver *yin*; calm the *shen*

A seven-year-old came for treatment after being diagnosed with attention deficit disorder. He had very little ability to listen to and respond to instructions at school or to remain focused on any task he was given. His father said that everyone in the family struggled to engage him or connect with him. This caused them all great sadness, even though the boy himself seemed content. I diagnosed him as having Phlegm misting the Mind. It took several months of weekly treatments, as well as dietary changes, but he gradually 'emerged' out of his own world and became more engaged at school and at home.

SUGGESTED TREATMENT

Kidney deficient children tend to be easily overstimulated, so no more than one or two points per treatment should be used.

Points

Ki 1 *yongquan*
Ki 3 *taixi*
Ki 6 *zhaohai*
Bl 23 *shenshu*
Ren 4 *guanyuan*
Liv 8 *ququan*

Method: tonification needle technique

Paediatric *tui na*

Heaven Gate *tianmen* (straight pushing)
Heart Gate *xinmen* (straight pushing)
Water Palace *kangong* (pushing apart)
Liver *ganjing* (straight pushing tonification)
Kidney *shenjing* (straight pushing tonification)
Inner Palace of Toil *neilaogong* (kneading)
Small Heavenly Heart *xiaotianxin* (tapping)
Two Men Upon a Horse *erma* (kneading)
Lower Back Bl 23 *shenshu* (strong rubbing)
Spinal Column *jizhu* (pinching from bottom to top)

Spleen *qi* and Heart Blood deficiency

Key symptoms

- difficulty concentrating and taking in information

- difficulty remembering facts

- mentally unfocused

- worse when tired and in the evenings

Other symptoms: may behave in an attention-seeking way, prone to worry, difficulty getting off to sleep

Pulse: deficient, thin, choppy

Tongue: pale

Treatment principles: tonify Spleen *qi* and nourish Heart Blood; calm the *shen*

SUGGESTED TREATMENT

One or two points per treatment, perhaps with moxa, is usually sufficient.

Points

St 36 *zusanli*
Sp 6 *sanyinjiao*
Sp 3 *taibai*
Bl 20 *pishu*
He 7 *shenmen*
Bl 15 *xinshu*

Needle technique: tonification

Other techniques: moxibustion may be applicable

Paediatric *tui na*

Heaven Gate *tianmen* (straight pushing)
Heart Gate *xinmen* (straight pushing)
Water Palace *kangong* (pushing apart)
Spleen *pijing* (straight pushing)
Heart *xinjing* (straight pushing)
Inner Palace of Toil *neilaogong* (kneading)
Small Heavenly Heart *xiaotianxin* (tapping)
Spinal Column *jizhu* (pinching from bottom to top)

> One ten-year-old girl with this pattern, who was struggling to focus on her school work, said, 'It's as if my worries find their way into my thoughts and gradually the thoughts fly away and I'm left only with my worries.'

A Five Element view of hyperactivity, inattention and learning difficulties

The reason a child is hyperactive or cannot concentrate is often related both to an imbalance in one or more of the Five Elements and an Organ/Pathogen pattern. The child's environment at home or at school exacerbates an emotion, the presence of which contributes to him being unable to focus or be calm. Treatment of both the Five Element constitutional imbalance and the Organ/Pathogen pattern often brings about a more profound and lasting change than does treating the Organ/Pathogen pattern alone.

The diagram below suggests ways of supporting each of the Elements in a child in the learning environment.

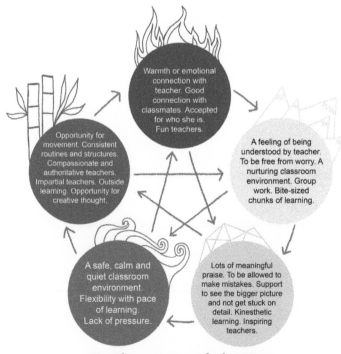

Five Element support for learning

Other treatment modalities

Shonishin

Core non-pattern-based root treatment.

Targeted tapping in the following areas if there is stiffness:

- LI 4 *hegu*
- Du 12 *shenzhu*
- Shoulder area
- Occipital area
- GB 20 *fengchi*

CASE HISTORY: EIGHT-YEAR-OLD BOY WITH AN ENORMOUS FEAR OF FAILURE

This case history illustrates:

- that treatment of a child's constitutional imbalance can have a profound impact on his ability to learn
- how *shonishin* stroking and tapping can be particularly effective when there is an imbalance in the Metal Element
- that sometimes it is necessary (but also adequately effective) to begin treatment with minimum intervention.

Jeremy was a bright boy who really struggled at school. He had one-to-one help from a teaching assistant throughout the school day. This was because of a strong tendency to become extremely anxious and not be able to engage in a task. Jeremy articulated clearly that he would 'rather not try than try and get it wrong'. He refused to ever read aloud to his parents, even though he was perfectly capable of it. He also refused to learn words for spelling tests. He was very clear that he could not take the risk of learning and then still get it wrong.

Jeremy was physically very healthy. His only symptom was a strong tendency to constipation. This had got somewhat better in the past few years but had been severe in his first years of life.

His mum reported that she was the only person Jeremy was happy to be touched by and that he generally eschewed any tactility.

Observations: Jeremy was exceedingly pale. His body was thin. He did not make any eye contact with me initially. His voice was very quiet and had a weeping tone to it. He seemed sensitive and vulnerable.

- Pulse: deficient, floating
- Tongue: normal

Diagnosis: I diagnosed Jeremy as having a constitutional imbalance in his Metal Element. I thought that he had a fragility to him that is characteristic of many children with this imbalance (see Chapter 18). I thought his enormous fear of failure and strongly self-critical voices were also a reflection of an imbalance in his Metal Element.

Treatment: I wanted to do a *shonishin* non-pattern-based root treatment on Jeremy first of all. I find this method especially beneficial for children with a Metal imbalance because the stroking movements on the skin are able to influence this Element via the *po*. Jeremy was reluctant to take his clothes off, so I did what I could by rolling up his sleeves and trousers, and lifting up his top.

I felt that Jeremy was much too vulnerable and deficient to be able to tolerate being needled. So I began by using the laser pen to tonify points on his Lung and Large Intestine channels.

By the third treatment, Jeremy was happy to take off his top and trousers and I taught his mother the *shonishin* to do at home daily. I continued to use the laser pen to strengthen the Lung and Large Intestine using a combination of distal points, and spirit points such as Lu 1 *zhongfu* and LI 18 *futu*.

Outcome: The first change Jeremy's mother noticed was that he started to read to her at home. She also noted that he began to allow his dad to hug him. At school, Jeremy gradually began to engage in tasks more easily and seemed to have less fear of failing at them. Jeremy was inherently a very sensitive and delicate boy but treatment helped him be the best that he could be and to find it a little easier to be in the world.

SUMMARY

» The Organs most commonly involved in problems with hyperactivity, inattention or learning difficulties are the Heart, the Liver, the Spleen and the Kidneys.

» The patterns most commonly seen are Heat in the Liver and/or Heart; Phlegm misting the Mind; Kidney and/or Liver *yin* deficiency; and Spleen *qi* and Heart Blood deficiency.

» Treating the child's Five Element constitutional imbalance, as well as any Organ/Pathogen patterns, is often very beneficial.

• Chapter 39 •

AUTISTIC SPECTRUM DISORDERS

• •

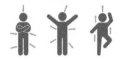

The topics discussed in this chapter are:

- The practicalities of treating a child with ASD

- Aetiology

- Organ/pathogen diagnosis of ASD

- A Five Element perspective of ASD

- Other treatment modalities

Introduction

Autistic spectrum disorder (ASD) is a condition that is now estimated to affect at least one in one hundred children in the UK. It is a spectrum disorder, meaning that it describes a wide range of behaviours, symptoms and, in some cases, disabilities. A child with an extreme version of ASD may never talk, become toilet trained, attend a mainstream school or be able to look after himself. Another child with ASD may attend a mainstream school, be very articulate and, in adulthood, support himself financially. However, one area that may provide challenges for all children with ASD, wherever they happen to be on the spectrum, is social interaction and relationships. The term therefore covers children who may bear little resemblance to each other at all in terms of symptoms or difficulties.* As one author wrote, 'Autism is both a disability and a difference. We need to find ways of alleviating the disability while respecting and valuing the difference.'[3]

In terms of making a Five Element and Organ/Pathogen diagnosis, there are a wide range of patterns, imbalances and pathologies that may be present in children with ASD, just as there could be in a neurotypical child. The process of treating a severely autistic child who is barely able to function in the world is obviously very different from treating a child who is high functioning and mildly aspergic. Most of my experience is in treating children who have ASD and are high functioning, and this is reflected in what I have written about the condition.

Why might a child with ASD come for treatment?

The aim when treating a child with ASD is not to somehow magically turn him into a neurotypical child. Rather, it is to make life for the child as easy as it possibly can be. In spite of the fact that society is slowly learning to accommodate difference better, the world is not geared towards the child with ASD. As a consequence of this, many children with ASD need more help and support to cope with life than a neurotypical child.

---

* There is an ongoing, heated debate in the autism community about the tension between identity and illness. Parents of some autistic children think that the idea that autism is not an adversity can seem insulting. Neurodiversity activists, on the other hand, speak of their children's difference in a positive light and reject any idea of interventions or 'treatments'.

A child with ASD, for example, may be prone to almost constant and sometimes extreme anxiety. He may not sleep well. He may struggle to regulate both his emotions and his behaviour. He is more likely to suffer from depression and other mood disorders. He may have difficulties eating a varied diet and present with symptoms related to digestion. Some of his symptoms may be part and parcel of ASD. Others may arise because of the stress of being ASD in a largely neurotypical world. The key point for us is that there is much we can do to make life a little easier. This may include treatment aimed at helping to reduce anxiety levels, regulate the emotions, promote good sleep and improve any accompanying physical symptoms.

Adolescent challenges

Adolescence is often a very tricky time for a child with ASD, whether he was diagnosed as a young child or more recently. Some of the reasons for this are the following:

- Adolescence is a time of enormous change, both within the child and in his environment. Change is often inherently stressful for a child with ASD.

- A smooth transition through puberty requires a strong basis of Kidney *qi*, which is commonly deficient in children with ASD.

- Puberty is also characterised by a surge of Kidney *yang*. A child with ASD often has an excess of pathological Heat in the system, and this surge of *yang* temporarily makes any symptoms associated with Heat more pronounced.

- Relationships outside the family become increasingly important around puberty. This may bring about further challenges for the child with ASD.

For all the above reasons, treatment during puberty can be beneficial for a child with ASD. It can make a difficult time less challenging.

The practicalities of treating a child with ASD

There are some challenges that are specific to treating children who have ASD. They should definitely be seen as obstacles to overcome rather than as reasons not to treat. Indeed, a small study carried out in 2014 confirmed that it is possible to administer acupuncture to a majority of children with ASD.[4]

Hypersensitivity to touch

Some children with ASD have a high degree of sensory hypersensitivity. Even the practitioner placing his fingers on the wrist to take the pulse or palpating the skin to feel for the point can feel too intense.

The key to managing this is to help the child relax as much as possible. A child with ASD can usually bear touch more easily when she is in a reasonably calm state. Each child needs a different approach in order to help her feel calm. It may take ingenuity and patience, but in nearly all cases it is possible to find a way of administering the treatment.

Some of the things I have found helpful are:

- giving the child 'stress balls' that she can hold before and during the treatment

- having a selection of soft, cuddly toys that the child can hold and stroke throughout the treatment

- asking the child to bring a favourite cuddly toy or comfort blanket

- when possible, putting a press-sphere on Du 12 *shenzhu* or ear *shenmen* before beginning treatment

- finding the part of the body where the child is least sensitive; for example, it may be that a child cannot tolerate her head being touched (this is common in ASD children because many have *qi* stagnation affecting the head) but she is happy to have her leg touched

- in a high-functioning autistic child, engaging her in a conversation about a topic that she finds interesting, which means her focus is taken away from her bodily sensations and treatment is easier to administer.

Fear of needles

A child with ASD often has a degree of Kidney deficiency and this may mean she has a genuine fear of needles. When this is the case, I usually turn to an alternative method of delivering the treatment, such as a laser machine. The combination of Kidney deficiency and *shen* disturbance means that needling may be counter-productive, at least initially.

Inability to stay still

A child with ASD, especially one with Full Heat, may struggle to stay still for any length of time. This means that it may not be possible to leave the needles in. The needle technique used on young children, which is described in Chapter 31, should be used if this is the case.

Extreme displays of emotion

Coming to a new place and having to interact with an unfamiliar person may sometimes be enough to trigger strong emotions in a child with ASD. She may typically be anxious, panicky or angry. The practitioner should be aware of her own internal state and remain calm and centred. A child with ASD may pick up on any stress in the environment. Running late and therefore trying to rush the appointment is a recipe for disaster. Sometimes it is worth allowing a longer appointment time when treating a child with ASD. Being flexible in your expectations of what you may be able to achieve during each appointment is also useful.

Managing expectations – both your own and the parent's

When treating a child for a relatively simple condition, there is often improvement within the first few sessions. Treating a child with ASD is not the same. For a start, it may take a few sessions to get to a point where you can administer much treatment at all. Before that, you may need to focus solely on gaining rapport with the child and letting him become familiar with the environment. Although one may be treating the relevant Element and Organs involved in the child's anxiety, he will still be exposed to the triggers of his anxiety on a daily basis. The aetiology remains. This means that there may be setbacks along the way.

Aetiology

The aetiologies laid out are not intended to be a complete description of the 'causes' of ASD. These aetiologies are present in many people's lives and yet not everyone has ASD. As with most diseases, autism arises when a particular set of aetiologies occur together in a susceptible child.

It was not that long ago that 'refrigerator mothers' were blamed for an autistic child. Thankfully, this theory has now been discarded. Even so, partly as a result of its prominence for a period of time, mothers of autistic children may be susceptible to guilt. The practitioner should bear this in mind when interacting with the parent of a child with ASD, particularly in reference to aetiologies that may have arisen in the womb. A particular set of circumstances may combine in a child to cause autism. It does not follow, however, that the mother or father are in any way to blame. The vast majority of the time parents are doing the best for their unborn baby or young child that they possibly can.

Inherited factors

Many recent studies have pointed towards the fact that there is a strong genetic element in the development of ASD. From the Chinese medicine perspective, there is often a degree of Kidney *jing* deficiency in a child with ASD, which manifests more at the level of the *shen* than it does the physical body. This deficiency is often something that the child has inherited in the pre-natal Essence (although of course it may not have manifested as ASD in either or both of his parents).

Womb Heat or Womb Poison

Heat is a very common pathogen present in many children with ASD. One possible source of this Heat may be that it developed whilst the foetus was growing in the womb. This may happen as a result of the mother having a lot of Heat herself, eating a very heating diet during pregnancy, consuming recreational drugs or alcohol, or taking a medication that is energetically Hot. Womb Heat and Womb Poison do not always cause ASD, however, and are unlikely to ever be the sole cause.

Problems during birth

A common pattern found in children with ASD is *qi* stagnation, which often particularly manifests in the head. A possible cause of this is a difficult delivery, especially one that involves the use of forceps. A prolonged second stage of labour may also result in the baby having *qi* stagnation in the head. This may be visible in the form of prominent blue veins somewhere on the head. A baby with *qi* stagnation is often an unhappy one, who cries a lot because he is probably in pain.

It is also possible that the *qi* stagnation in the head so often seen in a child with ASD comes about as a result of the baby or child finding himself in a world which feels sensorily overwhelming. As a result, *qi* rises to the head where it stagnates. *Qi* stagnation may therefore also arise due to the innate qualities of the baby, rather than anything connected with birth.

Absence of fevers

Chinese medical theory includes the concept of 'foetal toxins' which may develop *in utero* and which Flaws describes as 'deep-lying or hidden warm evils'.[5] Traditional childhood diseases, such as rubella and measles, would be an opportunity for these foetal toxins to be activated and then (all going well) to be expelled. Children rarely get febrile diseases these days either because they have been vaccinated against them or because any fever is quickly dampened down with medication. It is therefore possible that these 'deep-lying or hidden warm evils' remain in the system and agitate the *shen*, contributing to the symptoms experienced by some children with ASD.[*]

Shock

Vulnerability of the *shen* is a feature common to all children with ASD, as is discussed later in this section. Shock is a possible cause of a disturbed *shen*. Some parents feel that their child's symptoms become apparent after a traumatic event. Sometimes the shock may have occurred to the mother during pregnancy and been transmitted to the foetus.

---

[*] There is an interesting phenomenon called 'The Fever Effect' which has been reported by many parents of children with ASD. For many years, autism researchers have heard reports from parents who say that when their autistic child gets a fever, many of their autistic symptoms become much improved for the duration of the fever. They have noticed that they may make more eye contact, their communication abilities improve (sometimes quite drastically) and they become more able to show affection. When the fever subsides, then these improvements disappear too.

A child once came to the clinic who had been developing normally until he was attacked by a dog at the age of three. From this point onwards, he stopped talking and was later given a diagnosis of autism. The mother of another child with ASD told me that she had been in a bad car crash during the second trimester of her pregnancy and that she felt her child had 'been neither happy nor settled' since the day she was born. This was in stark contrast to her other two children.

Diet

Diet alone does not cause ASD but dietary factors may be a part of the picture. Dietary advice should be tailored to address the imbalance of the individual child, whether that be an excess of Heat or Blood deficiency, for example. Some parents have found that excluding gluten and casein (a protein found in dairy products) from their child's diet helps to manage some of the symptoms associated with ASD.

Managing the diet of a child with ASD is often challenging, however, and therefore it is important to work with the family to make sure that any dietary changes are genuinely worth making. Many children with ASD struggle to have a normal, healthy diet, let alone one that excludes many of the foods that form the basis of so many children's diets. This is because one of the symptoms of ASD is hypersensitivity to taste and smell, as the following quote illustrates:

> I was supersensitive to the texture of food, and I had to touch everything with my fingers to see how it felt before I could put it in my mouth. I really hated it when food had things mixed with it like noodles with vegetables or bread with fillings to make sandwiches. I could never, never put any of it into my mouth. I knew if I did I would get violently sick.[6]

Organ/pathogen diagnosis of ASD

Whichever Organ/Pathogen patterns may be present in a child with ASD, they all impact the *shen* (see Figure 39.1). Therefore, the treatment should always include addressing the *shen*.

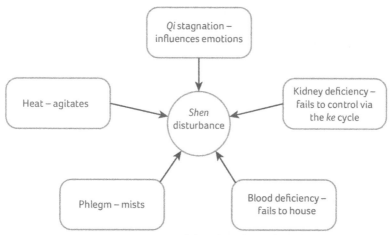

Figure 39.1 Causes of shen disturbance in ASD

How these patterns manifest in children with low-functioning and high-functioning autism

Phlegm and Heat are very likely to be present in a child who is low-functioning autistic. Many of the extreme symptoms associated with severe autism (such as not sleeping for night after night or cognitive challenges) are a manifestation of these pathogens. A high-functioning autistic child, on the other hand, may have some Phlegm or Heat but it is likely to be far less pronounced. Some children who are high-functioning autistic do not have any Heat or Phlegm at all. Their pathology is likely to consist of deficiency.

Below we consider:

- Full Heat
- Phlegm misting the Mind
- Kidney deficiency
- Blood deficiency
- *Qi* stagnation

Full Heat

Key symptoms

- agitation
- extreme insomnia (e.g. being awake for hours at a time in the night)
- sensory hypersensitivity
- outbursts of anger
- emotional volatility

Other symptoms: red face, thirst, constipation, dark and scanty urination

Pulse: overflowing and/or rapid

Tongue: red tongue, yellow tongue coating

Treatment principles: clear Heat; calm the *shen*

> **SUGGESTED TREATMENT**
> **Points**
> General points to clear Heat:
>
> > Du 14 *dazhui*
> > LI 11 *quchi*
>
> To calm the *shen*:
>
> > M-HN-3 *yintang*
> > Du 24 *shenting*
>
> **Method:** sedation needle technique
>
> **Paediatric *tui na*** to clear Heat and calm the *shen*
>
> > Heart *xinjing* (straight pushing sedation)
> > Liver *ganjing* (straight pushing sedation)
> > Heaven Gate *tianmen* (straight pushing)
> > Heart Gate *xinmen* (straight pushing)
> > Water Palace *kangong* (pushing apart)
> > Inner Palace of Toil *neilaogong* (kneading)
> > Small Heavenly Heart *xiaotianxin* (tapping)
> > Milky Way *tianheshui* (straight pushing)

Other symptoms and signs of Heat or Fire will relate to a specific Organ.

Heart Fire

- pronounced mental restlessness
- panic attacks
- dream-disturbed sleep
- excessive talking
- manic behaviour

Any of the following points should be added to the point prescription:

He 8 *shaofu*
Ren 14 *juque*
Bl 15 *xinshu*

Liver Fire

- rage attacks
- aggressive behaviour
- headaches
- red face and eyes
- dream-disturbed sleep

Any of the following points should be added to the point prescription:

Liv 2 *xingjian*
GB 38 *yangfu*
GB 43 *xiaxi*
Bl 18 *ganshu*

Stomach Fire

- intense thirst
- excessive hunger
- constipation
- mouth ulcers
- foul-smelling breath

The following point should be added to the point prescription:

St 44 *neiting*

Phlegm misting the Mind

Key symptoms

- disconnected
- hard to reach
- dulled senses
- lack of self-awareness

Other symptoms: excessive mucus, greasy skin, chronic cough, lethargy, dull headaches

Pulse: slippery

Tongue: thick sticky coat

Treatment principles: resolve Phlegm; clear the *shen*

> **SUGGESTED TREATMENT**
> One or two of the following points is usually sufficient:
>
> St 40 *fenglong*
> Pc 5 *jianshi*
> Lu 5 *chize*
> Ren 22 *tiantu*
> GB 13 *benshen*
> GB 41 *zulinqi*
>
> **Method:** sedation needle technique
>
> **Paediatric *tui na*** to resolve Phlegm
>
> Heaven Gate *tianmen* (straight pushing)
> Heart Gate *xinmen* (straight pushing)
> Water Palace *kangong* (pushing apart)
> Spleen *pijing* (straight pushing tonification)
> Eight Trigrams *bagua* (circular pushing anti-clockwise)
> Small Palmar Crease *zhangxiaowen* (straight pushing)
> Hand *yin yang shouyinyang* (pushing apart)
> Celestial Pillar Bone *tianzhugu* (straight pushing)
> St 40 Abundant Bulge *fenglong* (kneading)

> Heat and Phlegm often combine to form Phlegm-Fire. In this case, symptoms of Heat sometimes predominate and at other times symptoms of Phlegm. Phlegm-Fire is often an important component in sensory processing disorders, commonly seen in children with ASD. The Phlegm aspect mists the *shen*, making the child hyposensitive to some stimuli. The Fire aspect agitates the *shen*, making him hypersensitive to other sensory stimuli.

Kidney deficiency

Kidney deficiency may be either predominantly of *yin* or *yang*. In my experience, in children with ASD *yin* deficiency is more common.

Key symptoms

- agitation and restlessness
- unable to be still

- insomnia

- heightened sensitivity to the external environment

- poor sleep

- fearful and/or reckless

Other symptoms: feels hot in the evening and at night, malar flush, thirst, bedwetting, urinary frequency

Pulse: floating, empty

Tongue: red, may lack coating

Treatment principles: nourish Kidney *yin*; calm the *shen*

SUGGESTED TREATMENT

Two points per treatment is usually sufficient. The Kidney chest points are included because of their ability to calm the *shen*.

Points

Ki 3 *taixi*
Ki 6 *zhaohai*
Ki 23 *shenfeng*
Ki 24 *lingxu*
Ki 25 *shencang*
Sp 6 *sanyinjiao*
Ren 4 *guanyuan*
Bl 23 *shenshu*

Points to address *yin* deficiency of other Organs may need to be used:

Ren 12 *zhongwan* (for the Stomach)
He 6 *yinxi* (for the Heart)
Bl 18 *ganshu* (for the Liver)

Method: tonification needle technique

Paediatric *tui na*

Heaven Gate *tianmen* (straight pushing)
Heart Gate *xinmen* (straight pushing)
Water Palace *kangong* (pushing apart)
Kidney *shenjing* (straight pushing)
Two Men Upon a Horse *erma* (kneading)
Lower Back – area around Bl 23 *shenshu* (strong rubbing)
Spinal Column *jizhu* (pinching)

Blood deficiency

Key symptoms

- social anxiety

- vulnerability

- lack of emotional stability

- sleep problems

Other symptoms: no periods or light periods in girls, postural dizziness, floaters, blurred vision, awareness of the heartbeat

Pulse: thin or choppy

Tongue: pale, thin, dry

Treatment principles: nourish Blood; calm the *shen*

> **SUGGESTED TREATMENT**
>
> Points should be chosen according to which Organ or Organs the Blood deficiency stems from. Two points per treatment are usually sufficient.
>
> **Points**
>
> He 7 *shenmen*
> Pc 7 *daling*
> Bl 15 *xinshu*
> Bl 14 *jueyinshu*
> Bl 17 *geshu*
> Sp 6 *sanyinjiao*
> Ren 4 *guanyuan*
> Liv 8 *ququan*
>
> **Method:** tonification needle technique
>
> **Paediatric *tui na*** to tonify the *yin* Organs and calm the *shen*
>
> Heaven Gate *tianmen* (straight pushing)
> Heart Gate *xinmen* (straight pushing)
> Water Palace *kangong* (pushing apart)
> Kidney *shenjing* (straight pushing tonification)
> Spleen *pijing* (straight pushing tonification)
> Liver *ganjing* (straight pushing tonification)
> Two Men Upon a Horse *erma* (kneading)
> Knead the Navel *rou qi* (kneading anti-clockwise)
> Knead the Lower Abdomen *rou qihai* (kneading anti-clockwise)
> Lower Back – area around Bl 23 *shenshu* (strong rubbing)
> Spinal Column *jizhu* (pinching)

Qi stagnation

Qi stagnation in a child with ASD tends to especially affect the head, meaning that the symptoms tend to be predominantly mental/emotional ones.

Key symptoms

- excessive anger or aggression

- withdrawn and depressed

- emotional volatility and moodiness

- repeated banging of head

- inability to deal with change

Other symptoms: alternating constipation and diarrhoea, headaches, pre-menstrual syndrome in girls

Pulse: wiry

Tongue: normal

Treatment principles: move *qi*; calm the *shen*

SUGGESTED TREATMENT
Points

> GB 20 *fengchi* (this point is very important as the *qi* stagnation often affects the head)
> GB 34 *yanglingquan*
> GB 40 *qiuxu*
> Liv 3 *taichong*

Method: sedation needle technique

A Five Element perspective of ASD

Other symptoms of ASD, such as the inability to form intimate relationships or to read social cues, are more easily explained from a Five Element perspective.

The Fire Element

There are several aspects of the Fire Element that may be relevant when trying to understand and diagnose a child with ASD.

The shen and relationships

The *yin* Organs of the Fire Element are the Heart and the Pericardium. The Heart houses the *shen*, which is the most fundamental building block of a child's emotional world. At the core of the imbalance in all children with ASD is a vulnerability of the *shen*. Dechar[7] describes how the *shen* brings 'the gift of perception and consciousness' and also gives a child 'self-awareness and insight'. It is these qualities which are often lacking in a child with ASD, who may have little sense of the effect he has on those around him and may sometimes even appear disconnected from himself. Equally important, the *shen* enables him to form lasting, meaningful relationships with others. Struggles in both these areas may be at the core of the challenges a child with ASD may face.

One particular struggle in this realm is the difficulty a child with ASD may have in negotiating friendships. The Pericardium serves as a gateway to the Heart. As a child grows, he instinctively knows that he needs to have varying degrees of openness with the different people in his life. A child with ASD may confuse friendliness with friendship, and may be inappropriately open with people he has only just met. As a teenager, he may confuse friendliness with romantic interest. He may be somewhat socially naïve and trusting. His difficulties in relationships may mean that he has an even stronger desire to be loved and accepted than another child. This of course makes him extremely vulnerable to hurt and sometimes ridicule. At the opposite end of this spectrum, another child with ASD may not be capable of intimacy or showing love even to his parents or siblings. It seems that his Pericardium is locked tightly shut.

The Small Intestine is sometimes referred to as 'the separator of pure from impure'.[8] Not only does this Organ have the task of choosing to keep what is nourishing and discard waste on a physical level, it must do the same on a psychological level too. Attwood notes that children with ASD often have problems 'distinguishing the good guys from the bad guys'.[9] A child may be drawn into friendships with children who do not demonstrate good friendship skills, or who do not bring out his best sides. This may be because a weak Fire leaves the child with such a strong desire to be loved and connect with others. However, the Small Intestine may also play a role in the child's unconscious decisions about who to 'let in' and who to 'keep out'.

The Heart and anxiety

The anxiety that particularly pertains to the Fire Element is often centred around social interactions and what other people think of them. Situations which involve being around or interacting with others, especially large groups, may be one of the most stressful occasions for many children with ASD. A child with ASD whose Fire is imbalanced may also torment himself for days or even weeks about whether or not he said the right thing to somebody in a certain situation and worry about whether he made a fool of himself.

> One twelve-year-old girl with high-functioning autism came to the clinic one day and told me that she had been particularly anxious. When I asked about what, she said that she had not been able to stop thinking about an interchange she had had with a friend two weeks ago. She worried she had said the wrong thing and that the friend would not like her any more.

The Heart and language

Both the tongue and speech resonate with the Fire Element. Speech is one of the key ways in which a child reveals to other people who he is and the nature of his internal world. It is a means by which he connects with others. Many children with ASD have an unusual language profile. It may be that a child's language skills developed later than other children, or in severe cases that they have barely developed at all. Another child may have extremely well-developed language but, to the listener, his speech may sound unnatural or lack flow. A child with ASD may barely speak, or he may speak too much. He may use words or expressions idiosyncratically or speak in a way which sounds rather formal or pedantic. Table 39.1 summarises some common symptoms and behaviours that may be related to the Fire Element and its Organs (Heart, Small Intestine, Pericardium and Triple Burner).

Table 39.1 Symptoms and behaviour that may be related to the Fire Element and its Organs (Heart, Small Intestine, Pericardium and Triple Burner)

Physical symptoms	Behavioural symptoms
Sleep disturbances	Socially anxious
Agitation	Difficulty making eye contact
Speech difficulties	Difficulties with friendships

CASE HISTORY: THREE-YEAR-OLD GIRL WHO DID NOT SPEAK

Amy came to the clinic just after her third birthday. She had made lots of normal 'baby sounds' until she was eighteen months old. She then became almost totally silent. This change came about within a week of starting at nursery. She hated being left there and the nursery staff said that she rarely interacted with the other children. After a couple of months, her mum took her out of that nursery and she started at a different one where she was much happier. However, she remained almost entirely silent.

Amy slept very well and had a very happy disposition. She also ate well. She had no physical symptoms.

Interestingly, three times in her life, Amy had spontaneously spoken perfectly formed sentences. For example, when she and her mum had been visiting friends, she had suddenly said, 'I really want to go home now.' These three occasions were the only times she had ever spoken.

Observations: Amy made virtually no eye contact with me at all during the first two treatments. She then slowly began to look at me and her face would absolutely beam when she smiled. She rarely stayed still for any length of time, apart from when her mum held her chest to chest. She appeared to me to be extremely sensitive. I thought that she was hiding herself away because she felt so vulnerable being in the world.

Diagnosis

- Constitutional imbalance: Fire
- TCM diagnosis: Heart *yin*/Blood deficiency

Treatment

All points were treated with a laser machine.

Treatment 1

> *Yuan* source points: SI 4 *wangu*, He 7 *shenmen* (tonification technique)

I chose the *yuan* source points of the Element related to Amy's constitutional imbalance.

Treatment 2

> He 1 *jiquan*
>
> *Luo* connecting points: He 5 *tongli*, SI 7 *zhizheng* (tonification technique)

I chose to use a point that strongly affects the *shen*, followed by the *luo* connecting points because He 5 is indicated to affect speech and the tongue.

Treatment 3

> Ren 14 *juque*
>
> Tonification points: SI 3 *shaohai*, He 9 *shaochong* (tonification technique)

I chose Ren 14 *juque* because of its ability to strongly affect the spirit. I also chose it because of its location on the front torso. I had noticed that Amy was happiest when she was chest to chest with her mum, so I wanted to strengthen the *yin* aspect of her Fire (the front torso being the *yin* surface of the body).

Home treatment: At this point, I taught Amy's mum the *shonishin* non-pattern-based root treatment to do once a day at home.

Further treatments: I continued in this way using a range of points that affect the Heart and Small Intestine.

Outcome: Amy began making more sounds after the first treatment. Over several weeks, her sounds began to sound more like words. As I write, Amy is in her third month of regular treatments and has spoken whole sentences on several occasions. She is making much more eye contact and her nursery workers have commented that she is interacting with the other children much more.

The Earth Element

There are two key aspects of the Earth Element which may be relevant when trying to understand and diagnose a child with ASD.

Digesting the external environment

The *yin* Organ of the Earth Element, the Spleen, is responsible for transforming and transporting. In the physical sphere, this relates to digestion. In the emotional realm, it concerns a person's ability to 'digest' what is going on in the world around him. The Spleen is better able to absorb if it is presented with things in bite-sized chunks. If this aspect of the Spleen is impaired in a child with ASD, he may easily feel overwhelmed because he has difficulty digesting things on an emotional and/or intellectual level. For example, he may find it difficult to take in instructions when being asked to perform an exercise in class at school. Conversations involving several people at the same time may be stressful, as there is too much for his Spleen to digest all at once. A neurotypical child may take the expectations that are put upon him at any given age in his stride. For a child with ASD, the same expectations may feel overwhelming and he may have strong feelings of not being able to cope with what he has to do.

Separating and merging

The second aspect of the Earth Element which may be relevant in a child with ASD involves 'merging'. Five Element acupuncturists talk about a strong Earth Element enabling a child to stay centred and to maintain a sense of separateness from others. If this is not developed, one outcome is that the person feels as if he is 'merging' with people he comes into contact with. He takes on the feelings of the other person as if they are his own. This is a kind of over-empathising. At the opposite end of the spectrum, and perhaps a more commonly recognised trait of a child with ASD, is having no awareness at all of what another person is feeling. Baron-Cohen describes these two ends of the spectrum as 'mind reading' or 'mind blindness'.[10] Either one may stem from an imbalance in the Earth Element and may, for different reasons, cause the child to seek being alone. It should be remembered that these traits may also relate to other Elements, particularly Metal and Fire. In each instance, the practitioner should diagnose which Element the imbalance stems from, by using the key Five Element diagnostic skills of colour, sound, emotion and odour, as well as pulse diagnosis. Table 39.2 summarises some common symptoms and behaviours that may be related to the Earth Element and its Organs (Spleen and Stomach).

Table 39.2 Symptoms and behaviours that may be related to the Earth Element and its Organs (Spleen and Stomach)

Physical symptoms	Behavioural symptoms
Poor appetite	Obsessive and repetitive thoughts and speech
Picky eating	Merging with others
Strong sensitivity to tastes and smells	Lacking in empathy
Irregular bowel habits	Difficulty digesting information and instructions
Lethargy	
Clumsy gait and lack of coordination	

The Metal Element

There are two key aspects of the Metal Element which may be relevant when trying to understand and diagnose children with ASD.

The Corporeal Soul (po) and emotions

The *yin* Organ of the Metal Element, the Lungs, houses the Corporeal Soul (*po*). The *po* plays an important role in expression of emotion. Dechar explains:

> Emotions are intrinsically related to the sympathetic and parasympathetic nervous system. Emotions elicit involuntary instinctual responses at the level of the breath, the hormones, fascia and muscles, and these involuntary responses are all related to the movement of the *po* soul.[11]

It is exactly these instinctual, emotional responses that a child with ASD may find so challenging. He may find it hard to read these visceral movements and expressions of *qi* in others. For example, he may be unaware that his teacher is beginning to convey non-verbally the message that she is getting cross or that a friend is becoming bored of listening to him. He may also struggle to spontaneously produce these instinctual emotional responses himself. For example, on being given a present for his birthday, he may not show any of the normal signs of joy and excitement, and the lack of this may be wrongly interpreted as being 'rude'.

A child who lacks an ability to engage with the non-verbal, emotional aspects of human interaction may rely heavily on his intellectual abilities. These may be highly developed as a result of the fact he has spent a lot of time and energy pursuing facts. The protagonist in the novel *The Curious Incident of the Dog in the Night-Time*, who is an autistic boy, introduces himself in a way which demonstrates this very clearly: 'My name is Christopher John Francis Boone. I know all the countries of the world and their capital cities and every prime number up to 7507.'[12]

The *po* of a child with ASD may lack the fluid movement that helps emotions to flow through him. His expression of emotion may appear brittle as a result. There is an unspoken aspect to normal human interaction that helps the participants to feel connected to others and to the world around them. A child with ASD may struggle to be a part of this conversation or even to know that it is taking place. This may induce strong feelings of disconnection.

This difficulty in reading emotions also means that a child with ASD is having to work twice as hard as other children at school. Not only does he have to keep up with the academic work, but he has to expend an enormous amount of energy dealing with the social aspects. He may therefore feel that any enforced social interaction outside of school is just too much to deal with. As children grow and friendships become more and more central in their life, the child with ASD may become more isolated because he simply does not have the strength for friendships outside of school.

Defensive (wei) qi and interaction with the external world

Another function of the Lungs is to distribute defensive (*wei*) *qi* to the surface of the body. As well as helping to protect the body from Pathogenic Factors on a physical level, *wei qi* also provides a kind of semi-permeable membrane between the child and the emotional and psychic environment that he is in. If *wei qi* is being well distributed and is strong, a child can experience these aspects of life without becoming overwhelmed by them. A child with ASD may lack this membrane, which means that he has no way of filtering the emotions and psychic energy of other people. It may feel as if he is being bombarded. This may be another reason that a child with ASD chooses to spend time on his own rather than seek out the company of others. Table 39.3 summarises some common symptoms and behaviours that may be related to the Metal Element and its Organs (Lungs and Large Intestine).

Table 39.3 Symptoms and behaviours that may be related to the Metal Element and its Organs (Lungs and Large Intestine)

Physical symptoms	Behavioural symptoms
Bowel disturbances (inability to control the bowels, constipation, diarrhoea)	Cut off
	Emotionally inert
Immune dysfunction	Unable to pick up on non-verbal signals
	Hypersensitive to the external environment

The Water Element

There are two key aspects of the Water Element which may be relevant when trying to understand and diagnose children with ASD.

Kidney jing and ASD

As mentioned in the discussion on aetiology, there is commonly an inherited component to an autistic spectrum disorder. Although there may be a trigger early on in the child's life that activates or accentuates his autistic tendencies, the predisposition is something he will usually have been born with.

We often think of a person's *jing* as primarily determining his physical constitution. However, it has just as big an influence on a person's spirit. Sometimes, when with a child who has ASD, the practitioner may sense that in some ways the child is not really fully here in this world, and that being in the world is very difficult for him. Some common behaviours seen in an autistic child, such as counting obsessively or talking to himself, may be an attempt to ground himself in the physical world and also to try to reassure himself when frightened.

The Kidneys and fear/anxiety

The *yin* Organ of the Water Element is the Kidneys. The Kidneys house the *zhi*. The emotion resonant with the Water Element is fear. Fear encompasses many nuances of emotion from terror to anxiety. Anxiety is one of the most prevalent and disabling emotions that a child with ASD has to cope with. Attending school, going to a party, going on holiday or having a change in routine can all be things which provoke high levels of anxiety. A neurotypical child may barely blink an eyelid when he arrives at school to find he has a different teacher for the day. For a child with ASD, his immediate response may be increased levels of anxiety or even panic. A child who has heightened sensory sensitivity may be in a constant state of alert for the next trigger of pain. It may be the noise of a train, somebody bumping into him in a crowded place, the smell as he walks past a restaurant or a police siren. It may be that there are few times during the day when he is actually free from anxiety as he experiences the world as a place full of potential pain and threat.

THE DIFFERENCE BETWEEN KIDNEY ANXIETY AND HEART ANXIETY

Anxiety may stem both from Kidney imbalance and Heart imbalance. The quality of the anxiety is slightly different in either case.

When anxiety stems from Heart pathology, it is often focused on relationships, social interactions and 'what other people might think'. At the root of it may be a vulnerability the child has concerning the degree to which she is loveable and loved. There may be accompanying physical sensations in the chest, such as an awareness of the heartbeat.

When anxiety stems from Kidney pathology, it is often experienced as a fundamental distrust of the world in general and an unease about being in the world. The child may be focused on the possible dangers in almost every situation. He may be prone to catastrophising. The child may feel physically very on edge and find it hard to feel internally still.

Temple Grandin, who has written extensively on her own experience of being autistic, says that she 'experiences fear as her primary emotion and has an overdeveloped startle reflex of the kind that protects animals from predators'.[13] This is a wonderful description of the kind of anxiety that usually stems from a Kidney imbalance.

Sometimes both the Heart and the Kidneys are involved in anxiety. These two Organs ideally communicate with each other and provide a child with a deep sense in his core that he is all right and the world is a safe place.

The Kidneys and agitation

Many children with ASD have a strong tendency towards feeling agitated, both physically and mentally. This agitation may be due to a deficiency in the Water Element, in particular the Kidney *yin*, which provides a sense of internal stillness. Table 39.4 summarises some common symptoms and behaviours that may be related to the Water Element and its Organs (Kidney and Bladder).

Table 39.4 Symptoms and behaviours that may be related to the Water Element and its Organs (Kidney and Bladder)

Physical symptoms	Behavioural symptoms
Agitation and restlessness	Anxiety and fear
Frail physical body	Obsessive or repetitive behaviour
Incontinence	Phobias
	Aggressive when threatened

The Wood Element

Many common behaviours seen in a child with ASD may be related to an imbalance in the Wood Element and to its *yin* Organ, the Liver, in particular. Furthermore, it is often noticeable that signs of ASD become more pronounced at times of stress and change, as do most physical symptoms related to the Liver.

Expression of anger

The ability to regulate emotions comes, in part, from the smooth flow of Liver *qi*. The Liver is responsible, in particular, for the expression of the emotion of anger. For many children with ASD, one of their biggest challenges is in this area. A child with ASD may have a smaller emotional range or vocabulary than other children so that other emotions, such as sadness or fear, are expressed as anger. He may also experience a far greater number of frustrations on a daily basis than a neurotypical child and this in itself will be a strain on the smooth flow of Liver *qi*.

A child with ASD may be prone to rage attacks, which can sometimes be violent in their expression. The rapidity and intensity of his expression of anger may be extreme, going from being calm one second to raging the next. It is as if he only has two settings on his dial, either zero or ten, and he may go from one to the other in a flash.

Adaptability

A child's ability to be flexible and to adapt to the changes that inevitably occur in the world around him derive from the smooth flow of Liver *qi*. For example, many parents of a child with ASD will report that the transition from the school routine during the week to the home routine during the weekend is challenging for their child. The Liver is also responsible for a child's ability to plan. An adolescent child with ASD often struggles with the planning and organisational tasks that are expected of him. Table 39.5 summarises some common symptoms and behaviours that may be related to the Wood Element and its Organs (Liver and Gallbladder).

 Many of the behavioural challenges described here are also experienced by most neurotypical adolescents, whose brains are immature and highly affected by hormonal surges. In a child with ASD, these behaviours may be more extreme or long-lasting.

Table 39.5 Symptoms and behaviours that may be related to the Wood Element and its Organs (Liver and Gallbladder)

Physical symptoms	Behavioural symptoms
Headaches	Repetitive movements or head banging
Tense body	Rage attacks
Inability to be still	Moodiness and/or depression
Inability to deal with change	Irregular bowel movements

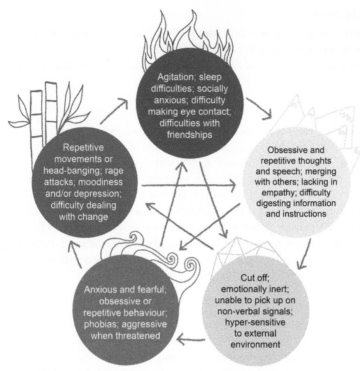

Common symptoms/behaviours of ASD and possible Element resonances

Note: It should be noted that some symptoms and behaviours may relate to more than one Element. The practitioner should primarily diagnose which Element is imbalanced based on colour, sound, emotion, odour and pulse (as described in Chapter 15) and use behaviour and symptoms as supporting evidence.

Other treatment modalities

Shonishin

Even though children with ASD are often hypersensitive to touch, I find that many accept the touch of *shonishin*. If it is possible to get the child to a point where *shonishin* treatment can be given, it may be enormously beneficial. It helps to bring *qi* downwards into the body, to counterbalance the tendency of it to rise up to the head. It can also support a child with ASD to establish firmer boundaries between herself and the external environment. It does this by 'activating' the defensive (*wei*) *qi*.

Press-spheres and retained needles

Press-spheres and retained needles are useful for a child with ASD to help manage symptoms between treatments. However, the practitioner should assess whether each child can be trusted not to fiddle with retained needles.

CASE HISTORY: THIRTEEN-YEAR-OLD BOY WITH HIGH-FUNCTIONING AUTISM

Ollie attended a mainstream school and was exceptionally bright, usually achieving top marks in all subjects. In the past year, he had developed some symptoms and behaviours that led his parents to bring him for acupuncture treatment. These were:

- severe anxiety, elicited by unfamiliar situations and social interaction
- obsessive compulsive disorder (OCD), specifically a phobia of touching anything that might be 'contaminated' by someone having touched it previously
- frequent 'rage attacks' at home, when he would become physically aggressive with his parents and younger sister.

He seemed to need very little sleep, taking a while to get off and usually waking early. He found it almost impossible to ever truly relax and feel calm.

Observations: Ollie looked like a rabbit caught in headlights when he first came to the clinic. It took about ten minutes for his mum to persuade him to even come in the door. I noticed that he had a blue-black colour to the side of his eyes. He was very pale-faced and his body was thin and extremely tense. When he spoke, his voice had a strong groan to it.

- Pulse: all positions thin and floating
- Tongue: red tongue body

Diagnosis

- Constitutional imbalance: Water
- TCM syndromes: Kidney *yin* deficiency

Treatment

- Ollie could not bear to be touched when I first met him. I began, therefore, by using a laser pen.

Treatment 1

> *Yuan* source points Bl 64 *jinggu*, Ki 3 *taixi*

This was to 'test' my hypothesis of Ollie's constitutional imbalance.

Treatment 2

> Ki 24 *lingxu*

> Tonification points Bl 67 *zhiyin*, Ki 7 *fuliu*

Having had a good response to the first treatment, I wanted to continue treating Ollie's Water Element and begin to address his spirit more directly.

Treatment 3

> *Shonishin* non-pattern-based root treatment

> Ki 25 *shencang*

> *Luo* junction points Bl 58 *feiyang*, Ki 4 *dazhong* (needles – not laser)

When Ollie came to the clinic for this session, he happened to meet my dog in the garden. I noticed that he immediately lay down on the ground and gave him a big cuddle. By the time he came into the treatment room, he was more relaxed than I had ever seen him. I decided to seize the moment and see if I could do some *shonishin* on him. Despite the fact he usually could not bear to be touched, he let me do the treatment and giggled uncontrollably as I did it. I suggested to him we try using needles instead of laser. He tolerated being needled really well.

Further treatments: From this moment on, Ollie began taking huge strides forwards. I taught his mum the basic *shonishin* non-pattern-based root treatment and she did it at home every day. I continued to treat a variety of points to strengthen his Water Element.

The first thing to change was that Ollie had far fewer rage attacks. By strengthening the Mother Element (Water), it helped the child (Wood). He began to wake up later in the mornings. His teachers noticed he made a lot more eye contact and was more vocal in class. Ollie continued to express aspects of OCD and to struggle with unfamiliar situations. However, with just occasional rage attacks and greatly reduced anxiety, life for him (and his family) became much less of a challenge.

SUMMARY

» Acupuncture may be used to treat some of the symptoms commonly seen in children with ASD, such as insomnia and anxiety.

» Although there can be challenges involved in treating a child with ASD, they can normally be overcome with patience and ingenuity.

» The patterns most commonly seen in children with ASD are Full Heat; Phlegm; Kidney deficiency; Blood deficiency; and *qi* stagnation.

» Treating the child's constitutional imbalance may also be beneficial in helping a child with ASD to cope more easily with a predominantly neurotypical world.

• Chapter 40 •

ANXIETY AND DEPRESSION
. . . .

The topics discussed in this chapter are:

- The building blocks of mental health

- Aetiology

- Key Organs involved in anxiety and depression

- Key pathogens involved in anxiety and depression

- Patterns

- The role of Five Element constitutional acupuncture in the treatment of anxiety and depression

Introduction

Had this book been written just a few years ago, it would have been very unlikely to contain a chapter on childhood anxiety and depression. A multitude of studies confirm what parents, teachers and anyone working with young people already know: that anxiety and depression are widespread in children and teenagers. Sometimes children as young as five or six come to the clinic with anxiety which is so extreme that it is having a significant impact on their lives. Children who are nine, ten or eleven seek acupuncture because they are unhappy or anxious. In teenagers, these conditions are amongst the most common reasons to seek acupuncture treatment.

Anxiety and unhappiness are, to some degree, a part of life and most children will experience them at times. Indeed, a child who escapes these emotions entirely may find himself less able to cope with the inevitable challenges of adult life. However, in some cases, the severity or frequency of the anxiety or depression that a child feels are such that they begin to get in the way of everyday life, affecting his schooling and relationships and even slowing down his development. Successful treatment with acupuncture can, therefore, have a profoundly positive impact on a child's life.

I have included anxiety and depression in the same chapter because they so often co-exist. There are also many overlaps in the patterns that cause them.

Anxiety

There is no one term in Chinese medicine that can be translated as anxiety. However, there are five ancient disease categories which all relate to the symptom of anxiety. They are:

- *jing ji* – fear and palpitations

- *zheng chong* – panic throbbing

- *fan zao* – mental restlessness

- *zang zao* – agitation

- *li ji* – internal urgency.

Some of the words that Maciocia uses to translate these terms are ones which describe well the varied nuances of anxiety.[14] One child may describe the state primarily as a particular bodily sensation, for example butterflies in his tummy, whilst another may describe it in terms of what goes on in his thoughts. The word 'anxiety' only gives us the big picture. The practitioner must fill in the detail by finding out as much as possible about what the individual child experiences.

Anxiety may be brought on by a wide variety of triggers. Sometimes anxiety is generalised and focused on everyday things, such as school-related activities or dealing with new situations. Sometimes it is focused on a specific area, such as in the case of social anxiety, where interactions and relationships induce anxious feelings. Anxiety may be a feeling that the child has to some degree most of the time, or it may be an acute episode, such as in the case of panic attacks.

Depression

Depression is a much-used term that covers an enormously wide range of emotional and psychological states. In common parlance, it is usually taken to mean unhappiness. From a medical perspective, however, it encompasses a wide range of feeling states and behaviours. Some of the most common are:

- agitation

- anger and irritability

- restlessness

- self-loathing

- a feeling of not being able to cope

- aversion to activity

- constant activity and an inability to rest and be still

- feelings of hopelessness.

The nature of depression, therefore, varies widely from child to child.

Traditionally, depression was always said to be caused by a full condition. In 1374, Zhu Dan Xi ascribed depression to one of the 'six stagnations', namely stagnation of *qi*, Blood, Dampness, Phlegm, Heat or Food. Whilst it is true that all chronic or intense emotions, even those that deplete *qi*, will always lead to some degree of stagnation, in the clinic today many cases of depression are also characterised by deficient pathologies.

What do young people become anxious or depressed about?

Some young people have a tendency towards feeling low and without hope. Others have a tendency to feel anxious. Many alternate between these two extremes. Some of the most common issues that lead to depression and anxiety in children and teenagers are shown below. Some of these evoke both depression and anxiety, whilst some may evoke one or the other.

COMMON FOCUSES FOR ANXIETY AND DEPRESSION

» Difficulties within the family

» State of friendships and relationships

» Academic achievement and exams

» Physical appearance

» The future

» World problems

> » Safety of family members
>
> » Separation from parents
>
> » Growing up
>
> » Getting things wrong
>
> » Social situations

When do anxiety and depression become pathological?

Anxiety

Most young people feel anxious from time to time. However, pathological anxiety may be characterised by the following traits:

- It is intense, unrealistic and uncontrollable.

- The child tends to catastrophise.

- The anxiety begins to shape the child's behaviour.

- The anxiety is not easily allayed by reassurance.

Depression

Feeling low is a normal reaction to a loss or some of life's struggles. However, it may be perceived as being pathological if the feelings:

- are overwhelming and intense

- are accompanied by physical symptoms, for example tiredness, digestive disturbances

- last for long periods of time

- prevent the young person from leading a 'normal', active life

- stop him from doing activities he previously enjoyed

- mean he cuts off from friends and/or family.

In whatever way anxiety and depression manifest in a child, and whatever triggers them, the practitioner must, as always, make a Chinese medicine diagnosis according to what she finds in the prevailing symptoms and signs, and treat the child accordingly. In some cases, the child may want to talk to the practitioner about her internal world and then the ensuing dialogue may become an important part of the treatment. However, in other cases, thinking and talking about the things that induce her anxiety or cause her to feel low are counter-productive to treatment, and the treatment should therefore focus only on the acupuncture itself. The practitioner should be led by what is best for the child. Treatment may be successful in either case.

Somatisation of feelings

Sometimes, the stated reason for a young person to seek treatment is anxiety or depression. Frequently, however, the child may present with a physical symptom which is, at least in part, an outward manifestation of his unhappiness or anxiety. It is also very common for a young child to somatise his unhappiness. This is because he will often lack the emotional insight and maturity, let alone the vocabulary, to express how he is feeling emotionally. He may also sense that the parent could not handle it if he began verbalising his unhappiness.* The most common example of this

---

* Please see Chapter 6 for a discussion of why a child may not feel it is 'safe' to express a particular emotion in front of one or both of his parents.

is a Monday-morning stomach ache. It is much easier for a child to say that he has a stomach ache than it is to say that he is worried about, or scared of, going to school. But many long-term, chronic physical symptoms, ranging from headaches to constipation, arise more as a result of somatised feelings than from any external trigger.

How can acupuncture help?

The effect of acupuncture on a child or teenager who is depressed, anxious or both is often enormously beneficial. Not only does it have the potential to help the child in the present, but it can have positive repercussions for the rest of his life. In a study by Kim-Cohen *et al.*, more than half of adults with mental health problems were diagnosed in childhood, and less than half of those were treated appropriately at the time.[15] The longer a person is anxious or depressed, the longer he is likely to go on being anxious or depressed. The longer a person is anxious or depressed, the more his self-confidence is eroded. Therefore, successful treatment in childhood or adolescence can potentially help him to avoid a lifetime of mental ill health.

When treating a child who is anxious and/or depressed, the practitioner should always have in mind what that particular child's individual 'optimum state' would be. Just like adults, some children are more prone to anxiety or depression than others. It may be an unrealistic goal for a particular child to become one who breezes through life, never worrying about anything. The aim of treatment is to facilitate a child to be the best that he possibly can, not to turn him into something that he is not.

 In some cultures, people are encouraged to avoid 'difficult' emotions such as sadness or anger. They are pushed under the carpet. The aim of treatment should be to help a child manage the wide range of emotions that are part of being a rounded human being. If a child is given the message that there is something wrong with him if he feels angry, sad or anxious at times, this only sets him up for failure and perpetuates the feelings.

The building blocks of mental health

A child's mental health is determined, broadly speaking, by several different components.

Jingshen

Jingshen has a slightly different meaning in different contexts but is a combination of physical constitution, inherited temperament and human individuality. It describes both the physical and emotional inheritance, including all aspects of the *shen* (i.e. the *shen* of the Heart and the other four spirits – the *yi*, *po*, *zhi* and *hun*). One description is '*Jing* represents any substance full of life, while *shen* represents the heavenly inspiration in each person. *Jing shen* expresses the origin and unfoldment of Heaven and Earth in man.'[16]

Just as a baby may be born with a strong or weak physical body, so may his spirit be robust or rather vulnerable. *Jingshen* is the most fundamental building block of a child's mental health. A good, strong *jingshen* will mean that a child is better equipped to deal with the trials and tribulations that will inevitably be a part of his life, to some degree or another.

Childhood

In the clinic the main areas of life that appear to impact most on the growing child are:

- family life (particularly the presence or absence of bonding with a main caregiver)
- school life (including both academic and social aspects)
- physical health (dealing with a severe or chronic health problem)

- the nature of the society the child grows up in (e.g. rich or poor, stable or war-torn)

- adolescence (a time of transition, when there are often added pressures).

Childhood can be regarded as a time to fill up a child's 'savings account' in terms of mental health. The more stable, loving and free of trauma it is, the more credit goes into the bank. Memories of love, warmth and security from childhood can be called upon in the future. The fuller the child's savings account, the more there is to draw upon when times get tough.

When a baby is born, his *shen* is immature. It is like an old-style photograph that has been taken but is yet to be developed. It is often possible to sense what the final picture will look like but parts of it are hazy and unclear. The process of developing the picture will have an impact on the final outcome. The same is true for a child. Everything that happens during the development stage, that is, the years of childhood, affects the nature of his *shen* when it fully emerges.

Trauma

The presence of a severe trauma in childhood or adolescence is likely to have a big impact on a child's mental health. Trauma may be a one-off event or something ongoing. It may be something unique to the child, or it may be happening at a societal level, for example a war or persecution. The *shen* of a child is immature and his ability to protect himself against his external environment is limited. Therefore, a 'major' traumatic event is likely to disturb the *shen* of any child to some degree.

Trauma may be something quite blatant, such as sexual abuse, the loss of a parent or a severe physical injury. It may also be something more subtle (perhaps going unrecognised as being at all traumatic), such as the birth of a younger sibling who is perceived to be more loved. The practitioner should never assume that because 'x' happened, the child will feel 'y'. There are many examples of adults who have not only survived but thrived in spite of horrific trauma in childhood, and of others who have been devastated and diminished by much less.

Coming through a trauma well may actually help a child to build his mental and emotional resilience. Conversely, burying trauma or an absence of the right kind of support at the time may cause a disruption of *qi* and *shen* that lasts for years to come. This may not lead immediately to depression or anxiety but instead may predispose the child to these conditions at some future point in time. This point usually occurs when he encounters a circumstance that triggers feelings that have been buried since the initial trauma. Figure 40.1 summarises the key factors that may build or erode a child's mental health.

An adult patient told me that her father died when she was seven. After she was told the news, it was never again mentioned within the family. She said that she suffered from depression throughout her teens and early adult life. She attributed this to the trauma of her father's death, and the lack of any support she received.

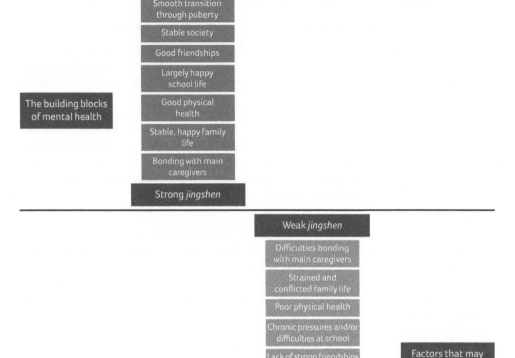

Figure 40.1 Factors that build or erode mental health

Aetiology
General aetiology

It is important when working with a young person who has anxiety and/or depression to get some sense of how and why the problem arose. It may be useful for the practitioner to gain an understanding of:

- the nature of the child's *jingshen*: a useful question to ask oneself may be, 'What would this child's emotional state be when he is at his best?'

- timing: at what stage during the child's life were the seeds of the problem sown and at what stages did the problem become more entrenched?

This not only helps to bring more clarity to the situation but can also inform the prognosis. This, in turn, helps the practitioner to have a realistic expectation of what she can do to help the child. The three following examples may help to illustrate this.

CHILD A: THIRTEEN-YEAR-OLD WITH ANXIETY AND DEPRESSION
Jingshen: Pronounced separation anxiety right up to adolescence. She slept in her parents' bed on and off until she was eleven years old. She was always a very sensitive child and easily knocked by small things.

Childhood: She had a loving, harmonious family, was in good health and adored her siblings. No major stressors.

Adolescence: She went to boarding school which she absolutely hated. She struggled to keep up academically. Her dad became very ill at the same time.

Prognosis: Child A's emotional constitution was slightly fragile, evidenced by her long-standing separation anxiety. Her untroubled childhood meant she had built up her emotional savings account. Her anxiety and depression were largely triggered by life becoming more difficult at adolescence. Although she may never be the most emotionally resilient child in the world, she had a relatively stable emotional place to get back to, so the prognosis was fairly good.

| Weak *jingsheng* (evidenced by sensitivity as a child) | **+** | difficulties in pre-pubescent phase | **=** | anxiety and depression |

Figure 40.2 Child A

CHILD B: ELEVEN-YEAR-OLD WITH DEPRESSION

Jingshen: Excellent *jingshen*. Emotionally robust throughout childhood, adapted to changes easily, resilient in school.

Childhood: Happy, stable family life, close to extended family members, no bereavements or major stressors.

One-off trauma: Aged nine, moved to the UK from Brazil. Hated leaving grandparents, aunts, uncles and cousins behind. Spoke no English, felt alone, struggled at school because of language. Mum became depressed because of difficulty adapting. Felt unable to talk about her feelings to her mum so kept them inside.

Prognosis: Child B had been so happy and emotionally resilient before the trauma of moving continents that the prognosis was positive. She had a benchmark of happiness to return to.

| One-off trauma that was internalised (moving to a new country) | **=** | depression |

Figure 40.3 Child B

CHILD C: FIFTEEN-YEAR-OLD WITH SEVERE ANXIETY AND DEPRESSION

Jingshen: Lots of time off school, constant tummy aches, never seemed to thrive physically or emotionally.

Childhood: Parents divorced when five years old, severely autistic older sibling, never enjoyed school or found it easy to make friends.

Adolescence: Life was more settled by then, had begun to enjoy school, lived with Mum and new partner, to whom she was close.

Prognosis: Not so good. Two big factors of a weak *jingshen* and a difficult childhood meant there was not much in the savings account of emotional resilience.

| Weak *jingshen* (rarely thrived as a child) | **+** | difficult childhood (parents divorced, autistic sibling, did not like school, struggled with friendships) | **=** | anxiety and depression |

Figure 40.4 Child C

Specific aetiology

The emotions of joy and anger are injurious to the spirit (shen). Cold and heat are injurious to the body.[17]

As the above quote illustrates, the internal causes of disease are more likely to underlie mental health conditions than are the external causes. Certain miscellaneous causes of disease may also create a predisposition to mental health problems. The causes of disease in children are described in detail in Part 1. Those which are most likely to come into play in anxiety and depression are:

- a distorted expression of any of the seven emotions (anger, joy, sadness, grief, overthinking or worry, fear and shock); any of these emotions that are repressed, felt with great intensity or present over a long period of time may lead to imbalance

- imbibing a dysfunctional emotional state from the mother, main caregiver or the atmosphere

- over-parenting

- lack of parenting

- a difficult 'fit' between the parents and the child

- growing up in a family under strain

- difficulties at school

- difficulties in friendships and relationships

- overstimulation

- 'addiction' to or problems in the online world.

Please see Part 1 for a detailed discussion of the above causes of disease.

Key Organs involved in anxiety and depression

The Organs that are most commonly involved in severe anxiety and/or depression are the:

- Heart

- Liver

- Kidneys

The Lungs and the Spleen may also be involved but, on their own, do not tend to cause severe mental health symptoms.

Heart

Su Wen Chapter 8 says, 'The Heart holds the office of lord and sovereign. The radiance of the spirits stems from it.'[18] The Heart is perceived to be of great importance because it governs all the other Organs. If the Heart, the lord and sovereign, is not settled and well, then there is no place for the *shen* to rest. The effect that this has on a child's well-being is profound. He may feel as if he has no internal stability or control, as if there is no firm ground beneath his feet. He may be prone to feelings of dread. This may make him want to cling to a parent or trusted adult because he feels so insecure inside himself. Figure 40.5 summarises the role of the Heart in anxiety and depression.

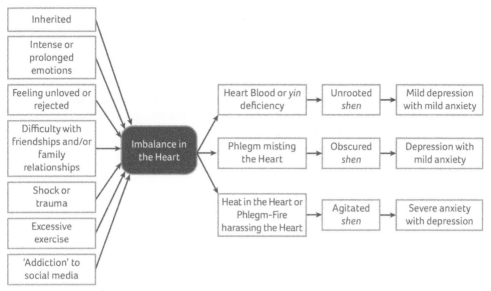

Figure 40.5 The role of the Heart in anxiety and depression

Liver

The Liver ensures the smooth flow of *qi* in order to create balanced emotions. The spirit housed by the Liver, the *hun*, helps to bring equilibrium to the child's emotional life. Both depression and anxiety are signs that this balance has been lost. An imbalance in the Liver may mean that a child is stuck in a hopeless depression or, alternatively, that his mood has no constancy and is forever changing. He may be chronically angry. A disturbance of the Liver often means there is chaos, confusion or both in the child's spirit. The child's capacity for clear thought and/or creativity may elude him. Figure 40.6 summarises the role of the Liver in anxiety and depression.

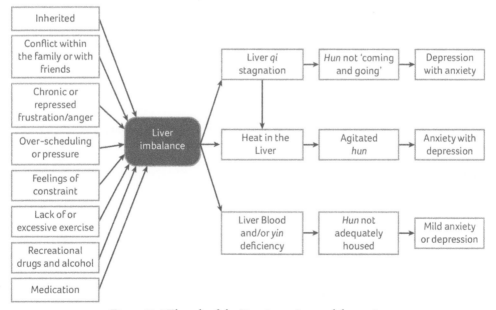

Figure 40.6 The role of the Liver in anxiety and depression

Kidneys

The spirit housed in the Kidneys, the *zhi*, enables a child to have a fundamental trust in the process of life. If the Kidneys are deficient the child may lose this innate trust and become prone to catastrophic fantasies. Trying to rationalise with a child who is in this state is rather like talking to him in a language he does not understand. His anxiety does not stem from the conscious mind but derives from the subconscious. Therefore, words will do little to alleviate it. Instead, the child needs to have adults around him who themselves have inner stability and who show by example that the world is a place that can be trusted and explored.

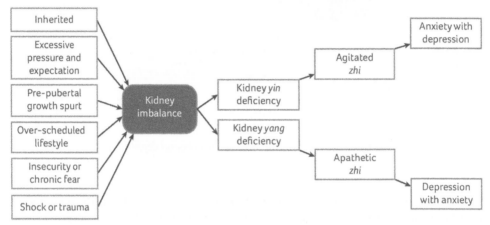

Figure 40.7 The role of the Kidneys in anxiety and depression

Key pathogens involved in anxiety and depression

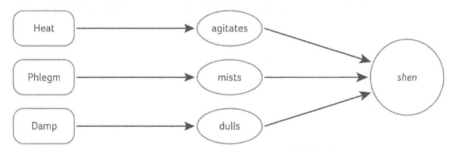

Figure 40.8 Key pathogens involved in anxiety and depression

Patterns

The patterns discussed below are:

- Liver *qi* stagnation
  - Liver *qi* stagnation leading to Heat
- Heart Fire Blazing
  - Heart and Liver Fire Blazing
  - Phlegm-Fire harassing the Heart
- Damp and Phlegm

- Heart and Kidney *yin* deficiency
- Liver and Kidney deficiency
- Spleen *qi* and Heart Blood deficiency
- Rebellious *qi* in the *chong mai*

Liver *qi* stagnation
Mental–emotional symptoms

- feelings of hopelessness
- cannot be bothered
- withdrawn
- sullen and moody
- occasional outbursts of anger
- mild anxiety often focused around the child's 'to do list'
- feels better with exercise and movement
- worse pre-menstrually in girls

Accompanying physical symptoms: headaches, bloating, belching, flatulence, alternating constipation and diarrhoea

Pulse: wiry Wood pulses

Tongue: may be normal

Treatment principles: smooth the Liver and move *qi*; calm the *shen*

Variation: Liver qi stagnation leading to Heat
In this case, as well as the symptoms above, there may also be mental–emotional symptoms: more pronounced anger, agitation and anxiety, insomnia, dream-disturbed sleep.

Pulse: wiry and overflowing Wood pulses

Tongue: red spots on the sides

SUGGESTED TREATMENT
Two or three points per treatment is usually sufficient.

Points

    Liv 2 *xingjian*
    Liv 3 *taichong*
    GB 40 *qiuxu*
    GB 34 *yanglingquan*
    Bl 18 *ganshu*

To calm the *shen*:

    M-HN-3 *yintang*
    Du 24 *shenting*

Plus points used specifically to treat the spirit described in Chapter 30.

Method: sedation needle technique

Heart Fire Blazing

Mental–emotional symptoms

- anxiety and panic attacks accompanied by a strong feeling of the heart pounding in the chest

- agitation and restlessness

- may become slightly manic or out of control when anxiety escalates

- child may tend to isolate himself because being around other people increases anxiety

Other signs/symptoms: poor sleep, may be awake for long periods, becomes red in the face when anxious, tendency to feel hot

Pulse: overflowing and full on the Fire pulses (left-hand side)

Tongue: red prickles on the tip of the tongue, tongue red, may have a yellow coating

Treatment principles: clear Heart Fire; calm the *shen*

Variation 1: Heart and Liver Fire Blazing
Heart and Liver Fire often co-exist. When the Liver is affected, the child is often prone to strong outbursts of anger and becomes anxious when overstimulated. Points to clear Liver Fire should be added to the point prescription.

Variation 2: Phlegm-Fire harassing the Heart
Fire in the Heart often condenses the fluids and leads to Phlegm-Fire harassing the Heart. This may cause alternating bouts of depression and anxiety, or the two may exist concurrently. Phlegm-Fire may also bring about confused thoughts and a feeling of disconnection. When this is the case, points to resolve Phlegm should be added.

> **SUGGESTED TREATMENT**
> It is usually sufficient to use one point to address the Heat, one to address the Phlegm and possibly another to calm the *shen*, per treatment.
>
> **Points**
> To clear Heat from the Heart:
>
> > He 8 *shaofu*
> > He 7 *shenmen*
> > Ren 14 *juque*
> > Bl 15 *xinshu*
>
> To resolve Phlegm:
>
> > Pc 5 *jianshi*
> > St 40 *fenglong*
>
> To calm the *shen*:
>
> > M-HN-3 *yintang*
> > Du 24 *shenting*
>
> Also points used specifically to treat the spirit, described in Chapter 30.
>
> **Method:** sedation needle technique

Damp and Phlegm
Emotional symptoms

- depression

- lethargy

- everything feels like an effort

- lack of vitality and spark

- somnolence

- disconnected

- confused thinking

Other symptoms and signs: slow speech, slow reactions, better with exercise and movement, a tendency to being overweight, greasy or puffy skin, heavy limbs, muzzy head, chronic cough

Pulse: slippery and/or wiry in middle positions or all over

Tongue: swollen; thick, sticky tongue coat

Treatment principles: resolve Damp and Phlegm; enliven the *shen*

SUGGESTED TREATMENT
It is usually sufficient to use two points per treatment.

Points
To resolve Phlegm:

> St 40 *fenglong*
> Pc 5 *jianshi*

To resolve Damp:

> St 8 *touwei*
> Sp 9 *yinlingquan*
> Sp 6 *sanyinjiao*
> Sp 3 *taibai*

Also points used specifically to treat the spirit described in Chapter 30.

Note: It may be necessary to address the underlying deficiency, most likely in the Stomach and Spleen, that has led to the accumulation of Damp and Phlegm.

Method: sedation needle technique

Heart and Kidney *yin* deficiency
Mental–emotional symptoms

- low-grade anxiety that may become more intense at times of stress

- easily feels insecure

- a generally fearful disposition

- prone to feelings of dread

- strong mental restlessness and agitation

- finds it hard to settle and feel calm

Other symptoms: anxiety accompanied by urinary or faecal urgency, takes a long time to get to sleep, wakes early in the morning and/or sleep may be interrupted throughout the night, has a tendency to feel slightly hot or thirsty in the evenings and at night

Pulse: floating and empty

Tongue: red prickles on the tip of the tongue

Treatment principles: nourish Heart *yin*; nourish Kidney *yin*; calm the *shen*

SUGGESTED TREATMENT

Combining one point to treat the Heart with one to treat the Kidneys is usually sufficient.

Points

To nourish Heart *yin*:

> He 6 *yinxi*
> He 7 *shenmen*
> Bl 15 *xinshu*
> Ren 14 *juque*

To nourish Kidney *yin*:

> Ki 6 *zhaohai*
> Ki 10 *yingu*
> Bl 23 *shenshu*
> Ren 4 *guanyuan*

To calm the *shen*:

> M-HN-3 *yintang*
> Du 24 *shenting*

Also points used specifically to treat the spirit described in Chapter 30 (the Kidney chest points are especially useful for this pattern).

Method: tonification needle technique

Liver and Kidney deficiency

This pattern is seen most commonly in children on the verge of puberty. Usually, this child was either born with a constitutional deficiency of the Kidneys or has been pushed hard throughout his childhood. His Kidney and Liver energy has become so depleted that he does not have enough reserves to call on to fuel him through puberty. The deficiency may be of *yin* or *yang* but more often is simply of *qi*.

Mental–emotional symptoms

- feels low, anxious or agitated
- grumpy and moody
- lacking in motivation and drive
- lacking in a desire for independence
- meek
- overly compliant

Physical symptoms
Delayed physical development, tired, lacking in vigour

Pulse: thin, deficient

Tongue: may be pale or red

Treatment principles: strengthen the Liver and Kidneys

> **SUGGESTED TREATMENT**
> **Points**
>
> > Bl 18 *ganshu*
> > Bl 23 *shenshu*
> > Du 4 *mingmen*
> > Ren 4 *guanyuan*
>
> Also points used specifically to treat the spirit described in Chapter 30.
>
> **Method:** tonification needle technique
>
> **Other techniques:** moxa may be applicable

Spleen *qi* and Heart Blood deficiency

Anxiety that stems from a Spleen imbalance is characterised by repetitive, fruitless thinking and tends to be less extreme than that which may arise from the Heart or the Kidneys.

Mental-emotional symptoms

- mild anxiety which is often worse at bedtime, when tired or when studying hard
- worry and overthinking
- pensiveness
- tendency to feel misunderstood and uncared for
- dysfunctional relationship with food
- feels emotionally vulnerable and easily hurt

Other symptoms: takes a long time to get to sleep, feels easily tired, abnormal appetite, loose stools, difficulty concentrating, easily startled

Pulse: thin or choppy in the front position on the left-hand side, overall deficient

Tongue: pale

Treatment principles: tonify Spleen *qi*; nourish Heart Blood

> **SUGGESTED TREATMENT**
> Two points per treatment are usually sufficient.
>
> **Points**
> To strengthen the Spleen:
>
> > St 36 *zusanli*
> > Sp 3 *taibai*
> > Bl 20 *pishu*

To nourish Heart Blood:

> He 7 *shenmen*
> Bl 15 *xinshu*

Also points used specifically to treat the spirit described in Chapter 30.

Method: tonification needle technique

Other techniques: moxibustion

Rebellious *qi* in the *chong mai*
Mental–emotional symptoms

- anxiety that begins around the time of puberty in girls
- anxiety may be relatively mild or there may be panic attacks
- degree of anxiety tends to wax and wane according to the phases of the menstrual cycle
- anxiety often worse pre-menstrually
- anxiety may be described as a feeling of 'internal urgency'
- a sense of anxiety rising up from the abdomen to the chest

Physical symptoms

Irregular periods or other menstrual difficulties, discomfort in the abdomen, tightness or discomfort in the chest, slight breathlessness, a feeling of a lump in the throat, a feeling of heat in the face, cold feet.

Pulse: the pulse picture will depend upon the underlying patterns, which may be a deficiency of Blood or Kidney deficiency, or a full condition such as Blood stagnation. In some cases, Rebellious *qi* in the *chong mai* occurs on its own without any underlying pathologies

Tongue: the tongue will depend on the underlying pathologies

Treatment principles: subdue Rebellious *qi* in the *chong mai*

> **SUGGESTED TREATMENT**
> **Points**
>
> > Sp 4 *gongsun* and Pc 6 *neiguan* (the opening and coupled points of the *chong mai*) with the sedation technique
> >
> > Ki 21 *yeomen*, Liv 3 *taichong* (needled with the sedation technique in order to calm and subdue the Rebellious *qi*)
> >
> > St 30 *qichong*, Ki 13 *qixue*, Ki 14 *simian* (needled with the tonification technique in order to strengthen the Lower Burner to 'hold down' the Rebellious *qi*)

Table 40.1 Defining characteristics of depression and anxiety according to pattern

Pattern	Depression	Anxiety
Liver *qi* stagnation	Feels hopeless	Mild anxiety
Liver *qi* stagnation leading to Heat	Feels hopeless with outburst of anger	Strong anxiety
Heart Fire Blazing	Needs constant stimulation or people contact to feel OK	Extreme anxiety

Liver and Heart Fire Blazing	As above plus outbursts of anger	Extreme anxiety
Phlegm-Fire harassing the Heart	Bouts of depression when cannot connect with others	Bouts of extreme anxiety
Damp and Phlegm	Extreme depression, low feelings and inactivity	Mild anxiety
Heart and Kidney *yin* deficiency	General feelings of lowness and insecurity	Anxiety worse before bedtime
Liver and Kidney deficiency	Lack of initiative and drive	Mild anxiety
Spleen *qi* and Heart Blood deficiency	Low mood, difficulty applying oneself	Mild anxiety worse at bedtime and during exams
Rebellious *qi* in the *chong mai*	May feel low at particular time of menstrual cycle	Anxiety worse around period time

The role of Five Element constitutional acupuncture in the treatment of anxiety and depression

Five Element constitutional acupuncture is invaluable in the treatment of anxiety and depression in children and teenagers. A child's constitutional imbalance is often the aspect of her that will have been most negatively affected by the challenges in her life. For example, even though there is not a Lung syndrome listed as a cause of anxiety, a constitutional imbalance in the Metal Element may still be at the root of the problem. A long-standing deficiency of Lung *qi*, often present in a child with a Metal constitutional imbalance, may over time lead to a deficiency of Heart *qi* that may at some point during childhood develop into Heart Blood or *yin* deficiency. If the child has a constitutional imbalance of Fire, Wood, Earth or Water, then the causation is more straightforward, as a pathology in the *yin* Organs of each of those elements may lead directly to depression and anxiety.

Aspects of anxiety and depression that may be related to the Fire Element

A balanced Fire Element will mean that a child is somewhere in the middle of the three spectra shown in Figure 40.9 most of the time. An imbalance in the Fire Element may manifest in one or more than one spectrum. It will mean a child tends to live at one end of the spectrum or the other, or alternates between both ends.

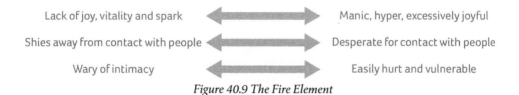

Lack of joy, vitality and spark ⟷ Manic, hyper, excessively joyful

Shies away from contact with people ⟷ Desperate for contact with people

Wary of intimacy ⟷ Easily hurt and vulnerable

Figure 40.9 The Fire Element

Other typical characteristics of an imbalance in the Fire Element are:

- social anxiety
- poor sleep
- mood lifts when with others and drops when alone.

Aspects of anxiety and depression that may be related to the Earth Element

A balanced Earth Element will mean that a child is somewhere in the middle of the three spectra shown in Figure 40.10 most of the time. An imbalance in the Earth Element may manifest in one or more than one spectrum. It will mean a child tends to live at one end of the spectrum or the other, or alternates between both ends.

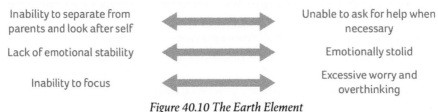

Inability to separate from parents and look after self	Unable to ask for help when necessary
Lack of emotional stability	Emotionally stolid
Inability to focus	Excessive worry and overthinking

Figure 40.10 The Earth Element

Other typical characteristics of an imbalance in the Earth Element may be:

- dysfunctional relationship with food
- feeling misunderstood and uncared for.

Aspects of anxiety and depression that may be related to the Metal Element

A balanced Metal Element will mean that a child is somewhere in the middle of the three spectra shown in Figure 40.11 most of the time. An imbalance in the Metal Element may manifest in one or more than one spectrum. It will mean a child tends to live at one end of the spectrum or the other, or alternates between both ends.

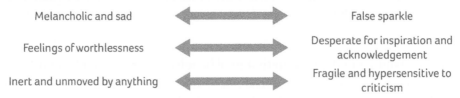

Melancholic and sad	False sparkle
Feelings of worthlessness	Desperate for inspiration and acknowledgement
Inert and unmoved by anything	Fragile and hypersensitive to criticism

Figure 40.11 The Metal Element

Other typical characteristics of an imbalance in the Metal Element may be:

- strong self-critical internal voices.

Aspects of anxiety and depression that may be related to the Water Element

A balanced Water Element will mean that a child is somewhere in the middle of the three spectra shown in Figure 40.12 most of the time. An imbalance in the Water Element may manifest in one or more than one spectrum. It will mean a child tends to live at one end of the spectrum or the other, or alternates between both ends.

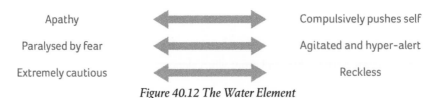

Apathy	Compulsively pushes self
Paralysed by fear	Agitated and hyper-alert
Extremely cautious	Reckless

Figure 40.12 The Water Element

Other typical characteristics of an imbalance in the Water Element may be:

- anxiety: as the emotion related to the Water Element is fear (*kong*), anxiety is an inherent part of a Water imbalance.

Aspects of anxiety and depression that may be related to the Wood Element

A balanced Wood Element will mean that a child is somewhere in the middle of the three spectra shown in Figure 40.13 most of the time. An imbalance in the Wood Element may manifest in one or more than one spectrum. It will mean a child tends to live at one end of the spectrum or the other, or alternates between both ends.

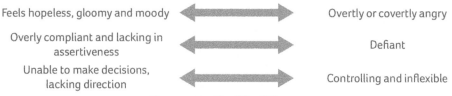

Feels hopeless, gloomy and moody ⟷ Overtly or covertly angry

Overly compliant and lacking in assertiveness ⟷ Defiant

Unable to make decisions, lacking direction ⟷ Controlling and inflexible

Figure 40.13 The Wood Element

Other typical characteristics of an imbalance in the Wood Element may be:

- anxiety focused on the young person's schedule/to do list.

CASE HISTORY: FOURTEEN-YEAR-OLD GIRL WITH SEVERE ANXIETY AND MILD DEPRESSION

This case history illustrates:

- that a weak *jingshen* means a shock or trauma may have more of an impact on a child's mental health than it otherwise would have

- the importance of having a sense of how a child would be when she is at her best, so as to manage expectations.

Signs and symptoms

- withdrawn, anxious, panic attacks, vulnerable in friendships, self-harming, difficulty coping with school, one suicide attempt

- physical symptoms: migraines, severe acne, takes hours to get off to sleep, vivid and disturbing dreams

Pulse: Wood overflowing, He/SI Choppy, Kidney pulse thin

Tongue: slightly red, very red sides and tip

What has led to this point?

The fact that Natasha was always an emotionally fragile child and that she wet her bed until she was eleven years old suggests there was a vulnerability and insecurity in her from a young age. The shock of witnessing a death and the difficulty of adjusting to secondary school (both of which occurred around adolescence) then tipped the balance from relatively good emotional stability to quite severe depression and anxiety.

Diagnosis

- Fire constitutional imbalance

- Heart Blood deficiency

- Kidney *yin* deficiency

- The fact that Natasha's *jingshen* was not very robust suggested that it might be difficult with treatment to reach a point where she had no triggers for her anxiety at all.

Treatment: Treatment addressed the constitutional imbalance and Organ/Pathogen syndromes described above. Natasha did well with treatment, gradually having fewer panic attacks and coping with the social and academic aspects of school more easily. However, at times of stress, her symptoms would return, albeit less severely. She continued coming for 'top-up' treatments monthly and more frequently during stressful periods.

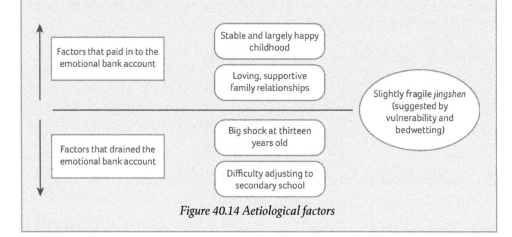

Figure 40.14 Aetiological factors

SUMMARY

» The practitioner should look at how anxiety and/or depression manifest in each individual, and treat it accordingly.

» Anxiety and/or depression that begin at puberty may be, at least in part, a result of circumstances in the child's life during earlier childhood.

» Developing an understanding of what factors have led a child to be anxious or depressed can help the practitioner to have realistic expectations of how treatment may help.

» The key Organs involved are: Heart; Pericardium; Liver; and Kidneys.

» The key pathogens involved are: Heat; Phlegm; and Damp.

» The patterns involved are: Liver *qi* stagnation (turning to Heat); Heart Fire Blazing; Phlegm-Fire harassing the Heart; Damp and Phlegm; Heart and Kidney *yin* deficiency; Liver and Kidney *yin* deficiency; Spleen *qi* and Heart Blood deficiency; and Rebellious *qi* in the *chong mai*.

» Treating the Five Element constitutional imbalance is of great value in the treatment of anxiety and depression.

• Chapter 41 •

EATING DISORDERS

· ·

The topics discussed in this chapter are:

*   Patterns that frequently arise as a result of an eating disorder
*   The Five Elements and eating disorders

Introduction

At some point, many people's relationship with food has somehow become incredibly disturbed. Many children are overweight, whilst others are deliberately starving themselves. There are many reasons why eating disorders in children and young people are on the rise, and this topic alone fills many books and is the subject of much contention and discussion. It is undoubtedly true that social media, television and films are full of heroines and heroes who are 'body perfect' and that there is a strong focus and value placed on looks and appearances. Girls in particular (but not exclusively) are often pushed to be perfect in terms of their performance, appearance and behaviour. Family dynamics may play a role for some children who have an eating disorder. There are usually many factors involved, some of which are poorly recognised or understood.

The phrase 'eating disorder' leads most people to think of either anorexia or bulimia. However, the most common eating disorder is Eating Disorder Not Otherwise Specified, or EDNOS. This covers a wide range of pathological eating habits, and the sufferer may manage to maintain a normal weight. There are yet more people who do not 'officially' have an eating disorder yet they live in a perpetual state of anxiety about food, experience intense feelings such as guilt, shame, anxiety or disgust when they eat, agonise about whether to eat or what to eat a lot of the time and do not like the way they perceive that they look.

Eating disorders affect children at many different ages. Research suggests that an increasing number of pre-adolescent boys and girls are suffering from them.[19] The youngest patient with an eating disorder I have treated was eleven. There are reports of children who are as young as eight or nine suffering from anorexia.

> **RED FLAGS: ANOREXIA**
> Anorexia has the highest mortality rate of any psychiatric disorder. It is therefore essential that any child with this condition is receiving appropriate medical interventions from other healthcare professionals.

What can we as acupuncturists do for people with eating disorders?

Before treating a teenager with an eating disorder, it is important to recognise that, although the condition may have become about food, it nearly always has deep and complex psychological roots. Unless the practitioner is also a trained psychotherapist with extensive knowledge in this area, her role is not to delve too deeply into the dark realms of the psyche.

Having said that, there is a lot that acupuncture can do to help a teenager who has an eating disorder. The key benefits of treatment are the following:

- Acupuncture treats the body, mind and spirit, and eating disorders are a disease of all three. Treatment has the potential to influence the thinking of the person, her physical health and her feeling state. This may precipitate recovery.

- Five Element treatment, in particular, can bring about profound changes in how a young person feels in herself and about herself. It may also change long-held emotional patterns, which may be an important part of recovery.

- Eating disorders take their toll on the physical body. Acupuncture can help to mitigate the effects. For example, anorexia sufferers are often *qi* and Blood deficient. By boosting *qi* and Blood we can help the person to remain healthier than she would otherwise be, until she begins eating better.

- The practitioner may be the only adult in a teenager's life who is not either questioning her about what she has eaten today, telling her what she must eat or feeling extreme anxiety about what she may not be eating. The practitioner does not need to see her food diaries that she has been told to keep or to weigh her. The weekly acupuncture appointment, therefore, may be a haven where she can escape from her illness for a while. This, together with a warm rapport with the practitioner, may help her to feel good about herself and reconnect her with 'normality'.

Patterns that frequently arise as a result of an eating disorder

The patterns listed below are by no means the only ones seen in young people who suffer from an eating disorder. However, they are the ones that commonly arise as a result of not eating, overeating or repeatedly inducing vomiting or using laxatives. Treating these patterns may alleviate some of the physical symptoms that arise as a result of an eating disorder. The symptoms present in some of the patterns, for example a feeling of fullness and distension in Liver *qi* stagnation, may also perpetuate a young person's resistance to eating.

Treating whichever patterns are present should be combined with treatment of the young person's constitutional imbalance.

 Although an eating disorder manifests in the body, the condition stems from the spirit. Therefore, treating the child's spirit should always be at the core of the practitioner's approach to treatment, whichever Organ/Pathogen patterns may be present.

The commonly observed patterns in eating disorders are:

- Spleen *qi* and/or *yang* deficiency
- Stomach *yin* deficiency
- Heart Blood and/or *yin* deficiency
- Liver Blood and/or *yin* deficiency
- Liver *qi* stagnation (invading the Stomach and/or Spleen)
- Phlegm misting the Mind

Spleen *qi* and/or *yang* deficiency
This pattern may be both a cause and a result of irregular eating patterns.

Key symptoms

- lack of desire to eat

- cravings for particular foods

- constant desire to eat

- irregular desire to eat

- obsessive thinking

Other symptoms: digestive symptoms such as irregular bowel movements and bloating, tired, weak limbs, feeling cold

Pulse: deficient

Tongue: pale, wet, normal

Treatment principles: tonify Spleen *qi*

> **SUGGESTED TREATMENT**
> **Points**
>
> Ren 12 *zhongwan*
> St 36 *zusanli*
> Sp 3 *taibai*
> Sp 6 *sanyinjiao*
> Bl 20 *pishu*
>
> **Method:** tonification needle technique
>
> Points to treat the spirit should also be used (see Chapter 30).
>
> **Other techniques:** moxibustion

Stomach *yin* deficiency

This pattern is particularly prevalent in children who induce vomiting as a result of bulimia nervosa.

Key symptoms

- diminished appetite

- snacks but does not eat full meals

- easily feels full

Other symptoms: constipation with dry stools, dull or slightly burning epigastric pain, dry mouth and throat which are worse as the day goes on

Pulse: floating and empty Earth pulses

Tongue: thin or no coat in the centre

Treatment principles: nourish Stomach *yin*

Points

> Ren 12 *zhongwan*
> St 36 *zusanli*
> Sp 6 *sanyinjiao*
> Bl 21 *weishu*

Method: tonification needle technique

Points to treat the spirit should also be included (see Chapter 30).

Variation: Stomach *yin* deficiency may predispose the child to Stomach Fire. If this is present, there may be a more intense burning epigastric pain, foul-smelling breath, bleeding gums and mental restlessness. It may mean that the child is hungry a lot of the time, which complicates the eating disorder. St 44 *neiting* should be used to clear the Fire from the Stomach, before treating the underlying *yin* deficiency.

Heart Blood and/or *yin* deficiency

This pattern commonly arises in a young person who has been restricting her food intake or depriving herself of Blood-nourishing foods for some time.

Key symptoms

- lack of sparkle

- anxiety or emotional agitation

- feels excessively vulnerable

- difficulty forming close connections with others

- tearful

Other symptoms: poor sleep (especially in the first half of the night), jumpy and easily startled, difficulty concentrating and poor memory

Pulse: thin or choppy, maybe floating

Tongue: pale or red, thin, dry, red spots on tip

Treatment principles: nourish Heart Blood and/or *yin*

SUGGESTED TREATMENT
Two points per treatment is usually sufficient.

Points

> He 6 *yinxi*
> He 7 *shenmen*
> Pc 7 *daling*
> Ren 14 *juque*
> Ren 15 *jiuwei*
> Bl 14 *jueyinshu*
> Bl 15 *xinshu*
> Bl 17 *geshu*

Points to treat the spirit should also be included (see Chapter 30).

Method: tonification needle technique

Liver Blood and/or *yin* deficiency

This pattern commonly arises in a young person who has been restricting her food intake or depriving herself of Blood-nourishing foods for some time. It may also come about as a result of over-exercise, which is a symptom of some eating disorders.

Key symptoms

- unhealthy relationship with anger which may be unacknowledged and repressed
- rigidity of thinking
- lack of direction
- feels 'lost', tearful and low

Other symptoms: absence of menstrual periods, postural dizziness, weakness

Pulse: thin, may be floating and empty

Tongue: pale, dry, thin

Treatment principles: nourish Liver Blood and/or *yin*

> **SUGGESTED TREATMENT**
> **Points**
>
> Liv 8 *ququan*
> Liv 3 *taichong*
> Ren 4 *guanyuan*
> Bl 18 *ganshu*
>
> **Method:** tonification needle technique
>
> Points to treat the spirit should also be included (see Chapter 30).

Liver *qi* stagnation (invading the Stomach and/or Spleen)

This pattern may arise due to repressed anger, which may be an underlying factor in some eating disorders.

Key symptoms

- unhealthy relationship with anger which may be unacknowledged and repressed
- rigidity of thinking
- inflexible eating habits
- obsession with exercise
- feeling full and distended even when has not eaten

Other symptoms: alternating constipation and diarrhoea, belching and nausea

Pulse: wiry

Tongue: normal, slightly purple or red on the sides

Treatment principles: smooth the Liver and move *qi*; tonify the Stomach and Spleen

> **SUGGESTED TREATMENT**
> **Points**
>
> > Liv 3 *taichong*
> > GB 40 *qiuxu*
> > GB 34 *yanglingquan*
> > Liv 13 *zhangmen*
> > Liv 14 *qimen*
>
> Points should also be included to tonify the Stomach and Spleen.
>
> **Method:** sedation needle technique

Phlegm misting the Mind

This pattern may be a part of the reason that a young person has a distorted image of her body in the midst of an eating disorder, especially anorexia nervosa.

Symptoms

- body dysmorphia
- disconnected from others
- hard to reach
- depressed and low
- dull eyes

Pulse: slippery or wiry

Tongue: thick, sticky coating, may be a Heart crack

Treatment principles: resolve Phlegm; open the Heart

> **SUGGESTED TREATMENT**
> **Points**
>
> > Pc 5 *jianshi*
> > St 40 *fenglong*
> > Ren 14 *juque*
> > Ren 15 *jiuwei*
>
> **Method:** sedation needle technique
>
> Points to treat the spirit should also be included (see Chapter 30).

The Five Elements and eating disorders

An eating disorder is a symptom of a deeper pathology which usually lies in the spirit. As one sufferer wrote, 'An eating disorder isn't caused by an external event: it is an expression of internal unhappiness and the trigger is a part of the illness. To claim otherwise is to confuse causation with symptoms.'[20]

Treating a young person's constitutional imbalance may have the effect of bringing her back into herself and helping her to become more aligned with her true nature. An imbalance in a particular Element may lead to a tendency to certain behaviours. However, when diagnosing the constitutional imbalance, the young person's colour, sound, emotion and odour should always be the prime methods used (see Chapter 15).

The Fire Element
Feelings of unlovability and vulnerability
Another emotion that is sometimes at the root of an eating disorder is a desperate feeling of unlovability and aloneness. The child or teenager is literally 'starving' for love, warmth and intimacy. She may feel too vulnerable to attempt to get this need met through other people and so turns to food instead. It is a safer bet to control her food intake than it is to try to trust another person, who may leave or reject her at any time.

The strength of this feeling of unlovability may be so great that it is too painful or overwhelming to fully acknowledge. Eating becomes a way of trying to 'feed' the need for love. If she eats, then the feelings of unlovability are temporarily vanquished. Of course, in the long run this strategy only exacerbates the feelings. A teenager who overeats and becomes overweight then feels even less lovable. A vicious circle is created.

Loss of insight and inspiration
A young person in the grips of an eating disorder has often lost insight into what she is doing and the reality of her situation. For example, she may believe she is overweight whereas in reality she is underweight. She may believe that she is 'in control' whereas the eating disorder has come to control her. The *shen* of the Heart enables a young person to have this kind of insight, and therefore a serious eating disorder is a reflection that the *shen* has lost its way.

A young person with an eating disorder may also feel and appear 'dead' in her spirit. It is as if the 'heart and soul' have gone out of her. She has become disconnected from anything that creates joy in her life. The obsession with food leaves no room for anything else, including true connection with other people.

The Earth Element
The ability to nurture oneself
At the heart of the Earth Element is the desire and ability to self-nurture. A balanced Earth Element will enable a child to look after her own basic needs and recognise when she needs to ask others for help. It will give her a balanced relationship to managing the conflicting needs of independence versus dependence.

Denial of need
A primary aspect of being independent is, obviously, the ability to feed oneself. In a child with an eating disorder, particularly anorexia, there is a part of her psyche that is denying she has any need or dependency, even the very basic dependency that all human beings have on food. Ironically, if the eating disorder is serious, then the child is inadvertently making herself even more dependent on others, who may in some cases need to take over the job of feeding her and control every aspect of what she eats.

Many young people with a constitutional Earth imbalance report that they feel guilty when they have eaten, especially if they have allowed themselves a treat. It is as if, in some way, the person is saying, 'I allowed myself to have a need and now I must deny that.' This may manifest in a disorder such as bulimia, where the child then takes laxatives or forces herself to vomit to get rid of the food she has just eaten.

Obsessive thought

In some eating disorders, there is a component of obsessive thought, which may stem from the Earth Element. If the *yi* is not strongly housed, then it may result in obsessional and repetitive thinking, when a person's thoughts just go around and around. Even though food is really just a symptom of the condition, it is characteristic of a young person with an eating disorder to become obsessive in her approach to food. She may obsess about what to eat, when she is next going to eat, what she has eaten and simply whether or not she should eat. A journalist who spent three of her teenage years in a psychiatric hospital with severe anorexia describes how, for 'twenty years, every bite of food was accompanied by endless miserable internal calculations'.[21] This is an example of the kind of obsessive thought that may stem from an imbalance in the Earth Element.

The Metal Element

Striving for perfection

A child or teenager who has an imbalance in her Metal Element may be constantly striving for perfection. This is a compensation for an internal sense of having no real worth or value. Nothing she does ever feels like it is quite good enough, so she then sets herself an even higher goal. If this pattern turns its attention to the realm of food, then it may contribute to an eating disorder. She believes that she will feel OK about herself once she has reached the desired weight or dress size, only to find that when she gets there that is not the case. So she then sets herself another target of a lower weight and a smaller dress size only to find that even that does not give her the desired feeling. This cycle may continue until the young person is at a dangerously low weight.

Craving purity

The *yang* Organ related to the Metal Element, the Large Intestine, is responsible for eliminating waste and impure *qi* both on a physical and emotional level. If this function is impaired, the person may feel as if she is 'polluted' or 'clogged up'. A response to this may be to try to cleanse her body by eating less, fasting or only eating very 'pure' foods. This may contribute to various types of eating disorder, a common one being when the teenager will only eat foods that she considers to be especially 'pure' or 'healthy'. She may do this under the guise of wanting to have a very healthy diet but in reality there is an obsessional quality to it which is driven by a deep desire to feel unpolluted, and this may dominate her emotional world and her every decision about what to eat or not eat.

> A thirteen-year-old girl had an eating disorder that manifested as only eating a narrow range of 'superfoods'. She spoke of feeling 'dirty' if she ate anything other than her chosen, narrow range of foods. She would rather not eat than be in a situation where she had to eat something she did not regard as 'clean' enough. Her constitutional imbalance was in Metal. Treatment to strengthen her Metal Element was a part of what enabled her to gradually eat a wider range of foods.

Disconnection from the physical body

The spirit of the Metal Element is the *po* (Corporeal Soul). One of the functions of the *po* is that it ensures a young person is connected with the wisdom of the body, with the minutiae of what it needs at any given moment. This is a process which goes on of which we have little conscious awareness. Dechar explains that 'problems at this level are expressed through dream images, irrational longings and obsessions, feelings of depression and anxiety, and especially bodily problems such as eating disorders, chronic tensions and psychosomatic distress'.[22] An eating disorder in a young person may result because she has become so divorced from the innate knowledge of what her body needs.

The Water Element

Excessive control

The spirit of the Water Element, the *zhi* (often translated as willpower), gives a young person an innate trust in the ebb and flow of life. It enables her to respond to the ever-changing world rather than attempting to shape it according to her needs and desires. One manifestation of an imbalance in the *zhi* is an attempt to excessively control some aspect of reality, which may be food and her body. This may be a response to a particular event, such as a bereavement or trauma, which meant she felt very out of control. Even puberty alone may, to some young people, feel like trauma. Or it may be a response to a more chronic feeling of life being chaotic. The only thing she then feels she has left to control is her own body.

Diminished instinct for survival

The *zhi* is also the foundation of our life force and our instinct to survive. When balanced, it helps a young person to make decisions that will keep her safe from danger and helps her to use her internal resources wisely so that she may both survive and thrive. When a young person becomes gripped by a very serious eating disorder, in particular anorexia, she is ultimately choosing death over life. Her will to live has become subsumed by her illness.

The Wood Element

Rigidity of thought and spirit

Some eating disorders are accompanied by a mental rigidity that may stem from an imbalance in the Wood Element. The *yin* Organ of the Wood Element, the Liver, ensures the smooth flow of *qi* for emotional regulation. If this function has broken down, then one manifestation may be a rigidity in the young person's thinking. For example, she may eat exactly the same thing at every meal and feel quite panicked by the thought of any change in this. Her life may become ruled by the need to keep to an incredibly strict routine in terms of what and when she eats. This lack of flexibility is symptomatic of a lack of smooth flow of Liver *qi*.

> One fifteen-year-old girl who was recovering from anorexia said that she felt really stressed if she went away or even went out for the day as it would mean she could not eat her 'normal' food. Her recovery took a step backwards after a week's holiday because she felt 'out of control' when forced to eat different food. With treatment to move her Liver *qi*, she became more flexible in her approach to food.

Unexpressed anger

The underlying emotions of a young person with an eating disorder are very different in every case. However, one possible scenario is that there is a large amount of denied and repressed anger. She is, for many varied reasons, unable to feel, let alone express directly, the anger inside, so she chooses not to eat, or to eat very little. This becomes her way of expressing her anger when she feels there is no other outlet for it. Or she may overeat or binge eat as a way of trying to numb these angry feelings.

Loss of direction and purpose

The *hun* enables a young person to have a vision of her journey towards her unique destiny. A serious eating disorder, however, may mean that a young person loses clarity concerning her direction and purpose in life. The goal of not eating or eating only certain foods gets in the way of her true goals. In severe cases, a young person may veer so far off her path that she loses touch with the point and purpose of her life.

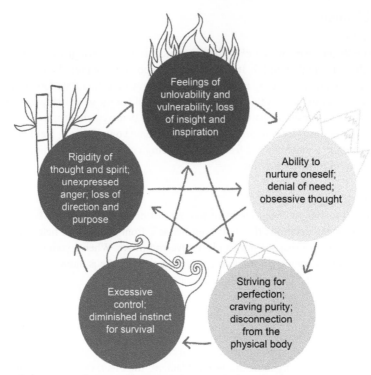

Imbalances in the Five Elements that may be involved in eating disorders

---

CASE HISTORY: THIRTEEN-YEAR-OLD GIRL WITH ANOREXIA

This case history illustrates how, when treating an eating disorder, it is useful to focus on the inner feelings of the child rather than on what she does or does not eat.

Iris was brought to the clinic because she had rapidly been losing weight over the past six months. She was controlling her food intake and going on one 'fad' diet after another. Her most recent was a 'clean' diet where she only ate fruit and vegetables. She refused to eat any carbohydrates, meat or fish. She had also taken up running, which she did every day after school.

Iris permanently felt cold and was severely constipated. She was relying on increasingly high doses of laxatives.

Iris was on the waiting list for a referral to the teenage mental health unit. She had begun seeing a counsellor at school a couple of months before coming to me.

Observations: Iris was exceedingly thin and physically frail. In contrast, she had a spirit of steel. Her eyes had a hardened look about them, as if she was about to go into battle. She was pale and dressed in lots of winter clothes even though it was a warm summer's day.

- Pulse: choppy on the Wood and Fire pulses; thin overall
- Tongue: orange sides, pale all over

She had a marked green colour around her mouth and her voice was noticeably shouting (in contrast to her small physical presence).

Iris expressed irritation and crossness with virtually everything her mother said during the initial case history taking.

Diagnosis: Based on colour, sound and emotion, I diagnosed Iris as having a Wood constitutional imbalance. In terms of Organ/Pathogen patterns, she had Liver and Heart Blood deficiency.

Treatment

It felt important to establish with Iris what she wanted to get out of treatment. Her mother obviously wanted her to start eating more, but Iris told me she did not think she had a problem with food at all. She did say, however, that she felt 'all knotted up inside' and that she did not feel she enjoyed the things she used to enjoy, such as being with her friends. So we agreed that I would focus on alleviating the feeling of being 'knotted up' and try to help her gain more joy in life again.

Treatment 1

> *Yuan* source points: GB 40 *qiuxu*, Liv 3 *taichong*
>
> Tonification needle technique

I started by needling the *yuan* source points on the channels associated with what I felt was Iris's constitutional imbalance. I used the tonification technique because her pulses reflected that there was a deficiency in the Wood Element. After needling these points, all the pulse positions felt less thin and the choppy quality on the Wood and Fire pulses was resolved.

Treatment 2

> Tonification/Water points: GB 43 *xiaxi*, Liv 8 *ququan* (tonification needle technique)

I chose these points because of their ability to bring more fluidity and flexibility to the Wood Element.

Treatment 3

> Back *shu* points of Liver and Gallbladder: Bl 19 *danshu*, Bl 47 *hunmen*, Bl 18 *ganshu* (tonification needle technique and moxa cones – seven on each point)

I chose these points to further strengthen the physical, mental and emotional aspects of the Wood Element.

Outcome: Treatment continued along these lines. After the first few sessions, Iris began to slowly unwind. It was as if she began to take a long, deep exhale. When I asked her about the knotted-up feeling, she said that it was coming and going a bit but may have been there less often.

I continued treating Iris for several months, seeing her every week or fortnight. After about three months, Iris had a birthday party. She came in the week after and said that she realised after it that she had genuinely enjoyed being with her friends in a way she had not for a long time. Her mother reported that she thought Iris was laughing more and was more relaxed when she was around the family.

Iris continued to resist eating more for quite a few months. However, she showed more flexibility in what she ate. After six months, she seemed to have abandoned her fad diets and showed more moderation in her approach to food.

Iris eventually got her referral to the teenage mental health unit eight months after she had first come to the clinic. However, by this time, both she and her mother agreed that her approach to food and eating was back to normal. She was now a healthy weight. She also began her periods four months into her course of treatment.

SUMMARY

» Acupuncture can be a helpful tool in the treatment of eating disorders, both to help the young person towards recovery and to minimise the physical impact of the illness.

» The patterns most commonly seen in eating disorders are: Spleen *qi* and/or *yang* deficiency; Stomach *yin* deficiency; Heart Blood and/or *yin* deficiency; Liver Blood and/or *yin* deficiency; Liver *qi* stagnation; and Phlegm misting the Mind.

» Treatment of the Five Element constitutional imbalance is a key aspect when working with a young person with an eating disorder.

• Chapter 42 •

SELF-HARM
. . . .

The topics discussed in this chapter are:

- Patterns involved in self-harm

- A Five Element approach to self-harm

Introduction

There is currently an epidemic of self-harm amongst young people in the developed world. Accurate statistics are almost impossible to obtain because it is a behaviour which is often hidden. However, it is thought that at least 10 per cent of young people self-harm.[23]

Why do children self-harm?

Self-harm is an outward manifestation of deep inner turmoil. The circumstances that have led to it are usually varied and complex. Some of the factors thought to lead to self-harm are:

- difficulties within the family

- difficulties with friendships (including bullying)

- pressures at school

- depression

- anxiety

- pressures associated with puberty or other transitions

- historical or current trauma

- alcohol or drug use.[24]

Self-harm may be a way to try to escape from overwhelming or unbearable emotional turmoil. It may arise because of an inability to express anger, which then gets turned inwards. It may also be a means by which the child or teenager punishes himself because he does not feel good enough in some way. His feelings of failure may be related to how he looks, friendships and relationships or academic achievement. Self-harm is thought to be an extremely addictive behaviour. The pain induced by self-harm is a kind of primitive, physical distraction from emotional distress.

Self-harm is very rarely a cry for attention. On the contrary, many teenagers who self-harm go to great lengths to hide it from family and friends. Self-harm is a form of expression, not of attention-seeking. It is not something that children get enjoyment out of. Even though there may be a short-lived high, it often piles shame and guilt on to a chaotic heap of negative emotions that have already proved overwhelming.

What forms does self-harm take?

Self-harm takes many different forms. Some of the most common ways of self-harming in children and teenagers are cutting, burning and pinching. Developing an eating disorder or abusing drugs or alcohol are also methods of self-harming. When working with a young person who is self-harming, it is usually more helpful to focus on what he is feeling rather than what he is doing to himself.

How can acupuncture treatment help a young person who is self-harming?

Acupuncture can help to balance emotions, helping the child to avoid intense or prolonged states of 'difficult' emotions such as anger, and promoting desirable feelings such as joy. This, in turn, reduces the need to self-harm.

Another way that acupuncture treatment can help a young person who is self-harming is that the treatment room may provide a space for him to find another way of expressing himself, rather than via self-harm. Good rapport with the acupuncturist is of course a crucial prerequisite in order for this to happen.

Thoughts on working with young people who are self-harming

- The focus of the treatment should be on how the child feels, not on the fact that he is self-harming. The self-harm is the *biao*, not the *ben*.

- A young person may feel a lot of shame about the fact that he self-harms. He may not be happy to expose the parts of his body where there are marks or scars, which may be parts of the body the practitioner would like to needle. The practitioner should be sensitive towards this. It is usually wise to find alternative points on another part of the body.

- It is helpful to ask the child (if he is willing and once rapport has been gained) how he feels after he self-harms. This may be diagnostically useful. For example, if he says he feels less angry and irritated, it may point towards a pattern of Liver *qi* stagnation.

- It is important to look out for the recurrence of symptoms as the child reduces his self-harm, which may be the reason he began to self-harm in the first place.[25] For example, if he begins to feel more anxious when he reduces his self-harm, this should be addressed with treatment to reduce the risk of setback.

- It is unwise for a child to reduce medication and reduce self-harming simultaneously. This is too big a withdrawal all at once. The practitioner should work with the child, his family and other healthcare professionals involved to develop a programme of withdrawal.

Patterns involved in self-harm[*]

The patterns which appear most regularly in children who self-harm are:

- Liver *qi* stagnation (leading to Heat)

- Full Heat in the Liver and/or Heart

- Phlegm-Fire harassing the Heart

- Phlegm misting the Mind and/or in the channels of the body

- Blood and/or *yin* deficiency

---

[*] Attwell-Griffiths and Bovey (2014) think that self-injury may be a form of self-treatment for any of the above syndromes. Self-injury may tonify Heart and Lung *qi* and *yang*; nourish Heart Blood; nourish Heart, Kidney, Liver, Lung and Stomach *yin*; clear Empty Heat; clear Heart, Liver and Stomach Fire; sedate the Liver; subdue Liver *yang*; disperse the Liver and regulate *qi*; resolve Phlegm in the Heart; open the Heart's orifices; and pacify the *shen*.

Liver *qi* stagnation (leading to Heat)

Some forms of self-harm are an attempt by the young person to move stagnant *qi*.

Mental–emotional symptoms

- cutting and pinching

- feeling low

- irritability and moodiness

- pre-menstrual syndrome in girls

- desire to self-harm may increase pre-menstrually in girls

Physical symptoms

Headaches, irritable bowel syndrome, painful periods

Pulse: wiry

Tongue: normal, red at the sides

Treatment principles: smooth the Liver and move *qi*; clear Heat (if necessary)

> **SUGGESTED TREATMENT**
>
> Two or three points per treatment, one of which should affect the spirit, are usually sufficient.
>
> **Points**
>
> Liv 3 *taichong*
> GB 40 *qiuxu*
> Liv 2 *xingjian*
> GB 38 *yangfu*
> Liv 14 *qimen*
> GB 24 *riyue*
>
> **Method:** sedation needle technique

Full Heat in the Liver and/or Heart

Cutting is essentially a form of blood-letting which has been an accepted way of releasing Heat in many traditional forms of medicine for many years.

Mental–emotional symptoms

- self-harm, especially cutting

- agitation and anxiety

- panic attacks

- poor sleep

Physical symptoms

Headaches, acne, excessive thirst, feeling hot

Pulse: overflowing Fire and Wood pulses

Tongue: red, especially tip and sides

Treatment principles: clear Heat from the Liver and Heart; calm the *shen*

> **SUGGESTED TREATMENT**
> Two or three of the following points per treatment are usually sufficient. A point to treat the spirit should be included.
>
> **Points**
>
> He 7 *shenmen*
> He 8 *shaofu*
> Ren 14 *juque*
> Liv 2 *xingjian*
> Du 24 *shenting*
> GB 9 *tianchong*
>
> **Method:** sedation needle technique

Phlegm-Fire harassing the Heart

Full Heat in the Heart is likely to condense the fluids and lead to the formation of Phlegm. In this case, the child may have bouts of agitation and anxiety, mixed with bouts of depression and disconnection. Points to resolve Phlegm, as well as points to clear Heat, should be used.

> **SUGGESTED TREATMENT**
> One point per treatment from each of the three groups are usually sufficient.
>
> **Points**
> To clear Heat:
>
> He 8 *shaofu*
> Ren 14 *juque*
>
> To calm the *shen*:
>
> He 7 *shenmen*
> Du 24 *shenting*
>
> To resolve Phlegm:
>
> Pc 5 *jianshi*
> St 40 *fenglong*
> GB 13 *benshen*
>
> **Method:** sedation needle technique

Phlegm misting the Mind and/or in the channels of the body

The presence of Phlegm may mean a child's experience of life is dulled and muffled. Self-harm may be a way of trying to create sharper and more intense sensations.

Symptoms

- self-harm, especially cutting, pinching and burning
- disconnected and in a world of his own
- depressed
- sleeps a lot

- slow responses

- muffled speech

- confusion

Pulse: wiry or slippery

Tongue: thick coating

Treatment principles: resolve Phlegm

SUGGESTED TREATMENT
Two of the following points per treatment is usually sufficient.

Points

> Pc 5 *jianshi*
> St 40 *fenglong*
> Ren 14 *juque*
> GB 9 *tianchong*
> GB 41 *zulinqi*

Method: sedation needle technique

Blood and/or *yin* deficiency

Agitation and anxiety are often a part of the picture in a child or teenager who is Blood or *yin* deficient. Self-harming can be a way of trying to allay these feelings. It temporarily induces a feeling of calm and relaxation.

Key symptoms

- self-harm

- worse when anxious or stressed

- anxiety and agitation

- feelings of vulnerability

- poor sleep

- difficulty relaxing

Other symptoms will depend on the Organ or Organs involved, which may be the Heart, Pericardium, Liver, Stomach, Lungs and/or Kidneys.

Pulse: thin, floating

Tongue: pale (if Blood deficiency predominates), red (if *yin* deficiency predominates)

Treatment principles: nourish Blood and/or *yin*; calm the *shen*

SUGGESTED TREATMENT
Points should be chosen according to which Organ or Organs are involved.

Points
To nourish Blood:

He 7 *shenmen*

Pc 7 *daling*

Liv 8 *ququan*

Ki 3 *taixi*

Ren 4 *guanyuan*

Sp 6 *sanyinjiao*

To calm the *shen*:

Du 24 *shenting*

Ren 14 *juque*

Method: tonification needle technique

Other techniques: moxibustion

A Five Element approach to self-harm

In my experience, the most effective way of helping a young person who is self-harming is to treat his constitutional emotional imbalance alongside any Organ/Pathogen patterns.

Fire constitutional imbalance

An attempt to alleviate feelings of unlovability/loneliness

When the Fire Element is out of balance, a young person may suffer from extreme feelings of unlovability. He may find it hard to make connections with other people because of his vulnerability. As a consequence, he may feel very alone. Sadly, this situation is common in children and teenagers. The main reasons are either bad family relationships, friendships at school not going well or romantic rejection in the teenage years. Teenagers these days have the added possibility of being 'rejected' on social media.

Treatment on the child's Fire Element, whether the imbalance is deficient or full in nature, can help a child to feel less vulnerable and therefore more able to make connections with other people. This will lessen his feelings of unlovability and, in turn, may reduce the need for self-harm. Figure 42.1 illustrates the role of the Heart in self-harm.

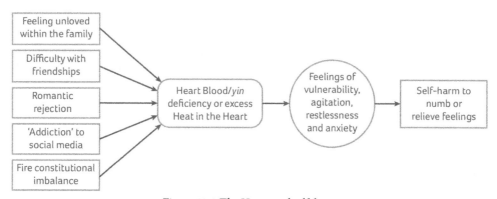

Figure 42.1 The Heart and self-harm

Earth constitutional imbalance

An attempt to 'unknot' qi

A child with an Earth imbalance may have a tendency for worry. At times of stress, such as before exams, the worry may become incessant and it may feel to the child that he cannot escape it. Worry knots the *qi*, which leads to a form of stagnation. Self-harm may be used as an attempt to escape from the spiralling, obsessive thoughts and to get the *qi* flowing again. Figure 42.2 illustrates the role of the Spleen in self-harm.

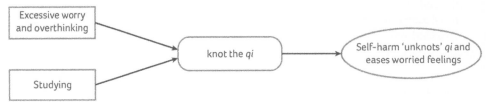

Figure 42.2 The Spleen and self-harm

An attempt to escape feelings of being misunderstood and uncared for

A child with an Earth imbalance may also have a tendency to feel misunderstood and uncared for. This is common during the teenage years, when a feeling that 'nobody understands me' or 'nobody gets me' may pervade. If the child is unable to come to terms with this, he may fall to self-harm as a way of dealing with the pain. Once again, when there is good rapport between the young person and practitioner, the treatment room may become a space where he can begin to verbalise these feelings, thereby lessening the need to self-harm. Figure 42.3 illustrates how the Earth Element may be involved in self-harm.

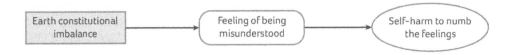

Figure 42.3 The Earth Element and self-harm

Metal constitutional imbalance

A form of self-punishment

A child with an imbalance in his Metal Element may have a tendency to be extremely self-critical and somewhat of a perfectionist. He may easily perceive that what he does, or simply who he is, is not good enough in some way. He may turn to self-harm to chastise himself for his perceived failings. Figure 42.4 illustrates how self-harm may be a form of self-punishment.

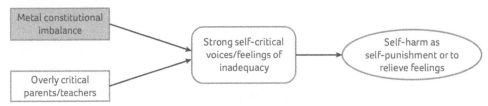

Figure 42.4 Self-harm as a form of self-punishment

Escaping painful feelings of grief

The emotion connected with the Metal Element is grief. If a child feels overwhelmed by grief, and is not able to find a way of expressing it, this may lead him to self-harm. Once again, when there is good rapport between child and practitioner, the treatment room may become a space where a child can begin to verbalise these feelings, thereby lessening the need to self-harm.

An attempt to alleviate feelings of numbness

The Metal Element has another particular relevance in children who are self-harming with methods that inflict injury or pain on the skin. The *yin* Organ related to Metal, the Lungs, is responsible for sending *wei qi* to the surface of the body, and it is via this that we connect with the external world. If the Metal Element, and therefore *wei qi*, are deficient, it may mean that the child feels cut off and is disconnected from everything. He may live his life in a rather numb state. Self-harm may be an attempt to induce strong sensations and feelings. Figure 42.5 illustrates how the Metal Element may be involved in self-harm.

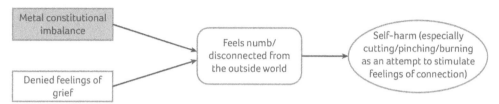

Figure 42.5 The Metal Element and self-harm

Water constitutional imbalance

Escaping intense feelings of fear

The emotion connected with the Water Element is fear. Fear and anxiety are extremely common emotions in children. The psyche of a young child is delicate. An image in a film or book, a taunt by an older sibling or an encounter with a barking dog may lodge in the child's mind and create ongoing fear or anxiety. In an older child, fear may be related to something he has read in the news or the responsibilities which come with growing up. A child may be prone to fear because of a constitutional imbalance in the Water Element or may become fearful due to overwork and lack of rest which depletes his Kidneys. Self-harm may be a way of trying to find some escape and respite from these unabating fearful and agitated feelings. Figure 42.6 illustrates how the Water Element may be involved in self-harm.

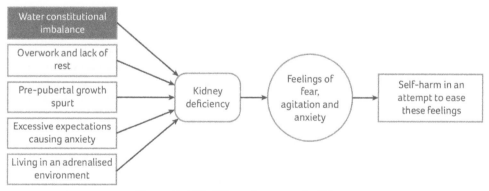

Figure 42.6 The Water element and self-harm

Recklessness and self-harm

A child with a deficient Water Element may also be prone to a higher degree of recklessness than another child. He may have a need for thrill and danger. A child who is 'over-parented' at home and allowed little freedom may seek out ways to feel alive and free. Self-harm may be an expression of thrill-seeking.

Wood constitutional imbalance

An attempt to alleviate unbearable feelings of anger

When the Wood Element is out of balance, the emotion that the young person usually finds the hardest to express smoothly is anger. Internalising anger or being chronically angry has the effect of stagnating Liver *qi*. Acupuncture treatment of the child's Wood element will help him to develop a healthier relationship with the emotion of anger. If a child begins to find a way to express his anger, or to let go of resentments and frustrations, his *qi* will flow more smoothly. This will reduce the need for self-harm. Figure 42.7 illustrates how the Wood Element may be involved in self-harm.

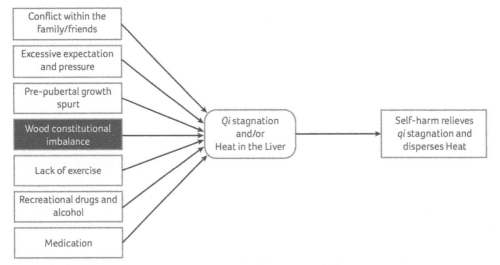

Figure 42.7 The Wood Element and self-harm

CASE HISTORY: HIGH-ACHIEVING ELEVEN-YEAR-OLD BOY

This case history highlights how bringing an underlying emotion into balance helps to reduce the need for self-harm.

Arthur had begun cutting his arms and abdomen for six months before coming to the clinic. His parents had become aware of this only recently, when a parent of one of Arthur's friends informed them they had overheard Arthur and their son talking about it. When asked, Arthur had eventually admitted to his parents what he was doing and said he did it because 'it's the only thing I know that makes me relaxed'.

Arthur was an especially bright boy who was preparing for an entrance exam to a top school. He also excelled at two musical instruments. He had lots of friends.

Observations: Arthur had a very red face, was dark under his eyes and had a dark blue/black colour to the side of his eyes. His voice was groaning. He fidgeted constantly as he spoke. Although he was smiley and confident, I saw occasional 'leaks' of fear flash across his face.*

- Pulse: overflowing Fire and Wood pulses, deficient Water pulses
- Tongue: very red tip, whole tongue body red

---

* Five Element acupuncturists look for 'leaks' of an emotion that are usually hidden. They may last less than a second but they are an excellent diagnostic clue indicating the constitutional imbalance.

Diagnosis: I diagnosed Arthur as having a Water constitutional imbalance, manifesting with Kidney *yin* deficiency, and Full Heat in the Liver and Heart. I thought that the combination of the Full Heat and the underlying deficiency of the Water Element created an enormous amount of agitation and anxiety in him, and that the self-harm was an attempt to allay this. Whilst on the surface Arthur was coping with the enormous academic pressure he was under, underneath it was taking a toll.

Treatment

Treatment principles: clear Full Heat in the Liver and Heart, calm the *shen*, strengthen the Water Element

Treatment 1

> Ren 14 *juque*, Liv 2 *xingjian* (sedation needle technique)

> Bl 64 *jinggu*, Ki 3 *taixi* (tonification needle technique)

Treatment 2

> He 8 *shaofu*, Liv 2 *xingjian* (sedation needle technique)

> Ki 24 *lingxu*, Bl 66 *zutonggu*, Ki 10 *yingu* (tonification needle technique)

I chose these distal points because, as the Water points on the channels of the Water Element, they have a particular ability to cool and calm the agitation that stems from Kidney *yin* deficiency.

I continued along these lines with a varied selection of points to treat Arthur's constitutional imbalance for six, weekly treatments. By this stage, Arthur said that he was feeling noticeably more relaxed and less anxious much of the time. He had not stopped cutting himself, but he said his compulsion to do so was less strong than it had been.

By this stage, the overflowing quality on the Fire and Wood pulses had gone. I therefore decided to focus the treatment purely on strengthening Arthur's constitutional imbalance. I wanted to treat his *zhi* in order to support his will to stop cutting himself. I found that Arthur had a particularly good reaction to the following points:

- Bl 52 *zhishi* (outer back *shu* point of the Kidneys)

- Bl 23 *shenshu*

- Ren 4 *guanyuan*.

Arthur continued to improve. During times of stress (usually when there was a school or music exam pending), he still resorted to cutting himself. I talked to his mother about pre-empting this and he came for more regular treatment when there was a particularly pressured time ahead. To date, Arthur has not self-harmed for an entire year.

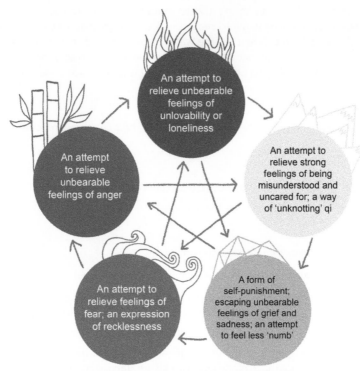

A Five Element perspective of self-harm

SUMMARY

» Self-harm is often an attempt to escape from intense feelings. Acupuncture may be used to help reduce the intensity of feelings, thereby reducing the need for self-harm.

» The patterns most commonly seen in young people who self-harm are: Liver *qi* stagnation turning to Heat; Full Heat in the Liver and/or Heart; Phlegm-Fire harassing the Heart; Phlegm misting the Mind and in the channels of the body; and Blood and/or *yin* deficiency.

» Treatment of the child's Five Element constitutional imbalance should always be considered when treating a young person who is self-harming.

• Chapter 43 •

SLEEP PROBLEMS

The topics discussed in this chapter are:

- The Organs involved

- Aetiology in babies and toddlers

- Patterns in babies and toddlers

- Other modalities for babies and toddlers

- Aetiology in school-age children and teenagers

- Patterns in school-age children and teenagers

- Sleep problems at different times of night

- Other modalities, for children of all ages

Introduction

Sleep problems fall somewhere between physical and mental–emotional disorders. In babies and toddlers, the root may be purely physical. In older children, it is more likely to be found in the emotional or psychological realm. For this reason, sleep is included under mental–emotional conditions.

Sleep problems are a common reason for children to come to the clinic. Sleep-disturbed nights lead to unhappy days. A child who has not slept well may be more emotionally volatile, is less likely to eat well, will cry more and need more attention. It is hard for a child who is consistently not sleeping well to thrive. She may become more prone to picking up infections and less physically robust.

The parents of a child who does not sleep often despair of ever getting an unbroken night's sleep again. Their health and mood suffer, which often means that their relationship and work also suffer. Even though parents may know a child is not sleeping badly 'on purpose', they may not be able to manage their feelings of exasperation with their child, so the parent–child relationship may also be impacted. Thus there is often a huge incentive for the whole family that a child sleeps well.

In some cases, there may not be any pathology present in the child who is not sleeping. The child's sleeping arrangements simply do not fit her individual nature. When this is the case, a simple suggestion of a change of approach may be all that is needed.

Approximate hours of sleep needed by babies and children at different ages

The hours in Table 43.1 are guidelines. Every baby and child is unique and some have sleep needs that are different from others of a similar age. However, if a child is getting a wildly different number of hours' sleep from the average for their age, it may indicate a pathology.

Table 43.1 Hours of sleep needed at different ages[26]

Age	Hours of sleep needed per 24 hrs	Daytime sleep	Night-time sleep
Newborns (0–3 months)	14–17 hours		
6 months	14 hours	3 hours	11 hours
1 year	13.5 hours	2.5 hours	11 hours
2 years	13 hours	1.5 hours	11.5 hours
3 years	11.5–12.75 hours	0–45 minutes	11.5–12 hours
4–9 years old	11–12.5 hours		11–12.5 hours
10–16 years old	9–12 hours		9–12 hours

Other matters to consider

What are the sleeping arrangements?

How parents choose to get their baby to sleep, and where he sleeps, is high up on the list of the most emotive topics parents discuss. Some have a strongly held belief that a baby should sleep on his own in a cot from day one and that doing otherwise will only 'create a rod for their own back'. Others believe passionately that a baby will not grow up with secure attachment unless he sleeps with the parents for the first three years of his life. It is only necessary to delve into this potentially fraught territory if we deem that the sleeping arrangements are a significant factor in why the baby is not sleeping well.

One situation that occurs relatively frequently is a mother and child co-sleeping and the child (usually a toddler) feeding frequently through the night. The baby is depleted because his sleep is interrupted, and his Spleen is strained because of a lack of breaks between feeds. At the opposite end of the spectrum is a baby who is sleeping in his own room and who wakes because he needs contact during the night in order to boost his *qi* and settle his *shen*.

Sometimes discussing sleeping arrangements with the parents can be helpful. It not only gives them permission to change, but helps them to develop more clarity on the matter. It is very hard, when in the middle of a situation and sleep deprived, to be able to do that oneself.

Is the baby or toddler 'overtired'?

Sleep begets sleep. Most young children sleep better at night when they are not overtired and have slept well in the day. When a baby or toddler is tired, his *qi*, Blood and *yin* become depleted so that his *shen* can no longer be well rooted. Consequently, he finds it harder to sleep.

The Organs involved

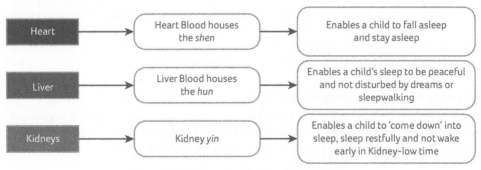

Figure 43.1 Organs involved in sleep problems

Aetiology in babies and toddlers

Babies and toddlers are, of course, affected by their emotions. If a baby feels anxious, insecure or angry, he is unlikely to sleep well. However, the sleep of babies and toddlers is influenced more strongly by what is going on in the physical body, particularly the digestive system. A baby may wake up because his supply of *qi* is dwindling and *qi* therefore fails to move Blood to the Heart. He needs a feed or contact with a parent to supplement his *qi*. He may wake up because food is accumulating in his digestive system and creating Heat, which then agitates the *shen*. Or he may be woken by the pain caused by Cold in his Stomach. Figure 43.2 summarises the key aetiologies of sleep problems in babies and toddlers.

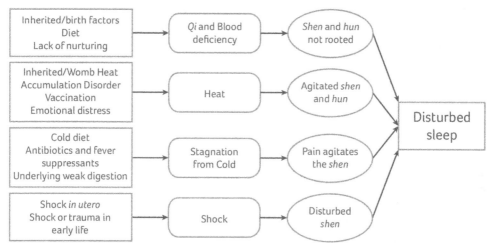

Figure 43.2 Aetiology of sleep problems in babies and toddlers

Patterns in babies and toddlers

- *Qi* and Blood deficiency

- Full Heat

- Stagnation from Cold in the digestive system

- Shock/Fright

 All the patterns listed above are commonly seen in the clinic. *Qi* and Blood deficiency is one of the most frequent causes of poor sleep in babies up until the age of about one or one and a half years old. Shock/Fright may co-exist with either *qi* and Blood deficiency or Full Heat.

Qi and Blood deficiency

Although it is the Blood that houses the *shen*, if *qi* is deficient then it does not adequately move Blood. As a result, the Heart does not receive enough Blood to house the *shen*. A child with this pattern may wake in the night because he needs some contact with a parent. He may be 'feeding' off the parents' *qi* in lieu of eating an appropriate amount of food.

Sleep symptoms

- wakes frequently during the night

- does not stay awake for long
- falls back to sleep after contact with parent, a drink or breastfeed
- falls to sleep easily in the evening

Other symptoms: pale, tires easily, poor appetite, quiet, loose stools

Pulse: deficient

Tongue: pale

Treatment principles: tonify *qi* and Blood

SUGGESTED TREATMENT

It is important to include a point on the Heart channel at each treatment because the *shen* is always involved in sleep problems. This may be combined with one or two other points to tonify *qi* and Blood.

Points

St 36 *zusanli*
Ren 12 *zhongwan*
Bl 20 *pishu*
Bl 21 *weishu*
He 7 *shenmen*

Method: tonification needle technique

Other techniques: moxibustion

Paediatric *tui na*

Heaven Gate *tianmen* (straight pushing)
Heart Gate *xinmen* (straight pushing)
Water Palace *kangong* (pushing apart)
Inner Palace of Toil *neilaogong* (kneading)
Heart *xinjing* (straight pushing tonification)
Small Heavenly Heart *xiaotianxin* (tapping)
Spleen *pijing* (straight pushing tonification)
Knead Ren 12 *zhongwan* (kneading anti-clockwise)
Spinal Column *jizhu* (pinching from the bottom to the top of the back)
St 36 *zusanli* (kneading)

Full Heat

This child has too much Heat in the system which rises up and disturbs the *shen* and the *hun*.

Sleep symptoms

- takes a long time to get off to sleep
- sleep is restless
- wakes and stays awake for several hours
- wakes up quietly but becomes afraid of the dark
- wakes early and is wide awake

- sleep is disturbed by dreams

- sleeptalks and sleepwalks

Other symptoms: feels hot, thirsty, red cheeks, finds it hard to settle, always on the go, tantrums or rages, clingy

Pulse: overflowing and rapid

Tongue: red or red tip

Treatment principles: clear Heat; calm the *shen*

> **SUGGESTED TREATMENT**
> It is usually sufficient to use one or two points per treatment. Points should be chosen according to which Organ is most strongly affected by the Heat. The Heart will always be involved because otherwise the Heat would not cause insomnia. It may be only the Heart that is involved, or other Organs too.
>
> **Points**
>
> He 7 *shenmen*
> He 8 *shaofu*
> Pc 8 *laogong*
> Liv 2 *xingjian*
> Liv 3 *taichong*
> LI 4 *hegu*
> St 44 *neiting*
>
> **Method:** sedation needle technique
>
> *Sifeng* may be used if the Heat derives from Accumulation Disorder.
>
> **Paediatric *tui na*** to clear Heat
>
> Heart *xinjing* (straight pushing sedation)
> Liver *ganjing* (straight pushing sedation)
> Heaven Gate *tianmen* (straight pushing)
> Heart Gate *xinmen* (straight pushing)
> Water Palace *kangong* (pushing apart)
> Inner Palace of Toil *neilaogong* (kneading)
> Small Heavenly Heart *xiaotianxin* (tapping)
> Milky Way *tianheshui* (straight pushing)

Stagnation from Cold in the digestive system

This pattern indicates the presence of full Cold in the digestive system. The pain this causes is the primary reason the child is waking. Only a full condition could cause the intensity of pain that accompanies this pattern. However, there may also be an underlying deficiency of *qi* and *yang*. The goal when treating this pattern is to enable the child's digestive system to work properly again.

Sleep symptoms

- wakes up in pain

- pulls legs up

- tight and contracted body

- clenched fists

- may sweat with pain

- may prefer to sleep on her tummy

Other symptoms: pale, poor appetite, loose stools. These symptoms will only be present if the child has an underlying deficiency of Spleen *qi* and *yang*.

Pulse: tight or wiry

Tongue: pale, may have a thick white coat

Treatment principles: expel Cold; tonify and warm the Stomach and Spleen

> **SUGGESTED TREATMENT**
>
> Moxa, together with approximately two points per treatment, is usually sufficient.
>
> **Points**
>
> St 36 *zusanli*
> Ren 12 *zhongwan*
> Sp 6 *sanyinjiao*
> Sp 4 *gongsun*
> Pc 6 *neiguan*
>
> *Sifeng* may be used to expel Cold when the underlying deficiency is not too great.
>
> **Method:** tonification needle technique
>
> **Other techniques:** moxibustion
>
> **Paediatric *tui na***
>
> Spleen *pijing* (straight pushing)
> Outer Palace of Toil *wailaogong* (kneading)
> Wind Nest *yiwofeng* (kneading)
> Three Passes *sanguan* (straight pushing)
> Knead the Navel *rou qi* (kneading clockwise)
> Spinal Column *jizhu* (pinching from bottom to top)

Shock/Fright

This is essentially a child's version of Heart Blood deficiency. The Heart Blood has been depleted by a shock, meaning that the *shen* is not settled. In the case of a prolonged or severe shock, the Kidneys may be affected too.

Sleep symptoms

- wakes up suddenly

- immediately frightened

- may resist going to sleep in the evening because of fear

- bad dreams

- cries out in sleep

- cannot settle himself on his own

Other symptoms: clingy, anxious and easily upset, bluish tinge on the bridge of the nose

Pulse: Heart pulse choppy and deficient, Kidney pulse deficient

Tongue: tip may be red

Treatment principles: clear shock; calm the *shen*

SUGGESTED TREATMENT

This pattern usually occurs in a sensitive child. Therefore, minimal treatment should be given. Often, just one point on the Heart channel is enough. It will only be necessary to treat the Kidneys in some children, who are likely to be anxious and fearful in the day as well as at night.

Points

> He 7 *shenmen*
> Ki 3 *taixi*
> Bl 15 *xinshu*
> Bl 17 *geshu*
> Ren 14 *juque*

Method: tonification needle technique

Paediatric *tui na*

> Heart *xinjing* (straight pushing tonification)
> Kidney *shenjing* (straight pushing tonification)
> Two Men Upon a Horse *erma* (kneading)
> Heaven Gate *tianmen* (straight pushing)
> Heart Gate *xinmen* (straight pushing)
> Water Palace *kangong* (pushing apart)
> Inner Palace of Toil *neilaogong* (kneading)
> Small Heavenly Heart *xiaotianxin* (tapping)

CASE HISTORY: EIGHTEEN-MONTH-OLD BOY WITH POOR SLEEP

This case history illustrates the importance of the mother–child link.

Robert was brought to the clinic by his mother when he was eighteen months old. The first thing that struck me was that both he and his mother looked exhausted. Robert was pale faced and calmly sat on his mother's lap whilst I took the case history. He didn't show any inclination to play. His mother said that he was waking up to feed every hour and had done since birth. He had never slept for more than an hour at a time. When he woke, he would have a short feed (he was sleeping with the mother and was breastfed) and then drop back off to sleep.

Robert ate a small range of solid foods but was not really interested and would always prefer to have some more breast milk. He had three or four bowel movements a day and his stools were usually not fully formed.

The birth had been very long and the mother had needed intravenous antibiotics. Although her husband was a doting father, he worked extremely hard and was away a lot. The family had only moved to the area just before Robert's birth, so had no family or friends nearby for support.

Diagnosis: *Qi* and Blood deficiency. I had a question mark in my mind as to whether the mother would need treatment too but, nevertheless, started off by treating Robert.

Treatment

- St 36 *zusanli*, Sp 3 *taibai* (tonification needle technique and moxa)
- He 7 *shenmen*, Bl 20 *pishu*, Bl 21 *weishu* (tonification, moxa on Bl 20 *pishu*)

> • Ren 12 *zhongwan*, St 36 *zusanli* (tonification, moxa)
>
> Treatment continued along these lines. I saw Robert twice a week for two weeks, and then weekly for four more weeks. He gradually began sleeping for longer stretches at a time. After the fourth session, his mother was slightly less fatigued and able to cope with a conversation about what she could perhaps do to help replenish herself. We talked about the importance of warming foods and she began to put Robert to sleep in his own cot for the first part of the night. This meant she could get a few hours of good-quality sleep before Robert woke up for his first feed. Her husband, when he was home, began tending to Robert if he woke. By the end of the tenth treatment, Robert was only waking once a night for a feed. He was eating more solids and his mother had begun to go out to mother and baby groups and build a network of friends and support.
>
> **Reflection:** This is an example of how much of a unit a mother and baby are. Robert and his mother had become stuck in a rut of depletion and tiredness and it needed one of them to have some kind of external boost (here in the form of acupuncture) for things to change. I believe it would have been equally effective had I treated the mother rather than Robert.

Other modalities for babies and toddlers

Shonishin

Core non-pattern-based root treatment.

Targeted tapping in the following areas:

- LI 4 *hegu*
- Du 12 *shenzhu*
- Shoulder area
- Occipital area
- Du 20 *baihui*

Aetiology in school-age children and teenagers

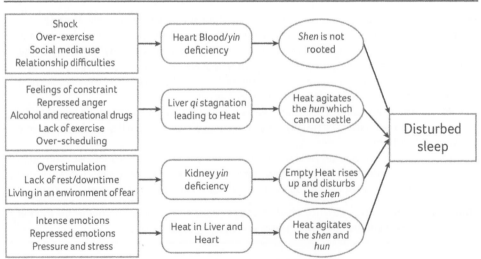

Figure 43.3 Aetiology of sleep problems in school-age children and teenagers

Other matters to consider

What goes on in the household in the evening?

Evening times may be stressful in a household with young children and tired parents. Nobody is at their best, and parents may be short of patience. If the energy of the household is frenetic, this may impact the child's ability to drop off to sleep. Cross words just before bedtime may mean a sensitive child feels insecure and this impairs her ability to sleep well.

Is the child struggling to separate from his mother to an age-appropriate level?

If the child wakes primarily because he needs contact with a parent, it may be that he is not getting what he feels to be enough contact during the day. Close contact with his mother just before bedtime can help.

It is always worth considering whether the mother is struggling to separate from her child. A child may pick up on his mother's struggle and, acting on an instinctive need to look after her, seek contact during the night. It may still be possible to help the mother and child through this phase purely by treating the child, however.

Is the child overstimulated and unable to wind down enough to sleep?

Too many activities and too little downtime may cause a child to be over-adrenalised and therefore unable to fall asleep. Making adjustments to the child's lifestyle, as well as treating the underlying pattern, is usually crucial.

What is the child or teenager doing in the hours before bedtime?

If a teenager is studying right up until the time when he goes to bed, it may disrupt his night's sleep. Apart from the fact that it may take him longer to drop off to sleep, it may also mean that his sleep during the night is more disturbed. It is essential that the *yi* and the *hun* are firmly rooted in the *yin* and Blood of their relevant Organs for sleep to be easy and peaceful.

If a child is using social media right up until he goes to bed, this may also interfere with sleep. If everything is going well in terms of his contact with friends, that is one thing (although even that may overstimulate some children). If he becomes upset, anxious or hurt by something a friend says to him or by somebody not replying to a message, this may be enough to knock his *shen*, which then disturbs his sleep. This is especially likely in a child or teenager who has Heart Blood deficiency.

Being on a screen of some kind, and especially playing fast-action video games, may also prove too stimulating for some children just before bedtime. This is particularly the case if the child has an imbalance in his Liver such as Liver *qi* stagnation or Liver Heat.

Patterns in school-age children and teenagers

- Heart Blood/*yin* deficiency

- Liver *qi* stagnation leading to Heat

- Kidney *yin* deficiency

- Heat in the Heart and/or Liver

All these patterns are commonly seen in the clinic. Heart Blood/*yin* deficiency is especially common in pre-pubescent girls. It often co-exists with either Kidney *yin* deficiency or Liver *qi* stagnation. Liver *qi* stagnation leading to Heat is commonly seen in girls and boys as they approach puberty.

Heart Blood/*yin* deficiency

Sleep symptoms

- takes a long time to get off to sleep
- lies awake with thoughts going around and around
- becomes anxious in the evening when more tired
- sleep tends to be light

Other symptoms: easily becomes tearful, feels vulnerable and easily hurt, easily startled, difficulty concentrating or struggles to retain facts

Pulse: thin or choppy Heart pulse and/or deficient Pericardium pulse

Tongue: pale

Treatment principles: nourish Heart Blood

> **SUGGESTED TREATMENT**
> Two or three points per treatment are usually sufficient.
>
> **Points**
>
> > He 7 *shenmen*
> > Pc 7 *daling*
> > St 36 *zusanli*
> > Sp 6 *sanyinjiao*
> > Bl 15 *xinshu*
> > Bl 44 *shentang*
> > Bl 20 *pishu*
> > Bl 49 *yishe*
>
> **Method:** tonification needle technique
>
> Liver Blood deficiency causes poor sleep too. Typically the sleep will be light and the child may feel that he never falls into a deep sleep, or that he is 'half awake, half asleep'. Liver Blood deficiency is especially common in girls who have started menstruating. If present, then points to nourish Liver Blood should be added (such as Liv 8 *ququan* and Bl 18 *ganshu*).

Liver *qi* stagnation leading to Heat

Sleep symptoms

- often wakes up between 1 and 3am in the morning
- takes a long time to get to sleep if goes to bed after midnight
- lies awake either feeling angry or making lists and plans
- sleep may be disturbed by dreams
- sleep is especially bad when has not had much physical activity

Pulse: wiry or overflowing Liver pulse

Tongue: may be red on the sides

Treatment principles: smooth the Liver and move *qi*; clear Heat from the Liver

Kidney *yin* deficiency

Sleep symptoms

- takes a long time to get to sleep in the evening

- wakes up early in the morning

- finds it harder to sleep the more tired he becomes

Other symptoms: prone to bedwetting, easily overstimulated, excessively fearful or alternatively rather reckless, intellectually precocious

Pulse: floating

Tongue: red

Treatment principles: nourish the Kidneys; bring *qi* downwards

SUGGESTED TREATMENT

Kidney deficient children are easily overstimulated, so no more than one or two points per treatment need to be used.

Points

    Ki 3 *taixi*
    Ki 1 *yongquan*
    Bl 23 *shenshu*
    Ren 4 *guanyuan*
    He 7 *shenmen*

Method: tonification technique

Heat in the Heart and/or Liver

Sleep symptoms

- light sleep with frequent waking during the night

- vivid dreams that often disturb sleep

- wakes up feeling anxious in the night

- may lie awake for hours at a time feeling hot and restless

Other symptoms: prone to irritability and tempers, or may suppress anger and become depressed, moodiness, may tend towards being slightly hyperactive or even manic, prone to anxiety or panic attacks

Pulse: overflowing in the Heart and Liver positions, rapid

Tongue: red tip, red sides, may have a yellow coat

Treatment principles: clear Heat from the Heart and/or Liver

> **SUGGESTED TREATMENT**
> **Points**
>
> > He 8 *shaofu*
> > He 7 *shenmen*
> > Liv 2 *xingjian*
> > GB 38 *yangfu*
> > Ren 14 *juque*
> > Du 24 *shenting*
>
> **Method:** sedation needle technique

Sleep problems at different times of night

Some of the patterns mentioned above have a tendency to cause problems with sleep during particular parts of the night. This is only really applicable in school-age children and teenagers. The sleep of babies and toddlers is so related to food and the need for contact that the guidelines in Table 43.2 do not really apply to them.

Table 43.2 Sleep problems at different times of night

Time of night	Possible patterns	Rationale
Difficulty getting off to sleep in the evening	Heart Blood deficiency Kidney *yin* deficiency	*Shen* is not housed Empty Heat agitates the *shen*
Waking up in the middle of the night	Liver *qi* stagnation turning to Heat	Hyperactivity in the Liver is worse during the time Liver *qi* is at its highest (i.e. 1am–3am)
Waking up early in the morning	Kidney *yin* deficiency	3am–7am is low Water time

Other modalities, for children of all ages
Retained needles or press-spheres

- A retained needle or press-sphere may be placed on Bl 17 *geshu*.

- A retained needle or press-sphere may be placed on any knots around Bl 15 *xinshu*.[27]

Auricular acupuncture

A press-sphere on ear *shenmen*.

> **CASE HISTORY: EIGHT-YEAR-OLD GIRL WITH DIFFICULTY FALLING TO SLEEP**
> This case history illustrates:
>
> - that a child often needs minimal intervention
>
> - how children are prone to absorbing the emotions of their main caregivers.

Rachel was not able to drop off unless there was somebody else in the room. She shared a room with her older sister but she wanted to move into a room of her own. She frequently woke in the night scared by noises that she heard in the house. She would wake up her parents or her sister and need reassurance before she was able to get back to sleep. She had no other health problems and a straightforward health history. She had a happy home life and enjoyed school. Her mother was devoted to her husband and children but experienced a lot of anxiety which had its roots in her childhood.

Rachel had strikingly red cheeks. She was a mix of rather coy and at the same time very engaging with an enormous smile. Her Heart pulse was slightly overflowing, whilst her Pericardium pulse was very thin and deficient.

Diagnosis

- Excess Heat in the Heart
- Fire Element constitutional imbalance

Treatment: Rachel was not willing to try needles. I began with some *shonishin* to help her relax and to try to bring down some of the excess *yang qi* from her head. Whilst doing *shonishin* on her back, I noticed that she had a pronounced, hard knot of muscle in the region of Bl 15 *xinshu*. I put a retained needle in the centre of the knot and gave her mother some spare ones with instructions on usage (see Chapter 33). I then used a laser machine to tonify the source points of Rachel's Pericardium and Triple Burner (Pc 7 *daling* and TB 4 *yangchi*).

Reaction to treatment: Rachel had a very strong reaction to her treatment, which was a useful reminder of how little intervention children usually need. She had gone home from her first session and had been upset by a minor scrap she had had with her sister. Her mother said she sobbed and sobbed in a way she had never seen before. She barely stopped sobbing until she went to sleep that evening. However, she dropped off to sleep very easily and did not wake up once during the night. For the rest of the week, she only woke up a couple of times, which was a big improvement.

Further treatment: At the second session, she voluntarily suggested that she was ready for her sister to move out of her room and try sleeping on her own. Her mother organised an audio book for her to listen to as she was trying to get to sleep. The knot around Bl 15 *xinshu* was much less pronounced so I suggested she stop using the retained needles. This time I tonified the *luo* connecting points (Pc 6 *neiguan* and TB 5 *waiguan*) with the laser machine. When she came back two weeks later, she was successfully sleeping in a room on her own and rarely waking at night.

Reflection: This case illustrates that sometimes children just need a tiny amount of intervention to make an enormous shift. I felt that Rachel had, during her lifetime, probably internalised some of her mother's anxiety and that this had led to a build-up of Heat in her Heart. Helping her to release this (as it was not really 'hers') and gently strengthening her Pericardium and Triple Burner was all it took for her to feel settled enough in herself to sleep alone and sleep soundly.

SUMMARY

» In babies and toddlers, sleep problems may have a physical cause.

» In older children, they are likely to have an emotional cause.

» The patterns most commonly seen in babies and toddlers are: *qi* and Blood deficiency; Full Heat; Cold in the digestive system; and Shock/Fright.

» The patterns most commonly seen in school-age children and teenagers are: Heart Blood/*yin* deficiency; Liver *qi* stagnation leading to Heat; Kidney *yin* deficiency; and Heat in the Heart and Liver.

TREATMENT OF PHYSICAL CONDITIONS

Chapter 44

INTRODUCTION TO THE TREATMENT OF PHYSICAL CONDITIONS

. . . .

Part 5 contains chapters on the treatment of physical conditions that commonly present in the clinic. It is by no means a definitive list. There are many other conditions that appear in children that can be successfully treated with acupuncture. It is my hope that the principles of diagnosis and treatment of children that run throughout the book will enable the practitioner to feel confident to treat most conditions.

Below, I outline a few points for the reader to bear in mind when using this part of the book.

Choice of Organ/Pathogen patterns

The patterns listed for each condition are the ones most commonly seen in an outpatient acupuncture clinic in a relatively affluent area in the UK. It is my hope that practitioners with experience of working with children in very different settings will share their findings.

A child may appear with a condition discussed but stemming from a different pattern to those given in this book. The practitioner should always be led first and foremost by her clinical findings and use this book, or any other, to support that, rather than the other way around.

Where applicable, I have noted how a pattern manifests across different age groups, and which patterns are most prevalent in children of different ages.

Description of Organ/Pathogen patterns

Patterns rarely occur in isolation, and therefore a child often presents with more than one of the patterns listed for each condition. Some patterns are on a continuum with one another, for example Spleen *qi* deficiency and Spleen *yang* deficiency. For example, a child may have many symptoms of Spleen *qi* deficiency and at times, in the winter perhaps, veer more towards Spleen *yang* deficiency. A teenage girl may have Liver *qi* stagnation only before her period. A toddler may have a tendency to Large Intestine Cold which manifests only when she eats ice cream. Patterns are a snapshot of a moment in time, whereas in reality the *qi* of a child is continually in flux.

Likewise, the symptoms and signs listed for each pattern are rarely all present. One child with Spleen *qi* deficiency may have several symptoms and signs, such as poor appetite, loose stools, tendency to worry and deficient Earth pulses. Another may only have deficient Earth pulses but the Spleen *qi* deficiency is causing other problems (such as scanty periods or constipation) that are not listed here. Each pattern will manifest slightly differently in each child depending on her constitutional nature and the circumstances of her life. The description of patterns, therefore, is a guide rather than something which is written in stone.

Treatment of the Organ/Pathogen patterns

When more than one pattern is present, the practitioner should endeavour to decide which is the predominant one and to treat that first. Treating too many aspects of a condition all at once is usually less effective. This is especially the case with children.

Suggested treatments

The treatments laid out are suggestions, not prescriptions that should be blindly followed. Practitioners should choose treatment modalities and techniques based on what is most suited to the individual child. Every practitioner will come to the treatment of children with their own unique experience and this will inevitably and rightly influence how they approach treatment.

Points

The acupuncture points listed, once again, are certainly not a definitive list. They are ones which the practitioner may especially consider using in the treatment of that condition. There may well be other points which will suit a particular child in a particular situation and which are not listed in this book. Each practitioner should evolve over time her own repertoire of points for particular patterns that she finds especially effective, and may prefer to use them rather than the points given here.

Paediatric *tui na* and *shonishin*

I have only included suggestions of paediatric *tui na* and *shonishin* for babies, toddlers and young children. Although these techniques are most used in this age group, this is not to say that either modality may not be used on older children. In particular, children who are especially sensitive or those who are developmentally delayed in some way may benefit enormously from these methods. Alongside acupuncture, they may be a useful adjunct to the treatment of any child.

Deliberate omissions

The reader will note that there are no definitive guidelines for how long a particular condition will take to treat. This is because, from experience, I do not believe this is possible to predict accurately. I hope that the case histories throughout the book will show that sometimes miracles do appear to happen in the treatment room and that, at other times, for reasons that are not always clear, acupuncture is unable to help a child. When parents ask how many treatments their child will need, it can be helpful for the practitioner to communicate that she feels optimistic that she will be able to help, and that, within approximately six treatments, she will be able to have a much clearer idea as to what degree and over what period of time.

Treatment of the constitutional imbalance

Treatment of the child's constitutional imbalance may be used in the treatment of any physical condition. Sometimes it is enough on its own to bring about the required change. At other times, it should be combined with treatment of the Organ/Pathogen patterns.

The case histories at the end of each chapter help to illustrate how treatment of the constitutional imbalance can be used in children and how it can be combined with treatment of the Organ/Pathogen patterns. Should a reader who is not trained in this style of acupuncture want further guidance, they are referred to the text *Five Element Constitutional Acupuncture* by Hicks, Hicks and Mole (2011).

Sources

- **Patterns:** The patterns listed for each condition are largely based on those described by Scott and Barlow, and Flaws.[1] I have adapted what these authors have written to include insights gained from my clinical experience. For those conditions not previously written about in English (such as paediatric chronic fatigue syndrome), I have looked at the adult literature on these topics, adapted it to children and included insights from my own clinical experience.

- **Paediatric *tui na* treatment:** My suggestions of paediatric *tui na* routines for each condition are based on the work of Dr Hongchun Yin (who I interned with), Fan Ya-li and Rossi.[2] They are ones that I have found to be effective. The practitioner should always adapt them to the particular child she is treating.

- ***Shonishin*:** My suggestions of *shonishin* treatment for each condition are based on those described by Birch.[3]

A final word

It is easy as a practitioner, when confronted with lots of information, to attempt to think one's way to a diagnosis or out of a difficult case. Whilst it is, of course, necessary for a practitioner to use her mind, when working with children the key to good diagnosis and treatment is often to feel the *qi* of the child. When the case is complex and seemingly full of contradictions, the practitioner should initially focus her treatment on one aspect that she *is* sure of, for example the child is deficient, or she has an Earth constitutional imbalance or her *qi* is rising upwards to her head. As treatment progresses, other aspects will, it is hoped, gradually emerge and become clearer.

• Chapter 45 •

PROBLEMS WITH EATING AND APPETITE

. . . .

Topics discussed in this chapter are:

* Organs involved

* Aetiologies prevalent in babies and toddlers

* Patterns in babies and toddlers

* Aetiologies in school-age children and teenagers

* Patterns in school-age children and teenagers

* Other treatment modalities

* A Five Element view of eating

Please note that the mental health condition of anorexia nervosa is discussed separately in Chapter 41, Eating Disorders.

Introduction

Many children are brought to the clinic by their despairing parents because of issues with eating and appetite. An infant or toddler may show little interest in solid food. A school-age child may eat only tiny quantities. Another child may be existing on pasta and chicken nuggets alone. How ironic that, at a time when those living in affluent countries are bombarded by the most enormous array of food choices, poor appetite should be such a prevalent condition amongst so many children. Sometimes, particularly with babies, the problem is related to a physical imbalance. In other cases, particularly with school-age children and teenagers, there may be an emotional component. Whatever the cause, acupuncture is very often an effective method of treatment.

Although a doctor once commented to me that children seem to be able to live off 'not much more than air and an apple once a month', having a poor diet over a period of months or years is obviously far from ideal. It greatly increases the chances of long-term deficiency of Spleen *qi*, Blood and the Kidneys.

A child who does not eat well may be the source of worry and stress within the family. Mealtimes may end in shouting or tears (both the child's and the parent's), and going to friends' houses or to restaurants may not be an option. Lovingly prepared packed lunches come home from school untouched. The problem may impact upon family life and relationships.

In babies and some young children, the problem of a poor or limited appetite may be helped purely by treating the Organ/pathogen pathologies with which the child presents. However, in other children (particularly those of school age), it may be helpful for the practitioner to understand a little bit about the context of the child's condition too. One of the problems for the parent of a child who barely eats is that this behaviour can evoke such strong emotions that it becomes difficult to step outside the situation, to see it clearly and then to make any changes that are necessary. As objective bystanders, we may be able to explore delicately what is going on in the family and help the parent and child to find a way through. Before looking at the Organ/ Pathogen patterns involved, I am therefore going to outline some of the key issues that may become entwined with the problem.

What is meant by 'abnormal appetite'?

Nearly all children have a phase when they are somewhat picky about food. 'Abnormal appetite' here refers to a problem that continues for months or is extreme in nature. An abnormal appetite manifests differently at different ages. For many children, an abnormal appetite only manifests in one sphere. For example, a child may eat vast amounts of pasta but *only* pasta. The manifestations described below rarely all occur simultaneously in one child.

- **Babies:** Lacks interest in feeding, loses interest or gets distracted during feeds, shows little interest in solids.

- **Toddlers:** Lacks interest in solid foods, wants to be fed rather than feeding himself, takes little interest in trying new foods, eats very small quantities of food, prefers just to drink milk.

- **School-age children:** Eats only a small range of foods, refuses to try new foods, shows little relish in eating, snacks but does not eat proper meals, 'comfort' eats.

- **Teenagers:** Snacks but does not eat proper meals, lives off junk foods and eats little by way of fresh, unprocessed foods, regularly skips a particular meal (often breakfast), shows little relish for food, 'comfort' eats.

The wider context of problems with eating and appetite

Food and emotions

Feeding a child is one way of expressing and demonstrating love. Most mothers have an inner glow of contentment when their young baby has finished a good breastfeed, or when their child has happily eaten a wholesome meal. The flip side of this is that if a baby fusses on the breast, or a child moans his way through mealtimes whilst simultaneously pushing his food around his plate, it may induce feelings of anxiety and even anger in the mother. As Bee Wilson puts it, 'One of the biggest things many children learn at the table is that our choice to eat or not eat unleashes deep emotions in the grown-ups close to us. We find that we can please our parents or drive them to rage, just by refusing dessert.'[4]

So, eating for a young child is rarely just about filling his stomach. It stirs intense emotions which then disturb his *qi*, often causing it to knot or stagnate, which does little to stimulate his appetite.

Food is good or bad

All food is not equal, and a child learns this from early on. The norm is to reward the eating of 'good' foods such as green vegetables with 'bad' foods such as sweets. A child may be being taught to eat as many 'good' foods as possible, whilst at the same time being given the implicit message that they are not generally very tasty – so he deserves a reward of a nice (but 'bad') food. It is all rather confusing. Eating up a good portion of greens, or even asking for seconds, is often highly praised. Eating too much dessert, or asking for more, is usually frowned upon. One minute, a child is told that he should eat up otherwise he will be hungry later; the next he is told to stop eating so much, otherwise he will feel sick.

All of this means that deciding what to eat and whether to eat can become a rather stressful business for a child. Any natural instinct simply to follow hunger cues or to want more of what his taste buds tell him is nice often becomes lost amid all this emotion and complexity.

How can acupuncture help?

 In babies and toddlers, a poor appetite or fussy eating is most commonly due to a physical dysfunction. In school-age children and teenagers, it is most commonly due to an emotional issue, although there may also be a physical problem.

Treating the child

Treating any imbalances present in the child's *qi* will optimise the chances of her eating well. For example, if a child has a lot of Damp or *qi* stagnation, it may reduce her appetite. Treating a child's constitutional imbalance often improves a child's well-being, which may also lead to an increase in appetite. On top of this, treating a young child may help to shift the dynamic between parent and child, sometimes miraculously. For example, if the child has Spleen *qi* deficiency, this may mean she is feeding off her mother's *qi* in lieu of eating.* Strengthening the child's Spleen *qi* will help to resolve this situation.

Giving information and reassurance

As well as guilt, many parents feel anxious if their child is not eating well. Providing a space where a parent can express her worries can, in itself, be a way of dissipating anxiety. If appropriate, the practitioner can reassure the parent that her child is essentially healthy. Giving the mother information about what would be considered 'normal' for a child of her age to eat can also be helpful. We can let her know, for example, that it is perfectly fine for a baby or toddler to have reduced appetite when she is teething (see Chapter 66).

WHAT DIETICIANS AND FAMILY THERAPISTS SAY ABOUT FEEDING CHILDREN

» Most dieticians agree that, from toddlerhood to adolescence, a parent should be responsible for 'what, when, where' and the child responsible for 'how much and whether'.

» A child should be offered a wide range of healthful foods, and should be given a lot of choice about which ones to eat and how much to eat.

» The best way for a child to learn to eat new foods is repeated exposure, that is, to offer different foods over and over again.

» Clear rules should be set around mealtimes. For example, even if the child is refusing to eat anything, he should sit at the table with the family.

---

* Scott and Barlow call this Hyperactive Spleen *qi* deficiency. Please see *Acupuncture in the Treatment of Children* (1999), pp.39–42.

Organs involved

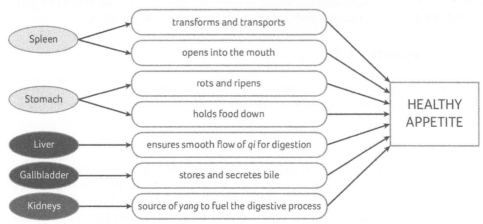

Figure 45.1 Organs involved in problems with eating and appetite

Aetiologies prevalent in babies and toddlers

A difficult start

Having a baby who does not show much interest in feeding may well induce anxiety in a mother. It is likely that midwives and health visitors will be stressing the importance of her baby putting on weight and growing according to the average of babies of his gender and age. The mother may be put under pressure to start feeding her baby formula milk rather than to continue breastfeeding. If the relationship between mother and child around food and feeding is characterised at this early age by anxiety, it may remain fraught with emotion for years to come. Other causes of problems with feeding, eating and appetite are shown in Figure 45.2.

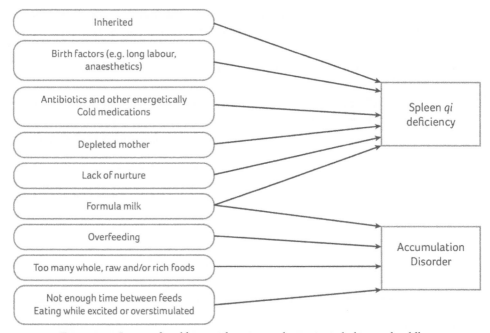

Figure 45.2 Causes of problems with eating and appetite in babies and toddlers

Patterns in babies and toddlers

- Spleen and Stomach *qi* deficiency
- Accumulation Disorder

Spleen and Stomach *qi* deficiency

Appetite

- shows little interest in solid foods
- eats very small amounts
- only eats a small number of foods
- often prefers 'simple' foods such as carbohydrates
- as a baby, breastfeeds little and often

Other symptoms: quiet, pale face, loose stools, wakes up regularly during the night

Pulse: deficient

Tongue: pale

Treatment principles: tonify Spleen and Stomach *qi*

> **SUGGESTED TREATMENT**
> It is usually sufficient to combine two points per treatment, together with some moxa.
>
> **Points**
>
> St 36 *zusanli*
> Sp 6 *sanyinjiao*
> Ren 12 *zhongwan*
> Bl 20 *pishu*
> Bl 21 *weishu*
>
> **Method:** tonification needle technique
>
> **Other techniques:** moxibustion on any of the above points
>
> **Paediatric *tui na*** routine to tonify and warm the Spleen, and stimulate the appetite
>
> Spleen *pijing* (straight pushing tonification)
> Stomach *weijing* (straight pushing tonification)
> Thick Gate *banmen* (straight pushing)
> Three Passes *sanguan* (straight pushing)
> Knead Ren 12 *zhongwan* (kneading anti-clockwise)
> Spinal Column *jizhu* (pinching from the bottom to the top of the back)
> St 36 *zusanli* (kneading)

Accumulation Disorder

Appetite

- phases of eating large amounts
- phases of not wanting to eat
- often shows an early interest in solid foods and eats a wide variety of them

- may not know when to stop eating

Other symptoms: red face, green mucus, loud and gregarious, distended abdomen, alternating constipation and diarrhoea

Pulse: full, slippery, wiry

Tongue: dirty, thick coating

Treatment principles: disperse accumulation of food

SUGGESTED TREATMENT
Points

    M-UE-9 *sifeng*

Needle technique: prick the *sifeng* points on one hand (and warn parents that the child may have several bowel movements over the next twenty-four hours: see Chapter 32)

Paediatric *tui na* routine to disperse accumulation of food

    Spleen *pijing* (straight pushing tonification)
    Stomach *weijing* (straight pushing sedation)
    Thick Gate *banmen* (straight pushing)
    Eight Trigrams *bagua* (circular pushing anti-clockwise)
    Four Wind Creases *sifengwen* (pinching)
    Abdomen Stimulation *fuyinyang* (pushing apart)
    Belly Corner *dujiao* (pinching)

In the clinic

- Treating the pattern of Spleen and Stomach *qi* deficiency may influence the relationship between the baby or toddler and her main carer, as well as improve her appetite. She may have been 'feeding' off the *qi* of a mother figure in lieu of eating. As she begins to eat more, she may make a developmental leap at the same time and become more independent in some way. She no longer relies so heavily on the *qi* of her mother figure.

- It is essential to give the appropriate dietary advice when treating Accumulation Disorder in order to avoid it recurring (see Chapter 27).

A COMBINATION OF ACCUMULATION DISORDER AND SPLEEN AND STOMACH *QI* DEFICIENCY

It is common for a child to start life as an excess child, who is prone to repeated bouts of Accumulation Disorder, due to his naturally large appetite. Over time, however, this gradually weakens his Spleen *qi*, so he alternates between the two patterns above. He may gradually become more and more Spleen *qi* deficient. Simultaneously, his appetite may gradually reduce.

It may also work the other way around. The Spleen of a child who is deficient may not have sufficient *qi* to digest even the relatively small amount of food he eats. This may then fester in his Stomach and Intestines, and lead to the development of Accumulation Disorder. This interaction between Spleen *qi* deficiency and Accumulation Disorder is illustrated in Figure 45.3.

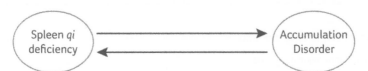

Figure 45.3 Interaction between Spleen qi deficiency and Accumulation Disorder

> **CASE HISTORY WHERE NO TREATMENT WAS NEEDED**
>
> This case history illustrates that:
>
> - sometimes, simply a piece of lifestyle advice is all that is needed for the child to regain health
> - the parent and child can benefit from the objectivity of the practitioner.
>
> Three-year-old Lucy was brought for treatment because she barely ate any solid food at all. A typical breakfast was half a banana, lunch was a plain rice cake and supper was three or four spoons of pasta. Her mother was desperate. She said Lucy refused to ever try new foods. Even when she went to parties and saw the other children eating, she would sit there pushing the food around her plate.
>
> At this point, I was perplexed. As her mother was telling me how little she ate, I was observing Lucy: she looked an appropriate size and height for her age, had rosy cheeks and seemed full of energy. She certainly did not look like a typical Spleen *qi* deficient child, the usual type to have so little interest in food.
>
> I then asked her mother what Lucy drank in a typical day. She told me that Lucy adored milk and she drank between four and six bottles of full-fat milk a day! Her mother said if she did not let her have the milk, she worried that she would be taking in virtually no calories at all.
>
> I suggested to Lucy's mother that, starting from today, she only allow Lucy one glass of milk a day. She should then let me know in a week if Lucy's appetite had improved. Sure enough, after a few tantrums at first, within a week Lucy had started eating much more solid food. Over the next few weeks, she began increasing her range of foods too.

Aetiologies in school-age children and teenagers

Unhappiness in the child or the family

Sometimes the way a child chooses to express an unhappiness is by not eating.

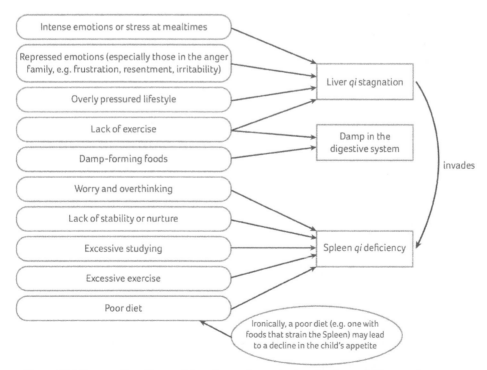

Figure 45.4 Causes of problems with eating and appetite in school-age children and teenagers

Patterns in school-age children and teenagers

- Spleen and Stomach *qi* deficiency

- Damp and Phlegm in the digestive system

- Liver *qi* stagnation (invading the Spleen or Stomach)

Spleen and Stomach *qi* deficiency is the most commonly seen of these patterns. It may be combined with either Damp and Phlegm and/or Liver *qi* stagnation.

Spleen and Stomach *qi* deficiency

Appetite

- rarely eats a large meal

- choosy about food

- avoids eating more complicated foods

- snacks a lot

- no appetite for breakfast

Other symptoms: pale, easily tired, loose stools, tummy aches, tendency to worry and overthinking, poor sleep

Pulse: deficient, thin

Tongue: pale

Treatment principles: tonify Spleen *qi*

> **SUGGESTED TREATMENT**
> It is usually sufficient to use approximately two points per treatment, combined with moxa. A poor appetite may be a manifestation of a deeper malaise. When this is the case, treatment of the child's constitutional imbalance is also useful.
>
> **Points**
> St 36 *zusanli*
> Sp 6 *sanyinjiao*
> Ren 12 *zhongwan*
> Bl 20 *pishu*
>
> **Method:** tonification needle technique
>
> **Other techniques:** moxibustion

Damp and Phlegm in the digestive system

Appetite

- often does not feel hungry

- finds it hard to eat in the mornings but may develop an appetite as the day goes on

- easily feels full and bloated

Other symptoms: puffy face, sluggish and lethargic, mucus in stools, sleeps a lot, may appear emotionally 'weighed down', resists exercise but feels better for it

Pulse: slippery

Tongue: swollen, thick sticky coat

Treatment principles: resolve Damp and Phlegm; tonify Spleen *qi*

> **SUGGESTED TREATMENT**
> The correct balance between clearing Damp and strengthening the Spleen must be found, based on the symptoms and signs of the individual child. If there is a lot of deficiency, sometimes treating just that enables the Spleen to start moving fluids and the Damp to disperse.
>
> **Points**
> To clear Damp:
>
> > Sp 6 *sanyinjiao*
> > Sp 9 *yinlingquan*
>
> To tonify the Spleen:
>
> > Ren 6 *qihai*
> > St 25 *tianshu*
> > St 36 *zusanli*
> > Sp 3 *taibai*
> > Bl 20 *pishu*
> > Bl 21 *weishu*
>
> **Method:** tonification needle technique
>
> **Other techniques:** moxibustion may be used too

Liver *qi* stagnation (invading the Spleen or Stomach)

Appetite

- a marked inflexibility towards what and when to eat
- food becomes a battle ground
- lacks hunger because of bloating and distension
- worse for a lack of physical activity

Other symptoms: irritability, moodiness, outbursts of anger, belching and flatulence

Pulse: wiry

Tongue: normal

Treatment principles: smooth the Liver and move *qi*; strengthen the Stomach and/or Spleen

> **SUGGESTED TREATMENT**
> Liv 13 *zhangmen* should be used if the child has irregular bowel movements, and Liv 14 *qimen* should be used if she has symptoms above the navel (in the epigastrium). Combining one of these points with two distal points is usually sufficient for one treatment.

> **Points**
>
> Liv 3 *taichong*
> GB 34 *yanglingquan*
> Liv 13 *zhangmen*
> Liv 14 *qimen*
>
> **Method:** sedation needle technique
>
> Also: additional points to strengthen the Stomach and Spleen if needed

Other treatment modalities

Shonishin

Light stroking down the arms, legs, back, abdomen and chest as in the core non-pattern-based root treatment.

Light tapping around the following areas or points:

- Bl 20 *pishu*

- Bl 21 *weishu*

- Ren 12 *zhongwan*

- around St 36 *zusanli*

A Five Element view of eating

A child's constitutional imbalance may manifest in the area of eating. Therefore, treatment focused on this imbalance may help to change a child's approach to food.

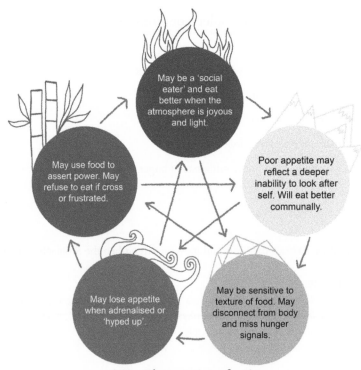

A Five Element view of eating

CASE HISTORY: SEVEN-YEAR-OLD BOY WITH LITTLE INTEREST IN FOOD

This case history illustrates:

- how the circumstances around birth can still have an influence years later
- how a lack of appetite can begin to affect all aspects of a child's health.

Jack came to the clinic because his mother was worried about his overall health. He was small for his age, skinny and generally lacking in vitality. He came down with every cough and cold that was going around. He regularly wet his bed at night. He was only interested in eating pasta and white toast, and he did not eat large quantities even of those. It was a struggle to get him to eat any fruit or vegetables.

Observations: Jack was pale, wan and had dark circles under his eyes. His pulse was deficient overall and his tongue was pale.

Aetiology: Jack's mum had taken prophylactic antibiotics throughout her entire pregnancy. She had had a previous late miscarriage due to a womb infection. Jack had been born three weeks early by c-section. Following an infection in her abdomen, his mother had further antibiotic treatment, this time intravenously. Jack was breastfed during this time.

Diagnosis: This was a clear-cut case of quite severe Spleen *qi* and *yang* deficiency, which had subsequently led to Kidney *yang* deficiency.

Treatment

I taught Jack's mum a paediatric *tui na* routine to strengthen the Stomach and Spleen, which she performed daily at home.

Treatment 1

St 36 *zusanli*, Sp 3 *taibai* (tonification technique with moxa cones)

Treatment 2

Bl 21 *weishu*, Bl 20 *pishu* (tonification technique with moxa cones)

Treatment 3

Ren 12 *zhongwan*, St 25 *tianshu*, Sp 6 *sanyinjiao* (tonification technique with moxa cones)

Treatment 4

Ki 3 *taixi*, St 42 *chongyang*, Sp 3 *taibai* (tonification technique with moxa cones)

Outcome: Weekly treatment continued along these lines and Jack's appetite, little by little, began to improve. There would be minor setbacks along the way, usually towards the end of a school term when Jack was especially tired. His mother showed great commitment to treatment, and Jack was treated either weekly or fortnightly for six months. By the end of this time, his appetite was greater and he ate a much wider range of foods. He had put on weight and looked much better. He had stopped bedwetting too. He continued to come for top-up treatments every month or so.

SUMMARY

- » An abnormal appetite may cause stress within the family and strain relationships.
- » In school-age children and teenagers, it often manifests as being picky about food.
- » In school-age children and teenagers, the practitioner should try to gain a sense of the dynamics in the family that may be related to the problem.
- » Any of the following Organs may be involved: Spleen, Stomach, Liver, Gallbladder and Kidneys.

» Common aetiologies for a poor appetite in babies and toddlers are: constitutional Spleen *qi* deficiency; difficulties around the birth; a difficult start with feeding; and overfeeding.

» The patterns that most commonly cause an abnormal appetite in babies and toddlers are Stomach and Spleen *qi* deficiency and Accumulation Disorder.

» The most commonly seen aetiological factors in school-age children and teenagers are: unhappiness; intense emotions around eating; insufficient exposure to a wide range of foods; stress and strain at school; and a poor diet.

» The patterns that most commonly cause an abnormal appetite in school-age children and teenagers are: Stomach and Spleen *qi* deficiency; Damp and Phlegm; and Liver *qi* stagnation.

» A child's constitutional imbalance may 'play out' in the area of eating.

Chapter 46

STOMACH ACHE AND ABDOMINAL PAIN (INCLUDING COLIC AND REFLUX)

The topics discussed in this chapter are:

- Organs that influence the abdomen
- Pathogens that may cause pain in the abdomen
- Diagnosis of abdominal pain in children
- Aetiology of abdominal pain in babies and toddlers
- Aetiology of abdominal pain in school-age children and teenagers
- Patterns that may cause abdominal pain
- Other treatment modalities
- Colic:
  - Aetiology of colic
  - Patterns that may cause colic
  - Advice for the mother of a baby with colic
  - Other treatment modalities

Introduction

Stomach ache is an almost universal childhood symptom. This is due to the fact that a child's digestive system is under constant strain because of the amount of food that needs digesting compared with the relative immaturity of the Stomach and Spleen.

Yet there is another reason so many children complain of stomach ache. A stomach ache may be a child's 'go to' symptom. It is something she has heard of and can easily express from a young age. A child may find it very difficult to articulate what is going on in her body and she may say her stomach hurts in lieu of having any other words to describe how she feels. To look at, babies and young children are almost all Middle Burner. Her stomach is often the part of herself to which she can most easily relate.

Stomach ache is also an archetypal psychosomatic symptom.* Menninger wrote that 'the gastro-intestinal tract mirrors the emotions better than any other body system'.[5] Emotions that are not expressed may be internalised and reveal themselves as a stomach ache. It is often much easier for a child to say 'I've got a stomach ache' than it is to say 'I am anxious about going to school

---

* The term 'psychosomatic' is often used pejoratively. It is not meant that way here. Just because a physical symptom has an emotional cause does not mean it is not real or that the sufferer is less deserving of our care.

today because I'm scared the teacher is going to shout at me'. This does not mean the child does not have a stomach ache or that the symptom should not be taken seriously. It simply means that one part of the reason for her stomach ache is an emotion that she is struggling to manage.

Whether there is a psychosomatic element to a child's stomach ache or not, treating both the Organ/Pathogen patterns and the Five Element constitutional imbalance in a child with stomach ache is often effective.

RED FLAGS: ABDOMINAL PAIN

Acute abdominal pain in a child may be a sign of a serious underlying condition which merits urgent referral to a conventional medical practitioner. This should be considered if:

✓ the abdominal pain is severe

✓ the pain is constant or colicky (coming in waves)

✓ there is rigidity, guarding or rebound tenderness.

As a general guideline, pain from an organic cause is likely to be near the navel or epigastrium and constant. Pain from a functional cause is likely to be further away from the navel or epigastrium and to move around.

Organs that influence the abdomen

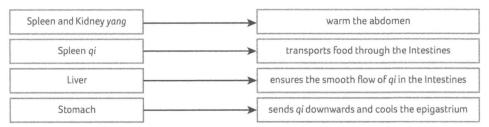

Figure 46.1 Organs that influence the abdomen

The Small Intestine and Large Intestine

The functioning of the Small and Large Intestines is largely determined by the condition of the *yin* Organs mentioned. It is not always necessary to treat these *yang* Organs directly. However, there are occasions when the practitioner should consider using points on these channels. For example, a child may have abdominal pain from Spleen *qi* deficiency with very few of the normal Spleen *qi* deficiency symptoms; the pattern is only affecting the Large or the Small Intestine. In this case, it is helpful to use points on the appropriate channel, and the back *shu* points, to affect the Intestines directly. This is also the case if the abdominal pain is severe (for example, in the case of Small Intestine *qi* pain).

How the different Organs relate to different areas of the abdomen

- A **Spleen** imbalance tends to affect the part of the abdomen below the navel.

- A **Stomach** imbalance tends to affect the part of the abdomen above the navel (the epigastrium).

- A **Liver** imbalance may affect either the lower or upper abdomen, as well as the hypochondrium (the area over the margin of the ribcage on either side).

Note: If there is pain in the hypogastrium (the area directly above the pubic bone), it usually indicates a Bladder problem. Urinary tract infections are discussed in Chapter 60.

Pathogens that may cause pain in the abdomen

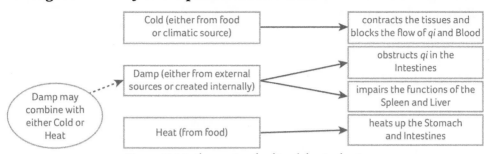

Figure 46.2 Pathogens involved in abdominal pain

Diagnosis of abdominal pain in children

When treating an adult with abdominal pain, the practitioner gleans a lot of diagnostic information from asking details about the nature of the pain, what makes it better or worse, etc. This is, of course, not possible at all in a pre-verbal child, whose parents may only know she is in pain because she pulls her legs up to her abdomen or holds her stomach. It is also quite common, however, for a much older child, or even a young teenager, to find it difficult to articulate the nature of pain.

The parent may, of course, be able to give useful information.* Other than that, the practitioner must rely on observation of the child, palpation of the abdomen and other signs and symptoms in order to make the diagnosis. If the child does not want her abdomen touched because it elicits pain, this is usually a reliable indication that the pain is full in nature.

Aetiology of abdominal pain in babies and toddlers

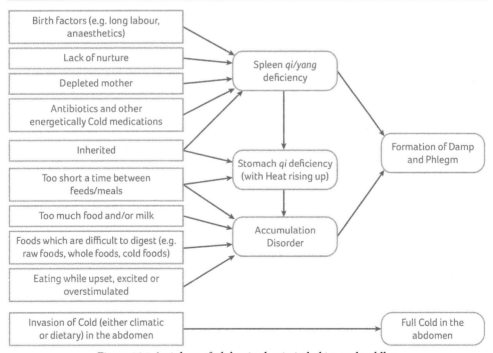

Figure 46.3 Aetiology of abdominal pain in babies and toddlers

---

* The child's evidence as to the location of the pain is usually more reliable than the parents, however.

Aetiology of abdominal pain in school-age children and teenagers

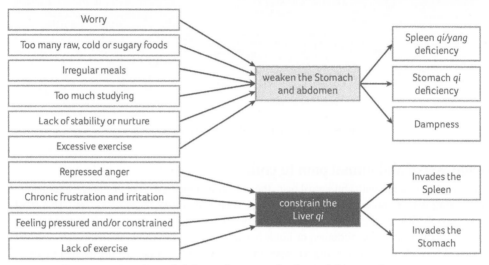

Figure 46.4 Aetiology of abdominal pain in school-age children and teenagers

Patterns that may cause abdominal pain

- Spleen *qi* and/or *yang* deficiency

- Stomach *qi* deficiency with Heat rising upwards

- Accumulation Disorder (babies and toddlers)

- External Cold (more common in babies and toddlers)

- Liver *qi* stagnation invading the Spleen or Stomach (school-age children and teenagers)

- Damp/Phlegm in the abdomen

External Cold and Accumulation Disorder are both common causes of abdominal pain in babies and toddlers. Spleen *qi* deficiency, often combined with Liver *qi* stagnation and/or Damp/Phlegm, are the patterns most commonly seen in school-age children and teenagers.

Spleen *qi* and/or *yang* deficiency

Pain

- dull, relatively mild pain below the navel which comes and goes

- child is likely to moan and whine rather than forcefully cry

- pain may get worse after food (especially cold food)

- worse after a bowel movement

- worse when the child is tired or has exerted herself

Other symptoms: loose stools which may contain undigested food, pale face, easily tired

Pulse: deficient

Tongue: pale, wet, swollen

Treatment principles: tonify and warm Spleen *qi* and/or *yang*

SUGGESTED TREATMENT

It is usually sufficient to needle two of these points per treatment on a baby or toddler. Sp 4 is particularly effective for stomach ache from whatever cause.

Points

> St 25 *tianshu*
> St 36 *zusanli*
> Ren 12 *zhongwan*
> Sp 3 *taibai*
> Sp 4 *gongsun*
> Ren 6 *qihai*
> Ren 8 *shenque*
> Bl 20 *pishu*

Method: tonification needle technique

Other modalities: moxa stick on the above points and over the abdomen

Paediatric *tui na* routine to tonify and warm the Spleen

> Spleen *pijing* (straight pushing tonification)
> Stomach *weijing* (straight pushing tonification)
> Thick Gate *banmen* (straight pushing)
> Three Passes *sanguan* (straight pushing)
> Knead the Navel *rou qi* (kneading anti-clockwise)
> Knead the Lower Abdomen *rou qihai* (kneading anti-clockwise)
> Spinal Column *jizhu* (pinching from the bottom to the top of the back)
> St 36 *zusanli* (kneading)

Stomach *qi* deficiency with Heat rising upwards

This pattern is commonly seen in babies with reflux. In adults, this pattern would be called Stomach *yin* deficiency. However, in children, it is not usually *yin* that is deficient, but simply Stomach *qi*. This leads to some local stagnation, which creates Heat, which then rises upwards.

Pain

- mild pain above the navel

Other symptoms: reflux after feed or meals, regurgitates milk after feeds

Treatment principles: tonify Stomach *qi*; subdue Heat rising upwards

SUGGESTED TREATMENT

It is usually sufficient to needle two of these points per treatment on a baby or toddler.

Points

To tonify Stomach *qi*:

> Ren 12 *zhongwan*

Ren 13 *shangwan*
Bl 21 *weishu*
St 36 *zusanli*

Method: tonification needle technique

To subdue Stomach Heat (if necessary):

St 44 *neiting*

Method: sedation needle technique

Paediatric *tui na* routine to tonify the Stomach and subdue Rebellious Heat

Spleen *pijing* (straight pushing tonification)
Thick Gate *banmen* (straight pushing)
Eight Trigrams *bagua* (circular pushing anti-clockwise)
Central Altar *shanzhong* (straight pushing)
Ren 12 *zhongwan* (kneading anti-clockwise)
Spinal Column *jizhu* (pinching from the bottom to the top of the back)
St 36 *zusanli* (kneading)

Accumulation Disorder

Pain

- strong pain

- pain worse with pressure

- pain better after a bowel movement or vomiting

Other symptoms: distended abdomen, irregular bowel movements, red cheeks, green colour around the mouth, foul-smelling flatulence, unhappy and restless

Pulse: wiry and/or slippery in the middle positions

Tongue: thick, sticky coating

Treatment principles: disperse accumulation of food

SUGGESTED TREATMENT
Points

M–UE-9 *sifeng*

Method: lightly prick the points on one hand (and warn the parent the child may have several bowel movements over the next twenty-four hours)

Paediatric *tui na* routine to disperse accumulation of food

Stomach *weijing* (straight pushing sedation)
Thick Gate *banmen* (straight pushing)
Eight Trigrams *bagua* (circular pushing anti-clockwise)
Four Wind Creases *sifengwen* (pinching)
Knead Ren 12 *zhongwan* (kneading clockwise)
Abdomen Stimulation *fuyinyang* (pushing apart)
Belly Corner *dujiao* (pinching)

Note: Accumulation Disorder may stem from a Spleen *qi* deficiency and therefore this needs to be addressed with treatment after the accumulation has been cleared.

External Cold

Although External Cold can cause acute abdominal pain, some children are prone to it, and therefore get repeated attacks. Cold may invade either the Spleen, causing pain below the navel, or the Stomach, causing pain above the navel.

Pain

- sudden onset of severe pain

- cries forcefully

- may arch back or pull legs up in pain

- sweating from pain

- pain comes on after eating cold foods

- often occurs during the night and wakes the child up

Other symptoms: diarrhoea after eating cold food, poor appetite, pale face, easily tires

Pulse: wiry or tight

Tongue: thick white coating

Treatment principles: expel Cold and move *qi*; warm and tonify Spleen *yang*

SUGGESTED TREATMENT

Sp 4 *gongsun* is probably the most effective point to treat stomach ache from almost any cause. In a baby or toddler, it is usually sufficient to combine it with one or two other points at each treatment. Liv 3 *taichong* need only be used in order to relieve the spasm when the child has acute abdominal pain.

Points

St 25 *tianshu*
St 36 *zusanli*
Sp 4 *gongsun*
LI 4 *hegu*
Liv 3 *taichong*

Method: sedation needle technique

Other techniques: moxa stick over the abdomen

Also: in between attacks of pain, it may be necessary to warm and tonify Spleen *yang*

Paediatric *tui na* routine to strengthen and warm the Spleen and expel Cold

Spleen *pijing* (straight pushing tonification)
Large Intestine *dachangjing* (straight pushing tonification)
Small Intestine *xiaochangjing* (straight pushing tonification)
Outer Palace of Toil *wailaogong* (kneading)
Wind Nest *yiwofeng* (kneading)
Three Passes *sanguan* (straight pushing)
Knead Ren 12 *zhongwan* (kneading anti-clockwise)

Liver *qi* stagnation invading the Spleen or Stomach

If Liver *qi* invades the Spleen, it will cause pain below the navel. If it invades the Stomach, it will cause pain and other symptoms above the navel.

Pain

- cramping abdominal discomfort which comes in waves

- worse with stress

- pain relieved by a bowel movement

Other symptoms: bowel movement may be urgent and stools loose, belching, flatulence, worse when angry/frustrated or stressed, irritability, outbursts of anger, repressed anger, may be worse pre-menstrually in teenage girls

Pulse: wiry

Tongue: normal

Treatment principles: smooth the Liver and move *qi*; tonify Spleen *qi*

> **SUGGESTED TREATMENT**
>
> When Liver *qi* stagnation is the primary pattern, it may not be necessary to treat the Spleen at all. When Spleen *qi* deficiency is the primary pattern, it may not be necessary to treat the Liver. In some cases, both Organs need to be treated. It is always preferable to keep treatment minimal and to find out what treating one Organ does before adding in treatment of another Organ. The pulse and nature of the symptoms will usually dictate which is the best place to start.
>
> **Points**
> To smooth Liver *qi*:
>
> Liv 13 *zhangmen* (for Liver *qi* invading the Spleen)
> Liv 14 *qimen* (for Liver *qi* invading the Stomach)
> Pc 6 *neiguan*
> Liv 3 *taichong*
> Ren 12 *zhongwan*
>
> **Method:** sedation needle technique
>
> To strengthen the Spleen:
>
> St 36 *zusanli*
> Sp 3 *taibai*
> Bl 20 *pishu*
> Bl 21 *weishu*
>
> **Method:** tonification needle technique

Damp/Phlegm in the abdomen

Damp/Phlegm may affect either the Spleen or Stomach, or both. If it is primarily in the Spleen, the pain will be below the navel. If it is primarily in the Stomach, the pain will be above the navel.

Pain

- dull, heavy or full feeling in the stomach

- may be worse in the morning or after eating

Other symptoms: poor appetite, child's tummy may look disproportionately big, nausea, intermittent vomiting of mucus

Pulse: wiry or slippery

Tongue: thick coat

Treatment principles: resolve Damp and Phlegm; tonify Spleen and Stomach *qi*

> **SUGGESTED TREATMENT**
> There is usually an underlying deficiency of the Spleen, which must also be addressed.
>
> **Points**
>
> Sp 9 *yinlingquan*
> Sp 6 *sanyinjiao*
> St 40 *fenglong*
> Ren 12 *zhongwan*
> St 28 *shuidao*
>
> **Method:** sedation needle technique
>
> Also: points to tonify and warm Spleen and Stomach *qi*

Other treatment modalities

Shonishin

Stroking and tapping core non-pattern-based root treatment.

Targeted tapping around the following areas or points:

- along the Stomach channel on the shins

- Bl 18 *ganshu* and Bl 20 *pishu* (if stiff)

- GB 20 *fengchi* and LI 4 *hegu* if the child is crying a lot[6]

CASE HISTORY: NINE-YEAR-OLD BOY WITH A STOMACH ACHE FROM 'FEAR'

This case history illustrates:

- how an unacknowledged emotion may be the cause of a physical symptom

- how it is not always necessary to treat the Organs most directly related to the part of the body the symptom is affecting.

Oli had been complaining of stomach ache on and off for the past six months. Sometimes the pain was mild, and sometimes it was so severe that he would lie down and scream. His appetite was unaffected, and his bowel movements were regular and unproblematic. Medical investigations had not revealed any organic cause.

Oli was an otherwise healthy child. Before the onset of the stomach ache, he had been happy, outgoing and generally enjoyed life. Over the past six months, he had become more and more inclined to want to just stay at home with his mum, and less keen to see his friends or play football.

Taking the case history: Oli's mum told me that he had been very anxious about coming to the clinic, so when he arrived I reassured him that I would not do anything without checking it out with him first. At first, Oli was reluctant to engage with me and he sat on his mum's lap looking away from me. This changed when he began to talk about Minecraft, his favourite computer

---

game. He gradually relaxed and I was able to then ask him more questions about his stomach pain and, more importantly, about his life.

Oli was telling me about school and I sensed a mix of enthusiasm but also anxiety in him. When I asked him about his teacher, he became really angry and said that he hated her. He was not able to express anything specific about why this was so. His mum confirmed that the stomach aches had started within a week of being in the class of that teacher.

Observations: Oli had a groaning voice and was dark by the side of his eyes. When he first arrived, he looked a little like a rabbit caught in headlights. He was almost paralysed by the fear and anxiety of coming to a new place. His tongue was unremarkable.

- Pulse: deficient and thin, especially in the left rear position. Wiry in the left middle position
- Tongue: normal
- Abdomen: he did not allow me to palpate his abdomen

Diagnosis: I diagnosed Oli as having a Water constitutional imbalance, due to his predominant emotion being fear, his groaning voice and the dark beside his eyes. I suspected that his stomach aches were due, at least in part, to a fear of his new teacher or something she had said or done.

Treatment
I treated Oli's constitutional imbalance by using a moxa stick and laser machine on points along the Kidney and Bladder channels.

Treatment 1

Yuan source points Bl 64 *jinggu*, Ki 3 *taixi*

Treatment 2

Tonification points Bl 67 *zhiyin*, Ki 7 *fuliu*

Treatment 3

Ren 6 *qihai*, back *shu* points Bl 28 *pangguangshu*, Bl 23 *shenshu*

Outcome: Oli's mum reported that, after the first treatment, he seemed to be in a kind of rage for the rest of the day, the likes of which she had never seen before. The following day, he was calmer and he had full attendance at school the whole week. He still complained of stomach ache on and off but it was not bad enough to stop him from doing anything. By the third treatment, Oli had been to school every day for three weeks and seemed back to his old, outgoing and happy self.

Reflection: Although I never found out what happened with Oli's teacher (and maybe he did not know either), I suspect his stomach aches were due to suppressed fear and anger. Strengthening his Water Element enabled the *qi* of the child Element (Wood) to flow. This in turn enabled the release of these emotions which had been stored up inside him.

COLIC

Colic tends to appear in newborn babies from the age of about two weeks onwards. It is characterised by periods of crying which can be hours long and tend to occur more frequently in the evening. Thankfully, it has usually passed by the age of about four months. It may be intensely stressful for the parents, especially first-time parents, who dread what is often referred to as 'baby witching hour'. Trying desperately to calm a screaming baby for hours every evening is exhausting, may put pressure on the marital relationship and can interfere with the bonding process between mother and baby.

Pulse and tongue are not included in the patterns that may cause colic. This is partly because it is hard to get accurate information from the pulse of such a young baby. On top of this, discerning which of the two patterns is causing the colic is usually possible just by careful observation of the baby.

Aetiology of colic

Constitutional Spleen *qi* deficiency

- **Baby feeds too often:** This strains the Spleen which then has a tendency towards becoming deficient and Cold. This can be the case even in breastfed babies.

- **Formula milk:** Tends to be energetically Cold and therefore weakens the Spleen *qi* of the baby.

- **Stress and anxiety in the mother:** As discussed in Chapter 2, a young baby will absorb the emotions around her. If she is breastfed, she may 'drink' in an energetic imbalance that is present in the mother and it will become her own.

- **Excess Heat in the mother:** In a breastfed baby, if the mother's energy is Hot this will be passed to the baby via the breast milk.

Patterns that may cause colic

- Hot Food stagnation (excess)
- Cold Food stagnation (deficient)

Hot Food stagnation (excess)

In this pattern, the baby consumes more milk than her Spleen is able to transform and transport. This leads to stagnation in the Intestines, and subsequently a build-up of Heat.

 KEY OBSERVATION
This baby will be red, hot and agitated.

Symptoms

- red face
- hot and agitated
- cry is loud and forceful
- feels warm or hot to the touch (especially hands and feet)
- strongly pulls legs up towards the abdomen
- stools are smelly and explosive
- flatulence
- bowel movement relieves pain

Treatment principles: disperse stagnation and clear Heat

SUGGESTED TREATMENT
Points

> M-UE-9 *sifeng*

Method: lightly prick the points on one hand

Paediatric *tui na* to disperse stagnation

> Stomach *weijing* (straight pushing sedation)
> Thick Gate *banmen* (straight pushing)
> Eight Trigrams *bagua* (circular pushing anti-clockwise)
> Four Wind Creases *sifengwen* (pinching)
> Knead the navel *rou qi* (kneading clockwise)
> Abdomen Stimulation *fuyinyang* (pushing apart)
> Belly Corner *dujiao* (pinching)

Cold Food stagnation (deficient)

At the root of this pattern is deficient Spleen *qi*. There is not enough *qi* to keep food moving through the Intestines. Although the stagnation must first be dispersed, the problem will not be cured unless the Spleen is then strengthened.

> ● **KEY OBSERVATION**
> This baby will be pale and her cry will lack force.

Symptoms

- pale face

- blue vein on bridge of nose

- prolonged crying without much force

- otherwise quiet

- lassitude

- cold hands and feet

- stools are not smelly

- likes to feed little and often

Treatment principles: disperse stagnation; tonify Spleen *qi*

SUGGESTED TREATMENT
If the baby comes to the clinic during an attack of colic, then treatment should focus on dispersing stagnation. Between attacks, treatment should focus on strengthening the Spleen.

Points
To disperse stagnation:

> LI 4 *hegu*
> Sp 4 *gongsun*
> Pc 6 *neiguan*

Method: sedation needle technique

To strengthen Spleen *qi*:

> St 36 *zusanli*
> Ren 12 *zhongwan*
> Bl 20 *pishu*

Method: tonification needle technique

Other techniques: moxa stick over Ren 8 *shenque*

Paediatric *tui na* routine to disperse stagnation of food and strengthen the Spleen

> Spleen *pijing* (straight pushing tonification)
> Large Intestine *dachangjing* (straight pushing tonification)
> Small Intestine *xiaochangjing* (straight pushing tonification)
> Thick Gate *banmen* (straight pushing)
> Eight Trigrams *bagua* (circular pushing anti-clockwise)
> Outer Palace of Toil *wailaogong* (kneading)
> Wind Nest *yiwofeng* (kneading)
> Three Passes *sanguan* (straight pushing)
> Knead Ren 12 *zhongwan* (kneading anti-clockwise)

Advice for the mother of a baby with colic

- The mother should be encouraged to leave gaps between feeds, so that the baby has the chance to fully digest one feed before the next one.

- In a breastfed baby, the mother's diet may need to be adjusted. The energetics of the food the mother eats will be passed on to the baby via the breast milk. So, in the case of a baby with a Cold and weak Spleen, for example, it is helpful for the mother to ensure her diet includes foods which warm and tonify the Spleen.

- The mother should be encouraged to call upon any support that is available to her. Having a baby with colic is extremely stressful, and the stress it creates for the mother may then perpetuate the colic in the baby.

- Ideally, the baby should be fed in a quiet and calm environment where she is not overstimulated and the mother is as relaxed as possible.

- Many parents find that their baby suffers worse from colic on a day when she has not slept so well or has become overtired. This is particularly the case in the deficient type of colic.

Other treatment modalities
Abdominal massage

The parent may perform the following massage on the baby twice a day as a preventive measure, and may also do it to relieve the symptoms during a bout of colic.

Following the flow of the Large Intestine: ascending the right side of the abdomen (ascending colon), across the top (transverse colon), descending the left side (descending colon) and across the bottom of the abdomen from left to right.

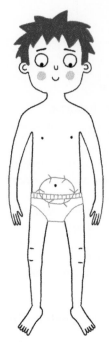

Abdominal massage for colic

If the colic is deficient, the parent should move her hand in small anti-clockwise circles as she massages, following the flow of the Large Intestine. If the colic is excess, the parent should move her hand in small clockwise circles as she massages following the flow of the Large Intestine.

SUMMARY

» The practitioner should be aware of the red flags of severe abdominal pain and refer the child to an orthodox medical practitioner when necessary.

» The following Organs may be involved: Spleen; Kidneys; Liver; and Stomach.

» The following pathogens may be involved: Cold; Damp; and Heat.

» In babies and toddlers, the cause of stomach ache or abdominal pain is most often dietary.

» In school-age children and teenagers, the cause is most often related to lifestyle and emotional constraint.

» The patterns involved may be: Spleen *qi* and/or *yang* deficiency; Stomach *qi* deficiency with Heat rising upwards; Accumulation Disorder; External Cold; Liver *qi* stagnation invading the Spleen; and Damp/Phlegm.

» Colic is either Hot and excess in nature, or Cold and deficient.

Chapter 47

CHRONIC LOOSE BOWELS

The topics discussed in this chapter are:

- Organs involved in loose bowels

- Aetiology in babies and toddlers

- Patterns in babies and toddlers

- Aetiology in school-age children and teenagers

- Patterns in school-age children and teenagers

- Other treatment modalities

Introduction

Loose bowels are characterised either by stools that are not properly formed or frequent bowel movements, or both.

Chronic loose bowels, although not a distressing or alarming symptom, is nevertheless one that should be treated. It is a sign that a child is not properly digesting his food. He will therefore not absorb all the nutrients which are vital for his development and ability to thrive. For a young baby, even a few days of loose bowels may have an impact on his overall health and vitality.

This begs the question of what constitutes loose bowels. The answer to this is very different depending on the age of the child. In the first six months of life, it is normal for a baby to pass unformed stools four or five times a day. By the age of about one, a toddler's stools will usually start to become more firm and less frequent. Of course, what is normal for one child will be different for another. Parents will usually have a sense of whether their child's bowel habits are healthy. A sudden change in bowel habits may be a sign of an imbalance.

When a parent brings her child for treatment with this problem, it is important to consider whether the child's bowel habits vary widely from what is the norm for his age. The practitioner should also look at the child's overall health to get a sense of whether he is becoming depleted by his abnormal bowel habits.

Organs involved in loose bowels

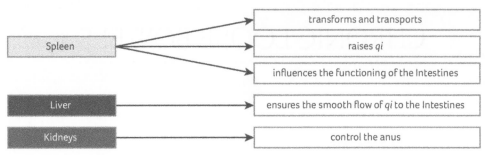

Figure 47.1 Organs involved in loose bowels

Aetiology in babies and toddlers

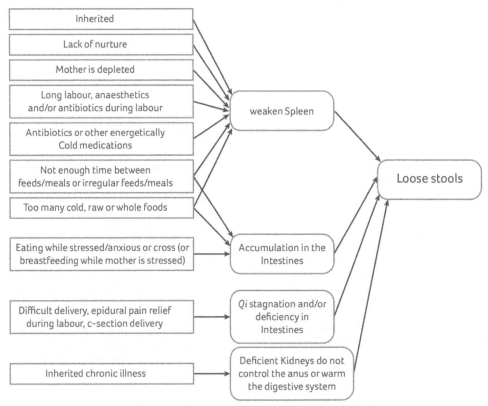

Figure 47.2 Aetiology of loose bowels in babies and toddlers

Patterns in babies and toddlers

- Spleen *qi* and/or *yang* deficiency
- Deficient and Cold Intestines
- Accumulation Disorder

These three patterns are all commonly seen in babies and toddlers. Spleen *qi* deficiency and Accumulation Disorder are frequently combined. Occasionally, there is also a deficiency of the Kidneys.

Spleen *qi* and/or *yang* deficiency

Bowel symptoms

- loose bowels
- frequent bowel movements
- bowel movement straight after eating
- undigested food in stools
- stomach ache after a bowel movement
- tired after a bowel movement
- worse when tired
- stools not smelly

Other symptoms: lethargic, pale, clingy, poor appetite, feels cold

Pulse: deficient

Tongue: pale

Treatment principles: tonify Spleen *qi*

> **SUGGESTED TREATMENT**
>
> In a baby or toddler, it is usually sufficient to needle two or three of these points per treatment, as well as using moxa.
>
> *Yang* deficiency may affect the Kidneys as well as the Spleen. In this case, the child may have more severe lassitude and be lacking in vigour. Moxa on Ren 8 *shenque* and Bl 23 *shenshu* should also be used.
>
> **Points**
>
> St 36 *zusanli*
> Sp 3 *taibai*
> Sp 6 *sanyinjiao*
> St 25 *tianshu*
> Ren 12 *zhongwan*
> Ren 6 *qihai*
> Bl 20 *pishu*
>
> **Method:** tonification needle technique
>
> **Other techniques:** moxibustion on any of the above points, and also on Ren 8 *shenque*
>
> **Paediatric *tui na*** routine to tonify and warm the Spleen
>
> Spleen *pijing* (straight pushing)
> Thick Gate *banmen* (straight pushing)
> Three Passes *sanguan* (straight pushing)
> Knead the Navel *rou qi* (kneading anti-clockwise)

> Knead Ren 6 *qihai* (kneading anti-clockwise)
> Spinal Column *jizhu* (pinching from the bottom to the top of the back)
> Seven Bound Bones *qijiegu* (straight pushing upwards)
> Turtle's Tail *guiwei* (kneading)
> St 36 *zusanli* (kneading)

Deficient and Cold Intestines

This is the same as the pattern above but the deficiency is confined to the Intestines. Apart from loose bowels, the child may be otherwise healthy and strong. Treatment should be the same as for the above syndrome, but improvement will generally be more rapid.

Accumulation Disorder

Bowel symptoms

- discomfort and pain which is relieved by a bowel movement

- stools are foul-smelling, explosive and may be green

- worse when teething

Other symptoms: grouchy and unsettled, green mucus, may have a big appetite, may vomit too. There may be none of the other usual signs of Accumulation Disorder if the child is having a bowel movement several times a day. This means that there is no time for the food to accumulate and so Heat does not develop.

Pulse: full

Tongue: may have a greasy, yellow coat

Treatment principles: disperse accumulation of food

> **SUGGESTED TREATMENT**
> **Points**
>
> M–UE-9 *sifeng*
>
> **Method:** the *sifeng* points on one hand should be quickly pricked with a needle
>
> **Paediatric *tui na*** routine to disperse accumulation of food
>
> Stomach *weijing* (straight pushing sedation)
> Thick Gate *banmen* (straight pushing)
> Eight Trigrams *bagua* (circular pushing anti-clockwise)
> Four Wind Creases *sifengwen* (pinching)
> Abdomen Stimulation *fuyinyang* (pushing apart)
> Belly Corner *dujiao* (pinching)

CASE HISTORY: EIGHTEEN-MONTH-OLD WITH LOOSE BOWELS

This case history illustrates:

- the vulnerability of the Spleen in babies and toddlers, both to dietary factors and the quality and consistency of nurture
- the small amount of intervention that is needed in straightforward cases in young children, both in terms of how many points are used and the number of treatments needed.

Nelly had been having between eight and ten bowel movements a day for the past three months. The stools were odourless and did not appear to cause her any pain. They were only partially formed and contained a lot of undigested food. Nelly was not particularly interested in food and ate little other than pasta and bananas.

During the consultation, Nelly sat quietly on her mother's lap. She looked pale. Her pulse was deficient and her tongue pale.

Diagnosis: My diagnosis of Nelly's condition was straightforward Spleen *qi/yang* deficiency.

Aetiology: About a month before the problem began, Nelly's mother had had a very bad dose of shingles. She had to abruptly stop breastfeeding Nelly as a result. Nelly had been looked after by various different friends and family members during this time. Her mother said that it was around this time her interest in food suddenly waned and that the loose bowels started shortly after that.

I thought that the combination of her mother's illness and the sudden halt in breastfeeding had depleted Nelly's Earth Element. This led to a decline in her appetite, and the problem was then perpetuated and exacerbated by her limited diet which further strained the Spleen.

Treatment

I gave Nelly's mother the following paediatric *tui na* routine to perform daily at home:

- Spleen *pijing* (straight pushing)
- Thick Gate *banmen* (straight pushing)
- Three Passes *sanguan* (straight pushing)
- Knead the Navel *rou qi* (kneading anti-clockwise)
- Spinal Column *jizhu* (pinching from the bottom to the top of the back)
- St 36 *zusanli* (kneading)

Treatment 1

St 36 *zusanli*, Ren 6 *qihai* (with tonification needle technique and moxa)

Treatment 2

St 25 *tianshu*, Sp 6 *sanyinjiao* (with tonification needle technique and moxa)

Treatment 3

Ren 6 *qihai*, St 36 *zusanli* (with tonification needle technique and moxa)

Treatment 4

Bl 20 *pishu*, Sp 4 *gongsun* (with tonification needle technique and moxa)

After the fourth treatment, Nelly was having two to three bowel movements a day, her stools were fully formed and she had begun to eat a wider range of foods.

Aetiology in school-age children and teenagers

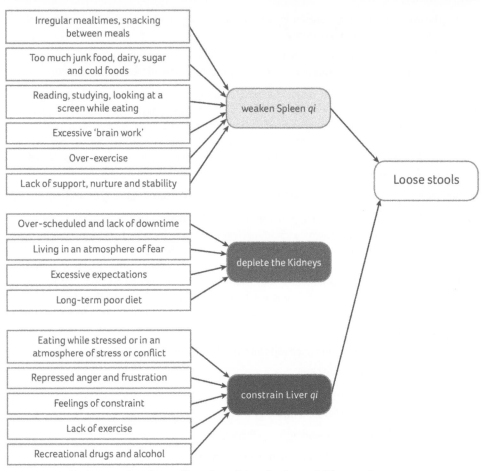

Figure 47.3 Aetiology of loose bowels in school-age children and teenagers

Patterns in school-age children and teenagers

- Spleen *qi* deficiency

- Liver *qi* stagnation invading the Spleen

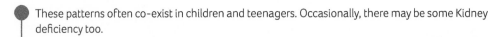

These patterns often co-exist in children and teenagers. Occasionally, there may be some Kidney deficiency too.

Spleen *qi* deficiency

Bowel symptoms

- loose bowels with some undigested food and mucus

- worse after lots of study, after exercise and when tired

Other symptoms: abnormal appetite, propensity to overthinking and worry, finds it hard to concentrate when studying, poor memory for facts, easily tires

Pulse: deficient

Tongue: pale, wet, swollen

Treatment principles: tonify Spleen *qi*

> **SUGGESTED TREATMENT**
>
> It is usually sufficient to choose a combination of two or three of the points suggested in each treatment. If there is Kidney deficiency too, points to address this should be added.
>
> **Points**
>
> St 36 *zusanli*
> Sp 3 *taibai*
> Sp 6 *sanyinjiao*
> St 25 *tianshu*
> Ren 6 *qihai*
> Ren 12 *zhongwan*
> Bl 20 *pishu*
> Bl 21 *weishu*
>
> **Method:** tonification needle technique
>
> **Other techniques:** moxibustion on any of the above points, and also on Ren 8 *shenque*

> The Stomach and Spleen are at their strongest between 7am and 9am. Therefore, a wholesome breakfast is an especially important meal for a child with Spleen *qi* deficiency. The Stomach and Spleen are at their lowest between 7pm and 9pm. Therefore, ideally the evening meal should be eaten earlier and the child should not study during this part of the evening.
>
> Modern research confirms Chinese medicine theory that breakfast is a crucial meal. Public Health England reviewed research which confirmed that children's school performance, as well as their long-term health, improves if breakfast is eaten and declines if it is skipped.[7]

Liver *qi* stagnation invading the Spleen

Bowel symptoms

- bouts of loose bowels or alternating constipation and loose bowels

- sudden need to defecate

- some abdominal pain before a bowel movement

- symptoms may be worse when stressed

- flatulence

Other symptoms: moodiness, irritability

Pulse: wiry Wood pulses, deficient Earth pulses

Tongue: may be pale or normal

Treatment principles: smooth the Liver and move *qi*; tonify Spleen *qi*

> **SUGGESTED TREATMENT**
>
> When Liver *qi* stagnation is the primary pattern, it may not be necessary to treat the Spleen at all. When Spleen *qi* deficiency is the primary pattern, it may not be necessary to treat the Liver.

In some cases, both Organs need to be treated. It is always preferable to keep treatment minimal and to find out what treating one Organ does before adding in treatment of another Organ. The pulse and nature of the symptoms will usually dictate which is the best place to start.

Points

To disperse Liver *qi*:

> Liv 3 *taichong*
> Liv 13 *zhangmen*
> GB 34 *yinlingquan*

Method: sedation needle technique

To tonify Spleen *qi*:

> St 25 *tianshu*
> St 36 *zusanli*
> Bl 20 *pishu*

Method: tonification needle technique

Other techniques: moxibustion may be used on the points to tonify the Spleen

Other treatment modalities

Shonishin

Core non-pattern-based root treatment.

Targeted tapping in the following areas:

- LI 4 *hegu*

- Du 3 *yaoyangguan* to Du 4 *mingmen*

- Du 12 *shenzhu*

- around St 36 *zusanli* and St 37 *shangjuxu*

- around the navel[8]

SUMMARY

» Prolonged loose bowels may become a cause of illness in a child and for this reason should always be treated.

» The Organs involved are: Spleen; Liver; and Kidneys.

» Dietary factors are the most common cause in babies and infants.

» The patterns in babies and toddlers are: Spleen *qi* and/or *yang* deficiency; deficient and Cold Intestines; and Accumulation Disorder.

» The cause of loose bowels in school-age children and teenagers is usually related to lifestyle and emotions, although diet may also still be involved.

» The patterns in school-age children and teenagers are Spleen *qi* deficiency and Liver *qi* stagnation invading the Spleen.

Chapter 48

CONSTIPATION AND STOOL WITHHOLDING

The topics discussed in this chapter are:

- Organs involved in constipation and stool withholding
- Pathogens involved in constipation
- Aetiology in babies and toddlers
- Patterns in babies and toddlers
- Aetiology in school-age children and teenagers
- Patterns in school-age children and teenagers
- Other treatment modalities
- Other things to think about

Introduction

Constipation and stool withholding are very common in young children. Life for the child and/or parent may revolve around when the last bowel movement was and when the next one will be. Like so many other childhood ailments, it causes anxiety that then perpetuates the condition. In a young child, the smooth working of the digestive system also plays a large role in determining her mood and demeanour. A child who is either constipated or withholding may be irritable and uncomfortable. In severe cases, she may not sleep well, is restless and loses her appetite.

A child may be considered constipated if the following occur:

- She has fewer bowel movements than normal. Constipation is often defined as having fewer than three bowel movements a week. The number of bowel movements may be different for each child. However, a change in what is normal for a particular child may signify an imbalance.
- She is passing stools that are hard and sometimes large.
- Her bowel movements are difficult or painful.

Orthodox medical treatment of constipation and withholding in childhood consists of laxatives, which may be osmotic or stimulant. Osmotic laxatives help by softening the stools, in comparison to stimulant laxatives which speed up the motility of the stool through the bowel. Faecal impaction may be treated with an enema. Children may become dependent on laxatives over time in order to have a bowel movement.

Constipation versus stool withholding

'True' constipation arises from an imbalance in the digestive system, which may have come about due to a variety of physical and/or emotional factors. Stool withholding, however, describes a condition when the child tries to stop himself from having a bowel movement. Although this does not stem from an imbalance in the digestive system, it often leads to one.

Stool withholding may be triggered by a one-off bout of constipation or anything else that causes a bowel movement to be frightening, painful or distressing for the child. The effort and straining is not actually a sign that the child is trying to poo, but that he is trying to hold on to his stool.

A child who is stool withholding usually lives under a cloud of fear. He is desperately trying to avoid the pain that he associates with a bowel movement. In so doing, he creates a different kind of pain and discomfort in his abdomen. He knows he cannot avoid the pain forever, and this may create anxiety. Figure 48.1 illustrates the interaction between constipation and stool withholding.

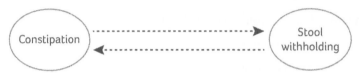

Figure 48.1 Constipation and stool withholding

Faecal impaction

Sometimes the stool that accumulates in the child's intestine becomes so dry and big that it is impossible to pass. This may result from either 'true' constipation or stool withholding. Some children are able to hold on to stools for days at a time. Faecal impaction may cause abdominal pain in some children.

Soiling (or encopresis)

Constipation or stool withholding may lead to and go hand and hand with soiling. Once a large, impacted stool has formed in the intestine, softer poo may tend to seep out around it. A child may be unaware that this is happening. In school-age children, it may be a cause of a lot of shame and anxiety.

RED FLAGS: CONSTIPATION AND STOOL WITHHOLDING
Referral to a paediatrician may be necessary in order to exclude a medical condition, such as hypothyroidism or Hirschprung disease, which may cause constipation in a child.

Organs involved in constipation and stool withholding

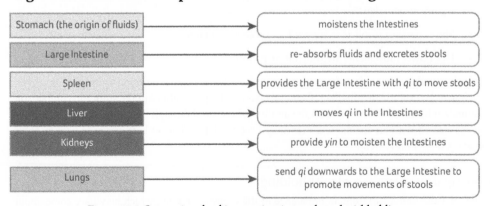

Figure 48.2 Organs involved in constipation and stool withholding

Pathogens involved in constipation

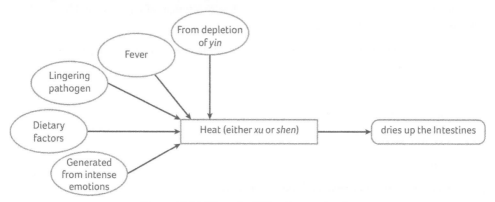

Figure 48.3A The role of Heat in constipation

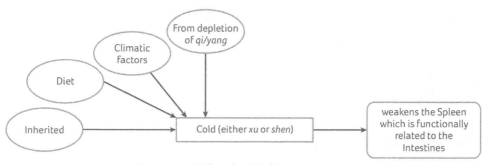

Figure 48.3B The role of Cold in constipation

Aetiology in babies and toddlers

Sometimes, the reason a child becomes constipated or withholds his stools is simply that he is fearful of a bowel movement being painful. Even a one-off bad experience can lead to weeks or months of problems.

Inherited

A baby may be born with weak Spleen *qi*. This may predispose him towards constipation as the Large Intestine is functionally related to the Spleen. If his constitutional imbalance is in Metal, he may have an inherent deficiency of the Large Intestine.

Birth factors

Epidural pain relief for the mother during labour may block the flow of *qi* to the Lower Burner, and consequently the Intestines, in the baby. A long labour or one that involved antibiotics may weaken the Spleen *qi* of the baby.

Depletion in the mother or a lack of nurture

Both of these factors may mean that the baby does not have enough *qi* to 'feed off', leaving her Spleen depleted.

Dietary factors

The following factors may cause imbalance in the digestive system of a baby or toddler, leading to any of the patterns which may cause constipation:

- too much cow's milk (calcium and certain proteins in cow's milk are thought to sometimes be a cause of constipation)

- lack of fibre in the diet

- not enough time between feeds

- too much food

- irregular mealtimes/feeds

- over-consumption of cold, raw and whole foods.

Emotions

There is a strong link between healthy bowel habits in a child and a relaxed emotional state. Intense or prolonged emotions affect the movements of *qi* in the body. The child's 'Achilles heel' may be her Intestines, which easily reflect an emotional imbalance. A baby or toddler may pick up on the stress in the family. Alternatively, he may feel stressed by toilet training and the pressure to 'succeed' at it. This impedes the flow of *qi* in his Intestines, which means a bowel movement is more difficult.

Patterns in babies and toddlers

- Spleen *qi* deficiency

- Large Intestine deficiency

- Accumulation Disorder

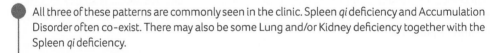

All three of these patterns are commonly seen in the clinic. Spleen *qi* deficiency and Accumulation Disorder often co-exist. There may also be some Lung and/or Kidney deficiency together with the Spleen *qi* deficiency.

Spleen *qi* deficiency

Bowel symptoms

- goes a long time without passing stools (sometimes a week or more)

- stools are usually soft and are not smelly

- complains of stomach ache and is tired after a bowel movement

Other symptoms: small appetite or picky eater, pale, quiet, may wake frequently during the night

Pulse: deficient

Tongue: pale

Treatment principles: tonify Spleen *qi*; promote bowel movement

SUGGESTED TREATMENT

It is usually sufficient to use two or three of these points at each treatment on a baby or toddler. One of these points should be local, for example Sp 15 *daheng*, Ren 6 *qihai* or Bl 25 *dachangshu*. There may also be some Kidney and/or Lung *qi* deficiency, in which case points to address this must be added.

Points

> St 36 *zusanli*
> Sp 15 *daheng*
> Ren 6 *qihai*
> Ren 12 *zhongwan*
> Sp 3 *taibai*
> Sp 6 *sanyinjiao*
> Bl 20 *pishu*
> Bl 25 *dachangshu*

Method: tonification needle technique

Other techniques: moxibustion

Paediatric *tui na* to tonify Spleen *qi* and promote a bowel movement

> Spleen *pijing* (straight pushing tonification)
> Large Intestine *dachangjing* (straight pushing tonification)
> Thick Gate *banmen* (straight pushing)
> Three Passes *sanguan* (straight pushing)
> Branch Ditch *zhigou* (TB 6) (kneading)
> Joining Valley *hegu* (LI 4) (kneading)
> Knead the Navel *rou qi* (kneading anti-clockwise)
> Spinal Column *jizhu* (pinching from the bottom to the top of the back)
> St 36 *zusanli* (kneading)
> Seven Bound Bones *qijiegu* (straight pushing)

Large Intestine deficiency

This pattern often arises because of a difficult birth, particularly one where the mother had epidural pain relief.

This is essentially the same as the Spleen *qi* deficiency pattern, but the deficiency only affects the Large Intestine. Treatment should be the same as for the Spleen *qi* deficiency pattern but improvement is usually quicker.

Accumulation Disorder

Bowel symptoms

- constipated for several days

- followed by stools which are often smelly and runny

Other symptoms: red cheeks, green nasal discharge, irritable, swollen abdomen, loud and makes his presence felt

Pulse: full

Tongue: may have a thick coat

Treatment principles: disperse accumulation of food

SUGGESTED TREATMENT
Points

M-UE-9 *sifeng*

Method: The *sifeng* points on one hand should be quickly pricked with a needle. Parents should be warned that the child may have several bowel movements over the following twenty-four hours.

Paediatric *tui na* routine to disperse accumulation of food

Large Intestine *dachangjing* (straight pushing sedation technique)
Thick Gate *banmen* (straight pushing)
Eight Trigrams *bagua* (circular pushing anti-clockwise)
Four Wind Creases *sifengwen* (pinching)
Seven Bound Bones *qijiegu* (straight pushing downwards)
Branch Ditch *zhigou* (TB 6) (kneading)
Joining Valley *hegu* (LI 4) (kneading)

Aetiology in school-age children and teenagers

Any of the aetiologies mentioned above under 'Babies and toddlers' may be relevant for a school-age child. However, there are some added factors in this age group, as shown in Figure 48.4.

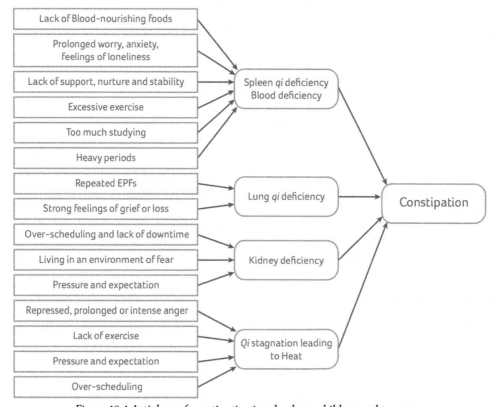

Figure 48.4 Aetiology of constipation in school-age children and teenagers

Other aetiological factors

- **Power struggles:** A child may hold on to a bowel movement as a way of fighting with a parent.

- **Busyness:** In order to function well, the bowels needs to be emptied regularly. A child may need to take her time when she is on the toilet and not be able to pass a stool if she feels rushed. Sometimes, a child's schedule is so busy that she is simply not given enough time to go to the toilet. Or she may have a large family with only one bathroom in the house and be rushed. When she is absorbed in an activity, she may ignore her body's signals.

- **Fear of public toilets:** A young child may only feel 'safe' having a bowel movement at home. She may hold on when she is out and about, or even when she is at school or in somebody else's house. This then causes stools to become hard, dry and impacted. The result is that her next bowel movement may be painful, so she then begins to dread going to the toilet.

Patterns in school-age children and teenagers

- Spleen *qi* deficiency
- Stagnation and Heat affecting the Intestines
- Blood deficiency affecting the Intestines

Spleen *qi* deficiency is the most commonly seen of these patterns in a school-age child. There may be some Lung and/or Kidney deficiency too. Blood deficiency becomes more common in teenagers, especially girls when they begin menstruation.

Purely treating the physical imbalance is rarely enough to cure the problem in a child of this age who has been constipated for a long time. Withholding stools becomes a habit. It also goes hand in hand with intense and prolonged emotions of fear and anxiety. Treatment of the child's constitutional imbalance can help to allay these emotions, relax the child and therefore break the habit.

Spleen *qi* deficiency

Bowel symptoms

- may go a long time without passing stools (sometimes a week or more)
- stools are usually soft and are not smelly
- stools may be long and thin
- incomplete evacuation of stools
- may complain of tummy ache and be tired after a bowel movement
- constipation is worse during term time or when tired

Other symptoms: small appetite or picky eater, pale, quiet, propensity to overthinking and worry, difficulty concentrating, poor memory for facts

Pulse: deficient

Tongue: pale

Treatment principles: tonify Spleen *qi*; promote bowel movement

---

SUGGESTED TREATMENT

It is usually sufficient to use two or three points per treatment on a school-age child. The practitioner should check whether or not the deficiency is also in the Kidneys and/or Lungs and add points accordingly.

Points

> St 36 *zusanli*
> Ren 12 *zhongwan*
> Sp 3 *taibai*
> Sp 6 *sanyinjiao*
> Sp 15 *daheng*
> Bl 20 *pishu*
> Bl 25 *dachangshu*

Method: tonification needle technique

Other techniques: moxibustion

Stagnation and Heat affecting the Intestines

This is essentially an older child's version of Accumulation Disorder. Either stagnation or Heat may predominate but the treatment in each case is virtually the same.

Bowel symptoms

- constipation for several days

- stools are likely to be smelly

- pellet-shaped stools

- feels agitated and uncomfortable before a bowel movement and better after

- unproductive desire to defecate

- belching and flatulence

- symptoms worse when stressed

Other symptoms: may be irritable and moody, may have disturbed sleep

Pulse: full or wiry

Tongue: red, yellow coat

Treatment principles: move stagnation; clear Heat from the Intestines

---

SUGGESTED TREATMENT

An excellent point combination for treating constipation from stagnation and Heat is Sp 15 *daheng*, LI 4 *hegu* and Liv 3 *taichong*. It is usually sufficient to use two or three points per treatment.

Points

> Sp 15 *daheng*
> TB 6 *zhigou*

Ren 12 *zhongwan*
GB 34 *yanglingquan*
LI 4 *hegu*
Liv 3 *taichong*
Liv 13 *zhangmen*

Method: sedation needle technique

Blood deficiency affecting the Intestines

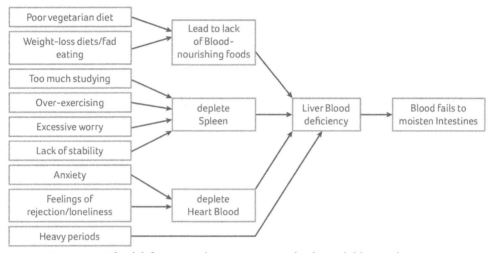

Figure 48.5 Blood deficiency and constipation in school-age children and teenagers

Bowel symptoms

- difficulty passing stools
- infrequent bowel movements
- dry stools

Other symptoms will depend on the Organ or Organs that the Blood deficiency stems from. Often, the most effective way to treat Blood deficiency is through the Organs of the child's constitutional imbalance.

SUGGESTED TREATMENT
Points
To affect the Intestines:

Sp 15 *daheng*
Bl 25 *dachangshu*
Sp 6 *sanyinjiao*

Method: tonification needle technique

Additional points to address Blood deficiency depending on the Organ or Organs from which it stems
Liver
Light-headed when stands up, imbalance in the expression of anger, blurred vision, floaters, dry eyes after a lot of studying, may get pins and needles easily

Points to affect the Intestines and additional points to nourish Liver Blood:

> Liv 3 *taichong*
> Liv 8 *ququan*
> Ren 4 *guanyuan*
> Bl 18 *ganshu*

Method: tonification needle technique

Kidney deficiency leading to Blood deficiency

Prone to anxiety, poor sleep (especially during the latter part of the night), physically unrobust, easily tires, dark circles under the eyes, late onset of periods in girls

Points to affect the Intestines and additional points to tonify the Kidneys:

> Ki 3 *taixi*
> Bl 23 *shenshu*
> Ki 13 *qixue*
> Ren 4 *guanyuan*

Method: tonification needle technique

Other techniques: direct moxibustion on any of the above points

Spleen deficiency leading to Blood deficiency

Small appetite, irregular eating, cravings for sugary foods or carbohydrates, prone to overthinking, easily feels overwhelmed, tearfulness, loose stools, easily tires

Points to affect the Intestines and additional points to tonify Spleen *qi*:

> St 36 *zusanli*
> Sp 3 *taibai*
> Sp 6 *sanyinjiao*
> Bl 20 *pishu*

Method: tonification needle technique

Other techniques: direct moxibustion on any of the above points

Other treatment modalities
Shonishin

Core non-pattern-based root treatment.

Targeted tapping to the following areas:

- Du 12 *shenzhu*
- Du 3 *yaoyangguan* to Du 4 *ming men*
- the navel
- St 25 *tianshu*
- Bl 25 *dachangshu*
- LI 4 *hegu*
- St 36 *zusanli* to St 37 *shangjuxu*[9]

Other things to think about

Toileting position

Teaching a child to sit on the toilet in a slightly different position can be helpful to reduce the pain of passing a large or impacted stool. The squatting position forces the rectum to relax and gets rid of a kink that naturally occurs just before the rectum. The easiest way to achieve this is to ask the child to put her feet on a low stool whilst sitting on the toilet.

Abdominal massage

The simple massage outlined below may be taught to parents. It can be used whenever the baby or child begins to show signs of constipation.

Massage the abdomen following the flow of the Large Intestine: up the right side of the abdomen (ascending colon), across the top (transverse colon), down the left side (descending colon) and across the bottom of the abdomen from left to right. If the constipation is from deficiency, move the palm in small, anti-clockwise circles. If the constipation is from excess, move the palm in small, clockwise circles. However, always follow the flow of the Large Intestine.

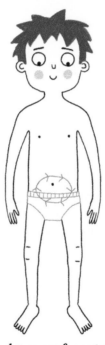

Abdominal massage for constipation

The above massage can either be done without oil or with castor oil. A small amount of the castor oil is absorbed by the Intestines and helps to promote peristalsis.

CASE HISTORY: INSECURITY AND EXCESSIVE EXERCISE CAUSING CONSTIPATION IN A SIX-YEAR-OLD BOY

This case history illustrates how:

- a young child may be affected by loss and a volatile emotional environment
- sometimes an ongoing aetiology impairs the effectiveness of treatment.

Tom was having a bowel movement approximately once a week when he first came to the clinic. His stools were soft and without smell. He was a shy and anxious boy who had no other physical symptoms of note.

Tom's parents had acrimoniously divorced when he was three, which was when the constipation began. His life was divided between three homes, that of his mother, father and grandmother. His father thought that exercise was good for boys so frequently took Tom out on runs of up to four miles.

Observations: Tom's pulse was deficient in all positions. His tongue was pale and had a very red tip. He had a weeping voice and was white by the side of his eyes. He smiled and twinkled but this felt like a mask, with little genuine joy underneath it.

Diagnosis: I diagnosed Tom as having a Metal constitutional imbalance due to the observations described above. This meant that he had reacted to the loss of his stable family life with feelings of sadness. This had depleted the *qi* of his Metal Element, in particular of the *yang* Organ, the Large Intestine. On top of this, the lack of a stable home and excessive exercise further weakened his Spleen *qi*.

Treatment
Treatment 1

Yuan source points LI 4 *hegu*, Lu 9 *taiyuan*

Treatment 2

Back *shu* points Bl 25 *dachangshu*, Bl 13 *feishu*

Treatment 3

Sp 15 *daheng*, Ren 6 *qihai*

Tonification points LI 11 *quchi*, Lu 9 *taiyuan*

Treatment continued with a range of points that affected the *qi* of the Lungs and Large Intestine, and the addition of points to tonify Spleen *qi* too.

Outcome: Tom's treatment seemed to take two steps forwards and then one step backwards. His father was adamant that he should continue exercising, and he continued to move between three houses during the week. His constipation continued, although less severely than before.

SUMMARY

» True constipation arises from an imbalance in the digestive system.

» Stool withholding is a condition where a child tries to prevent himself having a bowel movement.

» Constipation often leads to stool withholding.

» The Organs involved are: Stomach; Large Intestine; Spleen; Liver; Kidneys; and Lungs.

» The pathogens involved are: Heat and Cold.

» A baby or toddler may be constipated because of inherently weak Spleen *qi*, or a constitutional imbalance in his Metal Element. Birth, dietary and emotional factors are also common aetiological factors.

» The patterns involved in babies and toddlers are: Spleen *qi* deficiency; Large Intestine deficiency; and Accumulation Disorder.

» Emotional factors are commonly seen in constipation in school-age children and teenagers.

» Lifestyle factors such as too much sport or studying are also common.

» The patterns involved in school-age children and teenagers are: Spleen *qi* deficiency; stagnation and Heat affecting the Intestines; and Blood deficiency affecting the Intestines.

• Chapter 49 •

NAUSEA AND VOMITING
· ·

The topics discussed in this chapter are:

- Organs and pathogens involved in nausea and vomiting

- Patterns that cause nausea and vomiting

- Other treatment modalities

Introduction

Vomiting is common in babies and toddlers. A little bit of regurgitation of milk after a feed now and then, known as posseting, is of little concern. However, if a baby brings up what seems like an entire feed, and does so repeatedly over weeks or months, it is a sign of an imbalance that would benefit from being treated. It is both depleting for the baby and often a cause of anxiety in the parent.

When diagnosing the cause of vomiting in a baby or toddler, it is important to bear in mind that the pathology may be confined just to the Stomach. It is therefore necessary to differentiate the condition based almost entirely on the nature of the vomit and the vomiting. In older children, the pathology will usually be more generalised and there will therefore be accompanying symptoms that help to differentiate the pattern.

Babies and young children are prone to vomiting simply because of the fact that their digestive systems are small, weak and vulnerable and yet they have to deal with a large amount of milk or food relative to their size. In a child over the age of seven or eight years, this is no longer the case. Vomiting in an older child may derive from an imbalance that has become deeper because it was left untreated in his earlier years, or from a new aspect of life (e.g. worry associated with school) that is causing an imbalance.

As a general guideline, whilst in babies and toddlers nausea and vomiting often results from a physical imbalance in the digestive system, in older children there is very often an emotional component. The child may be unaware of certain emotions or unable to express them. He is literally 'sick' of something in his life that makes him angry, anxious, fearful or sad.

> **RED FLAGS: VOMITING**
> The following situations merit urgent referral to a conventional medical practitioner:
>
> ✓ Persistent vomiting (which lasts longer than twenty-four hours). This may lead to dehydration in a baby or young child. Dehydration may be indicated by a sunken fontanelle,* sunken eyes and dry nappies.
>
> ✓ Vomiting which is darkish green in colour (which may indicate intestinal blockage).
>
> ✓ Projectile vomiting in a small baby (which may be an indication of pyloric stenosis and may quickly lead to an imbalance of the salts and fluids in the blood).

---

* The fontanelles are soft areas at the top and the back of a baby's skull.

Organs and pathogens involved in nausea and vomiting

The key Organ involved in nausea and vomiting is, of course, the Stomach. Stomach *qi* normally descends. All cases of nausea and vomiting are due to Stomach *qi* rebelling upwards. This may happen either because of an underlying deficiency, or because a pathogen is blocking the descending movement.

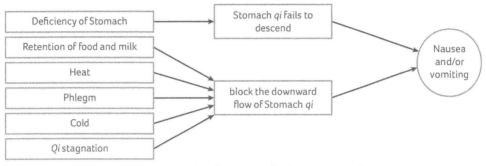

Figure 49.1 Organs and pathogens involved in nausea and vomiting

Maciocia[10] notes that nausea and vomiting may also be caused by Heart *qi* not descending. This is confirmed by the fact that young children sometimes vomit when they have experienced an intense emotion, which may cause a disturbance in the flow of Heart *qi*.

Patterns that cause nausea and vomiting

- Stomach and Spleen *qi* deficient and Cold

- Retention of Food and Milk

- Accumulation of Phlegm in the Stomach

- Accumulation of Heat in the Stomach

- Liver *qi* stagnation invading the Stomach

The most common patterns seen in babies and toddlers are Stomach and Spleen *qi* deficient and Cold, and Retention of Food and Milk. Accumulation of Phlegm is common in younger school-age children. In older children, Liver *qi* stagnation invading the Stomach is the most common pattern. Stomach and Spleen *qi* deficient and Cold, and Phlegm, are often seen together.

Please note that an acute bout of vomiting may be caused by Cold invading the Stomach. This pattern is described in Chapter 70, Treatment of Acute Conditions.

Stomach and Spleen *qi* deficient and Cold

This pattern may be localised, in which case the child will appear strong and healthy. Or it may be more generalised and accompanied by other symptoms and signs of Spleen *qi* deficiency.

Aetiology

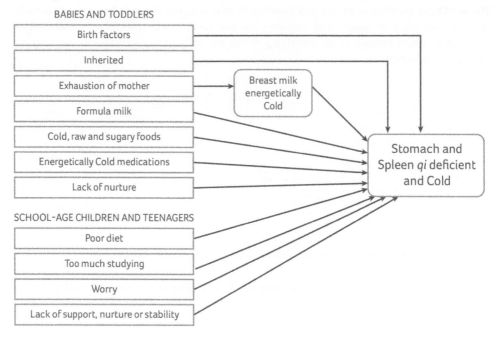

Figure 49.2 Causes of Stomach and Spleen qi deficient and Cold

Nausea and vomiting symptoms

- vomiting of undigested food and milk
- or may vomit clear, watery fluid
- vomit does not have a bad odour
- usually vomits only small amounts
- may become unhappy or tired after vomiting

Other symptoms: poor appetite, tiredness and lethargy, pale face

Pulse: deficient

Tongue: pale

Treatment principles: tonify Stomach and Spleen *qi*; restore descending of Stomach *qi*

> **SUGGESTED TREATMENT**
> When treating a baby or toddler, two or three points are usually sufficient.
>
> **Points**
>
> St 36 *zusanli*
> Sp 4 *gongsun*
> Ren 12 *zhongwan*
> Bl 20 *pishu*
> Bl 21 *weishu*
>
> **Method:** tonification needle technique

Other techniques: moxibustion

Paediatric *tui na* routine to tonify and warm the Stomach and Spleen

> Spleen *pijing* (straight pushing tonification)
> Thick Gate *banmen* (straight pushing)
> Eight Trigrams *bagua* (circular pushing anti-clockwise)
> Three Passes *sanguan* (straight pushing)
> Knead the Navel *rou qi* (kneading anti-clockwise)
> Spinal Column *jizhu* (pinching from the bottom to the top of the back)
> St 36 *zusanli* (kneading)

CASE HISTORY: THIRTEEN-MONTH-OLD GIRL VOMITING UP TO TWENTY TIMES A DAY

This case history illustrates:

- how, in a baby or toddler, a pathology may be localised (in this case, in the Stomach) and may not be reflected systemically

- when the pathology is localised, less treatment is needed for the child to fully recover

- the importance of relevant dietary advice.

Eve's mother was, understandably, at her wit's end when she brought Eve to the clinic. Eve had been vomiting multiple times a day since birth. Medical investigations could not find anything wrong and the family had been told by Eve's paediatrician that this was something she would eventually grow out of.

Eve vomited clear, watery fluid mixed with undigested food and milk after every single feed or meal. She showed few signs of distress and continued to have a fairly good appetite. She slept well and had a happy, calm disposition.

Eve ate a lot of bananas and raw vegetables.

Observations: Eve looked like a relatively robust baby. She was slightly pale.

Diagnosis: Localised Stomach *qi* deficient and Cold. Eve had no other significant signs of Stomach and Spleen *qi xu*.

Treatment

I used two points per treatment, selected from Pc 6 *neiguan*, Sp 4 *gongsun*, Ren 12 *zhongwan* and St 36 *zusanli*. These points were needled with the tonification technique, and a moxa stick was used on Ren 12 *zhongwan*. Eve's mother was advised to exclude bananas and any raw or chilled foods from Eve's diet.

Outcome: With these dietary changes, and three treatments, Eve had entirely stopped vomiting.

Retention of Food and Milk

Aetiology

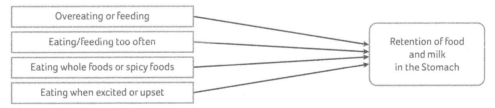

Figure 49.3 Causes of Retention of Food and Milk

Nausea and vomiting symptoms

- vomiting of curdled milk or undigested food
- sour-smelling vomit
- vomits a while after eating
- feels better for vomiting

Other symptoms: restless, unhappy, appears uncomfortable, foul-smelling breath, irregular, foul-smelling stools

Pulse: slippery or full

Tongue: thick, greasy coating

Treatment principles: remove retention of food; restore descending of Stomach *qi*

SUGGESTED TREATMENT

A typical treatment may consist of needling Pc 6 *neiguan*, St 36 *zusanli* and Sp 4 *gongsun*.

Points

Pc 6 *neiguan*
Ren 10 *xiawan*
St 36 *zusanli*
Sp 4 *gongsun*
Ren 22 *tiantu*

Method: sedation needle technique

Paediatric *tui na* routine to clear retention of food and milk, and descend Stomach *qi*

Spleen *pijing* (straight pushing tonification)
Stomach *weijing* (straight pushing sedation)
Thick Gate *banmen* (straight pushing)
Eight Trigrams *bagua* (circular pushing anti-clockwise)
Celestial Pillar Bone *tianzhugu* (straight pushing)
Knead Ren 12 *zhongwan* (kneading clockwise)
St 36 *zusanli* (kneading)

Accumulation of Phlegm in the Stomach

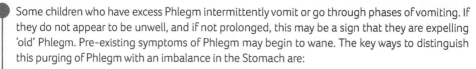

Some children who have excess Phlegm intermittently vomit or go through phases of vomiting. If they do not appear to be unwell, and if not prolonged, this may be a sign that they are expelling 'old' Phlegm. Pre-existing symptoms of Phlegm may begin to wane. The key ways to distinguish this purging of Phlegm with an imbalance in the Stomach are:

» vomiting is not associated with an illness and does not appear to cause any other symptoms

» the vomiting does not appear related to what the child has eaten

» it happens when the child is otherwise well or going through a growth spurt.

It can be helpful to give occasional treatments to strengthen the Stomach and Spleen during this process.

Aetiology

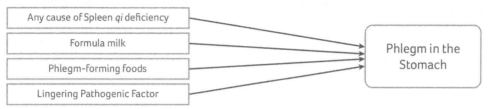

Figure 49.4 Causes of Phlegm in the Stomach

Nausea and vomiting symptoms

- vomiting of mucus or undigested food mixed with clear mucus

- vomits relatively infrequently

- variable appetite which increases after vomiting

- nausea

Other symptoms: tendency towards mucus in the nose and a congested chest, greasy skin

Pulse: slippery

Tongue: thick coating

Treatment principles: resolve Phlegm; descend Stomach *qi*

SUGGESTED TREATMENT

The practitioner needs to ascertain the balance between the strength of the Phlegm pathogen and the severity of the Spleen *qi* deficiency. In a baby or toddler, the symptoms and constitution of the child will usually reveal this. In an older child, the pulse may provide the key information. Treatment should be adjusted accordingly.

Points

> Ren 12 *zhongwan*
> Pc 6 *neiguan*
> Sp 4 *gongsun*
> St 40 *fenglong*

Method: sedation needle technique

Additional points to tonify the underlying Spleen *qi* deficiency (if necessary)

Paediatric *tui na* routine to resolve Phlegm, and descend Stomach *qi*

> Spleen *pijing* (straight pushing tonification)
> Stomach *weijing* (straight pushing sedation)
> Thick Gate *banmen* (straight pushing)
> Eight Trigrams *bagua* (circular pushing anti-clockwise)
> Celestial Pillar Bone *tianzhugu* (straight pushing)
> Knead Ren 12 *zhongwan* (kneading clockwise)
> St 36 *zusanli* (kneading)

Accumulation of Heat in the Stomach

Aetiology

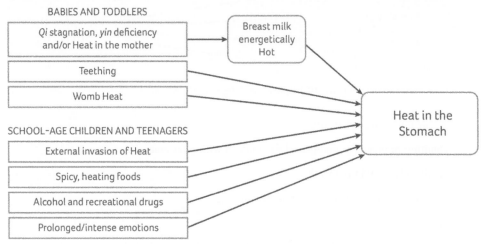

Figure 49.5 Causes of Accumulation of Heat in the Stomach

Nausea and vomiting symptoms

- vomiting of foul-smelling, yellow-coloured liquid
- vomits soon after eating
- projectile vomiting
- wants to eat again soon after vomiting
- restless and irritable before vomiting
- feels better after vomiting
- nausea

Other symptoms: constipation or foul-smelling stools, thirsty, red face, burning pain in stomach

Pulse: rapid

Tongue: red in the centre, yellow coat

Treatment principles: clear Heat from the Stomach; descend Stomach *qi*

> **SUGGESTED TREATMENT**
> St 44 *neiting* is the key point for clearing Heat in the Stomach. On a baby, it may only be necessary to use this point. On an older child, one or two other points usually need to be added.
>
> **Points**
> St 44 *neiting*
> LI 4 *hegu*
> Ren 12 *zhongwan*
> Pc 6 *neiguan*
> Sp 4 *gongsun*
>
> **Method:** sedation needle technique

Paediatric *tui na* routine to clear Heat, and descend Stomach *qi*

Stomach *weijing* (straight pushing from base to tip)
Large Intestine *dachangjing* (straight pushing from base to tip)
Thick Gate *banmen* (straight pushing)
Eight Trigrams *bagua* (circular pushing anti-clockwise)
Milky Way *tianheshui* (straight pushing)
Celestial Pillar Bone *tianzhugu* (straight pushing)
Ren 12 *zhongwan* (kneading clockwise)

Liver *qi* stagnation invading the Stomach

Aetiology

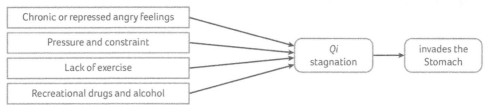

Figure 49.6 Causes of Liver qi stagnation invading the Stomach

Nausea and vomiting symptoms

- nausea and vomiting
- worse when stressed
- vomiting comes and goes
- feels better after vomiting
- belching and hiccuping
- worse pre-menstrually in girls

Other symptoms: moody, irritable or depressed

Pulse: wiry

Tongue: normal

Treatment principles: smooth the Liver and move *qi*; tonify Stomach *qi*

SUGGESTED TREATMENT

When Liver *qi* stagnation is the primary pattern, it may not be necessary to treat the Stomach at all. When Stomach *qi* deficiency is the primary pattern, it may not be necessary to treat the Liver. In some cases, both Organs need to be treated. It is always preferable to keep treatment minimal and to find out what treating one Organ does before adding in treatment of another Organ. The pulse and nature of the symptoms will usually dictate which is the best place to start.

Points

To move Liver *qi*:

Liv 14 *qimen*
Pc 6 *neiguan*

> Liv 3 *taichong*
> Ren 12 *zhongwan*

Method: sedation needle technique

To strengthen Stomach and Spleen *qi*:

> St 36 *zusanli*
> Sp 3 *taibai*
> Bl 20 *pishu*
> Bl 21 *weishu*

Method: tonification needle technique

Other treatment modalities

Shonishin

Core non-pattern-based root treatment.

Targeted tapping around the following areas and points:

- the navel

- Ren 12 *zhongwan*

- Stomach channel on the shins

- Bl 18 *ganshu* and Bl 20 *pishu*

- GB 20 *fengchi*, LI 4 *hegu* and over the shoulders if there is an emotional component

SUMMARY

» The practitioner should be aware of the red flags if a child is vomiting and refer to an orthodox medical doctor when necessary.

» All cases of nausea and vomiting inherently involve Stomach *qi* failing to descend. This may either be due to a deficiency or a fullness.

» In babies and toddlers, nausea or vomiting often arises due to a physical imbalance. In older children, there is very often an emotional cause too.

» The pathogens involved are: Heat; Phlegm; Cold; and *qi* stagnation.

» The patterns involved are: Stomach and Spleen *qi* deficient and Cold; Retention of Food and Milk; Accumulation of Phlegm in the Stomach; Accumulation of Heat in the Stomach; and Liver *qi* stagnation invading the Stomach.

Chapter 50

FOOD ALLERGIES AND INTOLERANCES
· ·

The topics discussed in this chapter are:

- What is a food allergy or intolerance?

- Treatment

- Aetiology

- Pathology

- The pathogen

- Underlying deficiencies

- Possible emotional responses to chronic food allergies according to Five Element constitutional imbalance

Introduction

There is barely a classroom in the Western world that does not contain at least one child who has to exclude a food or foods from his diet. There is a wide spectrum from, on the one hand, a child who gets a bit grumpy if he eats too much dairy to a child who goes into anaphylactic shock if he is near nuts. Although food allergies are largely thought to be a modern phenomenon, they were first written about by Hippocrates who lived in around 465 BCE. He noticed that, whilst most people could happily eat cheese and it was generally considered to be a healthy food, in some people just small amounts of it made them ill.

Many children who come to the clinic have food allergies. For some, it is their reason for seeking treatment. For others, it is secondary to their main complaint but becomes apparent whilst taking the case history. There are also cases where the practitioner may suspect a food allergy is present but the parent has not yet considered this. Conversely, there are other cases where the parent is convinced that a food allergy is at the root of their child's symptoms and the practitioner suspects that it is not.

Food allergies may have far-reaching ramifications. The child may not be able to eat his lunch at school with his classmates. He may not be able to attend parties and social occasions or, if he does, he needs to take his own food with him. Young children often hate to be different, and their allergies often mean they are perceived as being exactly that by their peers. Managing the allergy adds another layer of both practical and emotional complexity to family life.

Even more difficult, however, is the way that a severe food allergy in a child impacts his relationship with his parents. One or both of the parents has to take on the undesirable role of arbiter and controller. They must check every single piece of food or sip of drink that passes their child's lips. As the child gets older, but is not yet old enough to make these decisions himself, the parent must necessarily restrict his growing independence. The child may need to be accompanied to parties at a time when other children are beginning to enjoy the freedom of not always having a parent looking over their shoulders. One slip may lead to weeks of ill health and it is just not worth taking the risk. All of this means that the process of separating from a parent, and growing into independence, becomes even more challenging.

Thankfully, however severe the scenario, acupuncture can usually help. The reason for this is because the food is not really the problem. For a child to react to food in the way he does, there must be some underlying imbalance in his system. Treating the imbalance often means that, after some time, he is then able to tolerate the food either entirely or, at the very least, better than before.

What is a food allergy or intolerance?

A food allergy is a reaction in the immune system to a certain food or foods. It may affect numerous organs in the body, causing symptoms in the digestive system, on the skin, in the respiratory system or even in the entire circulatory system. An allergic reaction to a food may be relatively mild or life-threatening. There are two main types of food allergy (see Table 50.1 for a summary of symptoms).

Immediate onset (IgE-mediated) allergies

IgE-mediated allergies are characterised by their sudden onset. Within seconds of eating the culprit food, the child's body begins reacting. The response may be vomiting, diarrhoea, wheezing, hives or, at worst, anaphylactic shock. There is usually an element of itching or swelling involved. The symptoms are usually severe in nature.

Immediate onset allergies are relatively easy to diagnose with either skin prick or blood tests. Once the offending food or foods have been eliminated from the diet, the child may be in good health. Having said this, many children with immediate onset allergies also have chronic asthma and/or eczema.

> **AN EXAMPLE OF AN IMMEDIATE ONSET (IGE-MEDIATED) ALLERGY**
> Harry came for treatment when he was six years old. If he ate wheat or eggs, within seconds he would develop intensely itchy hives over the top part of his body and suffer from projectile vomiting. This was treated with antihistamine and, within a few hours, everything would have settled down, although the hives would take time to fade. He also had chronic asthma and eczema.

Delayed onset (non-IgE-mediated) allergies

Delayed onset allergies are also a 'true' food allergy but they do not involve a specific antibody reaction, as the immediate onset allergies do. They are characterised by a delayed reaction. Typically, a child will either eat or come into contact with a food and his symptoms will begin hours or even two to three days afterwards. Symptoms may be worsening of eczema, vomiting, diarrhoea, sleep disturbance, and mood symptoms (such as manic behaviour or lethargy). Non-IgE-mediated allergies are harder to diagnose because of this delayed response, but also because they are not diagnosable by skin prick or blood tests. They are usually diagnosed by a strict elimination diet and reintroduction of the suspect foods one at a time. A child with delayed onset allergies may be able to tolerate a small amount of the culprit food, but reacts to larger amounts.

> **AN EXAMPLE OF A DELAYED ONSET (NON-IGE-MEDIATED) ALLERGY**
> Eleanor was four years old when she first came for treatment. She was severely allergic to gluten, eggs, soya, dairy and oats. About thirty-six hours after exposure to one of the offending foods, her sleep would become severely disrupted and she would become very badly constipated. Her mood would oscillate between aggressive and manic one minute, then lethargic and disconnected the next. These symptoms would last for up to a month, gradually decreasing during this time.

Table 50.1 Immediate onset and delayed onset allergies

Immediate onset allergy	Delayed onset allergy
Rapid onset	Delayed reaction
Severe, immediate symptoms (may be followed by prolonged symptoms too)	May be severe but less acute
Often involves itching and swelling	Rarely involves itching and swelling
Usually short-lived	May last for weeks or months after exposure
Diagnosed by skin prick and blood tests	Diagnosed by elimination diets

Food intolerance

A food intolerance does not involve an immune response to the culprit food. It is generally understood to be caused by the body not being able to digest a food because of, for example, a lack of a certain enzyme. As with delayed onset allergies, the onset of symptoms is usually delayed and they do not begin to appear until hours after the food was eaten. Symptoms are generally less severe than with a true food allergy. They may range from mild digestive upset and bloating to headaches, tiredness, joint pain and a lack of concentration.

A child with a food intolerance may be able to tolerate a small amount of the culprit food but feels unwell if he eats large amounts. He may have an intolerance to additives in food, as well as to foods themselves. For example, some children do not tolerate sulphites, which are often found in dried fruits, or a flavour enhancer such as monosodium glutamate. A child with a food intolerance may find that he is able to eat a particular food sometimes and not suffer but at other times, usually when he is stressed or run down, he reacts to that food.

FOOD INTOLERANCE

Tom came for treatment when he was four because he had a bad night-time cough and wheeze. During the case history, his mother told me that he had an intolerance to dairy. If he ate too much of it, he would become tired and lethargic and complain of a tummy ache. His mum had noticed that after an illness or in the middle of winter he could barely tolerate any dairy. At other times when he was well and strong, he did not seem to react to it at all.

Treatment

The treatment of food allergies must be approached in different stages.

Stages of treatment

Acute stage

If the child comes for treatment when he is 'flaring', having come into contact with a trigger food, the focus of treatment is to soothe the allergic reaction. This involves treating the pathogen or pathogens that the allergic reaction has created or exacerbated (i.e. Heat, Phlegm or Damp, Wind, Cold).

RED FLAGS: ALLERGIES

Extreme bodily reaction, such as severe asthma, swelling and skin rash, may be signs of anaphylactic shock. In this case, orthodox medical treatment should be immediately sought.

Having an allergic reaction will, in itself, create more imbalance in the body. Just as it is common for somebody who has just had an invasion of Wind-Cold to be left with some residual Damp and Lung *qi* deficiency, so a child who has just had an allergic reaction will often come out of it with more imbalance than he went into it. Therefore, being able to treat a child during an acute reaction is extremely valuable. When a child has an acute illness, whatever it may be, his body will be in a state of openness and flux. A treatment during this time, as well as preventing further imbalance, can actually help a child to expel a pathogen that has been around for a long time. So, with appropriate treatment at this crucial time, a child may come through an allergic reaction healthier than he went into it.

> **EXTRA POINT FOR SYMPTOMATIC TREATMENT IN THE ACUTE STAGE OF AN ALLERGIC REACTION**
>
> *Uranaetei* ('below *neiting* St 44') may be treated with rice grain moxa bilaterally.[11]

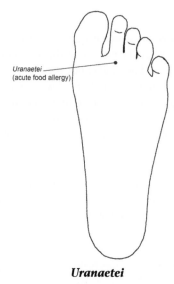

Uranaetei
(acute food allergy)

Uranaetei

Sub-acute stage

A child who has delayed onset allergies may have a reaction to a food that lasts many weeks. In some children it takes up to eight weeks for the reaction to subside completely. Treatments during this time of flare-up can help to reduce the severity of the symptoms and the time it takes for the child to return to health. Towards the end of the flare-up it may be appropriate to both clear the pathogen that still remains but also to start addressing the underlying deficiency of the digestive system.

In between flare-ups

When the child is well because he has not come into contact with any trigger foods, the aim of treatment should be to deal with the underlying imbalance. This usually involves strengthening an underlying deficiency of Spleen *qi*. It is also beneficial to treat the underlying constitutional imbalance at this time.

Repairing damage

PHYSICAL DAMAGE

A child's body may have sustained damage because of the severe symptoms caused by the food allergies. Most commonly, the damage will be to some part of the digestive system. For example, a child whose allergy resulted in inflammation of either the oesophagus or the small or large intestine (as in the case of eosinophilic disease) may be left with damage to this part of his body. The damage may manifest as pain or discomfort. It may equally manifest with a lack of sensation, such as a child who is not aware of a sensation when he needs to defecate. Treatment must be tailored to the specific case. However, below are points which may be useful:

- Damage to the small intestine: St 39 *xiajuxu*, Bl 27 *xiaochangshu*
- Damage to the large intestine: St 37 *shangjuxu*, Bl 25 *dachangshu*
- Damage to the rectum or anus: Bl 58 *feiyang*, Du 2 *yaoshu*
- Damage to the oesophagus: Ren 20 *huagai*, Ren 21 *xuanji*

EMOTIONAL DAMAGE

 Treatment of the child's Five Element constitutional imbalance may help to manage the enormous emotional impact that living with chronic food allergies may have.

There may be a significant, emotional impact on a child who has food allergies. Exactly how a child responds emotionally will depend to a large degree on his emotional constitution and character. Some common responses may be:

- anger and frustration
- fear
- lack of joy
- feeling hard done by.

Even after the physical symptoms have cleared, and the child is possibly able to tolerate the food or foods he was previously allergic to, the emotional patterns that severe allergies may leave in their wake can benefit enormously from treatment. A child's Fire energy, for example, may have been knocked by not having been able to enjoy as much carefree fun as his peers, and by activities with friends having needed to be restricted. The weakness in his Fire Element is just as much a part of his condition as any of the physical aspects of it. It could be argued that it is the one that may go on to have the biggest negative impact on his life, if left untreated. Deficiencies in the Organs of the Fire Element may lead to physical problems down the line but also have an impact on his ability to have happy, lasting and meaningful relationships during his life.

Is treatment working?

When starting to treat a child for a food allergy, it is preferable for him to exclude the culprit food or foods from his diet entirely. This will take the strain off his digestive system and mean that the treatment can work more quickly and be more effective. When it becomes clear that the treatment has had a pronounced effect (usually evidenced by an improvement in the pulse and tongue), then is the time to suggest a trial reintroduction of a food.

If a child's response to a food or foods is not very severe, and it does not stop him from leading a 'normal' life, the issue of when to reintroduce a food is not such a big one. For example, if a child develops mucus when he eats dairy, it is simple enough to try introducing a small amount of dairy into his diet and to see how he responds to it. If there are no adverse effects, then after a few days or a week a little more can be tried. Gradually, over a matter of weeks or months, larger amounts of the culprit food may be introduced and the times between the introductions reduced.

Reintroducing foods to which the child has had a severe response is another matter altogether. A food which has in the past caused a child to go into anaphylactic shock or cardiac shock or to projectile vomit should never be reintroduced in the home. Such children will normally be under the care of a doctor, who will set up a 'food challenge' when the offending food is reintroduced in a controlled and safe environment, and when medical care is to hand, should it be needed.

It is always worth mentioning to the parents that if, at any point in the future, their child seemingly begins to react badly to a food again, the food should be stopped immediately and he should be brought for treatment. This is most likely to happen when there is a stressful factor in the child's life, for example exams approaching or a big developmental leap taking place.

Some challenges when treating food allergies

- The child may crave the foods he is allergic to.

- Food and emotion may have become intertwined: because of the practicalities of living with food allergies, the whole issue of food and eating may have become one that is emotionally charged.

- Not everything is a food allergy: whilst there is no doubt that food allergies are prolific, they are not the cause of every physical, behavioural or emotional problem a child may have. It can be tempting to blame a problem on a food allergy rather than face a painful dynamic in the family that is the real problem.

Aetiology

There is a lot of speculation as to the reasons for the enormous rise in food allergies. The possible causes may be broadly divided into those which are 'global' and those which are related to the individual child.

Global factors

- **Consumption of non-local and non-seasonal food:** It is striking that food allergies are almost unheard of in unindustrialised societies, where people tend to eat food that has been grown locally, often soon after it is harvested. Perhaps it is simply too much of a strain for the digestive system of a child to have to deal with what may feel very 'foreign'.

- **Highly processed food:** Processing food is not inherently 'bad'. Some forms of processing, for example fermentation, may increase the nutritional content of food. However, other forms, for example those which involve the use of chemicals, may decrease the vitamin and mineral content of the food. The chemicals used in the process may themselves be harmful to the body. Many modern methods of food processing are thought to disturb the balance of the rich microbial flora of the intestines, which is fundamental to good digestive health.

- **Prevalence of antibiotic use:** Several studies have linked the use of antibiotics in children with an increased probability of the development of food allergies later in life. The use of antibiotics in farming is also thought to play a role in food allergies. From the Chinese medicine perspective, antibiotics deplete and chill the digestive system, impairing its ability to transform and transport foods.

- **Sanitation measures:** Some people believe that the modern obsession with hygiene leads to children not being exposed to a wide enough range of bacteria to keep their guts healthy. They advocate that children should play outside, in the dirt, as much as possible and eat a wide range of food grown in rich, bio-dynamic soil.[12]

Individual factors

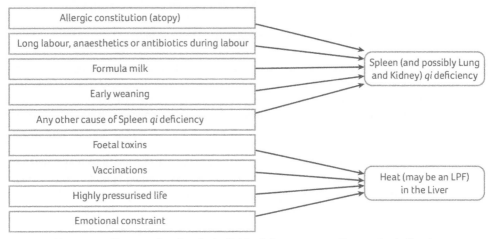

Figure 50.1 Factors related to the individual that may contribute to food allergies

Pathology

Looking at a young baby or toddler, it often appears that they are almost all tummy. Of the three Burners, the middle one is proportionally much bigger than either the upper or the lower. The first months of a baby's life are indeed governed by what goes on in the Middle Burner in terms of the digestive process.

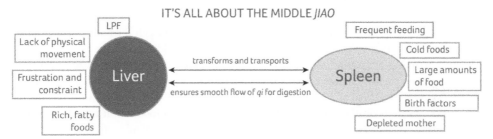

Figure 50.2 Dysfunction in the Middle Burner with food allergies

The two key aspects of food allergies

In order to accurately diagnose and treat food allergies, it is necessary to separate the pathology into two parts – namely:

- the particular pathogen that is created or exacerbated in the child by the offending foods

- the underlying imbalance.

The pathogen

In terms of the pathogen involved, it is not possible to say that dairy, for example, will always produce Damp or that sugar will always create Heat in the Liver. Depending on the child's constitution and pathology, he will respond to food in his own particular way. The pathogen created or exacerbated is not a reflection of the food itself but of the child's response to food.

Underlying imbalance (which may include both deficiency and/or fullness)	**+**	Food	**=**	Creation or exacerbation of pathogen

Figure 50.3 The role of pathogens in food allergies

 A food allergy may be likened to an over-sensitive car alarm. Ideally, a car alarm will only go off when somebody breaks into a car. Sometimes, it goes off when there is a strong gust of wind or a big lorry drives past. This is the kind of over-reaction that takes place in a child's body when he eats certain foods. The body reacts to something which should be innocuous. It is as if it is on red alert: hypersensitive, unsettled or inflamed.

The following pathogens may be involved in food allergies. Most of the time, a pathogen will be pre-existing in a child and become exacerbated when he eats an offending food. In this case, the pathogen can be said to be lingering. A Lingering Pathogenic Factor is akin to a rogue element in the system. It adds a degree of unpredictability to the picture. It blocks the healthy flow of *qi* in the body which may cause the child to respond to certain foods in an exaggerated way. This is what creates an allergic response. Sometimes, a pathogen is created in the body acutely as a reaction to a particular food.

- Wind

- Heat

- Damp and Phlegm

- Cold

Wind

Wind is a *yang* pathogen which arises quickly and moves swiftly through the body. It could only be such a pathogen that will, in a matter of seconds, turn a child from being absolutely fine to violently vomiting or gasping for air. The presence of Wind explains why an acute allergic response may affect so many different bodily systems so quickly. In some children, their respiratory and digestive systems, as well as their *shen*, become pathological, all within minutes.

Wind does not explain the entirety of the child's reaction to a food, but it accounts for the speed and the wide-reaching nature of the reaction. In TCM, external Wind is often said to invade primarily the Lungs. In the Five Element system, however, it is recognised that Wind resonates with the Liver. It is common, for example, for those with a Liver imbalance to feel out of sorts or agitated on a windy day. In the case of sudden onset food allergies, the culprit food agitates the Liver, which then generates internal Wind. The quality of this type of allergic reaction, with the sudden 'flaring-up', is very characteristic of Liver pathologies. Most commonly, the Wind generates Heat. The combination of the Wind and the Heat together causes the allergic symptoms.

 Wind accounts for the speed and wide-reaching nature of an acute reaction to food.

Symptoms

- sudden onset of allergy

- symptoms tend to affect the top part of the body

- symptoms move around

Pulse: floating and rapid

Tongue: may be unchanged or have a yellow coat and red prickles. In extreme cases, deviated

Treatment principles: expel Wind; subdue Liver *yang* rising or clear Liver Fire

> **SUGGESTED TREATMENT**
> **Points**
>
> > GB 20 *fengchi*
> > Du 20 *baihui*
> > Du 14 *dazhui*
> > LI 4 *hegu*
> > Liv 2 *xingjian*
> > Liv 3 *taichong*
>
> **Method:** sedation needle technique

Heat

If a child has a pre-existing condition of Heat, the body may react to certain foods by creating more Heat. For example, a child may naturally run hot, be slightly hyperactive and have a fiery temper. When he eats the offending food, he may then break out in a red rash and stop sleeping.

Heat is a commonly involved pathogen in many allergic responses, both those with a sudden onset and a delayed onset. This is apparent in the nature of the symptoms, which often include red rashes or hives, inflammation and 'Hot' digestive symptoms. Looking at the exact symptoms will guide the practitioner to where the Heat is in the body. In the case of anaphylactic shock, the Heat is often widespread and several Organs are involved.

 In babies and toddlers, Heat may come from Accumulation Disorder, in which case this needs to be cleared and the appropriate dietary advice given to the parent.

General symptoms of Heat

- looks red in the face
- red lips
- always feels hot
- hot to touch
- hypersensitivity
- reacts strongly to things (noises, smells, hectic situations)

Stomach Heat: vomiting, which may be projectile, foul-smelling and yellow in appearance

Liver Heat: manic, hyperactive or aggressive behaviour; disturbed sleep with bad dreams and sleeptalking

Heart Heat: manic behaviour, incessant talking, strongly agitated, very poor sleep, wakes up distressed in the night

Lung Heat: wheezing, restricted breathing, red skin rashes

Heat in the Intestines: violent diarrhoea, foul-smelling, yellow stools, burning anus, severe constipation

Pulse: rapid, overflowing

Tongue: red, yellow coating

Treatment principles: clear Heat

> **SUGGESTED TREATMENT**
> **Points**
>
> > Du 14 *dazhui*
> > Stomach: St 44 *neiting*
> > Liver: Liv 2 *xingjian*
> > Heart: He 8 *shaofu*
> > Lung: Lu 10 *yuji*
> > Intestines: LI 11 *quchi*
>
> **Method:** sedation needle technique
>
> If from Accumulation Disorder: M–UE-9 *sifeng* (pricked on one hand)
>
> **Paediatric *tui na*** routine to clear Heat
>
> > Any of the seven finger points, depending on which Organs are affected by Heat (straight pushing sedation)
> > Milky Way *tianheshui* (straight pushing)
> > Six *Yang* Organs *liufu* (straight pushing)
>
> If Accumulation Disorder is present:
>
> > Thick Gate *banmen* (straight pushing)
> > Eight Trigrams *bagua* (circular pushing anti-clockwise)
> > Four Wind Creases *sifengwen* (pinching)
> > Abdomen Stimulation *fuyinyang* (pushing apart)
> > Belly Corner *dujiao* (pinching)
>
> Hidden Heat: In some children the Heat is 'hidden' deep in the body. They may look pale, but when you look at their tongue, take their pulse and witness their behaviour, it is clear that they have Heat.

Damp and Phlegm

A child may be born with an excess of Damp or Phlegm or it may arise during the first years of life because of diet or an underlying Spleen deficiency. Certain foods may then trigger the production of more Damp or Phlegm.

 Thick Phlegm: If the Phlegm is very hard, it may not be visible at all. You will know it is there because of the hard nodules on the glands and the nature of the child's symptoms.

Symptoms of Damp or Phlegm in the body

- diarrhoea

- bloating

- stomach aches

- vomiting of mucus

- nasal discharge or blocked nose

- chronic productive cough

- glue ear

- snores and breathes through mouth
- needs to sleep a lot
- sleeps very deeply
- struggles to get going in the morning
- puffy face
- clammy skin
- chubby

Symptoms of Phlegm misting the Mind

- may appear very easygoing and not be perturbed by much
- hard to reach
- phases of 'zoning out'
- lacking in vitality and spark
- barely moves

Pulse: slippery or wiry

Tongue: thick, sticky coating, swollen

Treatment principles: resolve Phlegm; clear the Mind's orifices

---

SUGGESTED TREATMENT
Points

> Sp 9 *yinlingquan*
> Sp 6 *sanyinjiao*
> St 40 *fenglong*
> Pc 5 *jianshi*

Method: sedation needle technique

Paediatric *tui na* routine to resolve Damp and Phlegm

> Finger points (straight pushing) according to which Organs are affected
> Small Palmar Crease *zhangxiaowen* (straight pushing)
> Hand *yin yang shouyinyang* (pushing apart)
> Eight Trigrams *bagua* (circular pushing anti-clockwise)

When Phlegm is affecting the *shen*:

> Heaven Gate *tianmen* (straight pushing)
> Water Palace *kangong* (pushing apart)
> Heart Gate *xinmen* (straight pushing)

When a child reacts to a food, it is common for Phlegm and Heat to combine. At any given time, either the Phlegm or Heat will predominate. The child will oscillate between the symptoms of the two. This is similar to the *dian kuang*, which is seen in mental illness in adults.

Cold

Symptoms

- white face
- abdominal pain which tends to be strong and cramping
- wakes at night in pain
- watery diarrhoea without a smell
- tendency to clear or white mucus in the nose or chest
- may feel cold

Pulse: deep, maybe tight

Tongue: pale, may have a thick white coat

Treatment principles: expel Cold; tonify and warm Spleen *yang*

> **SUGGESTED TREATMENT**
> **Points**
>
> > Ren 12 *zhongwan*
> > St 25 *tianshu*
> > Sp 4 *gongsun*
> > St 36 *zusanli*
>
> **Method:** sedation needle technique
>
> **Other techniques:** moxibustion
>
> **Paediatric *tui na*** to tonify and warm the Spleen
>
> > Spleen *pijing* (straight pushing tonification)
> > Thick Gate *banmen* (straight pushing)
> > Three Passes *sanguan* (straight pushing)
> > Knead the Navel *rou qi* (kneading anti-clockwise)
> > Spinal Column *jizhu* (pinching from the bottom to the top of the back)
> > St 36 *zusanli* (kneading)

Underlying deficiencies

The underlying pattern that is present in nearly all cases of food allergies is Spleen *qi* and/or *yang* deficiency. The Spleen has an enormous influence in how efficiently and smoothly a child is able to digest his food. It is often a deficiency of the Spleen that makes a child susceptible to food allergies. It is sometimes not possible to immediately treat this deficiency because the child's allergies have led to the accumulation of a particular pathogen or pathogens in the digestive system. Strengthening the Spleen may therefore bring about an abnormal reaction to treatment. However, once these pathogens have been cleared, and after a period devoid of exposure to the trigger foods, strengthening the Spleen is crucial. It is often this that ultimately leads the child to be able to tolerate the foods to which he previously reacted.

Symptoms

- loose stools

- easily tires

- picky eater

- pale face

- quiet

Pulse: deficient

Tongue: pale, wet, swollen

Treatment principles: tonify Spleen *qi*; warm Spleen *yang* (if necessary)

SUGGESTED TREATMENT

Needling one or two points per treatment is usually sufficient, with moxa if necessary.

Points

St 36 *zusanli*
Ren 12 *zhongwan*
Sp 3 *taibai*
Sp 6 *sanyinjiao*
Bl 20 *pishu*
Bl 21 *weishu*

Method: tonification needle technique

Other techniques: moxibustion

Paediatric *tui na* routine to tonify and warm the Spleen

Spleen *pijing* (straight pushing tonification)
Thick Gate *banmen* (straight pushing)
Three Passes *sanguan* (straight pushing)
Knead Ren 12 *zhongwan* (kneading anti-clockwise)
Knead the Navel *rou qi* (kneading anti-clockwise)
Spinal Column *jizhu* (pinching from the bottom to the top of the back)
St 36 *zusanli* (kneading)

Possible emotional responses to chronic food allergies according to Five Element constitutional imbalance

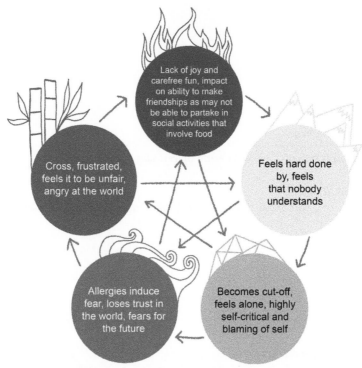

A Five Element perspective on the emotional impact of food allergies

---

CASE HISTORY: FOUR-YEAR-OLD GIRL WITH SEVERE DELAYED ONSET ALLERGIES TO VARIOUS FOODS

This case history illustrates:

- even in severe conditions, it is possible to get excellent results without using needles
- how to treat the different stages of food allergies.

Hermione had severe delayed onset (non-IgE-mediated) allergies to gluten, soya, dairy and eggs. If she ate a tiny amount of any of these foods, or even touched a crumb of gluten, she became severely ill for six to eight weeks. The main symptoms were:

- severe insomnia (awake for hours at a time every night)
- constipation and loss of bowel control (constipation and faecal soiling)
- mood changes: manic, aggressive behaviour, alternating with lethargy and disconnection.

Diagnosis

- Hot Lingering Pathogenic Factor in the Liver
- Phlegm in the body and Phlegm misting the Mind
- Spleen *qi* deficient and Cold

Treatment: When I first treated Hermione, her mother asked me if I could avoid using needles, because Hermione had been traumatised by some of the medical interventions she had received. The first thing I did was to use paediatric *tui na*, in order to clear Heat and Phlegm. This immediately began to help Hermione. After approximately three months, she readily accepted the use of needles.

These stages of treatment were not entirely linear. I went back and forth between them as Hermione's condition fluctuated. For example, if she showed signs of having a 'flare', I would focus more on clearing Heat from the Liver. In between flares, I would focus more on strengthening her Spleen.

Stage 1
Clear Hot LPF from the Liver using points such as:

- Liv 2 *xingjian*
- Liv 3 *taichong*
- Liv 13 *zhangmen*
- Bl 18 *ganshu*

(sedation needle technique)

Resolve Phlegm using points such as:

- Pc 5 *jianshi*
- St 40 *fenglong*

(sedation needle technique)

Stage 2
Tonify Spleen *qi* using points such as:

- St 36 *zusanli*
- Sp 3 *taibai*
- Bl 20 *pishu*
- Bl 21 *weishu*

(tonification needle technique)

Promote healing of nerve damage in the rectum with points such as:

- Bl 58 *feiyang*
- Du 2 *yaoshu*

(sedation needle technique)

Stage 3
Treatment of Five Element constitutional imbalance

Hermione had an Earth constitutional imbalance. Although I had already focused treatment on tonifying Spleen *qi*, I then directed the treatment more to the level of her *yi*. Examples of points used are:

- Sp 21 *dabao*
- Bl 49 *yishe*

● CHECKLIST TO DIAGNOSE AND TREAT A FOOD ALLERGY OR INTOLERANCE

» What pathogen is the allergy creating or exacerbating in the child's body? Is it Heat, Phlegm, Damp, Wind or Cold, or a combination of several pathogens?

» What is the underlying deficiency?

» What is the treatment priority? Is it to clear the pathogen created or to treat the underlying deficiency? Is it possible to do both simultaneously?

» What else needs to be treated? Is there any physical damage to the child's body? What impact has the allergy had on the child's emotional state?

SUMMARY

» Food allergies range from being life-threatening at one extreme, to causing occasional, mild symptoms at the other.

» Some food allergies are immediate, and others may come on some time after the culprit food is eaten.

» Food allergies may be due to a range of global and individual factors, all of which affect the *qi* of the Middle Burner and the Organs related to digestion.

» The symptoms of a food allergy are usually due to the creation or exacerbation of a pathogen.

» There is nearly always an underlying deficiency of Spleen *qi* involved too.

» The treatment of food allergies must be approached in stages, and includes treatment of any physical and emotional consequences of the allergy.

Chapter 51

MYALGIC ENCEPHALOMYELITIS/ CHRONIC FATIGUE SYNDROME (ME/CFS)

The topics discussed in this chapter are:

- Approaching the treatment of ME/CFS
- Aetiology
- Diagnosis and treatment
- Key symptoms of ME/CFS

Introduction

Myalgic encephalomyelitis/chronic fatigue syndrome (ME/CFS) is the name given to a complex and poorly understood condition, which is characterised by fatigue and involves a range of other symptoms. It may affect children as young as five years old, although it is more commonly seen in children from the age of thirteen upward. Many more girls are affected than boys. Young children are usually synonymous with vitality, enthusiasm and a strong life force. It is particularly heartbreaking to see a child in whom these qualities are diminished because of this illness.

 Some of the names this syndrome is known as are:

> chronic fatigue syndrome

> myalgic encephalomyelitis

> myalgic encephalopathy

> post-viral fatigue syndrome

> systemic exertion intolerance disease.

Historically, sufferers of ME/CFS were often thought of as malingerers and some doctors implied that the illness was all in the mind of the sufferer. To some degree, this attitude still prevails. ME/CFS can be a life-destroying illness for a child. The symptoms are not imagined, even though they are, in some cases, caused or exacerbated by an emotional or psychological factor. Many illnesses are caused by a mix of physical and emotional factors, whether this is generally recognised or not. Furthermore, just because no organic reason for an illness can be found, the sufferer is no less deserving of support and sympathy than one who has an illness with a recognised, physical cause.

It is more often possible to get 'complete' results when treating children with ME/CFS than it is when treating adults. The fact that the *qi* of a child is dynamic and not yet fully 'set' means that she is more responsive to acupuncture. In severe cases, it can be useful to combine acupuncture with other therapies and also dietary changes. For example, some children benefit from cognitive behavioural therapy (CBT) or other talking therapies. Others find cutting out a particular food from their diet for a period of time particularly helpful.

Table 51.1 The impact of ME/CFS on the child and the family

Child	Family
Lots of time off school	A parent may have to stop work
Affects ability to form and maintain friendships	Siblings may receive less care and attention
May affect physical development	May strain the relationship of parents
May affect emotional and psychological development	Therapies may be costly

Approaching the treatment of ME/CFS

As is the case with many long-term, complex conditions, the very existence of ME/CFS usually has ripples that spread far and wide. It is not just the illness that confronts the practitioner but also its consequences for the child and the family. Figure 51.1 illustrates the way the illness, the child and the family's response to it may interact.

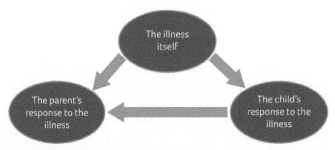

Figure 51.1 ME/CFS, the child and the family

Part of the role of the practitioner, therefore, is to be an objective voice and to try to interrupt this negative feedback loop. The simple action of truly listening to the child's and the parent's stories can begin this process. Many parents say that this is the first time they have been truly listened to.

Some ideas to bear in mind when treating a child with ME/CFS

- Avoid combining too many treatment principles at once: a child's *qi* is usually too volatile to cope well with treatments that are trying to do more than one or two things at the same time. Too many treatment principles will also mean that it becomes unclear what is helping and what is not.

- Avoid merely 'chasing the symptoms': the nature of CFS means that a child may have myriad symptoms and that the symptoms may change frequently. The most effective treatment is to address the root imbalance, rather than just focusing on the symptoms.

- The balance between fullness and deficiency should be reassessed at every treatment and the treatment principles adjusted accordingly.

- When possible, it is useful to treat during a flare-up of the LPF (when present). A flare-up may arise when the child becomes stronger, manifesting as a re-occurrence of the original illness. A treatment at this time helps to finally clear the LPF out of the body.

- The practitioner should be prepared for ups and downs when treating a child with ME/CFS. The road to recovery is rarely smooth. It is worth discussing this with the family at the start of treatment. This helps to lessen the disappointment if there should be a setback along the way.

Aetiology

Events that often precede the onset of ME/CFS

Reaction to one-off or repeated External Pathogenic Factors (including vaccination): Many parents report that their child's illness began after the child had a digestive or respiratory bug, which the child 'never really got over'. After the child seemingly recovered, he never really bounced back to his old self. In other cases, the child had a period of months when he had one bug after another. Sometimes parents notice that their child's symptoms begin within a week or two of the child having had a vaccination.

Exhaustion: In the run-up to the onset of the illness, the child may have experienced a period when he was especially tired and run down. The parent may have noticed that he was not firing on all cylinders and was becoming more tired than normal by his usual routine. Or, for example, there may have been a time when the child was having to push himself more than usual, because he had to prepare for exams or a particular sporting event.

Prolonged period of stress or unhappiness: It is common to hear that, preceding the onset of ME/CFS in a child, the child or the family experienced a particularly difficult time. It may be that the child was being bullied at school or the parents had separated. Or a 'happy' event, such as a younger sibling being born, meant that everybody was overtired and impatient so there was less love and attention available.

Trauma: A physical or emotional trauma may be a trigger for the onset of ME/CFS. For example, one girl who came to the clinic had become ill after banging her head badly in a fall. Another child's symptoms had begun a couple of months after the unexpected death of a cousin to whom he was very close.

Combination of factors: It is unusual for there to be only one trigger for this illness. In most cases, several events have occurred in a child's life at around the same time or in close succession which, together, tip the scales from health to illness. People often talk about being struck 'out of the blue' by an illness. However, if we question closely enough, we can frequently see how the ground was being laid in the weeks and months, or sometimes years, leading up to the person succumbing to an illness. The trigger is often actually the straw that broke the camel's back, rather than the sole cause of the illness.

Factors that may compound the illness

Stress or unhappiness: It is very hard for a child to physically thrive if she is struggling emotionally. The *qi* of a child so often reflects her external environment. If the home or school environment is not one where she feels she is nourished and supported, it will have a subtle but constant wearing-down effect on the child. This may be enough to stop her making the final leap back to health.

Family dynamics: Sometimes a child's illness serves a purpose within the family. Although it is unlikely that any family member will be aware of this kind of dynamic, it may exert quite a profound influence. A child who is ill, off school much of the time and in need of a lot of looking after may be a reason for the parents to avoid focusing on their relationship. For the child, it may be that she believes the illness is the only way she will get the attention which she desires. Being at home with Mum for a while may be a chance for a child to get what she missed out on earlier in her life because her mother was ill or depressed.

> I once treated an eleven-year-old boy who had been ill with ME/CFS for about four years. During the course of treatment, he would get to a point of being well enough to be back at school full time. Every time this happened, his mother would become anxious about a bug going around that she feared he would catch or that he was doing too much. This would become a self-fulfilling prophecy and, sure enough, within a matter of weeks the boy would become ill again and be off school. It became clear to me that his mother actually needed him to be ill and at home. She was very unhappy in her marriage and therefore relied heavily on her son for emotional closeness. She was also scared of having to face going back into work again. The boy, without even knowing it, felt responsible for his mother and was strongly driven to keep her happy. It was not until he went through puberty that this dynamic was finally broken and, with the surge of *yang* that is characteristic of this time, he managed to separate from his mother enough to become and stay well.

Dietary factors: When a child's *qi* is lowered, as it is with ME/CFS, she may be less able to tolerate a food or foods that have previously been unproblematic. Excluding that food takes a strain off the body, which allows it to heal more easily.

There are many ways that parents ascertain whether their child is intolerant to a particular food or not. Some will visit a nutritionist, or have blood tests. Others will try elimination diets or consult an applied kinesiologist. Some of these methods may be more reliable than others. There are children who have such a limited diet that it makes them truly miserable. It may be of dubious benefit anyway.

It can be helpful to work with parents and children to pinpoint whether the benefits of cutting out a particular food or foods are really greater than the stress and unhappiness the restrictions may cause. The foods which are most commonly problematic in children with ME/CFS are gluten, dairy and sugar.

Weak constitution: If a child who has a weak constitution gets a chronic illness such as ME/CFS, it is naturally more difficult for her to throw it off. She does not have the reserves of *qi* to call upon that a stronger child has. In this case, it may be necessary for the child to limit her activity for a period of time and to have a lot of regular treatment, and also possibly to take a herbal supplement. For a child who falls into this category, it may be that she needs to wait until she comes to the next seven-year cycle to become fully better.

Table 51.2 Factors that trigger and compound ME/CFS

Events that often precede the onset of ME/CFS	Factors that may compound ME/CFS
One or more External Pathogenic Factors or vaccination	Unhappiness
A period of being run-down or exhausted	Family dynamics
A period of stress or unhappiness	Dietary factors
Physical or emotional trauma	Weak constitution

Diagnosis and treatment

A child with CFS often has an enormous array of symptoms as well as conflicting signs. Furthermore, her condition may be changeable. The art of making a clear diagnosis is to find clarity amid what may appear to be confusion and chaos. In order to do this, it may be useful to take the following systematic approach.

Five key questions to ask oneself when diagnosing a child with ME/CFS

1. Is there a Lingering Pathogenic Factor (LPF) and, if so, what is its nature?

An LPF is present in the vast majority of children with ME/CFS. It may be that the child has always had this LPF, or at least has had it from an early age. It only begins to cause problems when the child is under particular stress or especially tired, or when she catches another illness. Alternatively, it may be that a child has had a recent acute condition that she has been unable to fully throw off, either because it was severe or because her *qi* was too deficient.

One indication is that she repeatedly succumbs to what appears to be the same acute 'illness'. This is often a respiratory or digestive condition, such as a sore throat or chest infection, but the quality and nature of it is very similar each time she gets it. The parents may believe that their child keeps catching 'another virus', but actually it is the same pathogen that she has been unable to throw off, raising its head time and again.

For a discussion of treating an LPF, please see Chapter 27.

2. What is the key deficiency? Which substance? Which Organ?

Pulse, tongue and symptoms will guide the practitioner to which Organ and substance the key deficiency lies in. There may be deficiency in several Organs and more than one substance. The practitioner should try to ascertain which deficiency is the longest standing and the most severe.

3. What is the relative strength of the LPF compared with the relative deficiency of the child?

The practitioner should ask herself whether the child has enough *qi* in order to be able to throw off the LPF, if present. In most cases, the reason the child has not yet been able to do this is because the underlying deficiency means she is unable to.

4. What is the child's constitutional imbalance and what is the state of her shen?

'When one applies medical treatment, one must, first of all, keep in mind the patient's spirit.'[13] As this quote suggests, if the child's *shen* is not vital, then it is unlikely that her body will be able to regain its vitality. If the practitioner deems that the state of the child's spirit is a key factor in her prolonged illness, this needs to be addressed with treatment.

5. What, if anything, is keeping the child ill?

For everything that is lost through illness, there may also be something that is gained. If the child has a secondary gain in being ill, it is rarely, if ever, conscious. Being ill may mean the child does not have to return to a school she hates or leave a mother whom she is worried about, for example.

> **FIVE KEY QUESTIONS TO ASK ONESELF WHEN DIAGNOSING A CHILD WITH ME/CFS**
>
> 1. Is there a Lingering Pathogenic Factor (LPF) and, if so, what is its nature?
> 2. What is the *key* deficiency? Which substance? Which Organ?
> 3. What is the relative strength of the LPF compared with the relative deficiency of the child?
> 4. What is the child's constitutional imbalance and what is the state of her *shen*?
> 5. What, if anything, is keeping the child ill?

Key symptoms of ME/CFS

ME/CFS may be defined as an 'overwhelming fatigue that has been present for at least six months, which is disabling and where there is no psychiatric illness or physical disease to explain it'.[14] Apart from fatigue, some of the most common symptoms that accompany the condition are:

- disturbed sleep
- muscle aches, pain, weakness or twitching
- sensory hypersensitivity
- feeling of overload
- mood symptoms
- digestive symptoms
- headaches.

The illness may be severe or mild. It can be relapsing and remitting or progressive.

The nature of fatigue

One of the key symptoms of ME/CFS is fatigue. It is important to define the nature of the fatigue, since this will help to differentiate it.

 It should be remembered that not all fatigue comes from deficiency.

Post-exertional fatigue or malaise

This is one of the hallmark symptoms of ME/CFS and means that a child will feel particularly tired or exhausted after either physical or mental exertion. The tiredness may come on immediately after the exertion but there may also be a delay. For example, the child may go to a birthday party one morning and feel fine for the rest of the day but wake up the next morning feeling shattered.

TCM differentiation: deficiency of *qi*, *yang* or Blood

> **SUGGESTED TREATMENT**
> **Points**
> Points should be selected according to which Organs and substances are deficient. For example:
>
> *Qi* deficiency:
>
> > St 36 *zusanli*
> > Lu 9 *taiyuan*
> > Ki 3 *taixi*
> > He 5 *tongli*
>
> *Yang* deficiency:
>
> > Any of the above points with moxa, as well as:
> >
> > Du 4 *ming men*
> > Du 14 *dazhui*
> > Ren 6 *qihai*
> > Ki 7 *fuliu*
>
> Blood deficiency:
>
> > Sp 6 *sanyinjiao*
> > Liv 8 *ququan*

> He 7 *shenmen*
> Bl 17 *geshu*
> Ren 4 *guanyuan*

Method: tonification needle technique

Brain fog

Brain fog is another hallmark symptom of ME/CFS. It means that a child will have trouble concentrating, thinking, coming up with words and being able to work things out. For example, she may try to do some maths homework that would normally be easy for her, but now she struggles to think clearly enough to do it.

> One bright child described the feeling of brain fog very articulately. She said, 'I just stare at the page and see lots of numbers but I can't work out how they are all connected or what I am supposed to do with them. It feels as if there is a barrier between my brain and the numbers.'

TCM differentiation:

- Damp or Phlegm in the channels of the head
- Spleen and/or Kidney *yang* deficiency failing to raise clear *yang*

Points

To resolve Damp or Phlegm in the head:

> St 8 *touwei*
> St 40 *fenglong*
> LI 4 *hegu*
> Sp 3 *taibai*
> GB 13 *benshen*

Method: sedation needle technique

To raise clear *yang*:

> Du 20 *baihui*
> Du 14 *dazhui*

'Molasses' or flu-like fatigue

This is characterised by a heavy feeling in the limbs. The child feels as if she has to drag herself around all the time. She may describe feeling as if she has to 'walk through treacle' or that it is an enormous effort to put one foot in front of the other in order to walk. The feeling of having flu becomes a chronic state. Everything is an enormous effort and the child often wants to sleep much of the time. This symptom may be worse in the mornings and on damp days. It may ease a little on mild exertion.

TCM differentiation: Damp or Damp-Heat in the muscles

Points

To resolve Damp and Damp-Heat:

> Sp 9 *yinlingquan*
>
> Sp 6 *sanyinjiao*
>
> LI 11 *quchi*
>
> GB 34 *yanglingquan*

Method: sedation needle technique

Wired but tired fatigue

It is common for a child with ME/CFS to feel exhausted but also agitated. She is really tired but cannot settle or sleep. Both she and her parents often have a strong feeling that, if only she were able to get proper rest, she would start to feel better. The more tired she becomes, the more wired she feels.

TCM differentiation:

- *yin* deficiency
- Full Heat with underlying deficiency

Points

To nourish *yin* should be chosen according to the Organs involved – for example:

Ki 1 *yongquan*
Ki 3 *taixi*
Ki 6 *zhaohai*
Ren 4 *guanyuan*
St 36 *zusanli*
Sp 6 *sanyinjiao*

Method: tonification needle technique

To clear Heat should be chosen according to which Organs are involved – for example:

Du 14 *dazhui*
Liv 2 *xingjian*
He 8 *shaofu*
TB 5 *waiguan*
St 44 *neiting*
Lu 10 *yuji*
LI 4 *hegu*
LI 11 *quchi*

Method: sedation needle technique

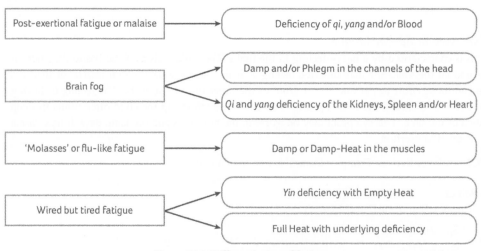

Figure 51.2 Differentiation of fatigue

Other symptoms

Problems getting a good night's sleep

Feeling tired or exhausted does not necessarily mean the child will sleep well. Unfortunately, the exact opposite is common and children with ME/CFS often struggle to have a regular sleep pattern. Obviously, this perpetuates the illness as sleep is vital for a child's health. Figure 51.3 summarizes the patterns causing different types of fatigue.

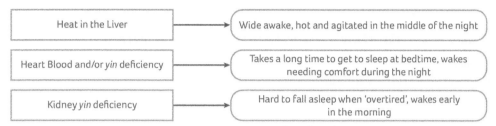

Figure 51.3 Patterns causing sleep disturbance

Points

To clear Heat in the Liver:

> Liv 2 *xingjiang*
> Liv 3 *taichong*
> GB 38 *yangfu*
> Du 24 *shenting*

Method: sedation needle technique

To nourish Heart Blood and/or *yin*:

> He 7 *shenmen*
> He 6 *yinxi*
> He 1 *jiquan*
> Bl 15 *xinshu*
> Ren 14 *juque*

Method: tonification needle technique

To nourish Kidney *yin*:

> Ki 3 *taixi*
> Ki 6 *zhaohai*
> Ki 10 *yingu*
> Ki 25 *shencang*
> Ki 1 *yongquan*

Method: tonification needle technique

Problems with muscles

It is common for a child with ME/CFS to have some kind of symptoms in her muscles, which may have a significant impact on her ability to carry out simple everyday tasks.

TCM differentiation

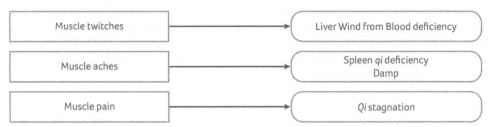

Figure 51.4 Patterns causing muscle twitches, aches and pains

Points

To treat Liver Wind from Blood deficiency:

> Liv 3 *taichong*
> Liv 8 *ququan*
> Bl 18 *ganshu*

Method: tonification needle technique

To treat Damp:

> Sp 9 *yinlingquan*
> Sp 6 *sanyinjiao*

Method: sedation needle technique, with additional points to strengthen the Spleen

To move *qi*:

> Liv 3 *taichong*
> GB 34 *yanglingquan*

Method: sedation needle technique

Sensory hypersensitivity

LIGHT AND SOUND

Many children with ME/CFS are hypersensitive to sounds. This obviously means that attending school can be very difficult. A child may also find it difficult to cope with noises around the home, such as the dishwasher being emptied or the vacuum cleaner being used. Less frequently, she may also find bright light difficult to bear. Even a particularly sunny day may leave her wanting to be in a darkened room.

TCM differentiation:

- **Liver Blood or *yin* deficiency:** Blood and *yin* act as the soundproofing in the body. A deficiency in either can mean that a child experiences any sounds as being magnified and she may feel as if the sound is 'bombarding' her senses.

- **Liver Heat:** The Liver is agitated by wind-like *yang* pathogens, which include sudden noises or flashing bright lights. If the Liver is too Hot, it will be more easily aggravated. Sounds and lights may stir up the Heat in the Liver, disturbing the *hun* and causing the child to feel agitated.

ODOURS

A child with ME/CFS may also have very strong reactions to odours. She may be left feeling quite sick or nauseous by cooking smells coming from the kitchen or by walking through a shop with a strong smell of cosmetics, for example.

TCM differentiation: Stomach *qi* or *yin* deficiency/Liver *qi* invading the Stomach: the Stomach sends *qi* downwards. If Stomach *qi* or *yin* is deficient, or if the Stomach is invaded by *qi* stagnation, it will mean *qi* rises, causing nausea or sickness. Figure 51.5 summarises the patterns that may be involved in sensory hypersensitivity.

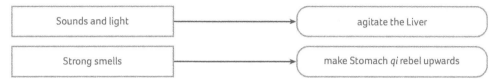

Figure 51.5 Patterns causing sensory hypersensitivity

Points

To nourish Liver Blood and/or *yin*:

> Liv 3 *taichong*
> Liv 8 *ququan*
> Bl 18 *ganshu*
> Ren 4 *guanyuan*

Method: tonification needle technique

To clear Heat from the Liver:

> Liv 2 *xingjian*
> GB 38 *yangfu*

Method: sedation needle technique

To tonify Stomach *qi* and/or *yin*:

> Ren 12 *zhongwan*
> Bl 21 *weishu*
> St 36 *zusanli*

Method: tonification needle technique

A feeling of overload

It is easy for a child with ME/CFS to feel overloaded by almost anything. For example, having to do more than one thing at a time or having to make decisions may both make her symptoms worse. It may even be that reading a book, watching television or listening to music feels like too much at times.[*]

> I treated a nine-year-old girl who had spent almost an entire year lying in bed, not doing anything. Each time she tried to look at a book, or even turned on some music, she would feel overloaded.

TCM differentiation

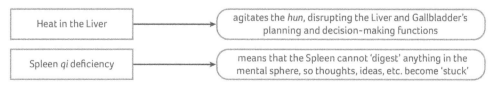

Figure 51.6 Patterns causing a feeling of overload

---

[*] A child with 'overload' from Heat in the Liver may feel like an adult who has a hangover. Any noise or light is too much to bear.

Points

To clear Heat from the Liver:

> Liv 2 *xingjian*
> GB 38 *yangfu*
> GB 9 *tianchong*

Method: sedation needle technique

To strengthen the Spleen:

> St 36 *zusanli*
> Sp 3 *taibai*
> Bl 20 *pishu*

Method: tonification needle technique

Mood symptoms

Unsurprisingly, a child will usually have strong emotions in response to the fact that she has an illness that is having such an impact on her life. There may be enormous sadness, frustration and worry arising from not being able to go to school or to play any sport, from having to miss out on fun activities or from having to repeat school years. However, most parents report that there are also certain emotional states, such as irritability or tearfulness, that seem to be a part of the illness itself, rather than arising as a response to the illness (see Figure 51.7).

TCM differentiation

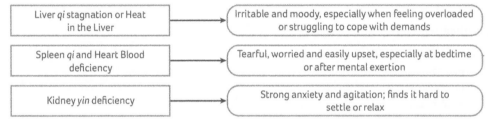

Figure 51.7 Patterns causing emotional symptoms

Points

To smooth the Liver and move *qi* and clear Heat from the Liver:

> Liv 2 *xingjian*
> Liv 3 *taichong*
> GB 43 *xiaxi*
> GB 40 *qiuxu*
> Liv 14 *qimen*

Method: sedation needle technique

To nourish Spleen *qi* and Heart Blood:

> He 1 *jiquan*
> He 7 *shenmen*
> Bl 20 *pishu*
> Sp 21 *dabao*
> Sp 6 *sanyinjiao*

Method: tonification needle technique

To nourish Kidney *yin*:

> Ki 23 *shenfeng*
> Ki 24 *lingxu*
> Ki 25 *shencang*

Ki 6 *zhaohai*
Ki 1 *yongquan*

Method: tonification needle technique

A twelve-year-old girl with ME/CFS became tearful and anxious whenever she did any school work. She often used to come home from school in tears, not because she had had a bad time, but simply from the exertion of having to study. Nourishing her Spleen *qi* and Heart Blood helped, as did advising her on diet.

Digestive symptoms

Digestive symptoms are very common in children with ME/CFS. As this function in a child may not yet be fully mature, it is particularly susceptible to imbalance. It is essential to the recovery of the child for her digestive system to be working properly. If it is not, then she will not be getting sufficient quality or quantity of post-natal *qi* from her food. This means she will struggle to recover from any of the deficiencies that may be present, or to be able to throw off a Lingering Pathogenic Factor.

TCM differentiation

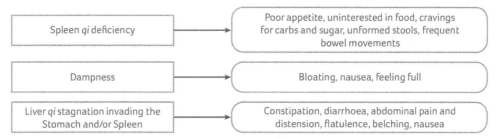

Figure 51.8 Patterns causing digestive symptoms

Points

To tonify Spleen *qi*:

Ren 12 *zhongwan*
Bl 20 *pishu*
St 25 *tianshi*
Sp 4 *gongsun*

Method: tonification needle technique

To resolve Damp:

Sp 9 *yinlingquan*
Sp 6 *sanyinjiao*
Ren 12 *zhongwan*

Method: sedation needle technique

To clear Liver *qi* stagnation invading the Stomach and/or Spleen:

Liv 14 *qimen*
Liv 13 *zhangmen*
Liv 3 *taichong*
Bl 18 *ganshu*

Method: sedation needle technique

One ten-year-old boy who had ME/CFS would wake up every morning with a stomach ache and show no interest in eating breakfast. He would feel lethargic and struggle to do anything other than lie around. He therefore missed a lot of school. He had a lot of Damp in his digestive system. Resolving Damp helped him to wake up feeling brighter and his appetite for breakfast returned. This meant he went to school more often, which helped him to re-engage with life. He made a rapid recovery from this point onwards.

Headaches
See Chapter 61 for the differentiation of headaches.

CASE HISTORY: NINE-YEAR-OLD GIRL WITH ME/CFS

The following case history shows the importance of keeping treatment simple, even in the face of complex symptoms and signs.

Philippa was nine years old when she arrived at the clinic. She had had phases during the previous year of being entirely bed bound. At these times she was too ill to read, intolerant to any noise and barely eating. During better phases, she was able to go for quite long walks in the countryside without any worsening of her symptoms. She suffered from severe migraines, a tremor in her left arm, brain fog and sleep disturbance. She had phases of extreme irritability.

Background: Philippa was a creative and sensitive girl. Her mother told me she had always struggled with the hubbub of the classroom and much preferred quieter environments. When she was seven, she had caught a strong respiratory virus, from which it took her a long time to recover. At aged seven and a half, she had fallen backwards on a tennis court and banged her head badly.

Her family were close and were coping extremely well with the stress and worry of Philippa's illness.

Observations: Philippa had a slight build and looked frail. She had a white colour beside her eyes and a green hue around her mouth. Her voice had a weeping tone to it. Her pulse was wiry and overflowing in the Wood position, and her Metal pulses were deficient. The sides of her tongue were red.

Diagnosis and treatment using the five key questions
1. Is there a Lingering Pathogenic Factor (LPF) and, if so, what is its nature?

Yes – Philippa had an LPF in her Liver causing recurrent migraines, a tremor, irritability and sleep disturbance. The LPF was Hot in nature, evidenced by the overflowing Wood pulse and red sides to the tongue.

2. What is the key deficiency? Which substance? Which Organ?

Philippa's main deficiency was Lung *qi* deficiency, linked to her constitutional imbalance which was Metal. Her Metal pulses were the most deficient, her voice was weeping and she was white beside her eyes.

3. What is the relative strength of the LPF compared with the relative deficiency of the child?

The symptoms caused by the LPF were severe, the Wood pulses very full. The fact that Philippa was able to go for long walks suggested that the LPF was more of a problem than the deficiency.

4. What is the child's constitutional imbalance and what is the state of her shen?

Philippa had a sadness to her but had coped remarkably well with being severely ill for several years. I felt her *shen* was in surprisingly good shape.

5. What, if anything, is keeping the child ill?

The Hot pathogen in Philippa's Liver was stopping her from sleeping and this was preventing her from fully recovering. I did not think there were any wider factors, in the family or in her life, which were keeping her ill.

Treatment: Treatment focused on clearing Heat from the Liver, and tonifying Philippa's constitutional imbalance in her Metal Element. A typical treatment would be, for example:

- Clear Heat: Liv 2 *xingjian*, GB 38 *yangfu* (sedation needle technique)
- Tonify Metal constitutional imbalance: LI 4 *hegu*, Lu 9 *taiyuan* (tonification needle technique)

Philippa came for treatment weekly or fortnightly for a year, over which time she went from barely being able to get out of bed to being back at school full time. There were ups and downs along the way. At one point, she went to London for the day and her symptoms worsened for a few weeks, which I assumed was due to the hubbub of the city. A key turning point was when Philippa reliably started to sleep better (which happened after about the first two months of treatment). At one point, she got a bad cold, followed by an outpouring of green mucus for several weeks. Many of her symptoms began to ease after this (in particular the migraines and the tremor in her arm). She occasionally comes back for a top-up now if she shows any signs of getting run down.

SUMMARY

» ME/CFS rarely arises due to one cause. Several factors usually occur which, when put together, lead to the child becoming ill.

» The picture of a child with ME/CFS is often a complex one. Therefore, one of the keys to diagnosis is to sift through the complexity and to prioritise treatment principles.

» Almost any pattern may appear in a child with ME/CFS. There is nearly always a mix of full and empty patterns.

» An LPF is present in the majority of children with ME/CFS.

» It is important to reassess the balance of full and empty at every treatment.

• Chapter 52 •

CHRONIC COUGH

· ·

The topics discussed in this chapter are:

- Organs and aetiology involved in chronic cough

- Patterns

- Other treatment modalities

- Treatment of the Five Element constitutional imbalance

Introduction

Cough is one of the most commonly seen conditions in the clinic. With luck, a cough will be a rare event and one that the child gets through relatively quickly and painlessly. Sometimes, however, it is something that a family begins to dread. A child may cough all night long, disturbing the whole family and getting very little sleep herself. Sometimes a cough precipitates other Lung conditions such as wheezing and breathlessness, and means a middle-of-the-night trip to the emergency department of the hospital. For another child, frequent coughs mean endless rounds of antibiotics which lead to more deficiency and hence more susceptibility to further coughs. A young child does not have the strength or ability to clear mucus from her chest, where it may therefore sit for many weeks. A child may go down with a cough in the autumn that lingers through the entire winter.

Acupuncture is effective at treating both chronic and acute coughs in children. Treatment can both help to clear a cough and also to strengthen a child so that she does not succumb to so many. It can hugely reduce the need for medication.

This chapter focuses on the treatment of chronic cough. Please see Chapter 70 for the treatment of acute cough.

Organs and aetiology involved in chronic cough

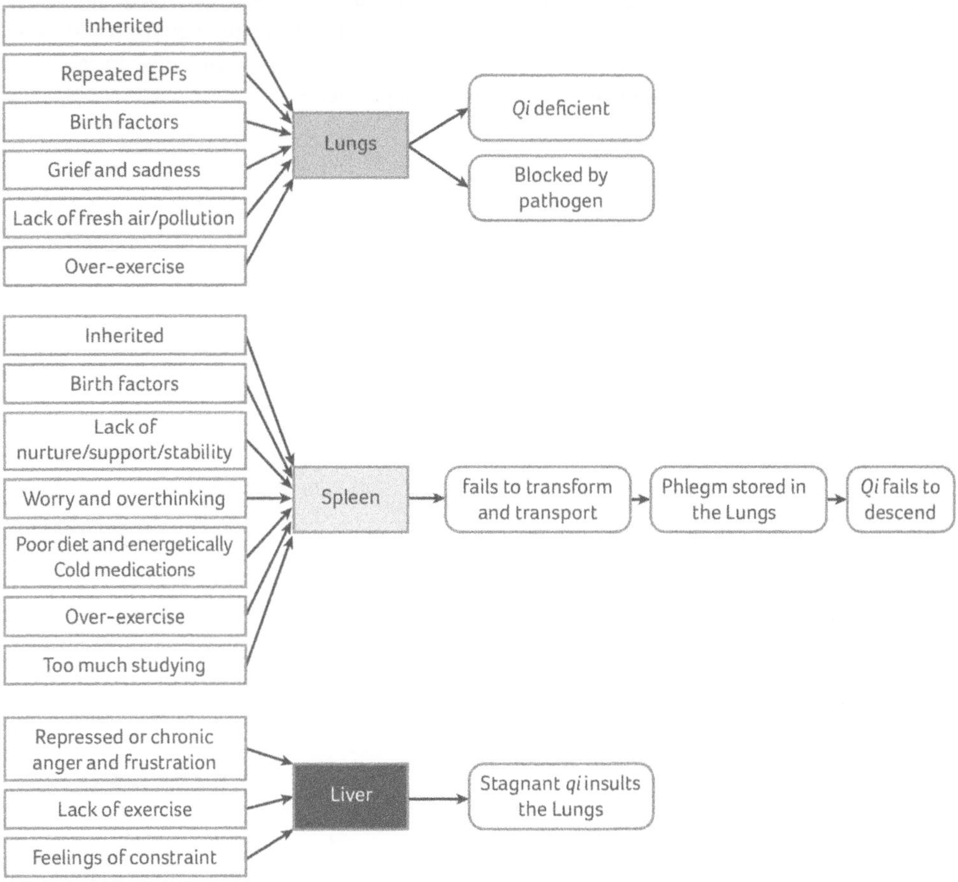

Figure 52.1 Organs and aetiology involved in chronic cough

The emotions and chronic cough

A chronic cough and grief

The emotion most closely connected with the Lungs is grief. As Maciocia writes, 'Sadness and grief constrict the Corporeal Soul, dissolve Lung *qi* and suspend our breathing.'[15] Sometimes, during treatment for a chronic cough, a child will have an outpouring of grief. This may even happen during the treatment, immediately on needling a point on the Lung channel. The child will start crying, initially saying that the needle hurt, but will just keep crying. This is normally a cathartic cry and sometimes, once the child starts crying, she will stop coughing. The cough was in lieu of crying. Treating the Lungs frees the constraint and lets the tears flow.

Phlegm as protection against the world

There may also be an emotional component to a chronic cough that is characterised by a lot of mucus. A very sensitive child will sometimes generate Phlegm as a kind of armour. It provides a veil between her and the world, making the latter easier to cope with. When the practitioner perceives this to be the case, ascertaining where the child's constitutional imbalance lies and treating it is crucial. It will enable the child to then feel robust enough to be in the world without needing the armour of Phlegm.

Damp-Phlegm and a heavy, depressed environment

Damp and Phlegm are heavy, lingering pathogens and are *yin* in nature. A child may mimic the emotional environment in which she lives. If that environment is characterised by depression and a lack of joy, then she may generate Phlegm as a response to that. It is often harder to resolve a mucousy cough in a child whose environment is an unhappy one.

Patterns

- Phlegm in the Lungs

- Lung and Spleen *qi* deficiency

- Lingering Pathogenic Factor (LPF)

- Constrained Liver *qi* affecting the Lungs

It is common to see two or three of these patterns together in a child with a chronic cough. Phlegm or a Lingering Pathogenic Factor in the Lungs is often present, together with Lung and Spleen *qi* deficiency.

It is vital in any child with a chronic cough to choose points on the back (such as Bl 13 *feishu*) and on the chest (such as Lu 1 *zhongfu*). Using distal points alone is not usually effective.

Phlegm in the Lungs

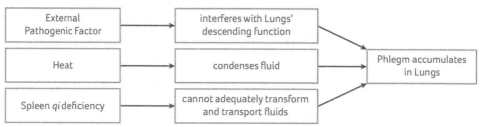

Figure 52.2 Phlegm causing chronic cough

Nature of cough

- cough which sounds as if the child's lungs are full of mucus

- cough often gets worse at night

- cough is often bad first thing in the morning

- child has prolonged bouts of coughing

- clear mucus which is relatively easy to expectorate

Other symptoms: blocked or runny nose, intermittently poor appetite. There may be other Phlegm symptoms such as glue ear or tummy ache

Pulse: slippery on the Metal and Earth pulses

Tongue: thick, sticky coating

Treatment principles: restore descending function of Lungs; resolve Phlegm

> Although only rarely an issue, it is important during the treatment of a cough in a young child to avoid stirring up mucus. This could result in the child being overwhelmed with mucus and struggling to breathe. To avoid this, first use points which descend the *qi* such as Ren 22 *tiantu* and Ren 17 *shanzhong*. Points such as St 40 *fenglong* and Lu 5 *chize* can be used later when the quantity of mucus has reduced.

Variations

- Phlegm-Heat in the Lungs will result in a barking cough with coloured mucus that is hard to expectorate, redness on the face and possibly other Heat symptoms.

- Phlegm and Accumulation Disorder: In babies and toddlers, the Phlegm may derive from Accumulation Disorder. In this case, there will be foul-smelling and irregular stools, irritability and a green colour around the mouth.

SUGGESTED TREATMENT

It is important to always use one or more points to descend *qi* when resolving Phlegm in the chest. A typical treatment may be Ren 22 *tiantu*, Lu 7 *lieque* and St 40 *fenglong*, followed by flash cupping on the upper back. The aim is to clear the Phlegm downwards, rather than upwards.

It may also be necessary to tonify the Spleen and/or Lungs in order to help the child move the fluids.

Points

Descend Lung *qi*:

> Ren 17 *shanzhong*
> Ren 22 *tiantu*
> Lu 7 *lieque*
> Bl 13 *feishu*

Resolve Phlegm:

> Lu 5 *chize*
> St 40 *fenglong*

Method: sedation needle technique

If Accumulation Disorder is present, this should be addressed first (using M-UE-9 *sifeng*).

Other techniques

> Gua sha or flash cupping over the area on the upper back, around Bl 13 *feishu*, can help to relieve congestion in the chest

> Stop coughing point (see below) treated with a press-sphere or retained needle

Paediatric *tui na* routine to resolve Phlegm, and descend Lung *qi*

> Lung *feijing* (straight pushing sedation)
> Spleen *pijing* (straight pushing tonification)
> Eight Trigrams *bagua* (circular pushing anti-clockwise)
> Small Palmar Crease *zhangxiaowen* (straight pushing)
> Hand *yin yang shouyinyang* (pushing apart)
> Central Altar *shanzhong* (pushing apart and straight pushing)
> Breast Sides and Breast Root *rupang and rugen* (kneading)
> Flanks and Ribs *xielei* (straight pushing)
> Lung Transport *jianjiagu* (pushing apart)
> Celestial Pillar Bone *tianzhugu* (straight pushing)
> St 40 Abundant Bulge *fenglong* (kneading)

Lung and Spleen *qi* deficiency

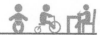

Nature of cough

- weak cough

- small amount of clear mucus which is relatively easy to expectorate

- cough gets worse when tired or after running around or in the cold

Other symptoms: quiet, dislike of going outside to play, fussy eater, pale face

Pulse: deficient Earth and Metal pulses

Tongue: pale

Treatment principles: tonify Spleen and Lung *qi*

> **SUGGESTED TREATMENT**
>
> A typical treatment may be a point to directly affect the Lungs, such as Bl 13 *feishu*, followed by one or two points to strengthen the Spleen, such as Ren 12 *zhongwan* and Bl 20 *pishu*.
>
> Lu 1 *zhongfu* is a particularly effective point for a cough from Spleen and Lung *qi* deficiency because the Spleen and Lung channels meet at this point.
>
> **Points**
> To tonify Spleen *qi*:
>
> > St 36 *zusanli*
> > Sp 3 *taibai*
> > Ren 12 *zhongwan*
> > Bl 20 *pishu*
>
> To tonify Lung *qi*:
>
> > Lu 1 *zhongfu*
> > Lu 9 *taiyuan*
> > Bl 13 *feishu*
>
> **Method:** tonification needle technique
>
> **Other techniques**
>
> > Moxibustion
> >
> > Stop coughing point (see below) treated with a press-sphere or retained needle
>
> **Paediatric *tui na*** to tonify the Spleen and Lungs and stop cough
>
> > Spleen *pijing* (straight pushing tonification)
> > Lung *feijing* (straight pushing tonification)
> > Knead Ren 12 *zhongwan* (kneading anti-clockwise)
> > Spinal Column *jizhu* (pinching from the bottom to the top of the back)
> > St 36 *zusanli* (kneading)
> > Central Altar *shanzhong* (pushing apart and straight pushing)
> > Breast Sides and Breast Root *rupang and rugen* (kneading)
> > Flanks and Ribs *xielei* (straight pushing)
> > Lung Transport *jianjiagu* (pushing apart)
> > Celestial Pillar Bone *tianzhugu* (straight pushing)

Lingering Pathogenic Factor (LPF)

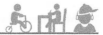

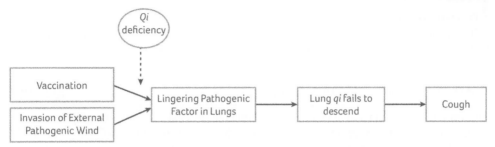

Figure 52.3 Lingering Pathogenic Factor causing chronic cough

Nature of cough

- hard, hacking cough which gets worse when tired

- cannot expectorate mucus

- cough may come and go a lot (may be absent for days at a time and then come back when the child gets tired or has an added stress in her life)

Other symptoms: hard glands in the neck, child 'not quite herself'

Pulse: full quality on Metal pulses; deficient in other positions

Tongue: if the LPF is Hot, there may be red points on the tongue in the Lung area

Treatment principles: loosen Thick Phlegm; resolve Phlegm; strengthen Lung and/or Spleen *qi*

SUGGESTED TREATMENT

Treatment will often move between the three stages outlined. At each treatment, the practitioner should reassess the child and decide which of the three principles is relevant. For further details of treating an LPF, see Chapter 27.

Points

To loosen Thick Phlegm:

> Bl 13 *feishu*
> M-HN-30 *bailao*

Method: sedation needle technique

To resolve Phlegm:

> Lu 5 *chize*
> Lu 7 *lieque*
> St 40 *fenglong*
> Ren 22 *tiantu*

Method: sedation needle technique

To tonify Lung and/or Spleen *qi*:

> St 36 *zusanli*
> Bl 20 *pishu*
> Lu 9 *taiyuan*
> Bl 13 *feishu*

Method: tonification needle technique

Other techniques: Stop coughing point (see below) treated with a press-sphere or retained needle

Paediatric *tui na*

Depending on the balance between fullness and deficiency, a combination of the *tui na* routines to resolve Phlegm and strengthen the underlying deficiency (see above) may be used.

Constrained Liver *qi* affecting the Lungs

This pattern is most common in older children (from the age of about seven or eight).

Qi stagnation often moves to the place in the body where there is most deficiency, as if to fill the void and act as a kind of protection. Therefore, it may also be necessary to strengthen Lung *qi* in this pattern.

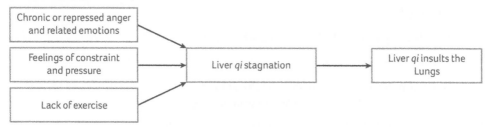

Figure 52.4 Constrained Liver qi affecting the Lungs causing chronic cough

Nature of cough

- bouts of violent, loud coughing
- tight chest
- cough triggered by stress or strong emotions
- better for relaxation or movement
- worse for inactivity

Other symptoms

- tight shoulders and upper back
- irritable, moody or depressed
- pre-menstrual syndrome in teenage girls
- abdominal distension

Pulse: wiry in the Wood position

Tongue: normal

Treatment principles: smooth the Liver and move *qi*; restore descending function of Lungs

> **SUGGESTED TREATMENT**
> **Points**
>
> Liv 14 *qimen*
> GB 34 *yanglingquan*
> Liv 3 *taichong*

Pc 6 *neiguan*
Ren 17 *shanzhong*

Method: sedation needle technique

Points to strengthen Lung *qi* if necessary

Paediatric *tui na* to promote the descending of *qi*

Lung *feijing* (straight pushing tonification)
Central Altar *shanzhong* (pushing apart and straight pushing)
Breast Sides and Breast Root *rupang and rugen* (kneading)
Flanks and Ribs *xielei* (straight pushing)
Lung Transport *jianjiagu* (pushing apart)
Celestial Pillar Bone *tianzhugu* (straight pushing)

Other treatment modalities
Stop coughing point

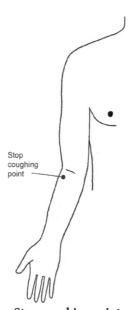

Stop
coughing
point

Stop coughing point

Location: The stop coughing point[16] is located approximately 0.5 cun distal and 0.5 cun lateral to Lu 5 *chize*. It is usually hard and tender on palpation.

Action: This point is used to calm a cough. It can be used in the treatment of both acute and chronic coughs, alongside other points addressing whichever patterns are involved.

Method of use: The point may be needled during a treatment. However, it is most useful in the common situation of a child who is kept awake coughing. The practitioner can mark the location of the point and give the parents some retained needles or press-spheres to place on the point at bedtime, with instructions to remove and safely dispose of them in the morning. Alternatively, the parent can be taught how to massage the point if the child wakes up coughing in the night.

Shonishin
Non-pattern-based core root treatment.

Targeted tapping around the following areas and points:

- supraclavicular fossa region
- Lu 1 *zhongfu*
- Ren 17 *shanzhong*
- Du 12 *shenzhu*

Gua sha

Gua sha over the upper back will help to relieve stagnation of Phlegm in the chest.

Retained needles may be used on the stop coughing point and Bl 13 *feishu*. See Chapter 33 for details on how to use retained needles.

Treatment of the Five Element constitutional imbalance

There is almost always an underlying deficiency of some kind and to some degree in a chronic condition. Even when the child's underlying constitutional imbalance is not in an Organ directly related to the Lungs, treating it can enable the child to throw off the chronic cough.

A Five Element perspective of chronic cough

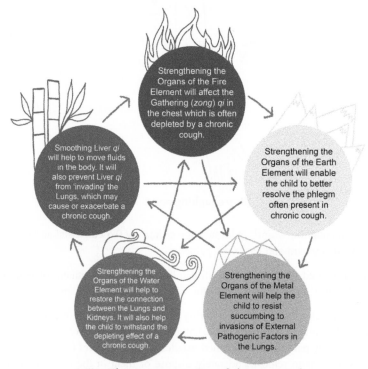

A Five Element perspective of chronic cough

CHECKLIST TO DIAGNOSE AND TREAT A CHRONIC COUGH

» Is the child coughing because Lung *qi* is deficient or because there is Phlegm blocking the descending of Lung *qi*? Or is it a mixture of both?

» What is the treatment priority? Is it to clear the Phlegm or to treat the underlying imbalance? Is it possible to do both simultaneously?

» What techniques can be used to help stop the cough in the short term whilst the underlying patterns of imbalance are treated?

» What is the child's constitutional imbalance and does this need to be treated?

CASE HISTORY: THREE-YEAR-OLD BOY WITH A CHRONIC COUGH

This case history illustrates an example of how to approach the treatment of a Lingering Pathogenic Factor.

Thomas had been coughing almost non-stop for three months when he came to the clinic. The cough had begun two weeks after he started going to nursery. He coughed all day but especially badly at night. Thomas looked in surprisingly robust health, but his family were exhausted.

Thomas's cough sounded like a harsh bark. He did not bring up any mucus. He had red cheeks, red lips and a puffy face. He had always had a voracious appetite, which had only slightly diminished since the cough had started.

- Pulse: slippery, wiry and full
- Tongue: red with a sticky coat

Diagnosis: Lingering pathogen of Phlegm-Heat in the Lungs

Treatments 1, 2 and 3: Loosen Thick Phlegm and descend Lung *qi*

I saw Thomas weekly for treatment.

M-HN-30 *bailao*, Bl 13 *feishu*, Ren 22 *tiantu* with sedation needle technique, flash cupping on upper back

I taught his mother a paediatric *tui na* routine focused on descending Lung *qi* and resolving Phlegm.

Treatments 4 and 5: Resolve Phlegm and descend Lung·*qi*

Thomas's cough had changed in nature. It was less barking and the mucus was looser.

Lu 5 *chize*, Ren 17 *shanzhong*, Bl 13 *feishu* (sedation needle technique)

I advised Thomas's mother to continue the *tui na* routine.

Treatment 6: Resolve Phlegm and descend Lung *qi*

Thomas had been coughing much less during the day but was still coughing a lot at night. The cough still sounded less harsh than it had originally and there was now less mucus apparent.

Lu 7 *lieque*, St 40 *fenglong*, Lu 1 *zhongfu* (sedation needle technique)

Thomas's mother was given a revised *tui na* routine to strengthen Spleen *qi* and descend Lung *qi*.

Treatment 7: Tonify Spleen *qi*

The cough was virtually resolved. Thomas's red cheeks had gone and he looked quite pale and tired. Treatment was to strengthen the Spleen to help Thomas recover from the ongoing cough.

St 36 *zusanli*, Bl 20 *pishu* (tonification needle technique)

SUMMARY

» Chronic cough is one of the most commonly seen complaints in the clinic.

» The key Organs involved are the Lungs and Spleen.

» Lung *qi* failing to descend is always an aspect of chronic cough. This may either be due to a deficiency or an excess.

» The most common causes of cough in babies and toddlers are: repeated invasion of External Pathogenic Factors; diet; and vaccinations.

» In older children, emotional causes, and excessive exercise and studying, are commonly seen causes.

» The patterns are: Phlegm in the Lungs; Lung and Spleen *qi* deficiency; Lingering Pathogenic Factor; and Liver *qi* stagnation insults the Lungs.

» There is often an emotional component to a chronic cough.

» Treatment of the child's Five Element constitutional imbalance is an important part of treatment in a child with a chronic cough.

• Chapter 53 •

ASTHMA

· · · · · · · · · · · · · · · ·

The topics discussed in this chapter are:

- Organs involved in asthma

- Aetiology, compounding factors and triggers

- Patterns

- Other treatment modalities

- The treatment of the child's Five Element constitutional imbalance in asthma

Introduction

Asthma in children is not only prevalent but, at its worst, life-threatening. It may have an impact on the child's ability to live a 'normal' life. Many parents are also aware of the well-documented side effects of the medication their child relies upon to manage his asthma.

Acupuncture can help an asthmatic child in several ways. At best, the disease can be successfully treated. At the very least, flare-ups may become less frequent and less severe. Treatment can also help a child to lessen his dependency on asthma medication and sometimes to eradicate his need for it altogether.

In most cases, the sooner after the onset of the asthma the child comes for treatment, the shorter the course of treatment needs to be. There may be setbacks along the way, but in many cases the parent and child will see some improvement early on. This will be an enormous relief and should inspire them to carry on treatment during the setbacks.

RED FLAGS: ASTHMA

An acute asthma attack is a potentially life-endangering situation. Any of the following signs indicate that the child should immediately receive orthodox medical intervention:

- ✓ rapidly worsening breathlessness

- ✓ very rapid breathing

- ✓ very rapid heart rate

- ✓ reluctance to talk because of breathlessness

- ✓ need to sit upright and still to assist breathing

- ✓ cyanosis.

Asthma medication

Most children with asthma manage the condition with two types of inhalers, often used with a spacer device.* Preventer inhalers are used on a regular basis, usually twice a day. Reliever inhalers are used when the symptoms worsen. The medication contained in both preventer and reliever inhalers often gives a child a burst of energy that makes her feel good. This can present problems when it comes to a child being weaned off her inhalers. She may feel temporarily awful and desperate for another puff. A conversation with the parent and child (depending on her age) about this problem beforehand can be useful. If the child then develops behaviour designed to ensure she gets her fix, it will be easier for the parent to resist.

Another issue that often arises when a child's asthma medication is being reduced is panic and anxiety. A child may become suddenly breathless and wheezy at the moment she realises she has left her inhaler at home. Therefore, it may be wise for a child to keep her inhaler with her for some time after she has stopped using it.

This chapter will describe the treatment of chronic asthma. However, see Chapter 70 for a guide to the treatment of a child through an acute asthma attack.

Organs involved in asthma

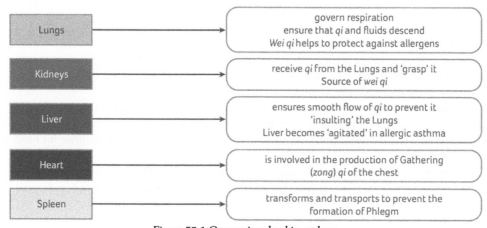

Figure 53.1 Organs involved in asthma

---

* Spacers are large, empty devices that may be used with an inhaler. They help to ensure the child gets the right dose of medicine and that it goes straight to the lungs.

Aetiology, compounding factors and triggers
Aetiology

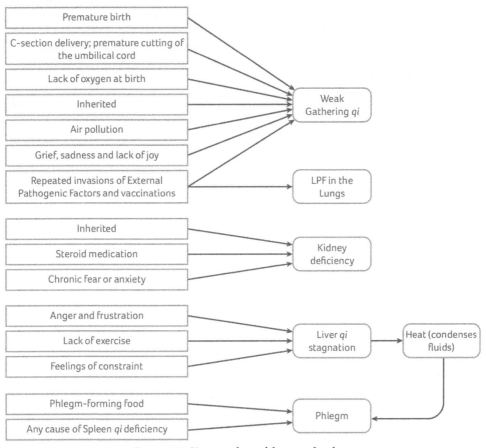

Figure 53.2 Key aetiological factors of asthma

Compounding factors

- **Lack of nurture:** Weakens the Spleen, possibly leading to the formation of Phlegm, which is a common component of childhood asthma.

- **Too much school work:** School work requires *qi* of the Spleen, Heart and Kidneys. Excessive amounts of study may mean the physical body suffers.

- **Over-scheduling:** A child who has every second of his day planned out for him, and who rushes from one activity to the next, often feels constrained and stressed. Depending on the child's nature, this may lead to his Liver *qi* being constrained and/or a depletion of his Kidney *qi*. Both of these patterns may be involved in asthma.

- **Foods which weaken the Spleen and produce Phlegm:** Many cases of asthma involve Phlegm which has derived from a Spleen *qi* deficiency and is lodged in the chest. It is very common for children to have diets containing cold foods, dairy products and sugar, all of which tend to weaken the Spleen or directly produce Phlegm in the body. Changing a child's diet, particularly in babies and toddlers, is sometimes enough in itself to bring about an enormous improvement.

- **Lack of running around outside:** It is such a simple thing for a child to have time running around outside in relatively clean and fresh air, yet so many children do not have this in their lives. This may be because they live in a polluted city, there are fears about 'stranger danger' or simply that lives are so structured that there is not enough time for it. Yet both using the Lungs and being outside strengthen Lung *qi* which helps to guard against the development of asthma. Once a child already has asthma, running around may be a trigger for an asthma attack. Even then, other outdoor activities can be helpful in strengthening the child's Lung *qi*.

- **Too much screen time:** Stooping over a computer, mobile device or even a book encourages bad posture. If the child's shoulders are hunched, he will not breathe properly and Lung *qi* will be weakened as a result.

Triggers

The following list describes triggers that may set off an asthma attack in a child. Once the underlying patterns are addressed with treatment, then the list of triggers for each individual child may become shorter, and the symptoms it triggers less severe.

- **High emotion:** This will have a particular impact on a child's asthma when the pattern of Liver *qi* or Liver Fire insulting the Lungs is involved.

- **Change in the weather or a sudden change in temperature:** This will also exacerbate any Liver pattern because the Liver, when imbalanced, has difficulty dealing with change. Sudden temperature changes (particularly when it suddenly becomes cold) may also be a problem when the Lung deficiency means there is insufficient *wei* (defensive) *qi* at the surface of the body.

- **Foods or food additives:** There is a wide range of foods which may trigger asthma in children. Some of the most common are milk and dairy products, eggs, nuts, seeds, shellfish, wheat and soya. Food additives, especially sulphites, tartrazine, monosodium glutamate and aspartame, may also be an asthma trigger. A child may respond to any of the above triggers by producing large amounts of Heat or Phlegm, for example.

- **Pollen, moulds and fungi:** A child may have a 'Heat response' to pollen which may worsen his asthma. A common reaction to moulds and fungi is for a child to produce a lot of Damp/Phlegm.

- **A cold or cough:** An invasion of Wind-Cold or Wind-Heat may exacerbate asthma symptoms because it disturbs the descending movement of *qi* in the Lungs. It may result in a Hot Lingering Pathogenic Factor, or lead to the production of Phlegm in the chest as the flow of fluids is interrupted.

- **Pollution:** Walking near heavy traffic, for example, may trigger an asthma attack, as the child's Lungs have to work hard to rid themselves of the pollutants in the air.

- **Smells** such as paint or cleaning materials may affect the Lungs via their sense orifice, the nose.

- **Animals:** It is common for asthma to be triggered by dogs, horses or cats.

- **Indoor triggers** such as central heating and house dust mites cause the Liver to 'flare', which may then affect the Lungs.

Table 53.1 Causes, compounding factors and triggers for asthma

Underlying causes	Compounding factors	Triggers
Premature birth	Lack of nurture	High emotion
Other birth factors	Too much school work	Changes in weather or temperature
Repeated chest infections	Over-scheduling	Food or food additives
Infections treated with antibiotics	Lack of running around	Pollen, moulds and fungi
	Lack of fresh air	Coughs and colds
Vaccinations	Too much screen time	Pollution
Inherited factors	A diet which does not support the Spleen	Smells
Emotional factors		Animals
		Indoor triggers

Patterns

- Lung *qi* deficiency (and possibly the Spleen, Heart and/or Kidneys)
- Damp-Phlegm in the Lungs (which may also be Hot)
- Thick Phlegm in the Lungs
- Constrained Liver *qi* affecting the Lungs

All of these patterns are commonly seen in the clinic. A common scenario is a child who has a combination of Phlegm or Thick Phlegm in the Lungs, with underlying deficiency of the Lungs, and possibly the Spleen, Heart or Kidneys too. Constrained Liver *qi* affecting the Lungs tends to be more common in older children. It may occur on its own or be combined with one of the Phlegm patterns.

Lung *qi* deficiency

Breathing symptoms

- shortness of breath
- worse on exertion
- worse when tired and when exposed to cold air

Other symptoms: pale face, easily tired by physical exertion, doesn't like the cold, clear nasal mucus, propensity to catching colds and coughs

Pulse: deficient

Tongue: pale

Treatment principles: tonify and warm Lung *qi*; restore descending function of the Lungs

Variations
There may also be:

- Spleen *qi* deficiency: in which case there may be poor appetite, loose stools and propensity to clear mucus.

- Kidney deficiency: in which case the child may struggle on the in-breath, urinate during or after an asthma attack, be easily overstimulated, struggle to drop off to sleep or wake up early. He may wet the bed and lack physical resilience. This is especially common in older children who have been on steroids for the treatment of their asthma.

- Heart *qi* deficiency: in which case the child may have poor sleep, be lacking in joy and easily upset.

SUGGESTED TREATMENT

Any point on the Lung channel may be used to strengthen Lung *qi*, when it is needled with the tonification technique. Typically, two points per treatment are usually sufficient.

Points

> Lu 9 *taiyuan*
> Lu 7 *lieque*
> Lu 1 *zhongfu*
> Bl 13 *feishu*

Additional points to strengthen the Spleen, Heart and/or Kidneys when necessary

Method: tonification needle technique

Other techniques: moxibustion on any of the above points

Paediatric *tui na* to strengthen Lung *qi* and promote the descending of *qi*

> Lung *feijing* (straight pushing tonification)
> Breast Sides and Breast Root *rupang and rugen* (kneading)
> Flanks and Ribs *xielei* (straight pushing)
> Lung Transport *jianjiagu* (pushing apart)
> Celestial Pillar Bone *tianzhugu* (straight pushing)
> Additional moves to strengthen the Spleen and/or Kidneys when necessary

Damp-Phlegm in the Lungs

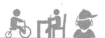

Key symptoms

- difficulty breathing because of large amounts of mucus

- cough with mucus which is easy to expectorate

- cough is bad when lying down and first thing in the morning

Other symptoms: clear or white nasal mucus, puffy skin, feels lethargic and heavy, tends towards feeling cold

Pulse: slippery

Tongue: thick, white coat

Treatment principles: resolve Phlegm; restore descending function of the Lungs

If there is already a substantial amount of mucus on the child's chest, do not use St 40 *fenglong*, which may stir up more mucus. Instead, use points to help descend the Phlegm. The most effective ones are:

> » Ren 22 *tiantu*

> » Lu 7 *lieque*

Variations

- Phlegm-Heat: If the Phlegm is Hot, there will be coloured mucus that is difficult to expectorate, redness somewhere on the face and a barking cough.

- Phlegm and Accumulation Disorder: In babies and toddlers, Phlegm may derive from Accumulation Disorder, in which case there will be irregular, foul-smelling stools, irritability and bad temper, and green around the mouth.

SUGGESTED TREATMENT

It is important to always use one or more points to descend *qi* when resolving Phlegm in the chest. A typical treatment may be Ren 22 *tiantu*, Lu 7 *lieque* and St 40 *fenglong*, followed by flash cupping on the upper back. The aim is to clear the Phlegm downwards, rather than upwards.

It may also be necessary to tonify the Spleen in order to help the child move the fluids.

Points

> Lu 5 *chize*
> Lu 7 *lieque*
> Lu 10 *yuji* (for Phlegm-Heat)
> Ren 22 *tiantu*
> St 40 *fenglong*

Method: sedation needle technique

Disperse Accumulation Disorder when present (using M-UE-9 *sifeng*)

Other techniques

Gua sha or flash cupping on the back may be used to open up the chest.

Paediatric *tui na* to resolve Phlegm and promote the descending of *qi*

> Lung *feijing* (straight pushing sedation)
> Eight Trigrams *bagua* (circular pushing anti-clockwise)
> Small Palmar Crease *zhangxiaowen* (straight pushing)
> Hand *yin yang shouyinyang* (pushing apart)
> Central Altar *shanzhong* (pushing apart and straight pushing)
> Breast Sides and Breast Root *rupang and rugen* (kneading)
> Flanks and Ribs *xielei* (straight pushing)
> Lung Transport *jianjiagu* (pushing apart)
> Celestial Pillar Bone *tianzhugu* (straight pushing)
> St 40 Abundant Bulge *fenglong* (kneading)

Thick Phlegm in the Lungs

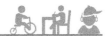

Symptoms

- difficulty breathing with a feeling of tightness in the chest

- wheezing

- no apparent mucus

- harsh-sounding cough

- may be an allergic component to the asthma

- asthma may occur when the child is particularly tired or stressed

Pulse: wiry

Tongue: may have a thick coat

Treatment principles: loosen and resolve Thick Phlegm; restore descending function of the Lungs; strengthen the underlying deficiency

The order in which these treatment principles should be addressed will depend upon the degree of underlying deficiency in the child. In most cases it is necessary to begin with strengthening the child.

> **SUGGESTED TREATMENT**
> It is usually necessary to alternate between the three treatment principles. See Chapter 27 for a further discussion of how to treat a Lingering Pathogenic Factor.
>
> **Points**
> To loosen Thick Phlegm:
>
> > Bl 13 *feishu*
> > M-HN-30 *bailao*
>
> **Method:** sedation needle technique
>
> To resolve Phlegm:
>
> > Lu 5 *chize*
> > Lu 7 *lieque*
> > St 40 *fenglong*
> > Ren 22 *tiantu*
>
> **Method:** sedation needle technique
>
> To tonify Lung and/or Spleen *qi*:
>
> > St 36 *zusanli*
> > Bl 20 *pishu*
> > Lu 9 *taiyuan*
> > Bl 13 *feishu*
>
> **Method:** tonification needle technique
>
> **Other techniques:** *Gua sha* or light cupping on the back may be used to open up the chest
>
> **Paediatric *tui na***
> It may be necessary to combine the two routines above (one to strengthen the underlying deficiency, the other to resolve Phlegm), or to begin with one and then move on to another.

Constrained Liver *qi* affecting the Lungs

This pattern is most common in older children (from the age of about seven or eight).

Qi stagnation often moves to the place in the body where there is most deficiency, as if to fill the void and act as a kind of protection. Therefore, it may also be necessary to strengthen Lung *qi* in this pattern.

Symptoms

- difficulty breathing with a tightness in the chest

- upper back and shoulders are tight

- breathing is worse when the child experiences intense emotions or when there are intense emotions in the environment

- asthma has an allergic trigger

- no signs of mucus

Pulse: wiry, especially on the Wood pulses

Tongue: normal or slightly red on the sides

Treatment principles: smooth the Liver and move *qi*; restore descending function of the Lungs

> **SUGGESTED TREATMENT**
> It is usually sufficient to use two or three points per treatment.
>
> **Points**
>
> Pc 6 *neiguan*
> GB 34 *yanglingquan*
> Liv 3 *taichong*
> Ren 17 *shanzhong*
>
> **Method:** sedation needle technique
>
> Points to strengthen Lung *qi* if necessary
>
> **Paediatric *tui na*** to promote the descending of *qi*
>
> Lung *feijing* (straight pushing tonification)
> Central Altar *shanzhong* (pushing apart and straight pushing)
> Breast Sides and Breast Root *rupang and rugen* (kneading)
> Flanks and Ribs *xielei* (straight pushing)
> Lung Transport *jianjiagu* (pushing apart)
> Celestial Pillar Bone *tianzhugu* (straight pushing)

Other treatment modalities
Shonishin
Core non-pattern-based root treatment.

Targeted tapping around the following areas and points:

- supraclavicular fossa region

- Lu 1 *zhongfu*

- Ren 17 *shanzhong*

- Du 12 *shenzhu*

Extra points

- **Asthma *shu* point:** The asthma *shu* point[17] is located slightly lateral and superior to Bl 17 *geshu*. It is very often tender and knotted on children who have breathing difficulties. Leaving a press-sphere or retained needle on this point may be helpful for a child with asthma.

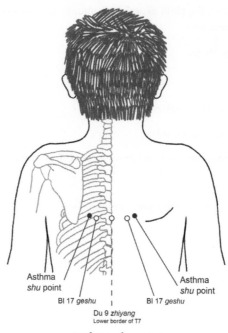

Asthma *shu* point

- **Stop coughing point:** Asthma often involves a cough. The stop coughing point is located slightly distal and lateral to Lu 5 *chize* (see Chapter 32).[18] The child will usually wince slightly when it is palpated, and it feels hard and knotted to touch. When a child's asthma manifests with a cough, this point can be needled or a press-sphere left on it.

- **M-BW-1 *dingchuan*:** This point is most commonly used in the treatment of acute asthma, and its use is described in detail in Chapter 32.

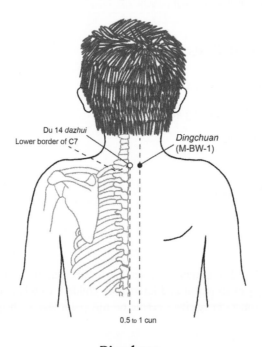

Dingchuan

The treatment of the child's Five Element constitutional imbalance in asthma

As practitioners of Chinese medicine, we are used to thinking of emotions as a cause of illness. Asthma, however, is a disease that has long been thought of by the orthodox medical profession as having an emotional component. The chairman of the British Lung Foundation, Dr Mark Britton, wrote, 'Asthma and a patient's personality and emotions are very intrinsically bound up with each other.'[19] It is also widely acknowledged, and recognised by many asthma sufferers, that intense emotions and stress may precipitate an asthma attack.

There is often a sense in a child with asthma that he is 'holding in' a lot of feelings, and that those feelings are sitting on his chest and make breathing difficult. The feelings may be of almost any variety.

A child's asthma often stems from the Organs associated with his constitutional imbalance. However, this is not always the case and so should not be assumed. When it is the case, treatment of the Element of the constitutional imbalance often produces the most profound and long-lasting improvements in the child's symptoms.

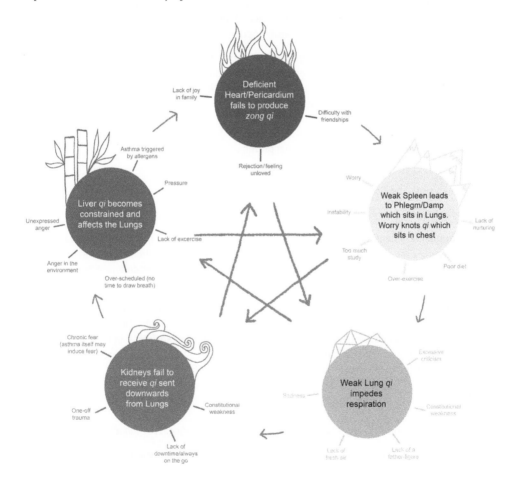

CHECKLIST TO DIAGNOSE AND TREAT ASTHMA

» Is there a pathogen involved that needs to be cleared? If so, what is its nature?

» Does the underlying deficiency affect only the Lungs? Or is there another Organ involved?

> » Which needs to be addressed first – the pathogen or the underlying deficiency?
>
> » What is the child's constitutional imbalance? What part does that play in the asthma?
>
> » Apart from acupuncture, what other modalities will be most useful to treat this child's asthma?

CASE HISTORY: ELEVEN-YEAR-OLD GIRL WITH ASTHMA AND A CONSTITUTIONAL FIRE IMBALANCE

This case history illustrates:

- how intense emotions in the family may become a cause of disease in children
- the importance of treating the constitutional imbalance in chronic disease.

Mel had been diagnosed with asthma at the age of three. She had relied heavily on both preventer and reliever inhalers ever since. Her asthma was triggered by stress, changes in the weather and certain allergens such as cats and pollens. She suffered from chronic wheezing and tightness in the chest, as well as occasional acute asthma attacks. She took a long time to get off to sleep and was prone to mild anxiety. She was otherwise in good health.

Observations: Mel was small for her age and had a thin body with a weak-looking chest. She seemed very lacking in joy, but her demeanour changed dramatically when she smiled and laughed. She would quickly sink back into a profound lack of joy. She had a lack of red colour around her eyes and her voice tone was flat.

Pulse:

- choppy Pericardium and Triple Burner pulses
- deficient Lung and Large Intestine pulses
- wiry Liver and Gallbladder pulses

Tongue: pale

Background: Mel's parents were in the process of divorcing when she first came for treatment. Her mother told me that Mel's father had rarely shown any interest in her, compared with her brother with whom he shared a lot of interests. She said that there had been an enormous amount of tension in the house for years.

Diagnosis: I diagnosed Mel as having a constitutional imbalance in her Fire Element, based on her lack of joy, lack of red colour and lack of laugh in her voice. I thought this had led to Heart Blood deficiency, evidenced by her mild anxiety and difficulty sleeping. This, in turn, had led to Lung *qi* (specifically *zong qi*) deficiency which was causing the shortness of breath. The allergic component to her asthma manifested as constrained Liver *qi* affecting the Lungs.

Treatment

Treatment 1

Yuan source points of Organs related to constitutional imbalance: TB 4 *yangchi*, Pc 7 *daling*

Needling these points with the tonification technique strengthened the pulse of the related Organs. It also reduced the wiry quality of the Wood pulse.

Treatment 2

Ki 24 *lingxu**** (to strengthen both the Fire Element and *zong qi* to help the asthma)

---

* Ki 24 *lingxu* treats the Fire Element as well as the Kidneys. The word *ling*, in the name of the point, is often translated as 'spirit'. It is thought of as the *yin* counterpart to the *shen*.

> *Luo* connecting points TB 5 *waiguan*, Pc 6 *neiguan* (to strengthen the Fire Element). Pc 6 has a particular effect on the *qi* of the chest.
>
> *Treatment 3*
>
> Bl 43 *gaohuangshu* to nourish the *qi* of all the Organs in the Upper Burner
>
> Tonification points TB 3 *zhongzhu*, Pc 9 *zhongchong* (to further strengthen the Fire Element). As tonification points, these points also helped to pull *qi* from the Wood Element into the Fire Element.
>
> Treatment continued along these lines and Mel's asthma became less and less of a problem. She also became less anxious and seemed to enjoy life more. Interestingly, I never needed to treat her Liver *qi* stagnation directly. Treating the Fire constitutional imbalance brought about harmony in all the other Elements.

SUMMARY

» Any of the following Organs may be involved in asthma: Lungs; Kidneys; Liver; Heart; and Spleen. The Lungs are always involved.

» There are usually a mix of aetiological factors combined with other factors which compound the condition and trigger the symptoms.

» The patterns involved are: deficiency of the Lungs; Phlegm in the Lungs; Thick Phlegm in the Lungs; and Constrained Liver *qi* affecting the Lungs.

» Treatment of the Five Element constitutional imbalance can be beneficial in the treatment of asthma.

Chapter 54

ECZEMA
. . . .

The topics discussed in this chapter are:

- Aetiology and pathology

- Pathogens involved in eczema

- Underlying deficiencies

- The pathology and treatment of itching

- Pulling it all together

- Eczema in babies and toddlers

- Eczema in school-age children

- Eczema in teenagers

Introduction

> On a bad night, we are up five, six, seven times. I am unable to soothe her. She screams, she writhes, she tears at her skin, her hand coverings, her clothing. Whatever I try doesn't help. We pace the floor together. We change her bandages. We try a bath. We try going outside. These are the nights I fear, when the bedclothes might be covered in blood, when she howls in agony, yelling, 'please make it stop'.[20]

This description by a mother of her daughter's eczema, albeit a particularly bad case, gives a powerful insight into the profound impact that a skin condition may have on both child and parent. For the child, the itching can be incessant and is often worse at night so it disturbs sleep too. For the parent, the feelings of helplessness can be hard to bear. For older children, there is the added component of the self-consciousness that a skin condition may induce.

Skin conditions are said to affect 10 per cent of all infants to some degree or another. The most common labels given are eczema, psoriasis or dermatitis. Whatever the particular nature of the condition, and whichever name it has been given, a diagnosis must be made according to which pathogens and Organs are involved.

Most authors agree that it is especially hard to predict the length of treatment needed and the possible outcome when treating a child with eczema.[21] There are usually ups and downs along the way, and a degree of perseverance may be required from parents. Treatment usually needs to be combined with some lifestyle and dietary changes. Whilst parents should be made aware of the fact that it may take time to bring about lasting changes, the potential rewards are enormous. When a bad case of eczema clears up, a child's spirit is able to blossom and life for the child and the family is irrevocably improved.

The orthodox medical approach to the treatment of childhood eczema is usually a regime of emollients, topical steroids and wet wraps. Many parents who bring their child to the clinic are, understandably, concerned about the long-term use of steroids.

Triggers

> I once wrote down the things that triggered Astrid's eczema: dust, animal hair, nuts, eggs, perfume, cleaning and laundry products, flour, soil, sand, bedding, pillows, cushions, soap, carpets, curtains, wool, synthetic fibres, paint, glue, leaves, seeds, wood smoke, petrol, the seams of clothing, lace trim, chlorine, soft toys, rope, firelighters, plastic cutlery, elastic, erasers, sea water, feathers, tree pollen, grass, plant sap, mould.[22]

As the above passage shows, the possible triggers for a child's eczema are almost limitless. For some children, it severely impedes their ability to live a full life. For others, there may only be one or two triggers and they are ones which are relatively easy to avoid. It is always useful for a parent to identify the triggers which make their child's eczema flare up if, indeed, there are any (in some children the eczema is just permanently there and does not vary much in its severity). However, the need to avoid these triggers should always be weighed up against the emotional cost that may result.

The aim of treatment should be to strengthen the underlying deficiencies of the child and clear the pathogens, so that she no longer reacts in the same way when she comes into contact with what were once triggers.

Aetiology and pathology
The Spleen

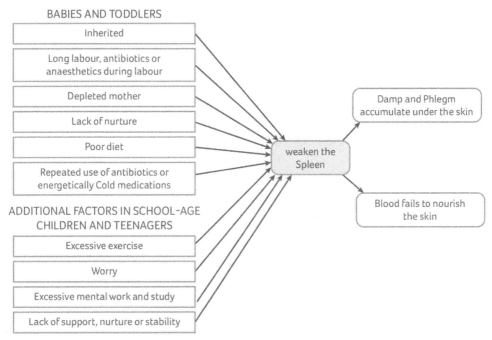

Figure 54.1 The Spleen and eczema

The Lungs

Inherited
Recurrent infections
Sadness and loss
Premature or difficult birth
Lung *qi* deficiency
Defensive (*wei*) *qi* fails to circulate and protect the skin

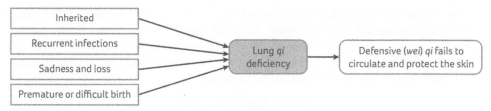

Figure 54.2 The Lungs and eczema

The Liver

BABIES AND TODDLERS
Inherited
Foetal toxins
Suppressed fevers
Accumulation Disorder
ADDITIONAL FACTORS IN SCHOOL-AGE CHILDREN AND TEENAGERS
Repressed anger and frustration
Pressure and constraint
Lack of exercise
Food additives
Drugs and alcohol
block smooth flow of Liver *qi*
Heat in the Blood which affects the skin

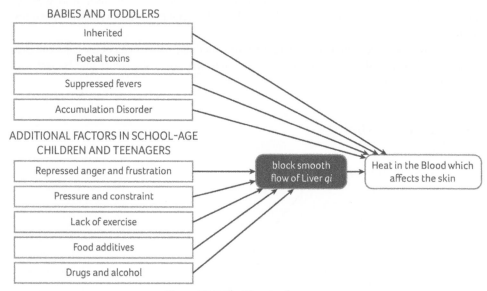

Figure 54.3 The Liver and eczema

The Kidneys

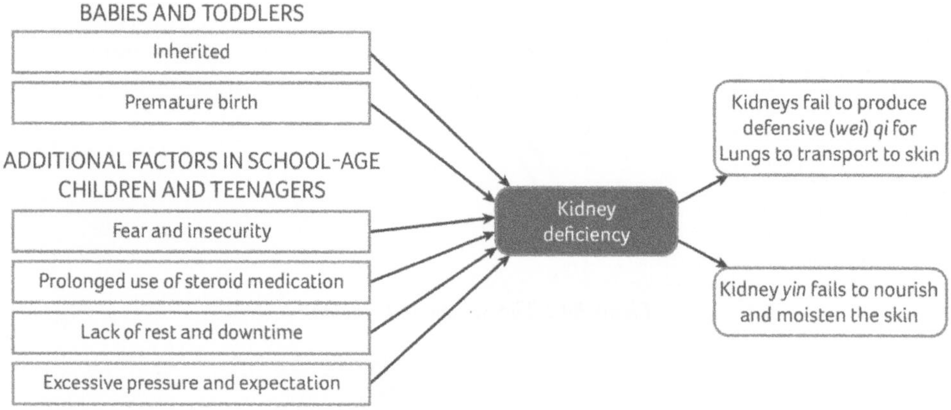

BABIES AND TODDLERS
Inherited
Premature birth
ADDITIONAL FACTORS IN SCHOOL-AGE CHILDREN AND TEENAGERS
Fear and insecurity
Prolonged use of steroid medication
Lack of rest and downtime
Excessive pressure and expectation
Kidney deficiency
Kidneys fail to produce defensive (*wei*) *qi* for Lungs to transport to skin
Kidney *yin* fails to nourish and moisten the skin

Figure 54.4 The Kidneys and eczema

The Heart

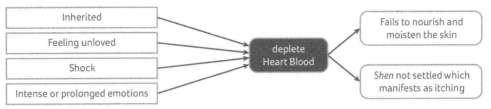

Figure 54.5 The Heart and eczema

A word about inherited tendency

Eczema is part of what doctors often refer to as an 'atopic triad', which also includes asthma and hay fever. It is very common for one or both of the parents of a child with eczema to have one of these conditions, or to have had it in the past. Maciocia understands this tendency in terms of a deficiency of the defensive (*wei*) *qi* system of the Lungs and Kidneys.[23]

Emotional factors

Prolonged or intense emotions distort the proper movements of *qi*. This may lead to a pathology in the particular Organ involved (as can be seen in Figures 54.1–54.5) which makes a child prone to eczema. There is, however, another aspect to the link between emotions and eczema. The very fact of suffering from eczema in itself creates prolonged and intense emotions. This is of course the case for many illnesses. However, skin conditions bring with them a particularly heavy emotional burden, especially in children who are old enough to have developed a level of self-consciousness. When I asked children in the clinic how having eczema made them feel, some of their replies were as follows: 'mad', 'itchy', 'sad', 'upset', 'different', 'frustrated', 'self-conscious', 'uncomfortable'.

Sometimes a child's emotional response to her eczema becomes habituated and continues even when the eczema becomes less of a problem. The effect that the particular emotion has on the child's *qi* then perpetuates the presence of her eczema. In this situation, treatment of the Element related to the emotion involved may have a beneficial effect.

Pathogens involved in eczema

In all cases of eczema, something is blocking the smooth flow of *qi* and Blood to the skin. Scott and Barlow write that, 'for eczema to occur, there must be something preventing good circulation of blood – or preventing circulation of good blood – to the skin'.[24] There are four possibilities as to what this might be, namely Damp, Thick Phlegm, Heat or Wind.

 These pathogens often combine in a child with eczema. For example, there may be Damp and Heat, or Wind and Thick Phlegm.

Damp

Whatever other patterns are present, there is nearly always a degree of Dampness under the surface of the skin involved in eczema. If Damp accumulates in the child's body, it may find a resting place in the *cou li*, the space between the skin and the muscles. The characteristics of eczema from Damp are:

- eczema is often localised, for example only on the wrists

- it oozes after scratching

- there may be vesicles or papules present.

The child will often have other symptoms of Damp, such as:

- mucus in the chest

- nasal discharge

- puffy skin.

Treatment principles: resolve Damp

> **SUGGESTED TREATMENT**
> **Points**
> When resolving Damp, it can be helpful to use points in whichever Burner the Damp is located in. The points here are focused largely on the Middle Burner. If there is Damp in the Upper Burner, Ren 17 *shanzhong* or Lu 7 *lieque* may be added. If Damp is in the Lower Burner, Ren 3 *zhongji* or Bl 22 *sanjiaoshu* may be added.
>
> Sp 9 *yinlingquan*
> Sp 6 *sanyinjiao*
> Ren 9 *shuifen*
> Ren 12 *zhongwan*
>
> **Method:** sedation needle technique

Thick Phlegm

If Thick Phlegm is lodged underneath the skin, this also prevents the flow of *qi* and Blood to the surface of the body. In this case, however, the child may have no other obvious signs of Phlegm or Damp. The Phlegm is thick and hard, so does not flow and produce overt symptoms. The eczema is usually dry and will not ooze, but may be very itchy. Other indications of the presence of Thick Phlegm in the system are hard nodules in the glands of the neck.

Treatment principles: soften and resolve Thick Phlegm

> **SUGGESTED TREATMENT**
> **Points**
>
> M-HN-30 *bailao*
> GB 34 *yanglingquan*
> Extra point *pigen*
> St 40 *fenglong*
>
> **Method:** sedation needle technique
>
> See Chapter 27 for a further discussion of the treatment of Thick Phlegm.

Heat

Heat is often present in atopic eczema. This is an inflammatory condition and is confirmed by blood tests which reveal a high level of IgE antibodies. Heat may disrupt the flow of *qi* and Blood to the skin. The characteristics of eczema from Heat are:

- redness

- eczematous patches that look and feel hot

- it is itchy and uncomfortable

- it bleeds on scratching.

Heat may be in the Lungs, Stomach, Liver or Heart. Symptoms will vary according to which Organ or Organs are affected. General symptoms and signs are:

- irritability and restlessness
- poor sleep
- red face.

However, Heat may just be in the Blood and therefore only affect the skin. In this case, the child will not have any other Heat symptoms.

Treatment principles: clear Heat; cool the Blood

> **SUGGESTED TREATMENT**
> **Points**
>
>> Sp 10 *xuehai*
>> LI 11 *quchi*
>
> Other points should be added depending on which Organ or Organs are affected.
>
>> Lungs: Lu 5 *chize* or Lu 10 *yuji*
>> Stomach: St 44 *neiting*
>> Liver: Liv 2 *xingjian*
>> Heart: He 8 *shaofu*
>
> **Method:** sedation needle technique

Wind

Chinese medicine talks of two types of Wind, namely external Wind (which causes colds and coughs, etc.) and internal Wind (which causes tremors and convulsions, etc.). However, there is a third type of Wind which is neither internal nor external, but is more closely related to external.[25] This Wind settles in the skin and can be a component of skin conditions. It causes the following characteristics:

- eczema which suddenly flares up, and continually changes in severity and location
- itching
- dryness.

Treatment principles: expel Wind

> **SUGGESTED TREATMENT**
> **Points**
>
>> Du 20 *baihui*
>> GB 20 *fengchi*
>> LI 4 *hegu*
>> Lu 7 *lieque*
>> Du 16 *fengfu*
>> Liv 3 *taichong*
>
> **Method:** sedation needle technique

No pathogen

If the child does not have any of the above pathogens, the pattern involved will usually be *qi* and Blood deficiency. The characteristics of the eczema are:

- dry and flaky skin

- eczema is relatively pale looking

- less intense itching

- no lesions

- may be worse at night

- relatively constant in severity and location.

Table 54.1 Pathogens involved in eczema

Pathogen	Nature of eczema
Damp	Oozing, clammy skin, swollen
Thick Phlegm	Dry, no oozing, very itchy
Heat	Red, hot, itchy, uncomfortable
Wind	Sudden flare-ups, eczema comes and goes, dry, itchy
No pathogen	Dry, flaky, not itchy, not red

Underlying deficiencies

As can be seen in the aetiologies and pathologies discussed, there may be a deficiency of any Organ in a child with eczema. The deficiencies that are most often seen in the clinic are:

- Spleen *qi* deficiency

- Blood deficiency

- Kidney and Lung defensive (*wei*) *qi* deficiency

Spleen *qi* deficiency

Symptoms

- loose stools

- pale

- easily tires

- poor appetite

Pulse: deficient

Tongue: pale

Treatment principles: tonify Spleen *qi*

> **SUGGESTED TREATMENT**
> It is usually sufficient to use one or two points per treatment.
>
> **Points**
>
> St 36 *zusanli*
> Sp 3 *taibai*
> Ren 12 *zhongwan*
> Bl 20 *pishu*

Method: tonification needle technique

Other techniques: moxibustion

Paediatric *tui na*

Spleen *pijing* (straight pushing)
Thick Gate *banmen* (straight pushing)
Three Passes *sanguan* (straight pushing)
Knead the Navel *rou qi* (kneading anti-clockwise)
Spinal Column *jizhu* (pinching from the bottom to the top of the back)
St 36 *zusanli* (kneading)

Blood deficiency

Key symptoms

- poor sleep

- easily upset

- tendency towards anxiety

- pale

Other symptoms and signs will depend on the Organ or Organs causing or most affected by the Blood deficiency.

Pulse: thin and/or deficient

Tongue: pale and maybe thin

Treatment principles: nourish Blood

SUGGESTED TREATMENT

Points should be chosen according to which Organ or Organs are causing the Blood deficiency. Bl 17 *geshu* is indicated if the eczema particularly affects the upper part of the body. Sp 10 *xuehai* is indicated if the eczema particularly affects the lower part of the body. Two or three points per treatment is usually sufficient.

Points

St 36 *zusanli*
Sp 6 *sanyinjiao*
Bl 20 *pishu*
He 7 *shenmen*
Ki 3 *taixi*
Liv 8 *ququan*
Bl 17 *geshu*
Sp 10 *xuehai*

Other points will depend on the Organ or Organs most affected by the Blood deficiency.

Method: tonification needle technique

Other techniques: moxibustion

Kidney and Lung defensive (*wei*) *qi* deficiency

This is often present in allergic (atopic) asthma.

Symptoms

- eczema starts in early childhood (often in the first six months of life)
- allergic eczema which flares when child comes into contact with allergens
- tendency towards allergies
- rhinitis
- asthma
- pale

Pulse: deficient

Tongue: pale or normal

Treatment principles: tonify and warm Kidney and Lung *qi*

SUGGESTED TREATMENT
Two points per treatment is usually sufficient.

Points

Lu 9 *taiyuan*
Lu 7 *lieque*
Ki 6 *zhaohai*
Bl 13 *feishu*
Bl 23 *shenshu*

Method: tonification needle technique

Paediatric *tui na* to strengthen the Lungs and Kidneys

Lung *feijing* (straight pushing tonification)
Kidney *shenjing* (straight pushing tonification)
Two Men upon a Horse *erma* (kneading)
Lower Back Bl 23 *shenshu* (strong rubbing)
Knead the Navel *rou qi* (kneading anti-clockwise)
Knead Ren 6 *qihai* (kneading anti-clockwise)

Cold inside, hot on the surface

A child with eczema will often appear to be red and hot. Yet it is important not to mistake how she appears on the surface with her internal state. The Spleen and Lungs are often inherently deficient and Cold in a child with eczema. This may be the cause of the build-up of Damp or Phlegm, which then causes local stagnation on the skin. So the local condition may be one of stagnation and Heat, but the internal condition is one of *qi* deficiency.

When this is the case, treatment needs to address both aspects of the condition. In most cases, until the child is stronger, it will be hard to begin to get the *qi* and Blood near the surface of the body moving, so it is often useful to tonify the underlying *qi* deficiency at first, and then begin to add in points to clear the pathogens afterwards.

The pathology and treatment of itching

Itching is not only unpleasant and sometimes disturbing for the child, but it also perpetuates the eczema by leading to scratching which breaks the skin and then prevents healing. Breaking the skin leads to an increased incidence of infection. Any point prescription used on a child who has significantly itchy eczema should include points which specifically stop itching.

The Heart

Chapter 74 of the *Su Wen* says, 'All pain [diseases with] itching and sores, without exception they are associated with the Heart.'[26] Some authors say that to treat itching one must treat the Heart channel.[27] Itching often gets worse when a child is anxious or agitated. Having intensely itchy skin can, on the other hand, cause a child to be agitated (see Figure 54.6).

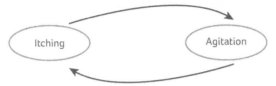

Figure 54.6 Relationship between itching and agitation

The Liver

When the Liver becomes imbalanced, it often manifests with agitation of some kind. In a child with eczema, this may result in itching. Heat in the Liver may cause red, inflamed, angry and itchy eczema. The Liver is often involved in eczema which gets worse when the child is emotionally upset or, in older children, when under stress. In teenage girls, the eczema often gets worse premenstrually.

The Lungs

Zhang Zie Bin said that 'the *po* can move and do things and [when it is active] pain and itching can be felt'.[28] This quote suggests that the *po* may also be involved in itching. This may especially be the case when itching is triggered by an external allergen, or a change in temperature.

> **Points**
> To calm itching:
>
> Sp 10 *xuehai*
> Bl 40 *weizhong*
> M-LE-34 *baichongwo* (1 cun above Sp 10 *xuehai*)
> GB 31 *fengshi*
> Extra point *zhiyangxue* (2 cun above LI 11 *quchi*)
>
> **Method:** sedation needle technique

Pulling it all together

The diagnosis and treatment of eczema should involve the following components:

- stop itching

- clear any pathogens present

- address underlying deficiency.

The degree to which the focus should be on clearing pathogens as opposed to addressing the underlying deficiency will, as always, be determined by symptoms and signs, especially the pulse.

Eczema in babies and toddlers

Accumulation Disorder

The Heat present in eczema in a baby or toddler may stem from Accumulation Disorder. If this is the case, the eczema will be hot and angry, the child red-faced and miserable. The Accumulation Disorder must be treated first by using M-UE-9 *sifeng*. Once the Accumulation Disorder has been dispersed, and the parents given advice on feeding to prevent it coming back, it is usually then necessary to strengthen the Spleen.

Treatment of eczema in babies and toddlers

Shonishin also has to be avoided if a child has extensive eczema as any stroking over the affected areas may exacerbate the condition. However, Birch recommends tapping around the lesions as a form of local treatment.[29] This seems to be effective in helping to clear up any particularly recalcitrant patches as it moves *qi* and Blood locally.

TWO CASE HISTORIES OF ECZEMA IN TWO-YEAR-OLDS WITH VERY DIFFERENT OUTCOMES

Eliza and Jimmy were both two years old when they were brought to the clinic. They had both suffered from eczema since they were a few months old. Eliza's eczema covered almost her entire torso and limbs, whilst Jimmy's was just in the elbow and knee creases. In both cases, the eczema was oozing and itchy.

Diagnosis: Eliza and Jimmy had the same diagnoses: Damp with a background of Spleen *qi* deficiency.

Neither had any other significant symptoms. They were both typically deficient children, evidenced by the fact they were quiet, compliant and rather picky about food.

Treatment: In both cases, I employed the following treatment principles:

- calm itching
- tonify Spleen *qi* deficiency
- resolve Damp.

In both cases, I gave the parents a *tui na* routine focused on addressing the patterns of pathology present. I also gave both parents advice on diet, in particular avoiding Damp-forming foods and incorporating foods to nourish and warm the Spleen.

Outcome: Both Eliza and Jimmy's eczema showed improvement early on in treatment. However, whilst Eliza went from strength to strength, Jimmy seemed to take one step forward and two steps backwards. This was in spite of the fact that his mother made all the necessary changes to his diet and followed the routine of *tui na* conscientiously. Eliza's eczema, which had been far more widespread than Jimmy's initially, showed an 80 per cent improvement after three months of treatment. Jimmy's, on the other hand, had shown no sustained improvement after six months of treatment.

Reflection: Jimmy and Eliza happened to arrive at my clinic around the same time. I was therefore acutely aware of the difference in their responses and reflected on why this should be. In the end, I put it down to the following.

Eliza very noticeably began to assert herself more as her *qi* became stronger with treatment. She became much less compliant and louder, and her mother told me that she had begun having tantrums that were perhaps typical of a child of her age. Jimmy, on the other hand, did not make the same developmental leap. He remained unusually quiescent and well behaved for a two-year-old in spite of treatments to tonify his *qi*. I suspected this may have something to do with

---

having stricter parents and a lack of opportunity for self-expression at home. I will never know for sure but believe it is probably the reason he did not respond so well to treatment.

Eczema in school-age children

All the basic patterns may cause eczema in school-age children. It is also possible for the deficiency to affect the Kidneys in this age group too. Kidney deficiency is more common in school-age children because of a busy school life and extra-curricular activities, which leaves them with little time to rest. The Kidneys play an important role in terms of nourishing and moistening the skin.[30]

Kidney deficiency
Key symptoms and signs

- long-term eczema
- nature of the eczema depends on the pathogens involved
- child is easily tired
- tendency to bedwetting
- may be small or slight for his age
- may lack physical robustness

Pulse: deficient

Other symptoms and signs will depend on whether the Kidney deficiency is more related to *yang* or *yin.*

> **SUGGESTED TREATMENT**
> **Points**
>
> Ki 3 *taixi*
> Ki 6 *zhaohai*
> Ki 7 *fuliu*
> Bl 23 *shenshu*
>
> **Method:** tonification needle technique

Eczema in teenagers

Eczema left untreated through puberty may then stay with the adolescent right the way through until adulthood. Treatment just before and during puberty makes use of a time of flux to potentially expel the pathogens involved and rectify the underlying deficiencies. This is obviously beneficial in terms of health. Equally importantly, it also saves the child from having to navigate the challenging teenage years with eczematous skin. The emotional impact of this can be detrimental and shape how a person feels about themselves.

Triggers for eczema in teenagers

- **The menstrual cycle:** A teenage girl with eczema may find that her skin gets better and worse at certain times of her menstrual cycle. This can help guide our diagnosis and treatment. For example, eczema that gets worse in the pre-menstrual phase often has a component of Heat. Eczema that is worse at the end of the period often has a component of Blood deficiency.

- **Stress:** In older children and teenagers, eczema often flares up during stressful times such as in the run-up to exams or when difficult friendship dynamics are being played out at school. It is important to ascertain which is the predominant emotion that is being triggered by the particular stress, and to treat the associated Organ and Element. For example, if a teenager has had her heart broken and the experience has left her feeling unloved and rejected, we may suspect that the Fire Element will be struggling. If this is confirmed by our findings on the pulse and other symptoms and signs, then the Fire Element should be treated.

HOME REMEDIES

Parents have reported finding the following helpful in the management of their child's eczema:

- » using cold-pressed or virgin coconut oil on the eczematous patches
- » neem cream
- » oatmeal baths.

SUMMARY

- » Any of the *yin* Organs may be involved in childhood eczema. The Spleen and the Lungs are those most commonly involved.
- » Atopic eczema usually involves a deficiency in the *wei qi* system of the Lungs and Kidneys.
- » Emotions may play a part in the pathology of eczema but also arise as a result of having to live with eczema.
- » The key pathogens involved in eczema are: Damp; Thick Phlegm; Heat; and Wind.
- » There may be underlying deficiencies of: Spleen *qi*; Blood; and Kidney and Lung *wei qi*.
- » The Organs involved in itching are: the Heart; the Liver; and the Lungs.
- » In babies and toddlers, Accumulation Disorder may be at the root of eczema.
- » Kidney deficiency is more likely to be present in school-age children with eczema.

• Chapter 55 •

ALLERGIC RHINITIS AND HAY FEVER

The topics discussed in this chapter are:

- Organs and aetiology

- Patterns

- Other treatment modalities

Introduction

Allergic rhinitis is a condition of inflammation of the nose. It is caused by the body over-reacting to certain airborne allergens. It may occur seasonally, when it is usually called hay fever and the child reacts to specific pollens. It may be present all year round, when the child also reacts to other allergens such as pet hair, mould or house dust mites.

The symptoms of allergic rhinitis usually affect the eyes and nose. For some children, the symptoms are more widespread. Figure 55.1 illustrates some of the most commonly seen hay fever symptoms.

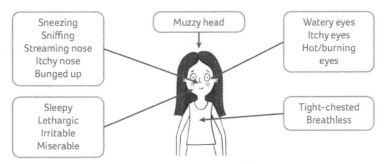

Figure 55.1 Symptoms of allergic rhinitis and hay fever

Although allergic rhinitis is relatively benign and a child often grows out of it, it can be hugely disruptive. The symptoms may make it hard for a child to concentrate in school. For a child in whom the symptoms are set off by pollen, the time of year when he is at his worst often coincides with school exams. It can prevent a child from being able to go outside and play in the summer months. However, many parents do not want their child to become reliant on anti-histamine medication.

There are two main aspects in the treatment of allergic rhinitis. The first is to ease the symptoms when they are present by treating the patterns that cause the manifestation (*biao*). The second is to treat the root (*ben*) in order to stop the symptoms from repeatedly occurring. The best time to address the root of the problem is in the months leading up to the time when the symptoms usually arise. If the allergic rhinitis is perennial, this is obviously not possible. In this case, the root and the manifestation need to be treated simultaneously.

As acupuncturists, we need not be too concerned with what the specific triggers are for a child's allergies. The focus of treatment is to bring about more balance in the child's body so that he no longer reacts to his environment in the same way. We cannot change the environment but we can change how the child responds to it.

Organs and aetiology
Liver

> **WHY IS THE LIVER SUCH AN IMPORTANT ORGAN IN ALLERGIC RHINITIS?**

  » The Liver resonates with springtime.

  » The Liver is responsible for dealing with change (in this case, of the seasons).

  » The Liver has a propensity to become Hot.

  » The *yang* of the Liver has a propensity to rise upwards.

  » The Liver opens into the eyes.

  » The deep pathway of the Liver channels goes to the tissues surrounding the eye and the back of the nose.

  » The Gallbladder channel starts at the outer canthus of the eye.

  » The deep pathway of the Gallbladder channel goes to the inner canthus of the eye.

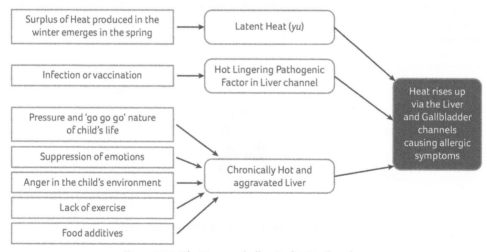

Figure 55.2 The Liver and allergic rhinitis/hay fever

Repressed feelings of anger and frustration

Repressed feelings of anger and frustration create imbalance in the Liver and Gallbladder. Scott and Barlow note that few children suffer from hay fever before the age of seven or eight, which they believe is also the age when a child is most likely to start suppressing emotions.[31] However, nowadays, many children as young as two or three experience hay fever symptoms (even though pollen levels are generally considered lower than they were a few decades ago). This suggests that younger children suppress their emotions and/or there are other factors which cause imbalance in the Liver and Gallbladder from an early age, such as the ones discussed.

Fever-reducing medication

Sometimes when a child has a fever, it is an opportunity for her body to expel Heat that has accumulated internally. If fevers are suppressed with medication, such as paracetamol, then this Heat often expresses itself in another way. One possible expression of Heat that has been suppressed is allergic symptoms. This is particularly true of allergies that appear in the springtime, when Heat that has laid dormant during the winter emerges.

Spleen

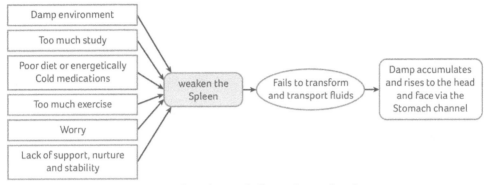

Figure 55.3 The Spleen and allergic rhinitis/hay fever

Lungs

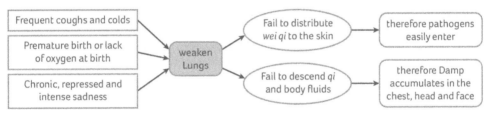

Figure 55.4 The Lungs and allergic rhinitis/hay fever

Patterns

- Heat in the Liver and Gallbladder rising upwards

- Wind-Damp in the channels of the face

- Spleen and Lung *qi* deficiency

> Children who come to the clinic with hay fever tend to fall into two broad categories. The first are 'Hot' children. In the hay fever season, the Heat is aggravated by exposure to pollen and causes hay fever symptoms. The second are children with Spleen and/or Lung *qi* deficiency who tend towards symptoms of Dampness in the head and face, which may present all year round or in damp weather.

Heat in the Liver and Gallbladder rising upwards

This pattern often corresponds to an acute attack of springtime hay fever. It may appear when the weather has just turned warmer. A child who has some chronic Heat in the Liver is especially prone to it. Exposure to pollen aggravates the Liver and Heat rises up to the face. The symptoms tend to affect the eyes more than the nose.

Symptoms

- itchy and irritated eyes and nose
- burning eyes
- red face
- feels hot in the face
- tight chest
- thirsty
- irritable
- flies off the handle
- often appears in spring

Pulse: wiry

Tongue: red sides

Treatment principles: clear Heat from the Liver and Gallbladder; soothe the nose and eyes

SUGGESTED TREATMENT

One local and one distal point per treatment is usually sufficient. GB 38 *yangfu*, the Fire and sedation point, clears Heat from the Gallbladder. GB 37 *guangming* particularly affects the eyes. If the child cannot tolerate LI 20 *yingxiang* being needled, a retained needle can be used on it during the treatment.

Points

LI 20 *yingxiang*
LI 4 *hegu*
GB 37 *guangming*
GB 38 *yangfu*
GB 43 *xiaxi*
Liv 2 *xingjian*
M-HN-3 *yintang*

Method: sedation needle technique

Paediatric *tui na* to clear Heat and ease the symptoms in the head and face

Heaven Gate *tianmen* (straight pushing)
Heart Gate *xinmen* (straight pushing)
Water Palace *kangong* (pushing apart)
M-HN-9 *taiyang* (kneading)
Bees Entering the Cave *huangfeng rudong* (kneading)
Wind Pond *fengchi* (kneading)
Big Bone Behind the Ear *erhou gaogu* (kneading)
LI 4 *hegu* (kneading)
Celestial Pillar Bone *tianzhugu* (straight pushing)
Eight Trigrams *bagua* (circular pushing anti-clockwise)

Wind-Damp in the channels of the face

A child with Spleen *qi* deficiency and chronic Damp is especially prone to this pattern. The symptoms tend to affect the nose more than the eyes.

Symptoms

- runny or blocked nose
- profuse mucus
- itchy nose
- head feels thick, heavy and 'bunged up'
- tiredness and lethargy
- puffy face and eyes

Pulse: slippery, floating

Tongue: may have a thick coat

Treatment principles: expel Wind; resolve Damp

SUGGESTED TREATMENT

One local and one distal point per treatment is usually sufficient. St 3 *juliao* helps to clear Wind-Damp from the face and is less painful than LI 20 *yingxiang*.

St 8 *touwei* also clears Damp from the head and helps with the symptom of a muzzy head.

Points

LI 20 *yingxiang*
LI 4 *hegu*
St 3 *juliao*
St 8 *touwei*
St 40 *fenglong*
Sp 3 *taibai*
Sp 9 *yinlingquan*

Method: sedation needle technique

Paediatric *tui na* to resolve Damp and ease the symptoms in the head and face

Heaven Gate *tianmen* (straight pushing)
Heart Gate *xinmen* (straight pushing)
Water Palace *kangong* (pushing apart)
M-HN-9 *taiyang* (kneading)
Bees Entering the Cave *huangfeng rudong* (kneading)
Wind Pond *fengchi* (kneading)
Big Bone Behind the Ear *erhou gaogu* (kneading)
LI 4 *hegu* (kneading)
Celestial Pillar Bone *tianzhugu* (straight pushing)
Eight Trigrams *bagua* (circular pushing anti-clockwise)

Spleen and Lung *qi* deficiency

This pattern causes a tendency to hay fever, rather than the acute symptoms. It is best treated during the winter months before the hay fever season begins.

Symptoms

- tendency to clear mucus

- allergies may be worse in the winter or during damp and humid weather

- easily tires

- poor appetite

- pale face

Pulse: deficient

Tongue: pale, wet, swollen

SUGGESTED TREATMENT

The underlying deficiency is best treated outside the hay fever season. If the child comes for treatment whilst he has allergic symptoms, the focus should be on easing the symptoms.

Of course, any point on the Lung or Spleen channel will strengthen the *qi* of that Organ. Those given here are some of the most effective and easily needled on a child. Usually, two or three points per treatment is sufficient.

Points

St 36 *zusanli*
Sp 3 *taibai*
Ren 12 *zhongwan*
Bl 20 *pishu*
Lu 7 *lieque*
Lu 9 *taiyuan*
Bl 13 *feishu*

Method: tonification needle technique

Other techniques: moxibustion

Paediatric *tui na* to tonify *qi* and ease the symptoms in the head and face

Heaven Gate *tianmen* (straight pushing)
Heart Gate *xinmen* (straight pushing)
Water Palace *kangong* (pushing apart)
M-HN-9 *taiyang* (kneading)
Bees Entering the Cave *huangfeng rudong* (kneading)
Spleen *pijing* (straight pushing)
Lung *feijing* (straight pushing)
Knead Ren 6 *qihai* (kneading anti-clockwise)
Spinal Column *jizhu* (pinching from the bottom to the top of the back)
Wind Pond *fengchi* (kneading)
Celestial Pillar Bone *tianzhugu* (straight pushing)
Big Bone Behind the Ear *erhou gaogu* (kneading)
Eight Trigrams *bagua* (circular pushing anti-clockwise)

Other treatment modalities

Shonishin

Core non-pattern-based root treatment.

Targeted tapping in the following areas:

- Du 22 *xinhui* to Du 23 *shangxing*
- Du 20 *baihui*
- GB 20 *fengchi*
- LI 4 *hegu*

Gua sha

Gentle *gua sha* on the upper back, in the region of the Lungs, helps to clear the stagnation of *qi* and fluids that has accumulated as a result of the Lungs failing to descend and disperse.

Auricular acupuncture

Press-spheres on the Lung and allergy points on the ear may help to relieve some of the acute symptoms.

CASE HISTORY: THREE-YEAR-OLD BOY WITH ALLERGIC RHINITIS

The following case history illustrates the importance of treating the underlying constitutional imbalance, and how that can improve seemingly unrelated physical symptoms.

Adam woke up between 4am and 5am each day and would sneeze repeatedly, his nose would pour with clear mucus and he would struggle to breathe easily because his chest was so full of mucus. Each of these symptoms would persist during the day, although not as severely as in the early hours of the morning.

Adam was very tired, partly because his sleep was so disturbed by the allergy. He had a poor appetite and was unusually placid for a boy of his age. He wanted to be carried a lot of the time, rather than walk himself.

Observations: The striking thing about Adam was that he never smiled or laughed. At his tender age, he looked as if he had the weight of the world upon his shoulders. The usual little games that would easily provoke laughter in most three-year-olds brought about no change in Adam at all. During treatments, Adam would sit quietly on his mother's lap. His face was pale and very puffy.

- Pulse: deficient
- Tongue: pale and swollen

Diagnosis

- Damp with underlying Spleen and Lung *qi* deficiency
- Fire constitutional imbalance

Treatment

The impact of Adam's allergic symptoms on his life was so great that I decided to start by treating them directly. The treatment principles during the first three or four sessions were:

Treatments 1, 2, 3 and 4

Tonify Spleen and Lung *qi* – with two of the following points per treatment: St 36 *zusanli*, Ren 12 *zhongwan*, Lu 9 *taiyuan*, Bl 13 *feishu* (Adam was a deficient child, so strengthening the underlying deficiencies was my primary treatment principle)

Resolve Damp and Phlegm – with one or two points per treatment, such as Sp 9 *yinlingquan*, St 40 *fenglong*, St 3 *juliao*, LI 4 *hegu*

After the fourth treatment, there was no change at all in Adam's symptoms.

At Treatment 5, I decided to address the other aspect of Adam's condition, namely his depleted Fire, which manifested in an extraordinary lack of spark and vivacity.

Treatment 5

Treat Fire constitutional imbalance: *Yuan* source points TB 4 *yangchi*, Pc 7 *daling*

Treatment 6

Adam's mother reported that, even though none of the allergic symptoms had changed, Adam had been noticeably more energetic, happy and vivacious since the last treatment.

Luo junction points: TB 5 *waiguan*, Pc 6 *neiguan*

Treatment 7

Adam's mother reported that, for the first time she could remember, he had been sleeping through until 6am or 7am. He was still full of mucus and sneezing during the day but was getting several hours' more sleep a night. His *joie de vivre* was going from strength to strength and he was running around in the playground in a way she had never seen before.

Treatment 8

I decided to continue treating Adam's Fire Element but to bring back the previous treatment principle of strengthening Adam's Spleen *qi* to try to alleviate some of the mucus.

St 36 *zusanli*, Sp 3 *taibai*

Back *shu* points: Bl 22 *sanjiaoshu*, Bl 14 *jueyinshu*

Adam continued to go from strength to strength and, after a total of twelve treatments, had significantly less mucus, sneezed only a handful of times a day and, most importantly, had seemingly begun to enjoy life.

Reflection: Strengthening Adam's Fire Element helped to alleviate the Damp and Phlegm. As his Fire grew stronger, it began to 'burn off' the Damp. Strengthening Adam's Spleen, and therefore the transformation and transportation function, aided this process.

SUMMARY

» The key Organs involved are: the Liver, Spleen and Lungs.

» The patterns that cause the acute symptoms are: Heat in the Liver and Gallbladder rising upwards; and Wind-Damp in the channels of the face.

» Lung and Spleen *qi* deficiency is the most common underlying deficiency.

» *Gua sha* and auricular acupuncture are helpful techniques in the treatment of allergic rhinitis and hay fever.

• Chapter 56 •

EAR CONDITIONS
· ·

The topics discussed in this chapter are:

- Organs involved in ear conditions

- Aetiology and components of ear conditions

- Other treatment modalities

Introduction

Few children get through childhood without, at the very least, the odd earache. A child may, however, be plagued by frequent, repeated attacks of pain in the ears. Another may live as if she has a veil between her and the world because her ears are so blocked. She cannot hear what is going on around her, and may be accused of not listening or being off with the fairies. Many a parent has had the experience of her child transforming from being miserable and cantankerous to happy and obliging once her hearing has improved.

Acute ear infections have usually been treated with antibiotics. However, new guidelines released by the National Institute for Health and Care Excellence (NICE) in 2017 now recommend the first line of treatment to be pain-relief medication.[32] Chronic ear problems that affect hearing (and therefore sometimes speech and development) are often treated with grommets. These are tiny tubes which are inserted into the eardrum.

Thankfully, there is so much we can do to help with acupuncture treatment. Ridding a child of pain and helping him to hear is usually relatively straightforward. Moreover, we can help to eliminate the need for repeated courses of antibiotics, which are the usual treatment for attacks of otitis media. Finally, successfully treating glue ear can mean a child avoids the need for a surgical procedure.

This chapter focuses on long-term treatment to reduce or entirely prevent recurrent ear infections and to eradicate glue ear. For symptomatic treatment during an acute infection, see Chapter 70.

Organs involved in ear conditions

As can be seen in Figure 56.1, there are many different Organs which affect the ears.

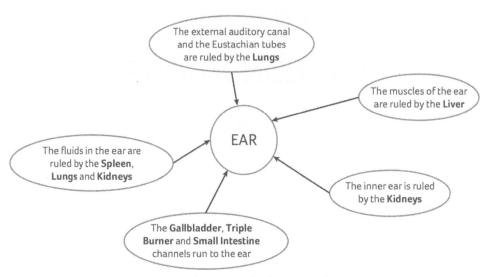

Figure 56.1 Organs involved in ear conditions

Aetiology and components of ear conditions

A combination of the factors shown in Figure 56.2 combine to cause ear conditions in children. There is often also an underlying deficiency in one or more Organs, in particular the Spleen, Lungs or Kidneys.

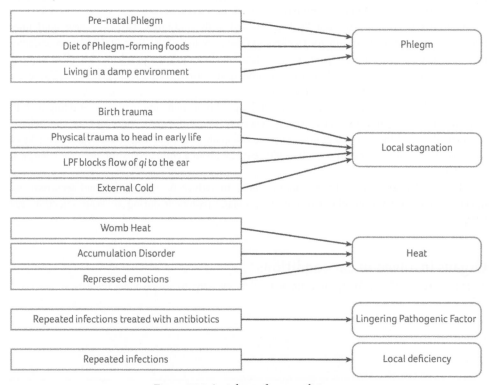

Figure 56.2 Aetiology of ear conditions

The practitioner should confirm or rule out the existence of each of these components in order to make a diagnosis.

> In the clinic, it is common to see:
>
> » a child who is Spleen *qi* deficient with an accumulation of Phlegm in the ears causing chronic glue ear
>
> » a child who is Lung *qi* deficient with local stagnation in the ears derived from a trauma, which causes recurrent earaches
>
> » a child with Accumulation Disorder, which leads to Heat which rises up and affects the ears
>
> » a child with an LPF of Thick Phlegm in the Gallbladder channel, which causes some loss of hearing and intermittent ear infections, which arise when there is a build-up of Heat.

Phlegm

Phlegm on its own tends to cause chronic diminished hearing. Therefore, it is not usually addressed during an acute episode of pain or infection.

Ear symptoms

- loss of hearing
- feeling of pressure
- ears feel blocked
- discharge from the ear

Other symptoms: chronic cough, blocked nose, vacant and disconnected, likes to sleep a lot

Pulse: slippery

Tongue: thick sticky coat, swollen

Treatment principles: resolve Phlegm; bring *qi* to the ears

SUGGESTED TREATMENT

It is usually sufficient to combine one local point with one or two distal points per treatment.

Points

To bring *qi* to the ear:

TB 17 *yifeng*
SI 19 *tinggong*
GB 2 *tinghui*

Method: tonification needle technique

To resolve Damp and Phlegm:

TB 5 *waiguan*
GB 34 *yanglingquan*
St 40 *fenglong*
Sp 9 *yinlingquan*

Method: sedation needle technique

Paediatric *tui na* to resolve Phlegm and descend *qi*

Lung *feijing* (straight pushing tonification)
Spleen *pijing* (straight pushing tonification)
Eight Trigrams *bagua* (circular pushing anti-clockwise)
Small Palmar Crease *zhangxiaowen* (straight pushing)
Hand *yin yang shouyinyang* (pushing apart)
Wind Pond *fengchi* (kneading)
Celestial Pillar Bone *tianzhugu* (straight pushing)
Big Bone Behind the Ear *erhou gaogu* (kneading)
St 40 Abundant Bulge *fenglong* (kneading)

CASE HISTORY: THREE-YEAR-OLD BOY WITH GLUE EAR

The following case history illustrates:

- how persistence is sometimes needed when treating Phlegm
- the changes that may take place in a child once he is less burdened with Phlegm.

Zach was three years old when he first came to the clinic. He had very poor hearing and his parents were considering whether to have grommets inserted or not. He had never had an ear infection and did not experience any pain or discomfort in his ears. He was also prone to a very snotty nose and a chesty cough. The mucus was either white or green. He snored a lot at night and was an exceptionally good sleeper. His appetite was relatively good. His stools were usually loose and contained undigested food. He was a very compliant but happy child. His tongue was swollen and pale but had a pronounced Stomach crack. His pulse was slippery.

Diagnosis: Phlegm, *qi* deficiency (both around the ears and systemically)

Aetiology: Zach was born with a lot of Phlegm. Even though neither his mother nor father appeared to be especially full of Phlegm, his grandmother who brought him for treatment one day told me that all her children had had glue ear when they were young and had all had grommets. So there appeared to be an inherited component to his condition. His diet was very good. His family lived on a canal boat for the first two years of his life, so the damp environment was also a factor.

Treatment principles
Resolve Phlegm; tonify Spleen *qi*; bring *qi* to the ears

Points used:

- Resolve Phlegm: GB 34 *yanglingquan*, St 40 *fenglong*, Sp 9 *yinlingquan* (sedation technique)
- Bring *qi* to the ears: TB 17 *yifeng* (tonification technique)
- Strengthen Stomach and Spleen: St 36 *zusanli*, Sp 6 *sanyinjiao*, Bl 20 *pishu*, Bl 21 *weishu* (tonification technique)

Other methods used: Paediatric *tui na* routine to resolve Phlegm and strengthen the Stomach and Spleen. The parents did this every night at home.

Lifestyle advice: Zach's mother tried taking him off gluten for about a month but there was no improvement in symptoms at the end of this. She also cut out dairy foods and this definitely helped. She noticed that if Zach had any dairy when he was at a party, for example, he would immediately become more mucousy.

Outcome: Zach improved quite quickly very early on in treatment, and became less mucousy and his hearing improved. He then went on a camping trip, when the weather was cold and damp, and came back full of snot and with a very persistent cough with profuse mucus. It took several months of treatment to entirely clear the cough and unblock his ears. During this time, I found that I got the best results from strengthening the Stomach and Spleen, and less good results from resolving Phlegm. Eventually, with admirable persistence from his mother, Zach got to a place where his hearing was consistently good, he avoided needing grommets and only occasionally became snotty.

Reflection: When I first saw Zach, he was in many ways a typically Phlegm-type child. He was very easy to treat and was totally unbothered by the needles (often a rather welcome result of too much Phlegm in the body which dulls the senses). As treatment progressed, he became more resistant to the needles. He also began to be more demanding at home as his *qi* became stronger. I explained to his mother that this was 'a good sign' and would pass in time. Thankfully, it did not deter her from continuing Zach's treatment. By the time I stopped treating Zach, he was four years old. It felt to me and his mother that Zach had blossomed and matured once he was unencumbered by Phlegm.

Stagnation

Localised stagnation is usually an aspect of an ear infection and therefore is commonly treated during the acute stage.

Ear symptoms

- pain

Other symptoms: moodiness, irritability or depression, alternating constipation and diarrhoea, pre-menstrual syndrome in teenage girls

Pulse: wiry (if stagnation is generalised)

Tongue: normal

Treatment principles: move *qi* in the channels of the ear

SUGGESTED TREATMENT
Points

> TB 17 *yifeng*
> TB 5 *waiguan*

Method: sedation needle technique

If there is generalised stagnation add:

> Liv 3 *taichong*
> GB 34 *yanglingquan*

Method: sedation needle technique

Paediatric *tui na* to move *qi* around the ear, descend *qi* and calm the *shen* (to help the child deal with pain)

> Heaven Gate *tianmen* (straight pushing)
> Heart Gate *xinmen* (straight pushing)
> Water Palace *kangong* (pushing apart)
> Wind Pond *fengchi* (kneading)
> Celestial Pillar Bone *tianzhugu* (straight pushing)
> Big Bone Behind the Ear *erhou gaogu* (kneading)
> Eight Trigrams *bagua* (circular pushing anti-clockwise)

Heat

Heat may cause an acute ear infection or recurrent attacks.

Key symptoms

- severe pain
- burning sensation in the ear
- outer ear may look red
- inner ear looks inflamed

Other symptoms: headache, fever, agitation, thirst

Pulse: rapid

Tongue: red, may have a yellow coating

Treatment principles: clear Heat

> **SUGGESTED TREATMENT**
> One local and one distal point per treatment is usually sufficient.
>
> **Points**
>
> TB 5 *waiguan*
> TB 17 *yifeng*
> GB 2 *tinghui*
> GB 41 *zulinqi*
> Liv 2 *xingjian*
>
> **Method:** sedation needle technique
>
> **Paediatric *tui na*** to clear Heat and bring *qi* downwards
>
> Milky Way *tianheshui* (straight pushing)
> Wind Pond *fengchi* (kneading)
> Celestial Pillar Bone *tianzhugu* (straight pushing)
> Big Bone Behind the Ear *erhou gaogu* (kneading)
> Eight Trigrams *bagua* (circular pushing anti-clockwise)

Deficiency

Qi deficiency is usually treated between ear infections rather than during an acute attack.

Local deficiency

Deficiency in the *qi* of the ears does not, in itself, cause a particular symptom. However, stagnation and Phlegm tend to settle where this is weakness, so it is important to treat.

Generalised deficiency

A systemic deficiency of Spleen, Kidney and/or Lung *qi* predisposes the child to chronic ear problems.

Symptoms

Symptoms depend on the Organ involved but will frequently include tiredness, poor appetite, lack of vigour and vitality, loose stools, being quiet, and prone to coughs and colds.

Pulse: deficient

Tongue: pale

Treatment principles: strengthen the *qi* of the ear

> **SUGGESTED TREATMENT**
> It is usually sufficient to use one local point and one or two distal points per treatment.
>
> **Points**
> Local points to strengthen *qi*:
>
> > TB 17 *yifeng*
> > SI 19 *tinggong*
> > GB 2 *tinghui*
>
> Distal points will depend on the Organs most involved in the deficiency:
>
> > Spleen: Sp 3 *taibai*, Sp 6 *sanyinjiao*, St 36 *zusanli*, Bl 20 *pishu*
> > Lungs: Lu 9 *taiyuan*, Bl 13 *feishu*
> > Kidneys: Ki 3 *taixi*, Bl 23 *shenshu*
>
> **Method:** tonification needle technique
>
> **Paediatric *tui na*** to tonify *qi* and bring *qi* to the ears
>
> > Spleen *pijing* (straight pushing)
> > Lung *feijing* (straight pushing)
> > Knead Ren 6 *qihai* (kneading anti-clockwise)
> > Spinal Column *jizhu* (pinching from the bottom to the top of the back)
> > Wind Pond *fengchi* (kneading)
> > Celestial Pillar Bone *tianzhugu* (straight pushing)
> > Big Bone Behind the Ear *erhou gaogu* (kneading)
> > Eight Trigrams *bagua* (circular pushing anti-clockwise)

Lingering Pathogenic Factor

Ear symptoms

An LPF in the ears is the most common cause of repeated ear infections.

Other symptoms: hard glands in the neck or groin, sudden collapses in energy, child is 'out of sorts' after an illness

Pulse and **Tongue** depend on the nature of the LPF and the underlying condition.

Treatment principles: soften Thick Phlegm; tonify *qi* to throw off the Lingering Pathogenic Factor

> **SUGGESTED TREATMENT**
> **Points**
>
> > Soften Thick Phlegm: M-HN-30 *bailao*
> > Local points: TB 17 *yifeng*
> > Distal points: GB 34 *yanglingquan*, St 40 *fenglong*
>
> **Method:** sedation needle technique
>
> Tonify *qi* to throw off LPF: Bl 13 *feishu*, Bl 18 *ganshu*, Bl 20 *pishu*, St 36 *zusanli*, Lu 9 *taiyuan*
>
> **Method:** tonification needle technique
>
> For a further discussion on the treatment of an LPF, see Chapter 27.
>
> **Paediatric *tui na*** to tonify *qi* and resolve Phlegm
>
> > Spleen *pijing* (straight pushing tonification)

> Lung *feijing* (straight pushing tonification)
> Small Palmar Crease *zhangxiaowen* (straight pushing)
> Hand *yin yang shouyinyang* (pushing apart)
> Three Passes *sanguan* (straight pushing)
> Knead the Navel *rou qi* (kneading anti-clockwise)
> Spinal Column *jizhu* (pinching from the bottom to the top of the back)

Accumulation Disorder

Ear symptoms

- repeated attacks of otitis media, usually hot in nature
- tend to occur most often when the child is teething

Other symptoms: red cheeks, green nasal mucus, foul-smelling stools, fractious and uncomfortable

Pulse: full

Tongue: thick, sticky and possibly yellow coat

Treatment principles: disperse accumulation of food

> **SUGGESTED TREATMENT**
> **Points**
>
> M-UE-9 *sifeng* on one hand
>
> **Method:** lightly prick the *sifeng* points of one hand with a needle
>
> In older children:
>
> Ren 12 *zhongwan*
> Sp 4 *gongsun*
> Pc 6 *neiguan*
> St 44 *neiting*
>
> **Method:** sedation needle technique
>
> **Paediatric *tui na*** to disperse accumulation of food and affect the ears
>
> Thick Gate *banmen* (straight pushing)
> Eight Trigrams *bagua* (circular pushing anti-clockwise)
> Four Wind Creases *sifengwen* (pinching)
> Knead Ren 12 *zhongwan* (kneading clockwise)
> Abdomen Stimulation *fuyinyang* (pushing apart)
> Belly Corner *dujiao* (pinching)
> Wind Pond *fengchi* (kneading)
> Celestial Pillar Bone *tianzhugu* (straight pushing)
> Big Bone Behind the Ear *erhou gaogu* (kneading)
> Eight Trigrams *bagua* (circular pushing anti-clockwise)

Other treatment modalities

Shonishin

Core non-pattern-based root treatment.

Targeted tapping in the following areas:

- TB 17 *yifeng*
- GB 12 *wangu*

- occipital area
- across the shoulders
- around the back of the ear

CASE HISTORY: SIX-YEAR-OLD GIRL WITH REPEATED EAR INFECTIONS

The following case history illustrates:

- how an LPF may have a profound effect on both the body and the spirit
- that not all cases fit into what it says in the textbooks!

Kathleen was six when she came to the clinic. She had had repeated ear infections since the age of six months. Her first bout coincided with her starting solid foods. Some had been treated with antibiotics. Her ears would become extremely painful, her hearing diminished and sometimes there was a greenish discharge too. She was otherwise a very healthy child. However, she hated school. Some days, she would protest so much at being left at school that she would vomit. On a few occasions she would hide under the car and refuse to come out unless her mother agreed to take her home.

Kathleen was a Hot child. She had a strong thirst and bright red cheeks. She had an enormous appetite.

Diagnosis: Hot LPF and stagnation in the ears

Treatment principles: Clear Hot LPF; move *qi* in the ears

Aetiology: Kathleen's first bouts of otitis media (OM) were triggered by Accumulation Disorder, which arose as a result of her enormous appetite and underlying Hot constitution. The Heat would build up in her Stomach and Intestines, and then travel up to the ears. As Kathleen became older, Accumulation Disorder became less of an issue, but the repeated treatment with antibiotics meant that she was left with a Hot LPF which would from time to time rise to the surface and cause another bout of OM.

Points used: TB 5 *waiguan*, GB 34 *yanglingquan*, TB 17 *yifeng* (sedation technique)

Outcome: Kathleen's treatment was straightforward and she responded quickly. She never had another bout of OM again after the first treatment. To her mother's surprise (and I have to say somewhat to mine too), she also went to school quite happily from the day she started treatment. The Hot LPF must have somehow been activated by the stress of leaving her mother, and the Heat rose up to affect her *shen*.

Reflection: Kathleen was unusual in that she showed virtually no signs of deficiency, despite having taken repeated courses of antibiotics. Her strong *qi* explains the fact that she was able to throw off the Hot LPF so quickly. Most children need to have their *qi* strengthened before they are able to do this.

SUMMARY

» Ear infections and glue ear involve one or more of the following components: stagnation; Phlegm and Damp; Heat; Accumulation Disorder; local *qi* deficiency; and Lingering Pathogenic Factor.

» Glue ear always includes an element of Phlegm.

» Acute ear infections which are characterised by severe pain usually include an element of Heat and/or stagnation.

» Treatment must include a combination of local and distal points.

• Chapter 57 •

SORE THROAT

• •

The topics discussed in this chapter are:

- Aetiology
- Patterns that cause acute symptoms
- Underlying patterns
- Other treatment modalities

Introduction

Recurrent or chronic sore throats are something which a child may be plagued by for years. At worst, the child's throat may be painful. Often, the tonsils are enlarged. Some children are caught in the vicious circle of recurrent bouts of sore throats treated with multiple rounds of antibiotics. These children are often tired and have digestive issues as a result of the antibiotic use.

Aetiology

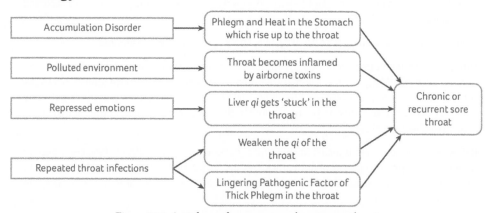

Figure 57.1 Aetiology of recurrent or chronic sore throat

Patterns that cause acute symptoms

A one-off sore throat may be caused by an invasion of Wind (see Chapter 70). However, recurrent or chronic sore throats in children may also arise as a result of an internal pattern.

Heat in Stomach

Throat symptoms

- swollen, red and painful throat

- yellow or white spots on tonsils

Other symptoms: thirst, constipation, scanty and dark urine, miserable and agitated

Pulse: rapid, overflowing

Tongue: red with a yellow coating

Treatment principles: clear Heat

Variations

- *Yangming* fever may be present with this pattern, in which case there will be high fever, severe thirst, copious sweating and an overflowing pulse. This pattern may stem from Accumulation Disorder in a baby or toddler.

SUGGESTED TREATMENT

These points are used during the acute stage. It is necessary afterwards to treat any underlying patterns to prevent recurrent attacks.

Points

LI 4 *hegu*
St 44 *neiting*
Lu 11 *shaoshang*
Ren 22 *tiantu*
SI 17 *tianrong*

Method: sedation needle technique

If Accumulation Disorder is present, this must be treated first (using M–UE-9 *sifeng*).

Paediatric *tui na* to clear Heat and promote the descending of *qi*

Lung *feijing* (straight pushing sedation)
Palace of Toil *laogong* (kneading)
Small Heavenly Heart *xiaotianxin* (kneading)
Milky Way *tianheshui* (straight pushing)
Six *Yang* Organs *liufu* (straight pushing)
Central Altar *shanzhong* (straight pushing)
Celestial Pillar Bone *tianzhugu* (straight pushing)

Underlying patterns
Retention of Thick Phlegm in the throat

This pattern is a type of Lingering Pathogenic Factor. In the Chinese texts, it is called 'stone tonsils'. It will cause intermittent symptoms, that tend to appear when the child is run down or stressed. See Chapter 27 for a further discussion of how to treat an LPF.

Symptoms

- chronic or recurrent bouts of severe sore throat

- tonsils are swollen

- throat is painful

- dry and hacking cough

Pulse: wiry or slippery

Tongue: colour of tongue will depend on underlying patterns

Treatment principles: loosen and resolve Thick Phlegm; move *qi* in the throat; strengthen underlying deficiency

> **SUGGESTED TREATMENT**
>
> This pattern may be present but only cause symptoms periodically. When symptoms are present, a selection of points should be used from those suggested. If symptoms are not present, the treatment should focus on strengthening the underlying deficient patterns.
>
> **Points**
>
> > M-HN-30 *bailao*
> > SI 17 *tianrong*
> > Ren 22 *tiantu*
> > LI 4 *hegu*
> > Ki 6 *zhaohai*
>
> If the Phlegm is Hot in nature, the following point can be added:
>
> > St 44 *neiting*
>
> **Method:** sedation needle technique
>
> Points to strengthen the underlying deficiency (see Spleen and Lung *qi* deficiency)
>
> **Paediatric *tui na*** to soften Thick Phlegm and promote the descending of Lung *qi*
>
> > Lung *feijing* (straight pushing tonification)
> > Eight Trigrams *bagua* (circular pushing anti-clockwise)
> > Small Palmar Crease *zhangxiaowen* (straight pushing)
> > Hand *yin yang shouyinyang* (pushing apart)
> > Milky Way *tianheshui* (straight pushing) if there is Heat
> > Central Altar *shanzhong* (straight pushing)
> > Celestial Pillar Bone *tianzhugu* (straight pushing)
> > St 40 Abundant Bulge *fenglong* (kneading)

Spleen and/or Lung *qi* deficiency

There is almost always some degree of underlying deficiency in a child who has chronic or recurrent sore throats. Both Scott and Barlow[33] and Flaws[34] discuss *yin* deficiency as a possible underlying pattern. However, this is not included here because it is so rare to see a child with true *yin* deficiency. By far the most common deficiency is that of Spleen and/or Lung *qi*.

Symptoms

- tired

- pale face

- loose mucus

- poor appetite

- loose stools

- colds and coughs often lead to a bout of sore throats

Pulse: deficient

Tongue: pale

Treatment principles: tonify Spleen and/or Lung *qi* deficiency

> **SUGGESTED TREATMENT**
> Two points per treatment are usually sufficient.
>
> **Points**
>
> St 36 *zusanli*
> Ren 12 *zhongwan*
> Bl 20 *pishu*
> Lu 9 *taiyuan*
> Bl 13 *feishu*
>
> **Method:** tonification needle technique
>
> **Other techniques:** moxibustion may be used
>
> **Paediatric *tui na*** to strengthen Lung and Spleen
>
> Lung *feijing* (straight pushing tonification)
> Spleen *pijing* (straight pushing tonification)
> Eight Trigrams *bagua* (circular pushing anti-clockwise)
> Knead the Navel *rou qi* (kneading)
> Spinal Column *jizhu* (pinching)

Other treatment modalities
Shonishin
Core non-pattern-based root treatment.

Targeted tapping around the following points:

- LI 18 *futu*

- St 9 *renying*

- Bl 11 *dazhu*

> SUMMARY

» An acute attack of recurrent sore throat is usually caused by Heat in the Stomach or Thick Phlegm.

» In recurrent sore throats, there is often a background of a Lingering Pathogenic Factor as well as Spleen and/or Lung *qi* deficiency.

» It is important to treat sore throats with a combination of local and distal points.

• Chapter 58 •

NOSEBLEEDS

· · · · · · · · · · · · · · · · · · · ·

The topics discussed in this chapter are:

* Patterns

* Other treatment methods to stop a nosebleed

Introduction

Nosebleeds are fairly common in children between the ages of about three and ten years old. Children who are brought to the clinic for nosebleeds may suffer from them every day, or even several times a day. Although they are usually a benign condition, they can be distressing for the child and difficult to manage at school. They are also, of course, a sign that the child has an underlying imbalance. For these reasons, they are definitely worth treating and generally respond well to acupuncture.

Patterns

* Full Heat in the Blood

* Spleen *qi* deficiency

Full Heat in the Blood

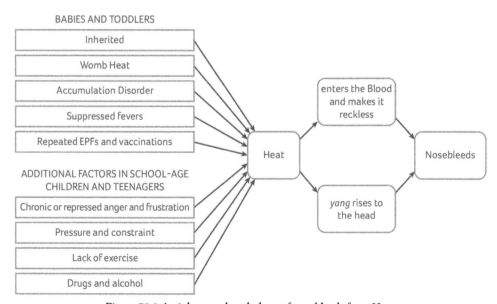

Figure 58.1 Aetiology and pathology of nosebleeds from Heat

There may be an underlying deficiency in conjunction with this pattern. In a child who is over-scheduled and exhausted, this is often of the Kidneys. When the Kidneys are deficient, *yang* tends to rise up to the head more readily.

Characteristics of nosebleeds

- profuse nosebleeds with fresh, bright red blood

Other symptoms: hot, restless, agitated, poor sleep, emotionally reactive

Pulse: rapid, overflowing

Tongue: red

Treatment principles: cool the Blood; stop bleeding

SUGGESTED TREATMENT
Points

> Sp 10 *xuehai*
> LI 4 *hegu*
> LI 20 *yingxiang*

Affecting the Lungs, worse during invasions of External Pathogenic Factors:

> Additional points: Lu 5 *chize*

Affecting the Stomach, brought on by eating or eating spicy foods:

> Additional points: St 44 *neiting*

Affecting the Liver, brought on by stress and anger suppression:

> Additional points: Liv 2 *xingjian*

Method: sedation needle technique

Between nosebleeds, treatment should focus on addressing the underlying deficiency which may be of any Organ, but is often either in the Kidneys or Organs related to the child's constitutional imbalance.

Paediatric *tui na* to clear Heat and to descend *qi*

> Heaven Gate *tianmen* (straight pushing)
> Heart Gate *xinmen* (straight pushing)
> Water Palace *kangong* (pushing apart)
> Wind Pond *fengchi* (kneading)
> Celestial Pillar Bone *tianzhugu* (straight pushing)
> Bees Entering the Cave *huangfeng rudong* (kneading)
> Eight Trigrams *bagua* (circular pushing anti-clockwise)
> Milky Way *tianheshui* (straight pushing)
> Six *Yang* Organs *liufu* (straight pushing)

Spleen *qi* deficiency

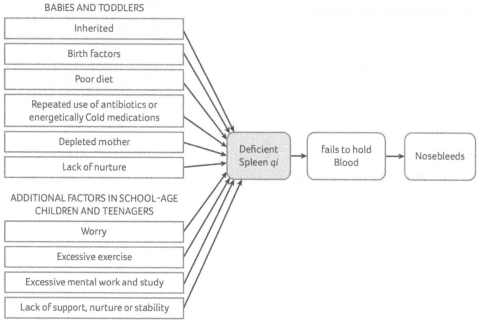

Figure 58.2 Aetiology of nosebleeds from qi deficiency

Characteristics of nosebleed

- nosebleeds with a light flow of blood
- pale, watery blood
- may come on when tired

Other symptoms: poor appetite, frequent bowel movements, picky eater, easily tires

Pulse: deficient

Tongue: pale

Treatment principles: tonify the Spleen to control Blood

Variation

There may also be a deficiency of any other Organ, particularly that which is related to the constitutional imbalance of the child.

> **SUGGESTED TREATMENT**
> **Points**
>
> > St 36 *zusanli*
> > Sp 1 *yinbai*
> > Bl 20 *pishu*
>
> **Method:** tonification needle technique
>
> **Other techniques:** moxibustion (especially on Sp 1 *yinbai*)
>
> **Paediatric *tui na*** to strengthen the Spleen and descend *qi*

Heaven Gate *tianmen* (straight pushing)
Heart Gate *xinmen* (straight pushing)
Water Palace *kangong* (pushing apart)
Wind Pond *fengchi* (kneading)
Celestial Pillar Bone *tianzhugu* (straight pushing)
Bees Entering the Cave *huangfeng rudong* (kneading)
Spleen *pijing* (straight pushing)
Eight Trigrams *bagua* (circular pushing anti-clockwise)
Three Passes *sanguan* (straight pushing)
Knead Ren 12 *zhongwan* (anti-clockwise)
Spinal Column *jizhu* (pinching from the bottom to the top of the back)
St 36 *zusanli* (kneading)

Other treatment methods to stop a nosebleed

- Gently pinch the soft part of the nose (just below the bony ridge) and keep pressure on this area, ideally for at least ten minutes after the bleeding has stopped.

- Moxa on Ki 1, or simply putting the child's feet in hot water (as hot as the child can comfortably stand), helps to draw down Heat from the head.

- The child should sit on the parent's lap, or on an upright chair, and her head should be tilted slightly forwards. Tilting the head backwards may mean the blood flows down the back of the throat and causes the child to gag, cough or vomit.

SUMMARY

» Profuse nosebleeds are due to Heat in the Blood. Mild nosebleeds are due to Spleen *qi* deficiency.

» The primary treatment principle should always be to stop bleeding.

» Underlying patterns may be addressed between nosebleeds.

• Chapter 59 •

BEDWETTING
. . . .

The topics discussed in this chapter are:

* Aetiology
* Patterns
* Other treatment modalities
* Other treatment considerations
* Advice

Introduction

Although bedwetting is a benign and self-limiting condition, it is a common reason for children being brought for acupuncture treatment. This is partly because there is very little that orthodox medicine can do to help. More importantly, any prolonged spell of bedwetting can have a profound impact on the family, as well as on the child.

Impact of bedwetting on the family

In the developed world, we live in a time where washing machines, tumble dryers and mattress protectors are ubiquitous. However, washing and changing the sheets every day can still feel to a parent like yet another chore in an already hectic routine. Every parent knows that their child is not wetting his bed intentionally, yet in the middle of the night or early in the morning when everybody is fractious and tired, irritation and despair may rise to the surface.

There is an association in the collective consciousness between bedwetting and insecurity (which may or may not be the case). Parents do not like to think that their child is insecure. All of this can put a strain on the relationship between parent and child. It may also place a strain on the parental relationship when one or other parent is required to get up, sometimes repeatedly, throughout the night to deal with wet pyjamas and sheets.

The child's emotional response to bedwetting

One child who comes to the clinic may seem surprisingly unbothered by the fact that she wets her bed. She may therefore be lacking the motivation to change. This in itself may provide a diagnostic clue. A lack of willpower and motivation may be a sign of a child whose Kidney *yang* energy is not strong. On the other hand, for another child, bedwetting induces intense feelings of shame and anxiety. Sleepovers and overnight school trips become a source of worry. This may also provide a diagnostic clue as these are the traits of an intense and competitive Kidney *yin* deficient child.

When a parent and a child who is bedwetting arrive in the clinic, they may bring with them strong and complex emotions that have arisen as a result of the condition and subsequently become a part of the problem. It can be really helpful to diffuse these emotions by explaining our understanding of the condition from a Chinese medicine perspective. Our explanation of this as a problem rooted in an imbalance in the child's *qi* can help to extract it from the intense emotions it has aroused. Guilt, shame, anxiety and worry begin to subside, which helps to begin turning things around. Most children become really proud of themselves when they start having dry nights. Change begets change. Once things start to improve, a child's confidence will begin to increase. This then further helps improvement since the child is less likely to go to bed fearful and anxious about whether she will have a dry night or not.

Bedwetting in children of different ages

The most common age bracket of children who are brought for treatment for bedwetting is five to eight years old. Children are often in nappies at night until the age of three. Parents do not usually start to worry about repeated bedwetting until a year or two after the child comes out of nappies.

If the child has gone through the first changeover of cycles that occurs around the age of seven or eight and is still bedwetting, it indicates a deeper pathology that may take longer to treat. However, treatment is still very helpful for this age group.

Aetiology

Many of the aetiologies shown in Figure 59.1 come into a child's life when she begins school, which is also a common time for a child to begin bedwetting.

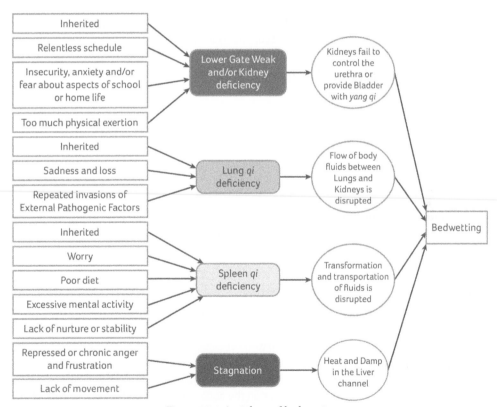

Figure 59.1 Aetiology of bedwetting

Lower Gate Weak refers to a type of Kidney deficiency, which manifests just in the area of urination. The Kidneys control the two lower orifices, the urethra being the one of significance here. If the urethra is not being held firm by strong Kidney *qi* then urine may leak out at the wrong time. It may arise when the *qi* of the Kidneys rises up to the head, which may be the case in bright children or in those who do a lot of mental activity from an early age. Lower Gate Weak may exist alongside more generalised signs of Kidney deficiency.

Bedwetting and insecurity

Bedwetting has long been associated with insecurity. Considering that there is always a degree of Kidney deficiency involved, this is often correct. However, the child does not need to have an overtly difficult aspect to her life that makes her insecure. A child who has a very stable and settled home and school life may be insecure too. Insecurity may come from something in her imaginary world, something she has seen in a film or, for example, because she is afraid of the neighbour's dog.

Patterns

- Lower Gate Weak with *yang* deficiency
- Lower Gate Weak with insubstantial *yin*
- Spleen and Lung *qi* deficiency (with Damp)
- Damp-Heat in the Liver channel

 Lower Gate Weak is present in all children who wet the bed. In some, this is the only pattern present. In others, it is combined with a deficiency of the Spleen and/or Lungs. In a child with Spleen *qi* deficiency, there may also be Damp blocking the water passages in the Lower Burner. Damp-Heat in the Liver channel is the least commonly seen pattern.

Lower Gate Weak with *yang* deficiency

Urinary symptoms

- bedwetting with large amounts of urine
- worse after lots of running around
- worse after getting cold
- worse towards the end of term when particularly tired

Other symptoms: easily tired, resists going outside and running around, lacking in motivation, timid and easily fearful, tendency to daydream, feels cold or cold feet, pale face and puffy skin

Pulse: deficient and may be deep

Tongue: pale

Treatment principles: strengthen the Lower Gate; bring Kidney *qi* to the Lower Burner; warm Kidney *yang*

SUGGESTED TREATMENT

It is usually sufficient to use one or two of these points and moxa, at each treatment. It is most effective to vary the points used, that is, points on the abdomen, points on the back, and distal points.

Points

> Bl 23 *shenshu*
> Bl 28 *pangguangshu*
> Ki 3 *taixi*
> Ki 7 *fuliu*

Ren 3 *zhongji*
Ren 6 *qihai*

Method: tonification needle technique

Other techniques: moxibustion

Paediatric *tui na* to tonify and warm the Kidneys

Kidney *shenjing* (straight pushing)
Two Men Upon a Horse *erma* (kneading)
Outer Palace of Toil *wailaogong* (kneading)
Wind Nest *yiwofeng* (kneading)
Three Passes *sanguan* (straight pushing)
Winnower Gate *jimen* (straight pushing from knee to groin)
Lower Back – area around Bl 23 *shenshu* (strong rubbing)
Spinal Column *jizhu* (pinching)
Du 20 *baihui* (kneading)

CASE HISTORY: EIGHT-YEAR-OLD GIRL WHO HAD NEVER BEEN DRY AT NIGHT

The following case history illustrates the wider benefits of treatment.

Meg came for treatment when she was eight years old. She had never been dry at night. She usually wet her bed soon after going to sleep and just before waking in the morning and sometimes one other time during the night. There were always huge amounts of urine. She was otherwise in very good physical and emotional health. She had good energy levels, a good appetite and was rarely ill.

Meg was a happy, carefree child, who enjoyed school and had lots of friends. Her mother said that she was unbothered by the fact that she wet her bed. She sometimes wore nappies at night because her mother felt she needed a break from changing the sheets. Meg didn't mind wearing nappies at all.

Meg's family life seemed happy and her life secure. The only alarm bell that rang was when her mother told me that Meg had to 'virtually bring herself up' because her older sister was incredibly demanding and complex. I held in my mind the possibility that night-time was the only time when Meg could get attention from her mother, who was very taken up with her older sister during the day.

Diagnosis: Meg had Kidney *yang* deficiency with weakness of the Lower Gate. She had a tendency towards feeling cold and all her pulses were slightly deep. Her tongue was pale. She had no signs of a Lingering Pathogenic Factor.

Treatment: Meg was slightly wary of needles, so I began by using a moxa stick on points to tonify the Kidneys and taught the mother a paediatric *tui na* routine.

Treatment 1: Moxa on Ki 3 *taixi* and Bl 23 *shenshu*

I taught the mother a paediatric *tui na* routine to warm and tonify Kidney *yang*.

Treatment 2: Moxa on Ki 3 *taixi* and Ren 3 *zhongji*

Treatment 3: First treatment using needles: Ki 7 *fuliu*, Bl 23 *shenshu* (tonification). Moxa on the same points.

Treatment 4: No change yet in symptoms but Meg announced that she never wanted to wear nappies at night again.

Ren 6 *qihai*, Bl 62 *shenmai*, Ki 6 *zhaohai* and moxa

After the fourth treatment Meg began having some dry nights. After the sixth treatment, she was dry six nights out of seven. There was a little bit of fluctuation after that, but after twelve treatments, still weekly, she had been consistently dry for three weeks.

Reflection: Whilst I have no doubt that warming and tonifying Meg's Kidney *yang* was the key to her becoming dry at night, I believe there was another story going on behind the scenes. Meg's older sister would always stay in the waiting room whilst Meg and her mother came into the treatment room. We would occasionally hear the older sister singing through the (supposedly) soundproofed walls. It seemed to me that she was always trying her best to draw her mother away from Meg to her. I felt that Meg particularly enjoyed coming for her treatments because they afforded what were otherwise rare moments, when she had her mother's undivided attention. Perhaps that was a part of the reason why she no longer needed to find ways of getting the attention during the night.

Lower Gate Weak with insubstantial *yin*
Urinary symptoms

- bedwetting which is worse when tired
- copious amounts of urine[*]
- more likelihood of wetting the bed after a late night or when overstimulated

Other symptoms: easily tired, becomes more excitable and 'hyper' the more tired she is, finds it hard to settle and be still, is competitive, driven, intellectually precocious, takes a long time to get to sleep, especially when overstimulated, wakes up early in the morning

Pulse: deficient

Tongue: normal or slightly red

Treatment principles: strengthen the Lower Gate; bring Kidney *qi* to the Lower Burner; nourish Kidney *yin*

> **SUGGESTED TREATMENT**
> Two points per treatment is usually sufficient. A Kidney *yin* deficient child is easily overstimulated.
>
> **Points**
>
> > Bl 23 *shenshu*
> > Bl 28 *pangguangshu*
> > Ki 1 *yongquan*
> > Ki 3 *taixi*
> > Ki 7 *fuliu*
> > Ren 3 *zhongji*
> > Ren 4 *guanyuan*
>
> **Method:** tonification needle technique
>
> **Paediatric *tui na*** to strengthen the Kidneys
>
> > Heaven Gate *tianmen* (straight pushing)
> > Heart Gate *xinmen* (straight pushing)
> > Water Palace *kangong* (pushing apart)
> > Kidney *shenjing* (straight pushing)

---

[*] Although in adults *yin* deficiency may cause scanty urine, in a child there is rarely enough Heat to condense the fluids. Both the Kidney patterns tend to cause more copious urine than the Spleen and Lung *qi* deficiency pattern.

Two Men Upon a Horse *erma* (kneading)
Winnower Gate *jimen* (straight pushing from knee to groin)
Lower Back – area around Bl 23 *shenshu* (strong rubbing)
Spinal Column *jizhu* (pinching)
Du 20 *baihui* (kneading)

Spleen and Lung *qi* deficiency (with Damp)

Spleen *qi* deficiency may also have led to Damp, which sinks downwards into the Lower Burner, blocks the water passages and contributes to the bedwetting.

Urinary symptoms

- bedwetting with relatively small amounts of urine

- wets the bed more often when tired and after an infection

- may not need to urinate very often during the day

- child may be chubby in the Lower Burner

Other symptoms: poor appetite or fussy eater, catches lots of coughs and colds, easily gets tired, pale faced, quiet

Pulse: deficient, may be slippery

Tongue: pale

Treatment principles: strengthen the Lower Gate; tonify Spleen and Lung *qi*; resolve Damp (if necessary); raise *qi*

SUGGESTED TREATMENT

Points should be chosen on the channels related to the Organ or Organs that have the greatest degree of deficiency in that particular child. Two or three points per treatment are usually sufficient.

Points

To tonify:

Bl 23 *shenshu*
Ki 3 *taixi*
Ren 3 *zhongji*
St 36 *zusanli*
Sp 6 *sanyinjiao*
Ren 12 *zhongwan*
Lu 9 *taiyuan*
Lu 7 *lieque*

Method: tonification needle technique

To resolve Damp (when necessary):

Sp 9 *yinlingquan*
Sp 6 *sanyinjiao*

Method: sedation needle technique

To raise *qi*:

Du 20 *baihui* – so that the child wakes up more easily when she needs to urinate

Method: tonification needle technique

Other techniques: moxibustion

Paediatric *tui na* to strengthen the Lower Gate, Spleen and Lungs

> Kidney *shenjing* (straight pushing)
> Spleen *pijing* (straight pushing)
> Lung *feijing* (straight pushing)
> Knead Ren 6 *qihai* (kneading anti-clockwise)
> Two Men Upon a Horse *erma* (kneading)
> Winnower Gate *jimen* (straight pushing from knee to groin)
> Lower Back – area around Bl 23 *shenshu* (strong rubbing)
> Spinal Column *jizhu* (pinching)
> Du 20 *baihui* (kneading)

Damp-Heat in the Liver channel

This is the least commonly seen cause of bedwetting in my practice. It should be remembered that Damp-Heat in the Liver channel may also be a cause of a urinary tract infection (UTI). If the bedwetting has had a recent, acute onset and the child urinates frequently during the day, consider that the child may have a UTI (see Chapter 60 for the treatment of urinary tract infections).

Urinary symptoms

- bedwetting with yellow and smelly urine

- painful urination

- inflammation of the urethra or vagina

- urinates little and often during the day

Other symptoms: irritable, easily flies into a tantrum, may be disruptive, may have red cheeks and/or a green colour around the mouth

Pulse: wiry and/or slippery on the Wood pulses, generally deficient

Tongue: may have a yellow tongue coating

Treatment principles: strengthen the Lower Gate; clear Heat and resolve Damp in the Liver channel

> **SUGGESTED TREATMENT**
> **Points**
> To clear Damp and Heat in the Liver channel:
>
> > Liv 8 *ququan*
> > Sp 6 *sanyinjiao*
> > Liv 5 *ligou*
>
> **Method:** sedation needle technique
>
> To strengthen the Lower Gate:
>
> > Bl 23 *shenshu*
> > Ki 3 *taixi*
>
> **Method:** tonification needle technique
>
> **Paediatric *tui na*** to tonify the Kidneys (the full aspect of the condition is best treated with acupuncture)

> Kidney *shenjing* (straight pushing)
> Two Men Upon a Horse *erma* (kneading)
> Winnower Gate *jimen* (straight pushing from knee to groin)
> Lower Back – area around Bl 23 *shenshu* (strong rubbing)
> Spinal Column *jizhu* (pinching)
> Du 20 *baihui* (kneading)

Any of these patterns may co-exist with a Lingering Pathogenic Factor which makes the picture somewhat more complex. In addition to any of the above symptoms, the child may:

» have swollen glands in the neck

» have emotional complexity

» be hard to read

» have sudden energy collapses or emotional meltdowns.

The pattern or patterns that accompany the Lingering Pathogenic Factor must be addressed. For how to approach treatment of an LPF, see Chapter 27).

Other treatment modalities
Shonishin
Core non-pattern-based root treatment.

Targeted tapping over the following areas:

- Du 12 *shenzhu*

- Du 3 *yaoyangguan* to Du 4 *ming men*

- lower abdomen

Extra points
There are two extra points which may be useful.

- **Hand bedwetting point** (called either *ye niao dian* or *shen xue*): This is located on the palmar surface of the little finger, in the middle of the transverse crease of the distal interphalangeal joint. It may be needled or a press-tack or press-sphere left on it.

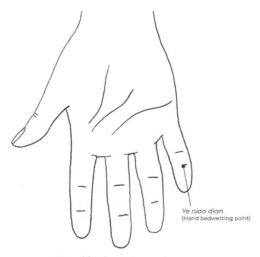

Ye niao dian
(Hand bedwetting point)

Hand bedwetting point

- **Foot bedwetting point** (*yi niao xue*): *Yi niao xue* is located on the sole of the foot, in the middle of the fifth metatarsophalangeal crease.[35] It may be needled although it is rather painful. Therefore, it is best treated with a laser pen or by leaving a press-tack or press-sphere on it.

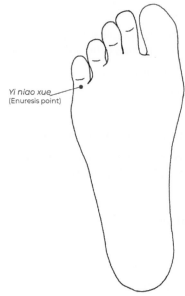

Yi niao xue
(Enuresis point)

Foot bedwetting point

Other treatment considerations
Kidney deficiency and fear of needles

Whatever other patterns may be involved, there is always some degree of Kidney deficiency present when a child is bedwetting. One of the symptoms of Kidney deficiency is being easily fearful, and this can mean that a child who is bedwetting may not take kindly to the prospect of being needled, at least at the start of her course of treatment. If this is the case, the following alternatives should be considered:

- The relevant acupuncture points can be stimulated with a moxa stick. This is a particularly good approach in a Kidney *yang* deficient child but can be used on children whose Kidney *yin* is insubstantial too, providing there are no significant signs of Heat.

- A laser pen may be used instead of needles.

Advice

- Japanese Kidney warmers (*haramakis*) are a fantastic way of protecting the Lower Burner from Cold and Damp. They can be found easily online and can be bought in children's sizes.

- One of the first steps on the road to dry nights may be the child deciding to stop wearing nappies. The decision to do this should come from the child and should generally be supported if it does. It is a sign that the child is mustering her *zhi* in order to face the issue!

- Parents often lift their child onto the toilet to urinate in the middle of the night in the hope of avoiding wet sheets and pyjamas in the morning. In most cases, this is not helpful, as the child may get used to not having to wake up when she needs to urinate.

CASE HISTORY: A NINE-YEAR-OLD WHO WAS NOT HELPED BY ACUPUNCTURE

The following case history illustrates how sometimes acupuncture is not enough when there is a strong, ongoing aetiology.

Lenny came for treatment at the age of nine. He had never been dry at night. He usually wet his bed once or twice during the night but often slept through it, despite very wet sheets and pyjamas. He was otherwise healthy with no other significant symptoms.

Background: Lenny's parents had had a very acrimonious divorce when he was three years old, during which time he had witnessed his father being violent towards his mother. He now lived between his parents. His mother was in a new relationship. Although her new partner did not live with them, he spent a lot of time with them.

Diagnosis: Lower Gate Weak with a Lingering Pathogenic Factor. Lenny's Water pulses were deep and weak. He had swollen, hard glands in his neck and would sometimes glaze over whilst I talked to him. He presented with a friendly exterior but I noticed flashes of anger through his eyes at times and sudden abruptness which seemed to come for no apparent reason.

Outcome: Although Lenny occasionally reported he had had a dry night, or had woken up when he needed to urinate at night, we never seemed to make any significant progress. After twelve treatments, I told his mother I didn't think there was anything else I could do to help, as I hadn't detected any significant change. She was very disappointed.

About six months later, I happened to bump into Lenny's mother. We stopped to talk and she told me that her relationship had ended. She had begun to realise that her partner, when she was not there, would often become aggressive towards Lenny and his sister. She told me that, within a week of ending the relationship, Lenny had become dry at night, every night.

Reflection: This was a case when the treatment did not appear to be enough to strengthen the child to withstand the emotional difficulties in his life. In other cases, it sometimes does. I wondered whether the fact that Lenny had witnessed violence against his mother at the age of three meant that the aggressive and threatening behaviour of his mother's new partner struck an even deeper chord in him than it otherwise would have done.

SUMMARY

» Most cases of bedwetting come from a deficiency, and therefore the key aetiological factors all relate to 'overdoing it' in some way (as well as inherited factors).

» All cases of bedwetting, whatever other patterns may be present, have an aspect of Lower Gate Weak involved. This is an imbalance in the Kidneys' function of controlling the two lower orifices (in this case the urethra).

» The key patterns are: Lower Gate Weak with *yang* deficiency; Lower Gate Weak with insubstantial *yin*; Spleen and Lung *qi* deficiency; and (albeit rarely) Damp-Heat in the Liver channel.

Chapter 60

URINARY TRACT INFECTIONS

The topics discussed in this chapter are:

* Aetiology

* Patterns

* Other treatment modalities

Introduction

Urinary tract infections (UTIs) are common in children. They can be difficult to spot in a pre-verbal child who cannot tell you how she is feeling. Unpleasant-smelling urine and intermittent, unexplained crying may be the only recognisable symptoms in this case. In an older child, diagnosis becomes easier. The child will need to urinate more frequently than usual, may complain that it hurts, may start wetting the bed at night and complain of stomach ache whilst holding her abdomen. A UTI may also be accompanied by a general malaise and sometimes a fever too.

Most children with a UTI are treated with antibiotics. Antibiotics deal with the acute phase of the problem but do not entirely eradicate it. They are cooling in nature and therefore tend to be effective at getting rid of the 'Hot' part of the infection. This means urination becomes less painful, the need for it less frequent and the child less feverish. However, antibiotics do not deal with the Damp aspect of the condition and, indeed, may exacerbate it. They weaken the Spleen, which then no longer keeps transforming and transporting fluids so efficiently, and so more Damp is created.[36]

A common presentation in the clinic is a child who has had several UTIs over a period of a few months, each of which has been treated with antibiotics. She seemingly 'gets better' after each course of antibiotics but, within days or weeks, another UTI begins to flare. From the Chinese medicine perspective, the original UTI is still in her system in the form of a Lingering Pathogenic Factor. When she becomes slightly more tired, depleted or stressed than usual, the lingering pathogen rears its head again, causing the urinary symptoms. More antibiotics further cool and deplete the system and a vicious circle begins. Acupuncture is very successful at breaking this cycle. Treatment that is aimed at both clearing the LPF and strengthening the underlying *qi* can eradicate the problem altogether.

Aetiology

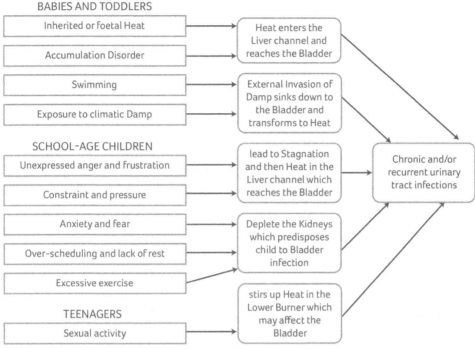

BABIES AND TODDLERS

| Inherited or foetal Heat |
| Accumulation Disorder |

→ Heat enters the Liver channel and reaches the Bladder

| Swimming |
| Exposure to climatic Damp |

→ External Invasion of Damp sinks down to the Bladder and transforms to Heat

SCHOOL-AGE CHILDREN

| Unexpressed anger and frustration |
| Constraint and pressure |

→ lead to Stagnation and then Heat in the Liver channel which reaches the Bladder

| Anxiety and fear |
| Over-scheduling and lack of rest |
| Excessive exercise |

→ Deplete the Kidneys which predisposes child to Bladder infection

TEENAGERS

| Sexual activity |

→ stirs up Heat in the Lower Burner which may affect the Bladder

→ Chronic and/or recurrent urinary tract infections

Figure 60.1 Causes of urinary tract infections

Emotions closely related to anxiety, such as jealousy, may also cause and be symptomatic of a Bladder pathology. Maciocia writes that 'an imbalance in the Bladder can provoke negative emotions such as jealousy, suspicion and the holding of long-standing grudges'.[37] Jealousy, such as that between siblings, is a common emotion for many children.

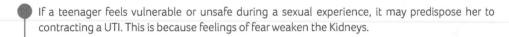

If a teenager feels vulnerable or unsafe during a sexual experience, it may predispose her to contracting a UTI. This is because feelings of fear weaken the Kidneys.

Patterns

- External pathogenic Damp-Heat in the Bladder

- Interior Damp-Heat in the Liver channel

- Spleen and Kidney *yang* deficiency

- Kidney *yin* deficiency

There are two common scenarios in children who have recurrent bladder symptoms. The first is a child with lingering Damp or Damp-Heat in the Bladder against a background of Spleen and Kidney deficiency. The second is a child who has some lingering Damp-Heat in the Liver channel against a background of Kidney *yin* deficiency.

External pathogenic Damp-Heat in the Bladder

This pattern usually originates when an external Damp-Cold pathogen invades the Bladder and then transforms into Damp-Heat. It describes an acute infection. If the pathogen is not properly cleared, it may lead to an LPF, which causes chronic, low-grade urinary symptoms. When this is the case, the treatment principles described here should be combined with tonification of the Organ or Organs in which the deficiency lies.

Urinary symptoms

- urinary urgency
- urinary frequency
- urine may be yellow or cloudy
- burning on urination
- difficulty in passing urine despite a feeling of urgency

Other symptoms: uncomfortable or painful lower abdomen, low-grade fever, clingy and unhappy, restless and/or lethargic

Pulse: slippery, possibly rapid

Tongue: there may be a slightly thick, sticky and possibly yellow coating

Treatment principles: resolve Damp and Heat in the Bladder

SUGGESTED TREATMENT

During an infection, three or four points should be used. Acute symptoms require slightly more intervention than do chronic symptoms. Bl 63 should be included when there is pain. Ren 3, as a local point, should always be included.

Points

Ren 3 *zhongji*
Bl 28 *pangguangshu*
Sp 6 *sanyinjiao*
Sp 9 *yinlingquan*
Liv 8 *ququan*
Bl 63 *jinmen*

Method: sedation needle technique

Paediatric *tui na*

Heaven Gate *tianmen* (straight pushing)
Heart Gate *xinmen* (straight pushing)
Water Palace *kangong* (pushing apart)
Eight Trigrams *bagua* (circular pushing clockwise)
Winnower Gate *jimen* (straight pushing from groin to thigh)
Milky Way *tianheshui* (straight pushing)
Three *Yin* Meeting Sp 6 *sanyinjiao* (kneading)

Interior Damp-Heat in the Liver channel

This pattern arises internally. It may cause acute symptoms or sub-acute symptoms that come and go.

Urinary symptoms

- painful or burning urination

- difficulty urinating despite the need to go
- urinary frequency
- yellow and scanty urine

Other symptoms: irritation and redness of the vulva in females, feels hot and restless, feverish, irritable and restless

Pulse: wiry Wood pulses

Tongue: yellow coating, possibly red sides

Treatment principles: clear Heat; resolve Damp in the Liver channel

SUGGESTED TREATMENT

A point on the Liver channel should be used in every treatment. This should be combined with a point which directly treats the Bladder. If there is a substantial amount of Damp, one of the Spleen points should be used too.

Points

Ren 3 *zhongji*
Bl 28 *pangguangshu*
Sp 6 *sanyinjiao*
Sp 9 *yinlingquan*
Liv 2 *xingjian*
Liv 5 *ligou*
Liv 8 *ququan*
Bl 63 *jinmen*

Method: sedation needle technique

Paediatric *tui na* to clear Heat and calm the *shen*

Heaven Gate *tianmen* (straight pushing)
Heart Gate *xinmen* (straight pushing)
Water Palace *kangong* (pushing apart)
Eight Trigrams *bagua* (circular pushing clockwise)
Winnower Gate *jimen* (straight pushing from groin to thigh)
Milky Way *tianheshui* (straight pushing)
Three *Yin* Meeting Sp 6 *sanyinjiao* (kneading)

The main difference between external Damp-Heat in the Bladder and interior Damp-Heat in the Liver channel is their origin. The first has an external origin, whilst the second arises internally. The treatment of them is very similar. In both cases, it is important to assess whether Damp or Heat predominates and adapt the points accordingly.*

Either of these two syndromes may cause a one-off acute urinary tract infection or a flare-up of a more chronic condition. It is especially beneficial to treat a child during an acute urinary tract infection. As well as possibly avoiding the need for antibiotics, it may help the child to throw off a pathogen which has been lingering for a period of time.

---

* Damp-Heat in the Stomach and Intestines may also cause a urinary tract infection. I am not including this pattern here as it is so rare, due to the fact it only arises after a *yang ming* fever.

Spleen and Kidney *yang* deficiency
Urinary symptoms

- bouts of urinary frequency
- urine may sometimes be cloudy
- bouts of difficulty urinating

Other symptoms: child is generally pale and lethargic, easily tires, has poor appetite, loose stools

Pulse: deep, weak and possibly slow

Tongue: pale, wet, may be swollen

Treatment principles: warm and tonify Spleen and Kidney *yang*

SUGGESTED TREATMENT

In each case, the practitioner should ascertain exactly which Organ or Organs the deficiency is in, and focus treatment accordingly. There will inherently always be a degree of deficiency in the Kidney and Bladder. This may have originated in those Organs or stem from another Organ. Two points at each treatment is usually sufficient.

Points

St 36 *zusanli*
Sp 3 *taibai*
Sp 6 *sanyinjiao*
Ren 12 *zhongwan*
Bl 20 *pishu*
Bl 23 *shenshu*
Ki 3 *taixi*
Ki 7 *fuliu*

Method: tonification needle technique

Other techniques: moxibustion

Paediatric *tui na* to warm and tonify Spleen and Kidney *yang*

Spleen *pijing* (straight pushing)
Kidney *shenjing* (straight pushing)
Two Men Upon a Horse *erma* (kneading)
Outer Palace of Toil *wailaogong* (kneading)
Wind Nest *yiwofeng* (kneading)
Three Passes *sanguan* (straight pushing)
Winnower Gate *jimen* (straight pushing from knee to groin)
St 36 *zusanli* (kneading)
Lower Back – area around Bl 23 *shenshu* (strong rubbing)
Spinal Column *jizhu* (pinching)

Kidney *yin* deficiency
Urinary symptoms

- bouts of urinary frequency
- bouts of painful and difficult urination

Other symptoms: finds it hard to settle, tends towards being hyperactive, takes a long time to get off to sleep and may wake early in the morning, driven and competitive

Pulse: floating, rapid

Tongue: red

Treatment principles: nourish Kidney *yin*

SUGGESTED TREATMENT

Two points per treatment is usually sufficient. A Kidney *yin* deficient child is easily overstimulated. Working on the lower part of the body in order to bring *qi* down from the head is important.

Points

Ki 3 *taixi*
Ki 7 *fuliu*
Bl 23 *shenshu*
Ren 4 *guanyuan*

Method: tonification needle technique

Paediatric *tui na* to strengthen the Kidneys and bring *qi* from the head down into the body

Heaven Gate *tianmen* (straight pushing)
Heart Gate *xinmen* (straight pushing)
Water Palace *kangong* (pushing apart)
Kidney *shenjing* (straight pushing)
Two Men Upon a Horse *erma* (kneading)
Winnower Gate *jimen* (straight pushing from knee to groin)
Lower Back – area around Bl 23 *shenshu* (strong rubbing)
Spinal Column *jizhu* (pinching)
Du 20 *baihui* (kneading)

In practice, a child often comes to the clinic with neither a clear-cut, acute UTI nor complete freedom from urinary symptoms. She may, for example, need to urinate very frequently but has no pain and does not wake up in the night needing to urinate. In this case, there is usually a lingering pathogen in the Bladder, combined with deficiency. The approach to treatment will either be:

» both to clear residual Damp and/or Heat from the Bladder and to tonify the underlying deficiency, *or*

» to tonify the underlying deficiency in order to give the child the *qi* needed to throw off the lingering pathogen.

It is not always an easy decision to make as to which approach is the right one. The practitioner should be guided by the pulse (particularly how deficient it is), the severity of the urinary symptoms and the overall picture of the child.

Other treatment modalities
Shonishin

Core non-pattern-based root treatment.

Targeted tapping in the following areas:

• Du 20 *baihui*

- occipital area
- Du 3 *yaoyangguan*
- lower abdomen

CASE HISTORY: SIX-YEAR-OLD GIRL WITH RECURRENT URINARY TRACT INFECTIONS

The following case history illustrates the power of treatment during a flare-up of a recurrent condition.

Leonie was brought to the clinic having suffered four UTIs in the past year. Each one had been characterised by painful, burning, frequent urination and a sharp abdominal pain. Leonie had taken antibiotics during each infection. The first one had come on after she had been swimming.

Observations: Leonie was a pale-faced and quiet child. Her mother said this was the only significant health problem she had experienced. She was a placid, easygoing child, who loved school and had a settled family life. During the infections, Leonie became extremely anxious and needed to sleep with her mum every night.

Diagnosis: Lingering Pathogenic Factor of Damp-Heat in the Bladder with underlying Spleen and Kidney *yang* deficiency.

Treatment
Treatment 1: the first time Leonie came for treatment, she was in the middle of an acute infection.

Liv 8 *ququan*, Sp 6 *sanyinjiao*, Bl 63 *jinmen*, Ren 3 *zhongji* (sedation needle technique)

Treatment 2: Leonie came for a second treatment the following day. The symptoms were abating but not yet gone.

Liv 8 *ququan*, Sp 6 *sanyinjiao*, Ren 3 *zhongji*, Bl 28 *pangguangshu* (sedation needle technique)

Treatment 3: Leonie's acute symptoms had cleared up after the previous treatment. She had no urinary symptoms at all when she came for her third treatment.

St 36 *zusanli*, Sp 3 *taibai*, Bl 23 *shenshu* (tonification needle technique)

I continued to tonify the Spleen and Kidney *yang*. I advised Leonie's mother that she should bring her to the clinic at the first sign of another UTI. This happened just once, about two months after Leonie first came for treatment. She began to develop symptoms whilst she was at her first 'sleepover' away from home without her parents. I treated Leonie through this infection and she avoided the need for antibiotics. She has not developed another UTI since.

SUMMARY

» It is common for a child to have ongoing, 'sub-acute' symptoms which are not as severe as those of an acute infection.

» In nearly all cases of chronic or recurrent UTIs, there is an underlying Kidney deficiency.

» The patterns involved in an acute infection are: external Pathogenic Damp-Heat in the Bladder; and interior Damp-Heat in the Liver channel.

» The underlying patterns are: Spleen and Kidney *yang* deficiency; and Kidney *yin* deficiency.

• Chapter 61 •

HEADACHES AND MIGRAINES

The topics discussed in this chapter are:

- Aetiology
- Common headache triggers in children
- Patterns
- Treatment of headaches

Introduction

It is estimated that up to half of all children will have experienced at least one headache before the age of seven, and that number increases to 80 per cent by the age of fifteen. Of course, children who have the odd headache now and then are not the ones who generally come for acupuncture treatment. The children we see in the clinic usually suffer from recurrent headaches, which may be frequent and severe. Western medical doctors may label headaches (for example, migraines or tension headaches), although in reality these labels are not sufficient to describe the almost limitless types of pain and discomfort. Thankfully, as acupuncturists, we practise a system of medicine that has the ability to differentiate headaches in a more thorough manner, and to treat them in a more individualised way.

Most of the children we see in the clinic with headaches are school-age children and teenagers. However, parents may suspect that their pre-verbal baby or toddler experiences a kind of headache. Behaviour such as sleeping with his head pushed hard up against the side of the cot, or even banging his head repeatedly against the wall, may be suggestive of pain that the child is trying desperately to relieve.

Headaches come in all sorts of different forms. However, there are some general differences in the way children tend to experience headaches compared with adults. Headaches may come on very suddenly in a child. Though they may be intense, they may be short-lived (although not always). A child will often recover from a headache more quickly than an adult.

Aetiology
Babies and toddlers

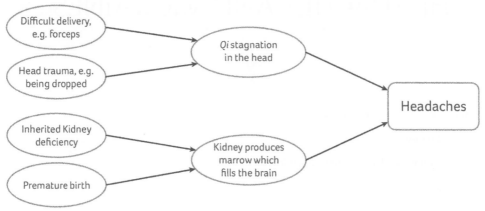

Figure 61.1 Headaches in babies and toddlers

School-age children and teenagers

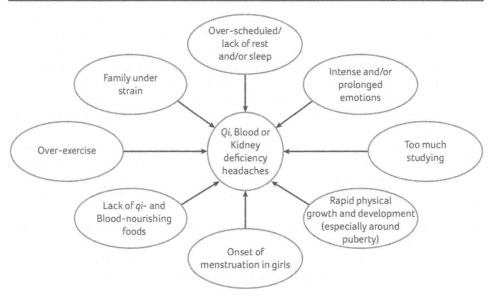

Figure 61.2 Deficiency headaches

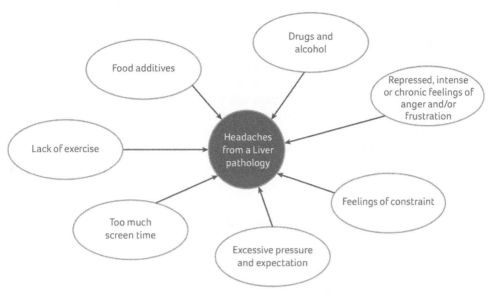

Figure 61.3 Headaches from a Liver pathology

As well as the specific aetiologies above, a factor which may be present in any child who suffers from recurrent headaches is simply spending too much time 'in his head'. Starting school at an early age, the pressure to excel academically and spending lots of free time on screens all draw a child's *qi* towards his head.

Common headache triggers in children

Although the parent and child will usually have thought long and hard about what triggers the child's headaches, it is always helpful for the practitioner, as an outsider, to help with this task. Some of the most common triggers for headaches in a child are:

- feeling stressed, worried or anxious

- internalising anger

- teething

- a cold or blocked sinuses

- losing sleep

- skipping a meal

- dehydration

- eating certain foods and drinks (e.g. ice cream, chocolate, alcohol)

- doing too much sport

- lack of movement and exercise

- in older children, poor posture when studying

- bright lights or smells

- prolonged time on a screen

- a change in the weather, particularly thundery and humid weather

- too much sun.

It is, of course, important to identify and eliminate headache triggers when possible. However, the fact that a child reacts to one or more of the above triggers by getting a headache is a sign of an imbalance. A child should be able to occasionally lose an hour or two of sleep or spend time outside in the sun without getting a headache. Therefore, diagnosis of the underlying imbalance should be made and treatment should be given accordingly. A true cure has been achieved when the same triggers no longer cause a headache in the child.

Patterns

- Liver *qi* stagnation (invading the Stomach and/or Spleen)

- Liver *yang* rising (or Liver Fire)

- Damp and Phlegm in the head

- *Qi* deficiency of the Stomach, Spleen, Lungs and/or Heart

- Blood deficiency of the Liver and/or Heart

- Kidney deficiency

In a very young child, there is often a Phlegm component to headaches. Liver pathologies are a common cause of headaches in children from the age of about seven or eight onwards. Blood deficiency and *yang* rising headaches are common in girls once they have started menstruating. Deficiency headaches are commonly seen in children who are over-scheduled. Full and empty patterns together often cause headaches, especially Blood or Kidney deficiency with Liver *yang* rising, or *qi* deficiency with Damp and Phlegm.

There may be a Lingering Pathogenic Factor in the Liver channel that is a component of either of the two Liver patterns (see Chapter 27 for a discussion of the treatment of a Lingering Pathogenic Factor).

Liver *qi* stagnation (invading the Stomach and/or Spleen)

The Stomach and Spleen are inherently weak in children, and the Liver tends towards excess. Therefore, this pattern is an extremely common cause of headache. In children with a history of head trauma, or who had a difficult birth, there may be local Blood stagnation as well as *qi* stagnation.

Symptoms

- intense, throbbing headache

- comes and goes and moves around to different parts of the head

- most commonly affects the temples or forehead

- better with movement or activity

- worse with stress, anxiety and humid weather

- Liver *qi* stagnation invades the Stomach: lack of appetite, nausea, vomiting, belching

- Liver *qi* stagnation invades the Spleen: abdominal pain, cramping, bloating, diarrhoea

Pulse: wiry Wood pulses, deficient Earth pulses

Tongue: may be pale or normal

Treatment principles: smooth the Liver and move *qi*; strengthen the Stomach and Spleen

> **SUGGESTED TREATMENT**
> In each treatment, it is usually sufficient to use one or two points to disperse the Liver, and one or two to strengthen the Stomach and Spleen.
>
> **Points**
> To smooth the Liver and move *qi*:
>
> > Liv 3 *taichong*
> > GB 34 *yanglingquan*
> > GB 20 *fengchi*
> > M-HN-9 *taiyang*
>
> **Method:** sedation needle technique
>
> To strengthen the Stomach and Spleen:
>
> > Ren 12 *zhongwan*
> > St 36 *zusanli*
> > Sp 3 *taibai*
> > Sp 6 *sanyinjiao*
> > Bl 20 *pishu*
> > Bl 21 *weishu*
>
> **Method:** tonification needle technique

Liver *yang* rising (or Liver Fire)

This type of headache often begins in the pre-adolescent phase. The surge of *yang* energy that occurs at this time causes the Liver to become Hot. Liver *yang* rising headaches are also common in children who are Kidney deficient, when *yang* is not sufficiently rooted.

Headache symptoms

- sudden, severe, intense headache

- pain may be throbbing, bursting or distending

- affects one or both sides of the head

- head may feel hot

Other symptoms: nausea, vomiting, visual disturbances, intolerance of noise, lights and smells

Pulse: wiry

Tongue: may be normal, there may be red spots on the sides

Treatment principles: subdue Liver *yang*; nourish Liver and/or Kidney *yin* or Blood

> **SUGGESTED TREATMENT**
> It will often be necessary to strengthen the underlying Liver and/or Kidney *yin* or Liver Blood deficiency too. This can normally only be done when the child does not have a headache. The

pulse will be the determining factor. If the Wood pulses are significantly wiry, this indicates that tonifying the underlying deficiency is not appropriate at that time.

Points

To subdue Liver *yang*:

> Liv 3 *taichong*
> Liv 2 *xingjian*
> GB 20 *fengchi*
> GB 43 *xiaxi*
> TB 5 *waiguan*

Method: sedation needle technique

To nourish Liver and/or Kidney *yin* or Liver Blood:

> Ki 3 *taixi*
> Sp 6 *sanyinjiao*
> Liv 8 *ququan*
> Bl 23 *shenshu*

Method: tonification needle technique

Damp and Phlegm in the head

Damp and Phlegm is a common cause of headache in children due to their inherently weak Spleens, and to the fact that many children have a heavily Damp-forming diet. The child may also produce Damp and Phlegm as a way of escaping from an aspect of reality that she finds too painful or difficult.

Headache symptoms

- thick, heavy, muzzy headache
- affects the forehead or the whole head
- often worse in the mornings or on damp days

Other symptoms: difficulty concentrating at school, muddled thinking, slightly disconnected, prone to a snotty nose or a chronic cough

Pulse: slippery

Tongue: thick, sticky coat

Treatment principles: resolve Damp and Phlegm

SUGGESTED TREATMENT

It will usually be necessary to strengthen the Stomach and Spleen as well as resolve Damp and Phlegm. Depending on the pulse picture, these two treatment principles may be done in the same treatment or on different occasions. If the pulses 'drop' and feel deficient after resolving Damp and Phlegm, it is probably necessary to immediately tonify the Stomach and Spleen. It may be enough to use one point per treatment to resolve Damp and Phlegm, and one or two points to tonify the Stomach and Spleen.

Points

> St 8 *touwei*

> St 40 *fenglong*
> Sp 9 *yinlingquan*
> Ren 12 *zhongwan*
> LI 4 *hegu*

Method: sedation needle technique

Additional points to strengthen the Stomach and Spleen

Qi deficiency of the Stomach, Spleen, Lungs and/or Heart

Key symptoms

- mild headaches
- worse in the mornings or when tired
- may be triggered by missing a meal, exercising or losing sleep
- persistent
- affect the whole head or just the forehead
- better with rest and food

Other symptoms will depend on the Organ which is predominantly affected but may include tiredness, poor appetite, pale face and tendency to coughs and colds.

Pulse: deficient; the position(s) affected will depend on the Organs involved

Tongue: pale

Treatment principles: bring *qi* to the head; tonify *qi* of the Lung, Heart, Stomach or Spleen as appropriate

> **SUGGESTED TREATMENT**
> **Points**
> Local points to bring *qi* to the head (should be chosen according to location of headache):
>
> > Du 20 *baihui*
> > Du 16 *fengfu*
>
> Points to tonify *qi* should be chosen according to the Organ or Organs most affected, but may include:
>
> > St 36 *zusanli*
> > Sp 3 *taibai*
> > Lu 9 *taiyuan*
> > He 7 *shenmen*
> > Bl 20 *pishu*
> > Bl 21 *weishu*
> > Bl 13 *feishu*
> > Bl 15 *xinshu*
>
> One or two points should be used at each treatment to address the deficiency.
>
> **Method:** tonification needle technique
>
> **Other techniques:** moxibustion

Blood deficiency of the Liver and/or Heart

Blood deficiency headaches are rarely seen in children until the teenage years. They are particularly common in girls and often begin soon after the onset of periods.

Headache symptoms

- mild, dull headaches

- often located on the top of the head or forehead

- worse with lots of studying, after exertion or after menstruation in women

- most commonly come on in the afternoon or evening

Other symptoms: mild anxiety, blurred vision, difficulty getting to sleep

Pulse: thin or choppy

Tongue: pale and dry; in extreme cases, may have orange sides

Treatment principles: nourish Liver and/or Heart Blood

> **SUGGESTED TREATMENT**
>
> Two or three points per treatment is usually sufficient. In all cases of Blood deficiency, the Organ or Organs that the deficiency stems from should be identified. This often coincides with the child's constitutional imbalance. Points along the channels connected with this Element and Organs should be chosen to address the Blood deficiency.
>
> **Points**
>
> Liv 8 *ququan*
> Liv 3 *taichong*
> Bl 18 *ganshu*
> He 7 *shenmen*
> Bl 15 *xinshu*
> Bl 17 *geshu*
> St 36 *zusanli*
> Sp 6 *sanyinjiao*
>
> **Method:** tonification needle technique
>
> **Other techniques:** moxibustion may be applicable

Kidney deficiency

Headaches caused by Kidney deficiency are generally seen either in children who are born with a congenital Kidney deficiency or those who are pushed excessively hard and become very depleted. The child may be small for his size or slow to develop. They are also seen in children going through puberty, or during an intense growth spurt at any age, when the Kidney *qi* is being taxed.

Headache symptoms

- vague headaches that the child may describe as being 'in their brain'

- a sensation of emptiness in the head

- worse during and after busy and stressful periods such as exam time

- worse when tired

- worse after exercise

- worse if does not get enough sleep

- prone to dark circles under the eyes

Other symptoms: bedwetting, hyperactivity, lethargy, easily overstimulated, lack of physical robustness

Pulse: deficient

Tongue: may be pale or red depending on the nature of the Kidney deficiency

Treatment principles: bring *qi* to the head; tonify the Kidneys

SUGGESTED TREATMENT

Kidney deficiency children are usually overstimulated, so no more than one or two points per treatment should be used.

Points

> Du 20 *baihui*
> Du 14 *dazhui*
> Bl 23 *shenshu*
> Bl 52 *zhishi*
> Ki 3 *taixi*
> Ki 7 *fuliu*
> Ren 4 *guanyuan*
> Ren 6 *qihai*

Method: tonification needle technique

Other techniques: moxibustion may be applicable if there is no Heat present

Treatment of headaches

Babies and toddlers

When a baby or toddler is brought for treatment with suspected headaches, it is usually because he appears to be in pain, is miserable most of the time and bangs his head or pushes it against the side of the cot. At this age, the cause of the headache is nearly always a difficult delivery or a trauma to the head. It may only be necessary to give local treatment to move *qi* and/or Blood in the head. Sometimes simply needling GB 20 *fengchi* is enough. At other times, it may be necessary to add in one or two distal points too.

It can be helpful to teach the parent some paediatric *tui na* in order to help move *qi* in the head too. The following routine will be helpful in all cases of headache, whatever the pattern, in a baby or toddler. Other moves may be added depending on the underlying pattern.

Heaven Gate *tianmen* (straight pushing)

Heart Gate *xinmen* (straight pushing)

Water Palace *kangong* (pushing apart)

Wind Pond *fengchi* (kneading)

Celestial Pillar Bone *tianzhugu* (straight pushing)

Big Bone Behind the Ear *erhou gaogu* (kneading)

Eight Trigrams *bagua* (circular pushing anti-clockwise)

CASE HISTORY: TWELVE-YEAR-OLD GIRL WITH VIOLENT AND PROLONGED MIGRAINES

The following case history illustrates that:

- emotions may be a cause of severe physical symptoms
- it is not always necessary to treat the Organ/Pathogen patterns for the child to get better.

Di had been experiencing migraines approximately every six weeks for the past year. When they came, she had to lie down in a darkened room and they were accompanied by vomiting. They would last for an entire week at a time.

The migraines had started when Di began secondary school. She had found the transition from primary school slightly challenging. None of her friends from primary school were in her class and, because it was such a big school, she could not necessarily find them during breaks. She had not yet made any new friends.

Di was otherwise a very happy, secure child who had a settled home life. She had never had any other emotional or physical issues at all before the migraines started.

Observations: Di had a large, warm smile and really twinkled as she was speaking. However, when she was not engaged in conversation, her face entirely changed and she looked very flat and sad. There was a lack of red colour on her face. She giggled a lot, even when she was talking about her difficulties at school.

- Pulse: Fire (TB/Pc) pulses were very thin and more deficient than the other pulse positions. Wood pulses were wiry.
- Tongue: normal

Diagnosis:

- Fire constitutional imbalance
- Liver *qi* stagnation invading the Stomach headaches

Treatment: Even though Di's headaches were due to a Liver pathology, I wanted to begin by treating the constitutional imbalance in her Fire Element. There was a very clear causal relationship between the headaches and her difficulties with friendships at school. I decided to treat the Triple Burner and Pericardium 'side' of Fire because the pulses of these Organs stood out as the lowest.

Treatment 1

Tonify Fire Element (TB and Pc)

Yuan source points: TB 4 *yangchi*, Pc 7 *daling* (tonification needle technique)

I noticed that, after needling these points, not only were the Fire pulses stronger, but the Wood pulses felt significantly less wiry.

Treatment 2

Di's mother said that she felt Di had 'got her spark back' since her treatment. She had not had any headaches, but since they only came intermittently, this was not significant.

Tonify Fire Element (TB and Pc)

Tonification points: TB 3 *zhongzhu*, Pc 9 *zhongchong* (tonification needle technique)

(I chose these points in order to draw the *qi* from the Mother Element (Wood) through to the Child Element (Fire).)

Once again, after needling these points, Di's Fire pulses felt stronger and her Wood pulse lost its wiry quality altogether.

Further treatment: I continued treating Di, using a selection of points to keep boosting her Fire Element. After she had gone for three months without a headache, I told her mother I thought we could stop treatment. I suggested she bring her back if she began to notice that her spark was going again, and obviously if she developed any more headaches.

Reflection: This case is a good example of how simple treatment of a child's constitutional imbalance may treat a symptom that is a result of an imbalance in entirely different Organs. If Di's Wood pulses had not become less wiry when I strengthened her Fire, I then would have treated her Wood directly. In this case, however, that was not necessary.

SUMMARY

» The cause of headaches in babies and toddlers is nearly always birth trauma or physical trauma early in life.

» Local treatment is often enough to cure headaches in a baby.

» The patterns involved in older children are: Liver *qi* stagnation; Liver *yang* rising or Liver Fire; Damp and Phlegm in the head; *qi* deficiency; Blood deficiency; and Kidney deficiency.

Chapter 62

SEIZURES

· · · · · · · · · · · · · · · ·

The topics discussed in this chapter are:

- Aetiology

- Diagnosis of seizures

- Weak seizures

- Strong seizures

- Further treatment considerations

- Dissociative seizures and the Metal Element

> **RED FLAGS: SEIZURES**
> A child who has had one or more seizures should always consult a Western medical practitioner so that any potentially dangerous causes can be excluded.

Introduction

> *The reason why seizures and tetany occur in very early childhood is always that visceral qi is not even.*[38]

Sun Simiao's words allude to the fact that because the *qi* of a young child is both *yang* in nature and has not yet settled into a smooth pattern, it easily moves in an uneven way. It could be likened to a toddler taking his first steps. At first he is unsteady, stops and starts and easily falls over. This kind of unsteadiness in the flow of *qi* can manifest in seizures, which are the epitome of a lack of smooth flow.

Seizures include the following conditions:

- epileptic seizures

- dissociative or non-epileptic seizures (NES)

- febrile seizures.

The *qi* of a child with seizures can sometimes feel very volatile and the seizures themselves can be understood as an outward expression of that volatility. During a seizure, a child switches from being apparently fine to losing both bodily control and consciousness. It may seem as if he has temporarily moved into a kind of parallel universe of which the onlooker is not a part. This may be a part of the reason why it is so hard for parents to see their child in this state. They feel as if they have entirely lost their connection with their child.

However, practitioners should not be discouraged from treating a child with seizures. In the case of epilepsy, acupuncture treatment has the potential to prevent the child being on heavily sedating medication for decades to come. Some children have such strong, prolonged and frequent seizures that they become brain damaged as a result. The implications of successfully treating a child with seizures are therefore profound. Parents should be warned that it may take some time. Changes in the child's medication along the way may muddy the waters and mean that the path to health has ups and downs.

The approach to the treatment of seizures should be almost the opposite of the disease itself, that is, simple rather than complex. Minimal intervention is often the best approach to the treatment of children. In the case of epilepsy, it is absolutely paramount. This is so as not to disturb the delicate and perhaps precarious balance of *qi* that the child has between seizures.

If the practitioner is able to discern the Element that is the child's constitutional imbalance and simply begin by treating this, it may provide a more stable foundation upon which more treatment principles may gradually be added.

Epileptic and non-epileptic seizures

Epileptic seizures are caused by a disturbance in the electrical activity of the brain. Non-epileptic seizures may have an organic cause, such as a brain tumour or a heart condition. They may also be psychogenic: in other words, they may be caused by mental or psychological processes. Both epileptic and non-epileptic seizures fall into the disease category *dian xian*, which was discussed in both the *Nei Jing* and the *Ling Shu*. *Dian xian* was called 'goat crying wind' because the noises patients sometimes make during a seizure were thought to resemble the bleating of a goat, and the movements they make were quick and erratic like wind. Underlying a condition of seizures, whether epileptic or non-epileptic, is usually a profound internal imbalance that the child was either born with or that has slowly been developing for years.

Febrile seizures

About five in one hundred children have a febrile seizure before the age of six. They most commonly occur between the ages of eighteen months and three years. They are rare in children aged under three months and over the age of six years. They are more common in boys than girls.[39] The convulsions are triggered by a high temperature, or a sudden rise in the child's temperature.

Although there is a slightly increased risk of epilepsy in a child with a history of febrile convulsions, the vast majority of the time they are considered to be a benign condition that the child will grow out of.

Emotions that may arise as a result of seizures

In Chinese medicine texts, epilepsy has historically been grouped together with mental health disorders. In the West today, epilepsy is considered a neurological disorder. However, seizures still often evoke a kind of fear, mistrust or awkwardness in many who are not familiar with them. This is partly, perhaps, because they trigger one of many people's deepest fears, namely the absolute loss of control of mind and body that is characteristic of a tonic-clonic seizure.

An older child with seizures may talk of extreme fear or anxiety associated with his seizures. Fear is actually considered a symptom of seizures for some children.[40] Parents may notice that their child becomes irritable or even aggressive when he is about to have a seizure. A child may find he feels anxious or low for days after he has had a seizure. The particular emotions that a child experiences in association with his seizures may help the practitioner to diagnose which Organs are particularly involved. Treatment may also help to lessen some of these emotions, making the condition easier to deal with for the child.

A child who has seizures in front of his schoolmates or in public sometimes finds himself also having to cope with others becoming distant or with being poorly understood. Over time, this may lead to intense feelings of one kind or another. Depending on the emotional constitution of the child, he may feel rejected, angry or fearful as a result of people's responses to his illness.

Types of seizures

Seizures may be divided into the following categories:

- **Absence seizures** (sometimes called petit mal): Absence seizures usually involve a brief loss and then return to consciousness. The child may or may not be aware of these absences and usually there is no after-effect.

- **Partial seizures** (sometimes called focal seizures): The child will remain conscious during a partial seizure. He may feel strange, intense emotions, become numb or stiff, or twitch in one part of his body and have visual disturbances or hallucinations.

- **Tonic-clonic seizures** (sometimes called grand mal): The child will lose consciousness, jerk and shake, his breathing may become difficult or noisy and he may have urinary incontinence.

- **Complex febrile seizures:** A 'complex' seizure is triggered by the rise in temperature during an invasion of Wind. It lasts longer than fifteen minutes, affects only one side or part of the body and/or recurs within twenty-four hours or during the same illness.

- **Simple febrile seizures:** A 'simple' febrile seizure is also triggered by the rise in temperature during an invasion of Wind. It lasts less than fifteen minutes and does not happen again during the same illness.

Aetiology

Even though a child may appear to have developed seizures overnight, in reality there have usually been several factors which have compounded over a period of time and have led to the development of the disease. Aetiological factors can be divided into those which affect primarily the body, and those which affect primarily the *shen* (see Figure 62.1).

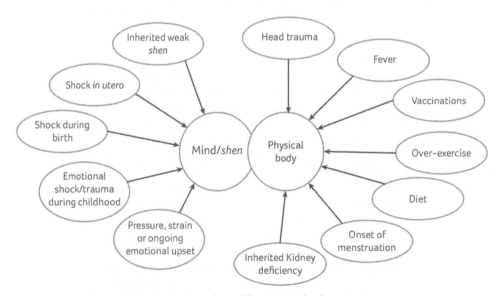

Figure 62.1 Aetiological factors involved in seizures

Triggers for seizures

There are many possible triggers for seizures and it can be helpful to work with the family to try to identify what these are. Some of the most common are:

- intense emotions: many children with epilepsy recognise that their seizures may be triggered, for example, by feeling upset, angry or anxious

- stress and pressure

- lack of rest or sleep

- over-exercise

- illness (such as a vomiting bug or a respiratory infection)

- skipping meals

- certain times of the menstrual cycle may be a trigger for seizures in adolescent girls

- changes in the dosage of medication

- bright or flashing lights

- being on a screen for too long

- over-excitement or overstimulation that makes the *qi* rise up

- fevers.

Diagnosis of seizures

The practitioner needs to be clear about two aspects of the child's condition, namely the underlying pattern and the pattern that actually causes the seizures: see Table 62.1.

Table 62.1 Patterns involved in seizures

Underlying patterns	Patterns that cause strong seizures	Patterns that cause weak seizures
Yuan qi and *shen* deficiency	Fright	Spleen (and Kidney) *yang* deficiency
Kidney deficiency	Phlegm	Phlegm
Phlegm	Blood stasis	
Blood stasis	Wind	
	Food	
	Invasion of Wind	

 Chinese medicine considers that every seizure will deplete the *yuan qi* of the growing child. Therefore, the primary treatment principle in all cases should be to prevent seizures.

Internal patterns which predispose a child to seizures

The four patterns below describe an internal predisposition to seizures. It then takes an external factor, such as one of those described above in Figure 62.1, for the seizures to develop.

- Deficient *yuan qi* and *shen*

- Kidney deficiency

- Phlegm

- Blood stasis in the brain and affecting the Heart's orifices

Deficient *yuan qi* and *shen*

This pattern describes a child who was born with a highly sensitive and delicate disposition. She is probably neither physically nor emotionally robust.

Original *qi* is Essence in the form of *qi* and therefore strongly related to the Kidneys. It relies on nourishment from post-Heavenly Essence. The treatment of it is best done through whichever Organ or Organs are primarily deficient in the individual child. This should be diagnosed according to the pulse, as well as other symptoms and signs present.

Key symptoms

- seizures often triggered by emotional upset or shock

- easily startled or upset

- strongly affected by the external environment (such as loud noises, crowds of people, emotional upset)

Other symptoms: in a young child clinginess, easily tires, pale face

Pulse: deficient

Tongue: may be pale, may have a Heart crack, lots of red spots on the tip

Treatment principles: strengthen original *qi*; calm the *shen*

> **SUGGESTED TREATMENT**
> Points should be chosen according to which Organ or Organs the deficiency stems from. Two points per treatment is usually sufficient.
>
> **Points**
>
> He 7 *shenmen*
> St 36 *zusanli*
> Ki 3 *taixi*
> TB 4 *yangchi*
> Lu 9 *taiyuan*
> Ren 4 *guanyuan*
> Ren 6 *qihai*
>
> **Method:** tonification needle technique
>
> **Other techniques:** moxibustion may be applicable if there is no Heat present
>
> **Paediatric *tui na***
> The following routine helps *qi* to descend and strengthens the child's constitution.
>
> Heaven Gate *tianmen* (straight pushing)
> Heart Gate *xinmen* (straight pushing)
> Water Palace *kangong* (pushing apart)
> Wind Pond *fengchi* (kneading)
> Celestial Pillar Bone *tianzhugu* (straight pushing)
> Big Bone Behind the Ear *erhou gaogu* (kneading)
> Eight Trigrams *bagua* (circular pushing anti-clockwise)
> Spinal Column *jizhu* (pinching)
> Knead the navel *roufu* (kneading)

Kidney deficiency

Key symptom

- weak or strong seizures which often come when the child is tired or has been ill

Other symptoms: physically un-robust, easily tires, dark circles under the eyes, tendency to bedwetting

Pulse: deficient

Tongue: may be pale or red depending on whether Kidney *yin* or *yang* deficiency predominates

Treatment principles: tonify Kidneys; stop seizures

SUGGESTED TREATMENT

One or two points per treatment is sufficient.

Points

Bl 23 *shenshu*
Bl 28 *pangguangshu*
Ki 3 *taixi*
Ki 7 *fuliu*
Ren 3 *zhongji*
Ren 6 *qihai*

Method: tonification needle technique

Paediatric *tui na* to tonify and warm the Kidneys

Kidney *shenjing* (straight pushing)
Two Men Upon a Horse *erma* (kneading)
Outer Palace of Toil *wailaogong* (kneading)
Wind Nest *yiwofeng* (kneading)
Three Passes *sanguan* (straight pushing)
Lower Back – area around Bl 23 *shenshu* (strong rubbing)
Spinal Column *jizhu* (pinching)

Phlegm

In seizures, Thick Phlegm inhabits the channels and blocks the flow of *qi*. It also mists the Mind, affecting consciousness and thinking. Phlegm may be an underlying condition in seizures, as well as causing both weak and strong seizures.

Dr Su Xin-ming[41] describes Phlegm as being the basis for all seizures. Once there is a background of Phlegm in the child, it may be stirred up by many other factors such as strong emotions or over-strain. The Phlegm is then carried upwards to the head by Liver-Wind. The Heart becomes misted by the Phlegm, which then means the *shen* has no resting place. This leads to either the absences or complete unconsciousness that are characteristic of many seizures.

Key symptoms

- tonic-clonic seizures

- absences

- vacant

- disconnected

- slow speech and movements
- needs to sleep a lot

Other symptoms: other physical signs of Phlegm such as a tendency to a snotty nose and cough

Pulse: slippery and/or wiry

Tongue: thick, sticky coat

Treatment principles: resolve Phlegm

> **SUGGESTED TREATMENT**
> **Points**
>
> > Pc 5 *jianshi*
> > St 40 *fenglong*
> > GB 13 *benshen*
>
> **Method:** sedation needle technique
>
> **Paediatric *tui na***
> The following routine resolves Phlegm and descends *qi*.
>
> > Spleen *pijing* (straight pushing)
> > Eight Trigrams *bagua* (circular pushing anti-clockwise)
> > Small Palmar Crease *zhangxiaowen* (straight pushing)
> > Hand *yin yang shouyinyang* (pushing apart)
> > Heaven Gate *tianmen* (straight pushing)
> > Heart Gate *xinmen* (straight pushing)
> > Water Palace *kangong* (pushing apart)
> > Wind Pond *fengchi* (kneading)
> > Celestial Pillar Bone *tianzhugu* (straight pushing)
> > Big Bone Behind the Ear *erhou gaogu* (kneading)
> > St 40 Abundant Bulge *fenglong* (kneading)

Blood stasis in the brain and affecting the Heart's orifices

Blood stasis may result from a traumatic birth or physical trauma early in life. The stagnation affects the Heart's orifices and the *shen* cannot be properly housed as a result.

Key symptoms

- strong, tonic-clonic seizures with complete loss of consciousness
- possible cognitive impairment or signs of brain damage

Other symptoms: habitual headaches in a fixed location, may press or bang head against the wall of the cot as a baby, poor sleep

Pulse: wiry or choppy

Tongue: purple or purple spots

Treatment principles: move stagnant Blood*

---

*   It is beneficial to combine acupuncture with another treatment, such as cranial osteopathy, when treating Blood stagnation in the head.

> **SUGGESTED TREATMENT**
> **Points**
>
> > Du 20 *baihui*
> > Du 14 *dazhui*
> > Local or *ahshi* points on the head if the site of the trauma is known
> > Liv 3 *taichong*
> > Bl 17 *geshu*
>
> **Method:** sedation needle technique
>
> **Paediatric *tui na***
> Paediatric *tui na* is not the treatment of choice for this pattern.

Weak seizures

The Excess patterns described above tend to cause strong seizures with violent shaking of the body and complete loss of consciousness. However, a child who has absences or mild, partial seizures may suffer from either a deficient pattern or Phlegm. The most likely is a deficiency of *yang* which affects the Spleen and possibly the Kidneys.*

Spleen and/or Kidney *yang* deficiency

Key symptom

* a tendency towards absences rather than tonic-clonic seizures

Other symptoms: easily tires, poor appetite, tendency to loose stools, pale and puffy face, may have a tendency to drool, easily feels cold

Pulse: deep, weak, deficient

Tongue: pale, wet, swollen

Treatment principles: warm and tonify Spleen and/or Kidney *yang*

> **SUGGESTED TREATMENT**
> Two points per treatment is usually sufficient.
>
> **Points**
>
> > St 36 *zusanli*
> > Sp 3 *taibai*
> > Sp 6 *sanyinjiao*
> > Bl 20 *pishu*
> > Ki 3 *taixi*
> > Ki 7 *fuliu*
> > Bl 23 *shenshu*
>
> **Method:** tonification needle technique
>
> **Other techniques:** moxibustion may be applicable if there is no Heat present
>
> **Paediatric *tui na***
> The following routine descends *qi* and warms Spleen and Kidney *yang*.

---

* Chinese books also describe Liver and Kidney *yin* deficiency as a pattern which may cause epilepsy. However, this is very rarely seen in the West because children do not tend to have strong, high fevers which deplete their *yin* to this degree.

Heaven Gate *tianmen* (straight pushing)
Heart Gate *xinmen* (straight pushing)
Water Palace *kangong* (pushing apart)
Wind Pond *fengchi* (kneading)
Celestial Pillar Bone *tianzhugu* (straight pushing)
Spleen *pijing* (straight pushing)
Kidney *shenjing* (straight pushing)
Three Passes *sanguan* (straight pushing)
Two Men Upon a Horse *erma* (kneading)
Outer Palace of Toil *wailaogong* (kneading)
Wind Nest *yiwofeng* (kneading)
Lower Back – area around Bl 23 *shenshu* (strong rubbing)
Knead the navel *rou qi* (kneading)
Spinal Column *jizhu* (pinching from the bottom to the top of the back)
St 36 *zusanli* (kneading)

CASE HISTORY: FIFTEEN-YEAR-OLD GIRL WITH EPILEPSY

The following case history illustrates:

- the importance of minimum intervention when treating epilepsy
- the difficulties of treating the condition when medication is being changed.

Alison had been diagnosed with juvenile absence epilepsy a few months before coming to the clinic. She had been having ongoing absence seizures and also two tonic-clonic seizures. She was already taking three anti-epileptic medications, the dosages of which were being regularly changed.

Alison's periods had stopped completely for the past eight months.

Alison tended towards feeling hot. She slept well, ate well and her digestion was good. She had had no poor health at all in her life before the epilepsy.

Alison was a very talented dancer. She trained for several hours a day, and had done since she was eight years old.

Observations: Despite being rather slender due to her intense dance training, Alison had quite a solid, robust body. She was extremely pale. Although articulate, she sometimes seemed to talk rather slowly or become muddled and pause mid-sentence. Her movements were rather slow.

- Pulse: extremely deep, weak and thin in all positions; slow (60 bpm); slippery on the Earth pulses. Metal pulses were the most deficient.
- Tongue: red

Basal body temperature (BBT): I asked Alison to record her daily temperature and to plot it on a BBT chart. Her temperature was consistently low – ranging between 35 and 36 degrees Celsius.

Her voice was weeping. She had a palpable sadness to her. Alison was unusually articulate for a girl of her age, yet she seemed entirely disconnected from any 'difficult' emotions such as sadness or anger. She appeared superficially to be unbothered by the development of her epilepsy.

Diagnosis: Alison's symptoms and signs were somewhat contradictory. Her tongue was red and she felt hot most of the time, yet her pulse was deep, weak and slow and she was pale and moved rather slowly.

I diagnosed her as having a Metal constitutional imbalance. In terms of Organ/Pathogen patterns, Alison had Kidney *yang* deficiency (confirmed by her BBT chart readings), Liver Blood deficiency and Phlegm.

Treatment: It took some time to establish the right way of treating Alison. Although it was at times difficult to know what was doing what because her medication was being changed so frequently, some treatments seemed to provoke a seizure. In the end, it proved to be two specific treatment principles that helped Alison:

- tonify Metal Element
- warm and tonify Kidney *yang*.

Alison's periods came back, and after a few months of treatment were regular again. After about six months, she stopped having tonic-clonic seizures. However, she still had absences approximately once a week over a period of a few hours or a day.

Aetiology: I felt that Alison's intense dance training over the past few years was the most significant factor in the development of her epilepsy. It had depleted her to an enormous degree. I spoke with Alison and her mother about this, but dance had become such a big part of Alison's identity and gave her so much pleasure that she chose to continue it.

Reflection: Treating Alison helped me to understand more deeply that the *qi* of a child who has epilepsy is, as Sun Simiao described, volatile and unsmooth. It takes very little to cause it to become unsettled, including an acupuncture treatment that is too strong.

Phlegm
Key symptoms

- absences rather than seizures
- vacant
- dulled responses
- slow speech and movements

Other symptoms: cough with mucus, blocked nose, lethargic

Pulse: slippery or wiry

Tongue: thick, sticky coat

Treatment principles: resolve Phlegm

For treatment, please see Phlegm under 'Internal patterns which predispose a child to seizures' above.

Strong seizures
There are six possible components that may be present in strong seizures. They rarely ever occur on their own and are nearly always seen in conjunction with each other.

Fright

Fright seizures, which only affect small children, describe a seizure which results from a shock. It may arise because the *shen* is weak, not yet strongly rooted, and because the child is not able to regulate himself (see Chapter 2).
    Sun Simiao said:

As for fright seizures, these begin with the patient crying loudly after being startled and frightened, after which the seizures occur. These are fright seizures. When fright seizures are still slight, hold the baby in a tight grip and do not let them be frightened again. It is possible that the seizures will stop on their own.[42]

Key symptom

- seizures triggered by a shock, such as a sudden, loud noise, an emotional upset, flashing lights or anything that scares the child

Other symptoms: tendency to anxiety, restlessness and agitated, poor sleep

Pulse: Heart pulse overflowing, rapid

Tongue: red, lots of red spots on the tip, Heart crack

Treatment principles: clear Heat from the Heart; calm the *shen*

SUGGESTED TREATMENT
Points

> He 7 *shenmen*
> Ren 14 *juque*
> Pc 6 *neiguan*
> Bl 15 *xinshu*

Method: sedation needle technique

Paediatric *tui na*
The following routine calms the *shen* and descends *qi*.

> Heart *xinjing* (straight pushing)
> Heaven Gate *tianmen* (straight pushing)
> Heart Gate *xinmen* (straight pushing)
> Water Palace *kangong* (pushing apart)
> Wind Pond *fengchi* (kneading)
> Celestial Pillar Bone *tianzhugu* (straight pushing)
> Palace of Toil *laogong* (kneading)
> Small Heavenly Heart *xiaotianxin* (kneading)

Phlegm

These seizures are triggered by an increase in Phlegm brought about by diet or the residual effect of an External Pathogenic Factor in the Lungs.

Key symptoms

- tonic-clonic seizures and/or absences

- vomiting of mucus

- clouding of the senses and loss of consciousness

- mental confusion

Other symptoms: profuse mucus, sound of mucus in the throat, mild spasms and contractions

Pulse: slippery and/or wiry

Tongue: thick, white coat

Treatment principles: resolve Phlegm

> **SUGGESTED TREATMENT**
> **Points**
>
> > St 40 *fenglong*
> > Pc 5 *jianshi*
> > GB 34 *yanglingquan*
> > GB 13 *benshen*
>
> **Method:** sedation needle technique
>
> **Paediatric *tui na***
> See Phlegm under 'Internal patterns which predispose a child to seizures' above.

Blood stasis

Key symptoms

- tonic-clonic seizures

- history of brain injury

- cognitive impairment

Pulse: wiry or choppy

Tongue: purple or purple spots

Treatment principles: invigorate Blood; stop seizures

> **SUGGESTED TREATMENT**
> **Points**
>
> > Du 20 *baihui*
> > Du 16 *fengfu*
> > GB 20 *fengchi*
> > *Ahshi* points on the head to the site of trauma if known
> > Liv 3 *taichong*
> > Bl 17 *geshu*
>
> **Method:** sedation needle technique

Wind

Wind seizures may come about in a child who suffers repeated or severe febrile convulsions. The convulsions themselves generate and stir up Wind.

Key symptoms

- sudden, tonic-clonic seizures

- very strong convulsions

- clenched teeth

- eyes staring upward

- stiffness and rigidity

Other symptoms: very hot, red face

Pulse: wiry, rapid

Tongue: stiff

Treatment principles: clear Heat and extinguish Wind

> **SUGGESTED TREATMENT**
> **Points**
>
> > Du 14 *dazhui*
> > GB 20 *fengchi*
> > Liv 2 *xingjian*
> > Liv 3 *taichong*
> > GB 43 *xiaxi*
>
> **Method:** sedation needle technique
>
> **Paediatric *tui na***
> The following routine clears Heat and descends *qi*.
>
> > Heart *xinjing* (straight pushing)
> > Heaven Gate *tianmen* (straight pushing)
> > Heart Gate *xinmen* (straight pushing)
> > Water Palace *kangong* (pushing apart)
> > Wind Pond *fengchi* (kneading)
> > Celestial Pillar Bone *tianzhugu* (straight pushing)
> > Palace of Toil *laogong* (kneading)
> > Small Heavenly Heart *xiaotianxin* (kneading)
> > Milky Way *tianheshui* (straight pushing)
> > Six *Yang* Organs *liufu* (straight pushing)

Accumulation of Food

Instead of being dispersed, food remains in the child's abdomen for a prolonged period of time, blocking the flow of *qi*. These seizures are most common in babies and very young children.

Key symptoms

- tonic-clonic seizures with spasms and tremors
- vomiting and diarrhoea

Other symptoms: seizures may be preceded by constipation, restlessness and a feeling of heat

Pulse: full

Tongue: thick, sticky coat

Treatment principles: disperse accumulation of food; resolve Phlegm; extinguish Wind

> **SUGGESTED TREATMENT**
> The *sifeng* points should not be used during a seizure because of the risk of temporarily releasing more Heat and Phlegm into the system.

Points

> *sifeng*

Method: prick the *sifeng* points lightly on one hand

or

> St 40 *fenglong*
> Ren 12 *zhongwan*
> Sp 4 *gongsun*

Method: sedation needle technique

Paediatric *tui na*

> Thick Gate *banmen* (straight pushing)
> Eight Trigrams *bagua* (circular pushing anti-clockwise)
> Four Wind Creases *sifengwen* (pinching)
> Knead the navel *roufu* (kneading clockwise)
> Abdomen Stimulation *fuyinyang* (pushing apart)
> Belly Corner *dujiao* (pinching)

Invasion of External Pathogenic Cold or Heat

This pattern is commonly a trigger for febrile seizures in young children. Traditionally, the sources of external Heat were said to be invasions of Wind-Cold or Wind-Heat, Summer Heat or 'epidemic pestilence' (i.e. a severe febrile disease such as meningitis). Today, invasions of Wind-Cold or Wind-Heat and the child's response to vaccinations are the ones routinely seen in the clinic.

Key symptoms

- strong spasms and tremor
- arched back, rigidity
- possible loss of consciousness

Other symptoms: fever, sore throat, headache, sweating

Pulse: floating, rapid

Tongue: thick yellow coating

Treatment principles: expel Wind; clear Heat; stop seizures

SUGGESTED TREATMENT

This treatment should be given as soon as the child shows signs of an invasion of a Pathogenic Factor. Ideally, the child should be treated every few hours in order to prevent a febrile convulsion. Liv 2 *xingjian* is included to prevent the Heat agitating the Liver, which then stirs up internal Wind.

Points

> Du 14 *dazhui*
> LI 11 *quchi*
> LI 4 *hegu*
> TB 5 *waiguan*
> Liv 2 *xingjian*

Method: sedation needle technique

> **Paediatric *tui na* to expel Wind-Heat and descend *qi***
>
> Heaven Gate *tianmen* (straight pushing)
> Heart Gate *xinmen* (straight pushing)
> Water Palace *kangong* (pushing apart)
> *Taiyang* (M-HN-9) (kneading)
> Wind Pond *fengchi* (kneading)
> Celestial Pillar Bone *tianzhugu* (straight pushing)
> Big Bone Behind the Ear *erhou gaogu* (kneading)
> Eight Trigrams *bagua* (circular pushing anti-clockwise)
> Lung *feijing* (straight pushing from base to tip)
> Two Panels Gate *ershanmen* (pinching or kneading)
> Milky Way *tianheshui* (straight pushing)

> Four-year-old Neil came for treatment because, every time he caught a cold, he had a short-lasting, febrile convulsion. He would lose consciousness and his whole body went into spasm. He had no other health problems but he was a frail child who always looked tired. His seizures were obviously triggered by an invasion of Wind. However, it was the underlying deficiency in his Kidneys that caused him to respond to the invasions with seizures. I began treatment by strengthening his Kidneys. His mother also brought him for treatment at the first sign that he was coming down with a cold. After three months of treatment he had a cold that did not trigger a seizure for the first time.

Further treatment considerations
Shonishin
Core non-pattern-based root treatment.

Targeted tapping around:

- Du 12 *shenzhu*
- the temples

Some important points in the treatment of seizures

- Du 26 *renzhong*: this is the principal point to restore consciousness; it can be pressed with the finger in a child who is having a seizure, but is also a helpful point to use between seizures, especially in a child who has frequent absences
- Pc 5 *jianshi*: resolve Phlegm misting the Heart
- St 40 *fenglong*: resolve Phlegm
- GB 20 *fengchi*: descend Wind-Phlegm
- Du 8 *jingsuo*: relieves spasms and contractions

Gua sha
Sun Simiao suggests that 'when you see these signs [of seizures], scrape the baby's yang vessels'.[43] Wilms suggests that this passage may be alluding either to the *yangming* vessel, or the *taiyang* Bladder channel of the back, or to the point Du 14 *dazhui*.

Ki 1 *yongquan* has the action of bringing excess *qi* down from the head. It can either be needled, massaged or treated with moxibustion.

Dissociative seizures and the Metal Element

Dissociative seizures can happen as a cut-off mechanism to stop bad memories from being relived. The child dissociates from her feelings about a particular experience because it is too difficult to cope with. The seizure happens almost in lieu of the child experiencing the intense feelings.

The ability to dissociate in this way brings to mind the spirit of the Metal Element, the *po* or Corporeal Soul. The *po* enables a child to stay connected with emotions and to the physiological responses in the body. An imbalance in the Metal Element may be involved in dissociative seizures in some children. Interestingly, Hammer[44] suggests that unexpressed grief (the emotion related to the Metal Element) may manifest as a form of epilepsy.

Strengthening the Metal Element can mean that a child gradually begins to connect with whatever has been repressed. In fact, it is common when treating a child's Metal to find that she generally becomes more in touch with her emotional world. In the case of seizures, this may mean that the need for seizures gradually disappears as the previously repressed emotions begin to emerge into the conscious mind.

SUMMARY

» There is usually a complex mix of aetiologies involved that affect both the body and the *shen*.

» The underlying patterns are: *yuan qi* and *shen* deficiency; Kidney deficiency; Phlegm; and Blood stasis.

» Patterns that cause strong seizures are: fright; Phlegm; Blood stasis; Wind; Accumulation of Food; and invasion of Wind-Cold or Wind-Heat.

» Patterns that cause weak seizures are: Spleen (and Kidney) *yang* deficiency; and Phlegm.

» An imbalance in the Metal Element may be involved in dissociative seizures.

Chapter 63

TICS

· · · · · · · ·

The topics discussed in this chapter are:

- Organs involved in tics

- Pathogens involved in tics

- Diagnosis and treatment of tics

- Patterns

Introduction

A tic is a brief, repetitive, purposeless, non-rhythmic, involuntary movement or sound. Tics that produce movement are called motor tics, whilst tics that produce sound are known as vocal tics. It is thought that one in five children will have a tic at some point during childhood. They may appear at any time, and tend to come in bouts.

Many children will, at one point or another during childhood, experience a transient, simple tic that often appears apparently out of nowhere, stays for a few weeks or months and then disappears. The children who are brought to the clinic with tics have usually had a simple tic for a prolonged period of time, have had several tics or have complex tics. The most severe manifestation of tics is Tourette's syndrome.

Strong tics may be extremely challenging for a child. First, a strong motor tic such as jerking of the body is, in itself, very tiring. It can be relentless and means the child is never still or relaxed. Second, a child with tics may be a target for unkind comments from other children or bullying. As a child gets older, he may feel embarrassed by his tics and struggle socially.

Acupuncture can be wonderfully effective when treating a child with tics.

Types of tic

Common motor tics

- blinking

- head jerking

- shoulder shrugging

- mouth grimacing

Common vocal tics

- throat-clearing

- grunting

- sniffing

- coughing

The tics described above are all known as 'simple' tics, which just involve one movement or one sound. A less common and more severe problem is 'complex' tics, which, in the case of motor tics, involve more than one muscle group. Complex vocal tics may mean the child utters phrases or that there is some linguistic meaning in her utterances.

Factors which affect tics

There are various factors which seem to make a child's tics better or worse. Some of the most common factors are listed below.

Factors which tend to exacerbate tics

- feeling under time pressure
- feeling stressed
- being overstimulated
- before and after tasks which require a lot of concentration
- tiredness
- being asked to suppress tics (with a delayed reaction)
- being talked to about tics

Factors which tend to ameliorate tics

- being distracted
- being engrossed in a task which is not stressful
- during a task which requires a lot of concentration
- being asleep
- being in a new and unfamiliar situation
- being asked to suppress tics (but only as an initial response)

Organs involved in tics

The Liver

The Liver easily becomes Hot. Children are said to have a pure *yang* constitution, which means that they have even more of a tendency to have a Hot, agitated Liver.

The sound associated with the Liver is shouting. If the *qi* of the Liver is Hot and in excess, this may lead to the child having a vocal tic which manifests as shouting sounds and utterances.

Liver Blood and *yin* may also be deficient in children. This often results from a deficiency of the Spleen leading to Blood deficiency. If Blood and *yin* are deficient, it leaves room in the channels for Wind to stir, causing a tic which may affect any part of the body.

The Heart

The Heart governs speech and may therefore be involved in the case of vocal tics. The Heart is affected by any intense emotion, especially fright. Once the Heart and the *shen* have become disturbed, they are more susceptible to being affected by Phlegm.

The Spleen

A deficiency of the Spleen, also common in children, may lead to a build-up of fluids in the body. If the Spleen does not efficiently transform and transport fluids, they may accumulate in the form of Damp. With the addition of Heat, this Damp then transforms into Phlegm.

Pathogens involved in tics

Internal Wind

Wind may either arise from an underlying deficiency of Liver Blood or from excess Heat in the Liver which stirs up Wind. Wind causes involuntary movements and tics. Wind tends to affect the upper part of the body, so is likely to cause tics that affect the face and head.

Phlegm

Phlegm may be formed when excess Heat dries and condenses the fluids. Phlegm rises up and may obstruct the Heart, meaning that utterances may be involuntary and uncontrolled.

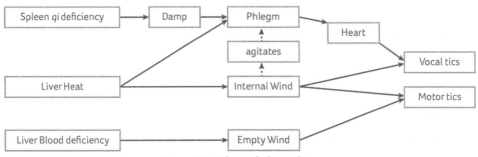

Figure 63.1 The pathology of tics

Diagnosis and treatment of tics

Broadly speaking, there are two different scenarios seen in the clinic. The first is a child who has a tic but none of the traditional Organ/Pathogen patterns described in Chinese medicine texts. The second is a child who has a tic that is related to an Organ/Pathogen pattern commonly ascribed to tics.

Tics not related to a specific Organ/Pathogen pattern

Some children who suffer from mild tics do not have any pathology related to internal Wind or Phlegm. In these cases, the tics often appear after the child has become stressed. Very often, there is an obvious correlation. The parents report that the tic began, for example, soon after the child changed schools, fell out with a friend, witnessed an upsetting incident or lost her grandmother.

However, sometimes the trigger is not obvious. The tic seems to literally appear out of the blue. In these cases, it is not that there was not a trigger (there always is) but that the trigger is not apparent to either parent or child. It may be that the child suddenly realised that her parents will one day die, or that there are people in the world who do nasty things, or that one day she will have to work really hard for exams as her big sister does. It is as if the child was happily going on enjoying life and then something she read, saw or heard forced her into a developmental leap for which she was not quite ready. This puts a strain on her, and the outward manifestation of the strain is a tic. Of course, most of the time, the child is totally unaware that this is what has happened.

Treatment of tics not caused by an Organ/Pathogen pattern

There are two possible approaches to the treatment of these tics:

- They are often caused by an imbalance in the Heart, which must be confirmed by the pulse. It is as if the child has had a type of shock and the tic manifests as a result of that. Speech tics, including stuttering, often fall into this category. The point of choice in this case is He 5 *tongli*.

- If the Heart pulse does not reveal any pathology, treating the constitutional imbalance of the child is often effective. Gentle support of the relevant Element will help the child to release the strain that is causing him to tic. It may take some time, but in nearly all cases, the tic will gradually fade.

Patterns

- Liver Wind and Phlegm-Heat stirring within
- Liver Blood and/or *yin* deficiency with Empty Wind stirring within

Liver Wind and Phlegm-Heat stirring within

Key symptoms

- strong tics
- twitching of any limb or part of the body
- facial tics such as blinking or sniffing
- tics become worse when stressed or with heightened emotions
- worse from inactivity and having to sit still

Other symptoms: may have febrile convulsions, hyperactive, flares with anger, moodiness or irritability, disturbed sleep, red face

Pulse: wiry, slippery, rapid

Tongue: red, sticky yellow coat

Treatment principles: expel Wind; clear Heat; resolve Phlegm

> **SUGGESTED TREATMENT**
> It is usually sufficient to use two or three points per treatment. Points should be chosen according to which pathogen predominates. The combination of LI 4 *hegu* and Liv 3 *taichong*, known as the Four Gates, is especially effective at extinguishing Wind.
>
> **Points**
> To extinguish Wind:
>
> > GB 20 *fengchi*
> > Du 20 *baihui*
> > LI 4 *hegu*
> > Liv 3 *taichong*
> > Liv 2 *xingjian*
> > St 40 *fenglong*
> > Pc 5 *jianshi*

Method: sedation needle technique

If Accumulation Disorder is present, this should be treated by pricking the M-UE-9 *sifeng* points of one hand.

Paediatric *tui na* to clear Phlegm and Heat and descend *qi*

> Spleen *pijing* (straight pushing tonification)
> Eight Trigrams *bagua* (circular pushing anti-clockwise)
> Small Palmar Crease *zhangxiaowen* (straight pushing)
> Hand *yin yang shouyinyang* (pushing apart)
> Milky Way *tianheshui* (straight pushing)
> Six *Yang* Organs *liufu* (straight pushing)
> Heaven Gate *tianmen* (straight pushing)
> Heart Gate *xinmen* (straight pushing)
> Water Palace *kangong* (pushing apart)
> Wind Pond *fengchi* (kneading)
> Celestial Pillar Bone *tianzhugu* (straight pushing)
> Big Bone Behind the Ear *erhou gaogu* (kneading)
> St 40 Abundant Bulge *fenglong* (kneading)

Liver Blood and/or *yin* deficiency with Empty Wind stirring within

Key symptoms

- mild tics

- worse when tired and towards the end of the day

- blinking eyes

Other symptoms: mild anxiety, poor appetite, easily tires, pale face

Pulse: thin or deficient; Wood pulses slightly wiry

Tongue: pale

Treatment principles: extinguish Wind; nourish Liver Blood/*yin*

SUGGESTED TREATMENT
Points
To extinguish Wind:

> GB 20 *fengchi*
> Du 20 *baihui*

Method: sedation needle technique

To nourish Liver Blood/*yin*:

> Liv 8 *ququan*
> St 36 *zusanli*
> Sp 6 *sanyinjiao*
> Bl 18 *ganshu*
> Bl 20 *pishu*

Method: tonification needle technique

Local points should be added depending on which part of the body the tics are in.

Paediatric *tui na* to strengthen the underlying deficiency

Spleen *pijing* (straight pushing from tip to base)
Kidney *shenjing* (straight pushing from tip to base)
Liver *ganjing* (straight pushing from tip to base)
Knead the Navel *rou qi* (kneading anti-clockwise)
Spinal Column *jizhu* (pinching from the bottom to the top of the back)
St 36 *zusanli* (kneading)
Bl 23 *shenshu* (strong rubbing)

CASE HISTORY: FOUR-YEAR-OLD GIRL WITH A SNIFFING TIC

This case history illustrates:

- how Accumulation Disorder may be the source of Phlegm and Heat in the body
- the importance of dietary changes.

Lou came to the clinic because she sniffed virtually constantly. The sniff was loud and came every few seconds she was awake. The only time it would stop was if she was engrossed in an activity. It had started quite suddenly a few months previously. At first her family thought she had a cold, then put it down to an allergy, but finally came to the conclusion it was a tic.

Lou had a voracious appetite, lots of energy and bright red cheeks. She had a distended tummy and her stools were sometimes irregular and particularly smelly. Her mother said she had a very strong temper.

Her pulse was full and her tongue had a yellow, sticky coat.

Diagnosis: Accumulation Disorder leading to Phlegm-Heat

Treatment
Treatment 1

M-UE-9 *sifeng* points pricked on one hand

I chatted to Lou's mother about her diet, which contained a lot of red meat, spicy foods and whole foods. I advised switching the red meat to chicken and fish, cutting down on spices and giving Lou white rice instead of brown. I also warned Lou's mother to expect a big 'clear-out' after the treatment.

Lou indeed had a big clear-out of her bowels after the first treatment. Her mother said that she had almost entirely stopped sniffing for a whole day, but the sniff had then come back just as strongly as before. Lou's mum had struggled to make some of the dietary changes – particularly switching to white rice – as she was unconvinced that this could be a part of the problem. I explained further about the difficulty a child's immature digestive system may have in processing whole foods.

Treatment 2

M-UE-9 *sifeng* points pricked on the other hand

I also taught Lou's mum the paediatric *tui na* routine described earlier to resolve Phlegm and Heat, and also to disperse accumulation of food.

Lou had another big clear-out of her bowels after the last treatment. This time her sniff stopped for three days, but again came back. Lou looked much less red-cheeked than she had beforehand and her tummy was much less distended.

Treatment 3

Liv 3 *taichong*, LI 4 *hegu* (sedation needle technique)

This time Lou's sniff did not stop entirely for any length of time, but her mother said it came and went a lot more and seemed to have lost some of its intensity. She also said that she and her husband really did not want to make the dietary changes I had suggested as that was the kind of food their family had always eaten and thrived off.

Treatment 4

LI 20 *yingxiang* (with laser pen), LI 4 *hegu*, St 40 *fenglong* (sedation needle technique)

Lou's mother emailed me after the fourth treatment to say that Lou was still sniffing but much less than before. She did not come back for further treatment.

SUMMARY

» The Organs most commonly involved in tics are: the Liver; the Heart; and Spleen.

» The pathogens most commonly involved in tics are: internal Wind; and Phlegm.

» The patterns that may cause tics are: Liver Wind and Phlegm-Heat stirring within; and Liver Blood and/or *yin* deficiency with Empty Wind stirring within.

» Tics are commonly seen in children without either of these patterns. In this case, the pathology is usually related to either the Heart or the Organ related to the child's constitutional imbalance.

Chapter 64

CONJUNCTIVITIS

The topics discussed in this chapter are:

- Aetiology
- Treatment
- Patterns

Introduction

Chronic and recurrent conjunctivitis is a benign yet disruptive complaint. It rarely causes serious problems but is unpleasant and interferes with life.

It usually manifests with a pus-like discharge in the eye, which often feels sore and may look bloodshot. Western medicine sees conjunctivitis as being caused by either a bacterial or viral agent, or as an allergic reaction. In chronic conjunctivitis, the eye may rarely be totally clear but there will be times when the symptoms flare up and times when they recede.

Aetiology
Underlying weakness of the eyes (*ben*)

One reason that a child may be prone to conjunctivitis is because her eyes are inherently weak.

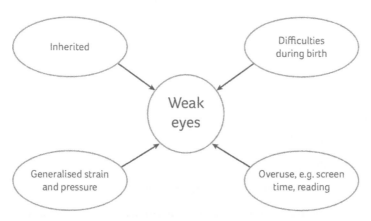

Figure 64.1 Causes of weak eyes

Manifestation (*biao*)

Once the eyes are weakened, the following factors may then 'target' the eyes and cause conjunctivitis:

- **Accumulation Disorder:** Excess Heat and Phlegm in the digestive system rise up to the eye via the Stomach channel.

- **Lingering Pathogenic Factor:** Owing to the connection between the Liver and the eyes, an LPF in the Liver channel may manifest as chronic or recurrent conjunctivitis.

Treatment

The treatment of chronic conjunctivitis should combine local and distal points. Any of the following local points may be used:

- GB 1 *tongziliao*
- M-HN-9 *taiyang*
- Bl 2 *zanzhu*
- St 1 *chengqi*

Although the points around the eye tend not to be particularly tender when needled, a child may be nervous at the prospect. If it is not possible to needle them, it is usually effective for the parent to massage the points on a twice-daily basis at home. This brings *qi* to the eyes. A combination of strengthening the eyes and treating the underlying patterns is usually sufficient to cure the conjunctivitis.

Patterns

- Damp-Heat in the Liver and Gallbladder rising up
- Stomach Heat rising up

 Damp-Heat in the Liver and Gallbladder channel is commonly seen against a background of Spleen *qi* deficiency. Conjunctivitis from Stomach Heat is commonly seen in excess-type babies who are prone to Accumulation Disorder.

Damp-Heat in the Liver and Gallbladder rising up

This pattern may either cause an acute bout of conjunctivitis, or intermittent symptoms. Recurrent bouts of conjunctivitis from this pattern often involve an LPF.

Key symptoms

- conjunctivitis
- eye looks red
- eyes are sore and itchy
- green pus in the eye

If the Damp predominates, the discharge will be abundant.

If the Heat predominates, there may be less discharge but the redness and irritation will predominate.

Other symptoms: irritability, ear infections

Pulse: slippery and wiry on the Wood pulses

Tongue: may be red or with red spots on the sides, may be a sticky coat

Treatment principles: resolve Damp; clear Heat from the Liver and Gallbladder

SUGGESTED TREATMENT

It is usually sufficient to use one local point and one distal point per treatment. If the child comes for treatment when free of symptoms, the treatment should address any underlying deficiencies.

Points

> Liv 2 *xingjian*
> GB 37 *guangming*
> GB 20 *fengchi*
> LI 4 *hegu*
> M-HN-9 *taiyang*
> GB 1 *tongziliao*

Method: sedation needle technique

Paediatric *tui na* to clear Heat and descend *qi*

> Heaven Gate *tianmen* (straight pushing)
> Water Palace *kangong* (pushing apart)
> M-HN-9 *taiyang* (kneading)
> Celestial Pillar Bone *tianzhugu* (straight pushing)
> Liver *ganjing* (straight pushing from base to tip)
> Milky Way *tianheshui* (straight pushing)

Stomach Heat rising up

In babies and toddlers, Stomach Heat often has its origins in Accumulation Disorder.

Key symptoms

- conjunctivitis

- eye and particularly the eyelids are red

- sore and itchy eyes

Other symptoms: constipation, bad breath, frequently hungry and thirsty

Pulse: overflowing on the Earth pulses, rapid

Tongue: may have a yellow coat

Treatment principles: clear Stomach Heat

SUGGESTED TREATMENT

These points should be used when the child has symptoms. Between bouts of conjunctivitis, treatment should address any underlying deficiencies.

Points

> St 44 *neiting*
> LI 4 *hegu*
> M-HN-9 *taiyang*

If Heat in the Stomach derives from Accumulation Disorder, the *sifeng* points may be used.

Method: sedation needle technique

Paediatric *tui na*

> Heaven Gate *tianmen* (straight pushing)
> Water Palace *kangong* (pushing apart)

M-HN-9 *taiyang* (kneading)
Celestial Pillar Bone *tianzhugu* (straight pushing)
Large Intestine *dachangjing* (straight pushing from base to tip)
Eight Trigrams *bagua* (circular pushing)
Thick Gate *banmen* (straight pushing)
Milky Way *tianheshui* (straight pushing)
Six *Yang* Organs *liufu* (straight pushing)

CASE HISTORY: TWO-YEAR-OLD GIRL WITH CHRONIC CONJUNCTIVITIS

This case history illustrates:

- how, on a young child with a simple condition, the smallest amount of intervention may be enough
- how a child may be born with a Lingering Pathogenic Factor passed to her whilst in the womb.

As soon as I met Rani, I noticed that both eyes were oozing a green, gloopy fluid. Her mother said that they had been like that since the day she was born. Despite treatment with antibiotic eye drops and oral antibiotics, they never seemed to get better. Rani's mum also said that her daughter was often grouchy and miserable and that she sensed this was connected with her eyes.

She had no other health problems. She slept well, ate fairly well and had good digestion.

The only other history of note was that, during the pregnancy, Rani's mum had contracted hepatitis A after eating out at a restaurant. She was poorly with it for a few weeks, during which time she rested a lot.

Diagnosis: Rani had a Lingering Pathogenic Factor in her Liver channel, contracted when she was in the womb from her mother when she had hepatitis.

Treatment: Massage on GB 1 *tongziliao*; needle with the sedation technique on GB 37 *guangming* and Liv 2 *xingjian*.

I taught Rani's mother a paediatric *tui na* routine to clear Heat and descend *qi*.

When Rani came back for the second treatment, her mum told me that, miraculously, Rani's conjunctivitis had cleared up almost immediately and stayed away.

Reflection: I was somewhat surprised myself at the speed with which Rani got better. On reflection, I concluded that this was probably due to several reasons. First, Rani was young and otherwise strong. Second, everything else in her life was supportive of her health (her diet, her daily schedule, a happy home life, etc.). Even though it had caused her to have a permanent symptom, it felt to me that the LPF had never really taken hold. It was like a visitor who had never quite settled and then decided to go on their way.

SUMMARY

» Recurrent or chronic conjunctivitis usually involves both an underlying weakness in the *qi* of the eye as well as Heat or Damp-Heat that then 'targets' the eyes.

» The patterns involved are: Damp-Heat in the Liver and Gallbladder; and Stomach Heat. In babies and young children, the Heat may arise from Accumulation Disorder.

» Whatever the pattern, it is important to always use a local point as well as distal ones.

• Chapter 65 •

MOUTH ULCERS
······································

The topics discussed in this chapter are:

- How do mouth ulcers arise?

- Patterns

Introduction
Most children get the occasional mouth ulcer at some point in the first few years of life. Some children, however, are plagued by repeated, painful ulcers. At worst, this means they do not want to eat because it is so painful and they cannot sleep well. Therefore, although usually benign and short-lived, mouth ulcers are well worth treating. They usually respond to acupuncture treatment quickly and well. Whichever patterns are present, the key is always to strengthen the digestive system.

How do mouth ulcers arise?
The mouth is related to the Stomach and Spleen
The state of the mouth is largely determined by the state of a child's digestive system. Therefore, if a child is prone to mouth ulcers, the practitioner should immediately suspect that there is something awry in the digestion.*

This digestive imbalance may, broadly speaking, be characterised by Heat or Cold.

The tongue is the offshoot of the Heart
Whilst the mouth itself is a reflection of the Stomach and Spleen, the Heart is reflected in the tongue. Therefore, if the child has ulcers not only on the mucous membranes but also on the tongue, this is an indication that the Full Heat has entered the Heart. The cause of this is usually intense, prolonged emotions.

Patterns

- Full Heat in the Stomach and Spleen

- Cold-Damp in the Stomach and Spleen**

- *Yin*-Fire flaring upwards

---

* The *Zhu Bing Yuan Hou Lun* described a condition called 'goose mouth', which equates to oral thrush and was said to be caused by the mother eating too much sweet food when pregnant.

** Scott and Barlow (1999, p.162) identified this second syndrome which is common in children in the West but is not given in Chinese books.

> The most common scenario in the clinic is a child with a combination of Spleen *qi* deficiency and either Damp-Cold or Damp-Heat. *Yin*-Fire is most commonly seen in older children.

Full Heat in the Stomach and Spleen

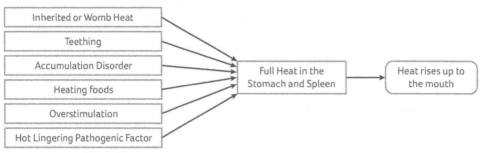

Figure 65.1 Mouth ulcers from Full Heat in the Stomach and Spleen

Key symptoms

- ulcers and sores in the mouth which are white but with red borders
- mouth is very painful

Other symptoms: child is agitated and miserable, does not want to eat, may be constipated, may have bad breath

Pulse: Earth pulses overflowing, rapid

Tongue: yellow coat

Treatment principles: clear Heat

Variations

- There may also be an element of Damp involved with the Heat in the Stomach and Spleen. In this case, the child may have foul-smelling stools instead of being constipated and will have a thick, sticky tongue coating.

- If the ulcers are on the tongue as well, then Heat should also be cleared from the Heart as well as from the digestive system.

- If the Heat arises from Accumulation Disorder, then the *sifeng* points may be used.

SUGGESTED TREATMENT
Points

St 44 *neiting*
LI 4 *hegu*
Ren 23 *lianquan*

Method: sedation needle technique

If the Heat arises from Accumulation Disorder, then M-UE-9 *sifeng* points should be pricked lightly on one hand.

Paediatric *tui na* to clear Full Heat and descend *qi*

Heaven Gate *tianmen* (straight pushing)

Heart Gate *xinmen* (straight pushing)
Water Palace *kangong* (pushing apart)
Wind Pond *fengchi* (kneading)
Celestial Pillar Bone *tianzhugu* (straight pushing)
Big Bone Behind the Ear *erhou gaogu* (kneading)
Stomach *weijing* (straight pushing sedation)
Large Intestine *dachangjing* (straight pushing sedation)
Small Intestine *xiaochangjing* (straight pushing sedation)
Thick Gate *banmen* (straight pushing)
Eight Trigrams *bagua* (circular pushing anti-clockwise)
Milky Way *tianheshui* (straight pushing)
Six *Yang* Organs *liufu* (straight pushing)

Cold-Damp in the Stomach and Spleen

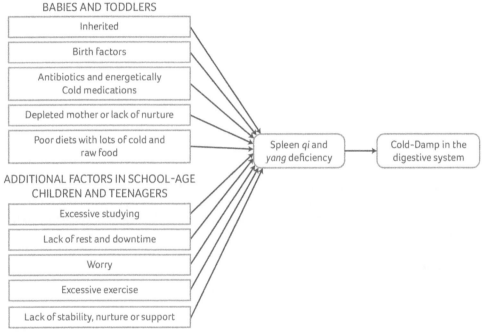

Figure 65.2 Mouth ulcers from Cold-Damp in the digestive system

Key symptoms

- white ulcers

- white, slimy coating on the mucous membranes in the mouth

- mouth is uncomfortable but not painful

Other symptoms: loose stools, poor appetite, pale face

Pulse: deficient

Tongue: pale

Treatment principles: resolve Damp; warm the Stomach and Spleen

> **SUGGESTED TREATMENT**
> **Points**
> To affect the mouth:
>
>> LI 4 *hegu*
>> Ren 23 *lianquan*
>
> **Method:** sedation needle technique
>
> To address the deficiency:
>
>> St 36 *zusanli*
>> Ren 12 *zhongwan*
>> Bl 20 *pishu*
>
> **Method:** tonification needle technique
>
> **Other techniques:** moxibustion
>
> **Paediatric *tui na*** to warm and tonify the Stomach and Spleen
>
>> Spleen *pijing* (straight pushing tonification)
>> Stomach *weijing* (straight pushing tonification)
>> Thick Gate *banmen* (straight pushing)
>> Eight Trigrams *bagua* (circular pushing anti-clockwise)
>> Three Passes *sanguan* (straight pushing)
>> Knead Ren 12 *zhongwan* (kneading anti-clockwise)
>> Spinal Column *jizhu* (pinching from the bottom to the top of the back)
>> St 36 *zusanli* (kneading)

Yin-Fire flaring upwards

True *yin* deficiency arises as a result of a severe febrile disease. This is uncommon in the West. More often, this pattern manifests as a deficiency of the *yuan qi* of the Stomach and Spleen, which means that Empty Heat rises upwards. It usually occurs in children who have been doing too much and who are exhausted.

Key symptoms

- small, white ulcers in the mouth with red borders

- not particularly painful

Other symptoms: child is very tired but struggles to get enough sleep, feels cold in her body but has a hot face

Pulse: deficient, slightly floating

Tongue: pale or red

Treatment principles: strengthen the *yuan qi*; clear Heat from the mouth

> **SUGGESTED TREATMENT**
> **Points**
> To affect the mouth:
>
>> LI 4 *hegu*
>> Ren 23 *lianquan*
>
> **Method:** sedation needle technique

To address the underlying deficiency:

St 36 *zusanli*
Sp 3 *taibai*
Ren 4 *guanyuan*
Bl 23 *shenshu*

Method: tonification needle technique

Paediatric *tui na* to tonify the Spleen and descend *qi*

Celestial Pillar Bone *tianzhugu* (straight pushing)
Spleen *pijing* (straight pushing)
Thick Gate *banmen* (straight pushing)
Three Passes *sanguan* (straight pushing)
Knead the Navel *rou qi* (kneading anti-clockwise)
Spinal Column *jizhu* (pinching from the bottom to the top of the back)
St 36 *zusanli* (kneading)

CASE HISTORY: EIGHTEEN-MONTH-OLD GIRL WITH BOUTS OF SEVERE MOUTH ULCERS

This case history illustrates that minimal treatment is often all that is needed in a young child with a straightforward condition.

When Amy came to the clinic, she had had five bouts of mouth ulcers that spread throughout her mouth and throat. Each bout had lasted for at least a week, during which time she had barely eaten and woke up frequently at night because of the pain. The other significant symptom was that she had strong-smelling and loose stools.

When she was free from ulcers, Amy was a placid and happy girl who ate well and slept well.

Observation: Amy was a quiet toddler with pale skin and slightly red cheeks. Her pulse was deficient. She did not want me to look at her tongue.

Diagnosis: Damp-Heat in the Stomach and Spleen with underlying Stomach and Spleen *qi* deficiency

Treatment
Treatment 1

LI 4 *hegu* (sedation) to clear Heat

St 36 *zusanli* (tonification) to strengthen the Stomach and Spleen

Home treatment: I taught Amy's mum a paediatric *tui na* routine to clear Heat and strengthen the Stomach and Spleen.

Treatment 2

LI 11 *quchi* (sedation) to clear Heat

Bl 20 *pishu*, Bl 21 *weishu* (tonification) to strengthen the Stomach and Spleen

Amy's mum reported that her stools were now formed almost all the time and had become much less smelly.

Treatment 3

Ren 12 *zhongwan*, St 36 *zusanli*, Sp 3 *taibai* (tonification) to further strengthen the Stomach and Spleen

Outcome: I suggested to Amy's mum that she bring Amy back if there were any recurrence of her symptoms. She actually came back to the clinic three years later, when she had just begun school. Amy had not had any more mouth ulcers but had started getting stomach aches. The underlying weakness in her Earth Element was obviously still there, and starting school, with all the associated stresses and strains, had meant it began manifesting a pathology again. This time Amy had weekly treatments for almost three months. At the end of this, she was free from stomach aches and loving school.

SUMMARY

» The mouth reflects the state of a child's digestive system.

» The Organs that may be involved in mouth ulcers are: the Stomach; the Spleen; and the Heart.

» The patterns seen are: Full Heat in the Stomach and Spleen; Cold-Damp in the Stomach and Spleen; and *Yin*-Fire flaring upwards.

» Treatment should involve points to directly affect the mouth, as well as distal points.

Chapter 66

PROBLEMS WITH TEETH AND TEETHING

The topics discussed in this chapter are:

- The different aspects of teething
- Treatment of teething problems
- Advice for the parent of a child who is teething
- Teeth as a diagnostic sign

Introduction

Teething is, of course, a physiological process and an inherent part of childhood. It is an example of what Sun Simiao termed transformations and steamings (*bian zheng*) (discussed in Chapter 3) and which he understood as times of intense growth and development. In some children it is also, unfortunately, the cause of suffering. Whilst one child may sail through the teething process, another may suffer a wide array of symptoms. Some of the most common are:

- pain in the gums
- excessive mucus in the nose and chest
- disturbed sleep
- restlessness and agitation
- diminished appetite
- diarrhoea
- vomiting
- fever
- febrile seizures.

An outward sign that a child is teething is that one cheek, on the side that the tooth is coming through, is red.

The different aspects of teething

There are several different aspects to the teething process. Understanding what these are helps to clarify why teething causes the problems it does in some children.

An increase in Kidney *yang*

The process of a tooth rising up and breaking through the gum is driven by heightened activity in the *ming men.* Just as athletes need to warm up in order to be able to run at their fastest pace, so the child's body needs to summon its *qi* in order for the tooth to be able to break through.

Disruption to the digestive system

The channels of the Stomach and Large Intestine run through the gums. When a tooth is in the process of pushing through, the *qi* in these channels temporarily stagnates and becomes disrupted. This explains why a child may go off her food during teething. This is an instinctive and healthy response to the fact that her digestion cannot cope with as much food as usual.

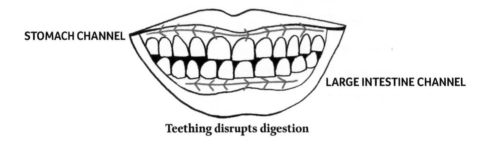

STOMACH CHANNEL

LARGE INTESTINE CHANNEL

Teething disrupts digestion

Why do some children suffer with teething and others not?

Looking at these two aspects of teething, it is easy to see which children may suffer with it:

- children who have a lot of pre-existing Heat in the body

- children who already have stagnation in their digestive system (often manifesting as Accumulation Disorder).

Why do some children produce a lot more mucus when they are teething?

Some children have runny noses and coughs whenever they are teething. There are two possible reasons for this. The first is that, in Hot children, the extra Heat condenses the fluids and results in green or yellow phlegm. This is usually resolved if the excess Heat is cleared.

The second reason is that the extra activity in the *ming men* that is characteristic of teething provides Cold and deficient children with the opportunity to expel Phlegm/Damp that may have been lingering in the system. This will most likely result in clear or white nasal mucus and a cough with loose mucus.

Treatment of teething problems

There are two aspects to the treatment of teething problems. The first is preventive, and the second is to treat the child during the acute phase.

Treatment between episodes of teething

Based on the description of the teething process above, there are two aspects to preventing problems.

Clear excess Heat

If the child already has too much Heat in his system, the rising up of Kidney *yang* during teething may mean that the degree of Heat becomes pathological.

> **SUGGESTED TREATMENT**
> One or two points per treatment is usually sufficient.
>
> **Points**
>
> > LI 4 *hegu*
> > St 44 *neiting*
> > He 8 *shaofu*
> > Liv 2 *xingjian*
> > Du 14 *dazhui*
>
> **Method:** sedation needle technique
>
> **Paediatric *tui na*** to clear Heat, descend *qi* and promote the flow of *qi* in the digestive system
>
> > Heaven Gate *tianmen* (straight pushing)
> > Heart Gate *xinmen* (straight pushing)
> > Water Palace *kangong* (pushing apart)
> > Wind Pond *fengchi* (kneading)
> > Celestial Pillar Bone *tianzhugu* (straight pushing)
> > Palace of Toil *laogong* (kneading)
> > Small Heavenly Heart *xiaotianxin* (kneading)
> > Thick Gate *banmen* (straight pushing)
> > Eight Trigrams *bagua* (circular pushing)
> > Milky Way *tianheshui* (straight pushing)
> > Six *Yang* Organs *liufu* (straight pushing)

Disperse accumulation of food in the digestive system

The most effective way to disperse accumulation of food in the digestive system is by using *sifeng* (M-UE-9). However, Accumulation Disorder will keep returning unless the appropriate dietary changes are made. It is essential that the child does not overeat and does not eat foods that are too difficult to digest, and that his feeds/meals are appropriately spaced.

Treatment during the acute phase

If a child comes for treatment during the acute phase, this means that there is already stagnation in the digestive system and too much Heat.[*]

> **SUGGESTED TREATMENT**
> **Points**
>
> > LI 4 *hegu*
> > St 44 *neiting*
>
> **Method:** sedation needle technique
>
> **Paediatric *tui na*** to disperse accumulation of food and descend *qi*
>
> > Celestial Pillar Bone *tianzhugu* (straight pushing)
> > Thick Gate *banmen* (straight pushing)
> > Eight Trigrams *bagua* (circular pushing anti-clockwise)
> > Four Wind Creases *sifengwen* (pinching)
> > Knead the navel *roufu* (kneading clockwise)
> > Abdomen Stimulation *fuyinyang* (pushing apart)
> > Belly Corner *dujiao* (pinching)

---

[*] Scott and Barlow in *Acupuncture in the Treatment of Children* (1999) advise against using *sifeng* in this situation as it may release more Heat in the system which runs the risk of causing convulsions in the child.

It can also be useful to add in a local point (which can be massaged when it is not possible to needle it):

SI 17 *tianrong* – for the lower teeth

SI 18 *quanliao* – for the upper teeth

Method: sedation needle technique

Advice for the parent of a child who is teething

Diet

It is best to avoid coaxing a teething child into eating more than he wants. It is natural for parents to worry when an infant loses appetite. Explaining to the parent a little about the teething process (as described above) is helpful. It will usually reassure her that their child's lack of desire for food at this time is an appropriate response to the process taking place.

Foods should be kept simple and light during teething. This means avoiding foods that are heating (e.g. red meat, spicy food), or heavy and rich (e.g. cheese, sugary products). This is the one time in a child's life when it may be appropriate for him to have quite cooling foods for a short period of time, such as yoghurt, which may help to soothe his gums and cool his Stomach.

The child must have breaks between meals in order to lessen the chances of stagnation and accumulation forming in the digestive system.

Rest

As mentioned, teething is seen as an outward manifestation of a strong developmental phase in a child. Therefore, when possible, allowing the child to rest, be in a quiet environment and be nurtured by his main caregiver is helpful. This means he will come through the developmental stage more smoothly.

Home remedies

Different children respond in different ways to the following home remedies. It is worth the parent exploring which one seems to particularly suit her child.

- Homeopathic chamomilla, in the form of a powder or a dissolvable sugar pill, works wonders in many children.

- Mix ground cloves into a paste with butter or water and rub onto the gums.

- Keep a supply of chopped-up pieces of frozen fruit in the freezer that can be given to the baby to chew. If the baby is still milk fed, a flannel soaked in chamomile tea works just as well.

Teeth as a diagnostic sign

- Late teething, when combined with other symptoms and signs, may reflect an underlying Kidney deficiency.

- Teeth which are very prone to decay, despite a good diet, may be a reflection of Kidney deficiency.

- Teeth which are spaced apart may be a sign of Kidney *yin* deficiency.

SUMMARY

» Teething problems are usually rooted in excess Heat and stagnation in the digestive system.

» Treatment may be used both to prevent teething problems and also to ease the symptoms when they do occur.

» Eating the right diet is often enough to prevent and cure teething problems.

» A propensity to problems with the teeth is often rooted in a Kidney deficiency.

• Chapter 67 •

GROWING PAINS
··

The topics discussed in this chapter are:

- Aetiology

- Patterns

Introduction

'Growing pains' is the term used to describe pain which occurs intermittently, usually in the thighs, calves or behind the knees. It affects the muscles rather than the joints. It is most common in children between the ages of three and five years old, and those eight to twelve years old. The sensation may range from mild discomfort to pain. It is most commonly felt by the child in the late afternoon, evening and during the night.

Medically speaking, there is no known explanation for growing pains. Growth is not considered to cause pain, and the pain does not tend to occur at times of rapid growth or in areas of the body that are growing at a particularly fast rate. But although the term 'growing pains' may be somewhat misleading, it is a very real problem for some children and their families. This is, not least, because it often disrupts sleep night after night.

Aetiology

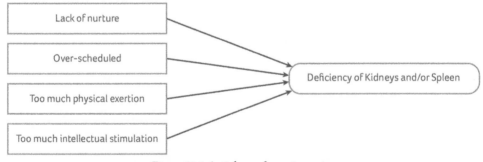

Figure 67.1 Aetiology of growing pains

Although each child experiences growing pains in a slightly different way, there are some aspects that are almost universal and that provide clues as to what causes these mysterious pains.

- Growing pains tend to be worse in the latter part of the day and are often more pronounced on days the child has been particularly athletic. This points towards there being a **deficient** aspect to the condition.

- Most children feel better if the painful area is touched or massaged. This also points towards a **deficient** aspect to the condition.

- Growing pains also commonly arise at night, when the child is obviously not moving. This points towards some **local stagnation**, as conditions of stagnation tend to get worse at rest.

Patterns

- Spleen *qi* deficiency

- Kidney deficiency

- Damp in the channels of the legs

- *Qi* stagnation in the channels of the legs

In nearly all cases, growing pains are caused by a mix of local stagnation or fullness with an underlying deficiency. In young children, the most common deficiency is of Spleen *qi*. In older children, there is more likely also to be a Kidney deficiency. The most commonly seen combinations of patterns are Spleen *qi* deficiency with Damp, and Kidney deficiency with *qi* stagnation.

Spleen *qi* deficiency

Key symptom

- Growing pains that are worse after lots of physical and/or mental activity

Other symptoms: poor appetite, easily tired

Pulse: deficient

Tongue: pale

Treatment principles: tonify Spleen *qi*

SUGGESTED TREATMENT

Two or three points per treatment is usually sufficient. Other points on the Stomach and Spleen channels can be chosen according to where the child feels the worst of the pain.

Points

St 36 *zusanli*
Sp 3 *taibai*
Sp 6 *sanyinjiao*

Method: tonification needle technique

Other techniques: moxibustion

Paediatric *tui na*

Spleen *pijing* (straight pushing)
Thick Gate *banmen* (straight pushing)
Three Passes *sanguan* (straight pushing)
Knead Ren 12 *zhongwan* (kneading anti-clockwise)
Spinal Column *jizhu* (pinching from the bottom to the top of the back)
St 36 *zusanli* (kneading)

Kidney deficiency

Key symptom

- Growing pains which are worse after exertion or when generally tired

Other symptoms: dark circles under the eyes, easily tired, bedwetting

Pulse: deficient

Tongue: pale

Treatment principles: tonify the Kidneys

> **SUGGESTED TREATMENT**
> **Points**
>
> Ki 3 *taixi*
> Ki 7 *fuliu*
> Bl 23 *shenshu*
>
> **Method:** tonification needle technique
>
> **Other techniques:** moxibustion may be applicable
>
> **Paediatric *tui na*** to tonify and warm the Kidneys
>
> Kidney *shenjing* (straight pushing)
> Two Men Upon a Horse *erma* (kneading)
> Outer Palace of Toil *wailaogong* (kneading)
> Wind Nest *yiwofeng* (kneading)
> Three Passes *sanguan* (straight pushing)
> Lower Back – area around Bl 23 *shenshu* (strong rubbing)
> Spinal Column *jizhu* (pinching)

Damp in the channels of the legs

Symptoms

- growing pains that feel achy and heavy

- pain better for movement

- pain bad at night

Pulse: slippery

Tongue: pale tongue, swollen, sticky tongue coat

Note: Pulse and tongue will be determined by whether or not the Damp is systemic and what the underlying deficiencies are.

Treatment principles: resolve Damp in the channels

SUGGESTED TREATMENT

Points must be chosen according to the channels affected. One or two points per treatment (combined with one or two points to treat the underlying deficiency) is usually sufficient.

Points

Stomach channel:

> St 32 *futu*
> St 34 *liangqui*
> St 40 *fenglong*

Gallbladder channel:

> GB 31 *fengshi*
> GB 34 *yanglingquan*

Distal points:

> Sp 9 *yinlingquan*

Method: sedation needle technique

Qi stagnation in the channels of the legs

This pattern may occur in a child who has a very full schedule which is depleting, but at the same time does not do enough physical activity.

Symptoms

- growing pains which are throbbing

- pains worse at night and with inactivity

- pains come and go

Pulse: may be wiry

Tongue: may be normal, may reflect any underlying deficiencies

Treatment principles: move *qi* in the channels

SUGGESTED TREATMENT

Points must be chosen according to the channels affected.

Points

Stomach channel:

> St 32 *futu*
> St 34 *liangqui*
> St 40 *fenglong*

Gallbladder channel:

> GB 31 *fengshi*
> GB 34 *yanglingquan*

Distal points:

> Liv 3 *taichong*

Method: sedation needle technique

CASE HISTORY: EIGHT-YEAR-OLD BOY WITH GROWING PAINS

This case history illustrates:

- how in some children the Kidney *qi* is unequally distributed between the head and the body

- the importance of recognising children's differing constitutions.

Luke struggled to get to sleep because his legs were painful. He said his legs ached strongly and also felt 'fidgety'. This had been happening on and off for a couple of years. It always seemed to be better in the school holidays and worse towards the end of a school term.

Luke had no other symptoms but was generally frail. He became tired easily. His mother noted that the more tired he was, the more hyperactive he became. He would 'crash' for a week or so at the end of term and needed time at home doing very little.

Luke was bright and was always top of his class in every subject. He had begun reading at three and his hobby was to do difficult maths equations.

Observations: Luke was small, had a thin body and was rather nervous. His mother told me he was anxious about coming to the clinic. His pulse was thin and deficient, his tongue was normal. He was dark around his eyes. His voice was groaning.

Diagnosis: I diagnosed Luke as having a Water constitutional imbalance, with quite pronounced Kidney deficiency. The Kidneys had done an exceptional job of nourishing his brain, but his body had not done so well. Even though there was some local stagnation in Luke's legs, the priority was to begin strengthening his Kidneys.

Treatment

Luke was too nervous to try needles so I began treating him with a moxa stick and a laser pen.

Treatment 1

Bl 64 *jinggu*, Ki 3 *taixi*: *yuan* source points to treat Luke's constitutional imbalance and strengthen the Kidneys

Treatment 2

Bl 67 *zhiyin*, Ki 7 *fuliu*: tonification points

Treatment 3

Bl 65 *shugu*, Ki 1 *yongguan*: Wood points to continue treating the constitutional imbalance; Ki 1 *yongguan* helps to draw *qi* downwards

Treatment 4

Ren 4 *guanyuan*, Du 4 *ming men*: to strengthen the Kidneys and bring *qi* to the Lower Burner

Treatment 5

Bl 28 *pangguanshu*, Bl 23 *shenshu*: to treat the constitutional imbalance and strengthen the Kidneys

Treatment continued along these lines, using a variety of different points to strengthen the Water Element and the Kidneys. Slowly but surely, Luke began to feel less pain in his legs. After the tenth treatment, Luke was ready to try needles for the first time and took to them well. After three months of near-weekly treatment, Luke was reliably falling asleep easily without pain in his legs. He continues to come for top-ups when he feels things are slipping, which is invariably in the last weeks of term. Since he began treatment, his mother has noticed that he has become more confident and has lost the need to push himself so hard academically.

SUMMARY

» Growing pains usually have a deficiency at their root but also a full aspect.

» It is necessary to address the full aspect of the condition with local points, as well as treat the underlying deficiency.

» The patterns involved are: Spleen *qi* deficiency; Kidney deficiency; Damp in the channels of the legs; and *qi* stagnation in the channels of the legs.

» The most important piece of advice is that the child needs to reduce his schedule and/or rest more.

Chapter 68

TEENAGE MENSTRUAL PROBLEMS

The topics discussed in this chapter are:

- TCM physiology of puberty
- Aetiology and pathology
- Commonly seen menstrual problems in teenagers
- Patterns involved in menstrual problems

Introduction

Treating a teenage girl during the time when she is becoming a woman feels like a privilege. Acupuncture can play an enormous part in establishing a healthy menstrual cycle that may save a woman years of monthly pain and difficulties.

Many women feel at the mercy of their menstrual cycles. Painful, heavy or irregular periods are seen as something that just have to be tolerated, certainly not spoken about, and sometimes considered 'part of being a woman'. Many teenage girls are introduced to their menstrual cycle solely in terms of sexual intercourse and the dangers of unwanted pregnancies. Few are given any guidance and help in understanding the wider aspects of the cyclic menstrual rhythm, its different phases and the menstrual wisdom that can help it to become something which enhances a woman's life rather than blights it. The more a young woman is armed with knowledge of the workings of her uterus, fallopian tubes and ovaries, the less she feels powerless in the face of it.

There is a worrying trend amongst teenage girls to escape the very existence of periods at all. Advertisements on television and in magazines sell sanitary products wrapped up in prettily coloured paper, and with menstrual blood depicted by a light blue liquid. They proclaim that life can go on as normal during period time. According to these advertisements, you might even choose to go hiking in the mountains in tight, white jeans during the heaviest days of your period.

On the other hand, and at the same time, there is a strong message in our culture that pain should be avoided at all costs and there are over-the-counter medications freely available to try to ensure this happens. Doctors are sometimes willing to prescribe contraceptive methods such as an implant or injection that may stop a woman from having periods altogether. Many teenagers think nothing of taking the contraceptive pill without a break so that the inconvenience of bleeding can be avoided. All of this is perhaps a reflection of a general ethos that *yang* is good and *yin* is a weakness that needs to be denied and overcome. This makes it extremely difficult for a teenage girl to embrace the beginning of her menstruating life.

Of course, we cannot, as acupuncturists, stop this trend. We can, perhaps, help the teenage girls who come to us for treatment to feel empowered by their menstrual cycle and hope that this will proliferate outwards into society.

What is 'normal' for a teenage girl in the first year of menstruation?

A teenage girl may have little idea of whether the nature and timing of her periods are within the realm of normal. It is easy for her to assume that what she experiences is similar to what her friends are experiencing. Conversely, if she does talk to her mother or another trusted adult about concerns, they may worry unnecessarily because they have forgotten how irregular menstruation can be when it starts.

The following are considered normal menstrual cycles in adolescent girls.[45]

Table 68.1 Normal menstrual cycle facts for adolescent girls

Menarche (median age)	12.43 years
Mean cycle interval	32.2 days
Cycle interval	21–45 days
Menstrual flow length	7 days or less
Menstrual product use	3–6 pads or tampons per day

The benefits of treating an adolescent girl as she begins her menstrual life

There are many benefits to treating a girl at this time:

- It is easier to steer the menstrual cycle towards balance and health whilst the body is still in a state of flux than it is to correct an imbalance years down the line.

- A balanced menstrual cycle helps to promote overall physical and emotional health.

- The time prior to and at the start of menstruation is characterised by emotional turmoil for some girls. Treatment over this time helps to smooth the process of change that is occurring.

- It is common for girls to develop physical symptoms at this time, such as acne or headaches. Treatment can address these symptoms before they have time to take hold.

- Many girls particularly benefit from a good therapeutic relationship at this time. Having an adult other than a parent to chat to may feel supportive and ease the transition to womanhood. Psychologist Steve Biddulph identifies the presence of 'aunties' (in the loose sense of the word) as one of the secrets of well-being for girls, especially during puberty.[46]

TCM physiology of puberty

The time leading up to the first menstrual period is a time of preparation. The girl's body is gathering in the resources it needs to make it through the enormous changes that lie ahead. *Yang* increases and is the fuel that is needed for this transition. Yet, until the first period, this abundance of *yang* cannot be discharged. It is like a river which has had a dam put across it. All the water is building up on one side of the dam with nowhere to go. The water usually becomes rough, with whirlpools and eddies forming. A pre-pubescent girl's physiology is similar. It is changing. There is a sense of expansion and increase. Along with this usually comes some turbulence and chaos. Periods beginning are akin to the sluice gates of the dam opening. After some time, a new harmony and monthly rhythm can be found.

How can this process become pathological?

In a **deficient** child, or one who has too many demands placed upon her, the increase in *yang* is not sufficiently great. The fire of the *ming men*, which stems from the Kidneys, is being consumed by the demands of her daily life rather than being available to fuel the physiological changes that should be taking place. Other Organs may be affected by this. The Spleen may not adequately produce *gu qi* and Blood therefore becomes deficient. In most cases, the girl's body diverts its resources towards ensuring the physical changes associated with puberty do indeed happen. However, something else in her body suffers. She begins getting headaches, loses vitality or becomes depressed, for example. It may be that her periods are light or her cycle very long. In extreme cases, it means that she does not go through the many physical changes associated with puberty, and menstruation does not begin. In this scenario, the treatment principles should be to tonify the deficiencies.

In an **excess** child, *qi, yang* and Blood increase but have nowhere to go. The result of this is that there is an abundance of energy 'trapped' in the body. This may show itself in physical symptoms such as headaches or insomnia, and also emotional symptoms such as outbursts of anger and rage. In this scenario, the treatment principle should be to move *qi* and Blood (and perhaps clear Heat that comes from the stagnation).

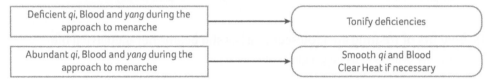

Figure 68.1 Two basic pathologies in the approach to menarche

In clinical practice, of course, it is often the case that there is both some deficiency and some stagnation, and both treatment principles should be combined.

The *chong mai* (penetrating vessel) and the *ren mai* (directing vessel) at puberty

> Now, at fourteen years old, the superabundance of essences and blood have enough fertility and life for the *ren mai* to offer the uterus a rich blood, and the *chong mai* is able to make this blood circulate, arrive in the uterus and be so full of life that it has the ability to make and sustain a new life.[47]

It is the 'filling up' and 'activation' of the *chong mai* and the *ren mai* that enables menstruation to begin. These two extraordinary vessels are fuelled by Kidney *qi* in order to reach this stage of maturity. In the years leading up to the arrival of menstruation, this almost imperceptible yet profound process is taking place behind the scenes. It comes to fruition with the arrival of the girl's first period.

The function of the *ren mai* at this time is to ensure that the Uterus becomes replete with good-quality Blood. The function of the *chong mai* is to ensure that menstruation occurs regularly, with the right quantity of blood and without pain.

Aetiology and pathology
A girl's relationship to her menstrual cycle

At certain stages in history and in certain cultures, menstruating women have been considered taboo. Although less overt in the present day in the West, shadows of this feeling still persist. A girl may be handed down generations' worth of shame when she begins menstruating. The message is often implicitly or explicitly given that periods are something to be hidden away and are a nuisance or even 'a curse'.* One author asks women to imagine:

---

*   I have several times heard mothers in the treatment room tell their daughters that they will have, for example, heavy or painful periods 'just like I have always had'. The power of suggestion is enormous and this may become a self-fulfilling prophecy.

How might it have been different for you if, on your first menstrual day, your mother had given you a bouquet of flowers and taken you to lunch, and then the two of you had gone to meet your father at the jeweller's, where your ears were pierced, and your father bought you your first pair of earrings, and then you went with a few of your friends and your mother's friends to get your first lip colouring; and then you went,

> For the very first time,
>
> > To the Women's lodge,
> >
> > > To learn
> > >
> > > > The wisdom of women?

How might your life be different?[48]

A girl's menstrual cycle will be strongly shaped by how she feels about leaving her girlhood behind, her sexuality and becoming a woman. How a young woman really feels about her menstrual cycle often lays deep in her unconscious mind. It is not something that can be changed overnight. However, providing a space to talk about it can be of enormous therapeutic value.

The Liver and menstruation

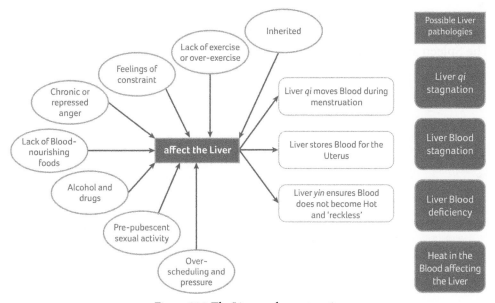

Figure 68.2 The Liver and menstruation

The Kidneys and menstruation

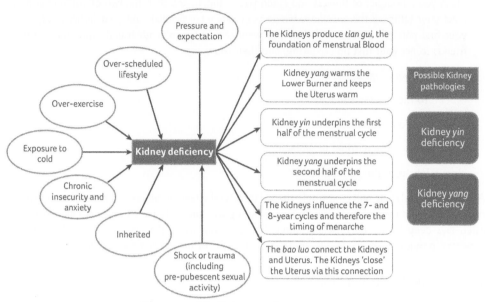

Figure 68.3 The Kidneys and menstruation

The Spleen and menstruation

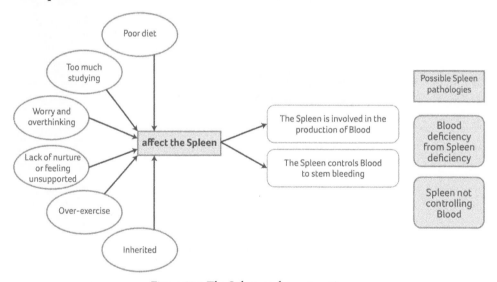

Figure 68.4 The Spleen and menstruation

The Heart and menstruation

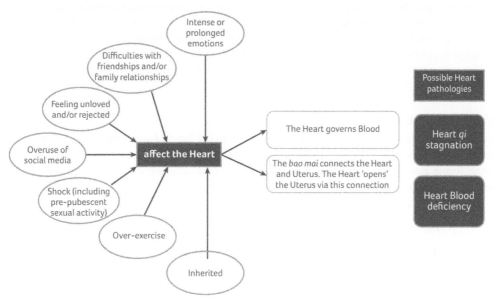

Figure 68.5 The Heart and menstruation

> Any of the aetiological factors that affect the Kidneys may have an impact on the functioning of the *ren mai* and the *chong mai*. In particular, shock or trauma (including sexual abuse) may cause Blood to stagnate in the *chong mai*. Over-exercise and an overly demanding schedule may consume *yin* and Blood so that the *ren mai* is not able to supply the Uterus.

Commonly seen menstrual problems in teenagers

Irregular periods

As previously mentioned, some irregularity in the periods is normal for the first year or so. If a girl's cycle is three weeks one month and then five weeks the next, as long as there are no other symptoms it is probably not something to worry about. However, there are degrees of irregularity. If a girl has a period approximately every month for a few months, and then does not have one for three months, it is a sign of imbalance. Similarly, if she has periods every two weeks, this needs to be rectified. Even though it may be one that will naturally sort itself out in the course of time, there are good reasons to treat the imbalance.

Irregular periods may be due to:

- *qi* stagnation

- Blood stagnation

- Cold stagnation

- Kidney *yin* deficiency

- Kidney *yang* deficiency.

(See 'Patterns involved in menstrual problems' below.)

> Blood or Cold stagnation will tend to make the menstrual cycle longer. *Qi* stagnation can make the cycle either longer or shorter. Kidney deficiency tends to make the cycle shorter.

A fifteen-year-old girl came for treatment because, since starting her periods two years earlier, she had been getting periods anywhere from every two weeks to every three months. Her periods were very painful. I diagnosed Cold stagnation against a background of Kidney *yang* deficiency. She had many other symptoms of Cold. I used a moxa box on her abdomen at every treatment, as well as points to tonify and warm Kidney *yang*. We talked about the importance of keeping her Lower Burner protected from the cold and she began wearing a haramaki. After four months of weekly or fortnightly treatments, her cycle was regular.

Painful periods

Period pain ranges from something that is a mild inconvenience to something that is feared and causes havoc in the girl's life. The patterns discussed below are excess patterns which all tend to cause strong pain. Deficient patterns may cause pain too but it is not usually strong enough to bring a girl to acupuncture.

Painful periods may be due to:

- *qi* stagnation
- Cold stagnation
- Blood stagnation.

(See 'Patterns involved in menstrual problems' below.)

Strong period pain is most commonly caused by Cold stagnation in teenage girls. There is often a background of Kidney *yang* deficiency. Moderate pain that comes in waves is due to *qi* stagnation. Cramping pain that is alleviated by Heat is due to Cold stagnation. Severe, stabbing and fixed pain is due to Blood stagnation.

Heavy periods

Heavy periods may be distressing for a teenage girl. They may lead to her feeling anxious about how to cope if her period falls during a school residential trip, on an exam day or when she is competing in a sporting event. For this reason alone, it is a symptom that is well worth treating. It is also important to prevent a girl's periods being chronically heavy because this, over the years, will lead to Blood deficiency.

Heavy periods may be due to:

- Heat in the Blood
- Spleen *qi* deficiency
- Blood stagnation.

(See 'Patterns involved in menstrual problems' below.)

Both Spleen *qi* deficiency and Heat in the Blood are commonly seen in the clinic, causing heavy periods. They often co-exist. Heat in the Blood tends to cause profuse, gushing bleeding. Spleen *qi* deficiency tends to cause periods that start heavy, become lighter but then drag on for days. Blood stagnation tends to cause heavy periods with clots and pain.

CASE HISTORY: FIFTEEN-YEAR-OLD GIRL WITH HEAVY PERIODS

The following case history illustrates:

- the strong link between the menstrual cycle and emotions
- how heavy bleeding may sometimes result from unexpressed emotions.

Freya came to the clinic because she was struggling to manage her heavy periods. They only lasted four days but, for two or three of those days, Freya had to change her sanitary protection at least once every hour, day and night. She said it felt as if the blood just 'gushed out'. It was bright red with some small, red, clots. There was no pain. Her period came every three weeks.

Freya also had bad acne, which had started six months before her periods. The whole of her face was covered in red, angry-looking spots. Freya was self-conscious about this.

Freya's doctor had suggested she go on the pill, which he thought would help both with her heavy periods and acne. Freya desperately wanted to do this. Her mother, however, was keen to avoid it as she worried about the long-term effects of the pill. They had agreed they would give acupuncture a try for three months and then make a decision.

Background: Freya was a high-achieving girl, who excelled both academically and musically. She attended a demanding school and had four or five extra-curricular musical activities each week.

Observations: Freya was an exceptionally polite and articulate fifteen-year-old. It appeared to me, however, that she was giving me a performance. I was unable to get her to reveal more of her feelings. I suspected she never really did this and had little awareness of what they were. The best phrase to describe her was 'pent up'.

Freya had a green colour around her mouth, and her voice was shouting in tone. Her Wood pulses were wiry and overflowing. Her tongue was red on the sides.

Diagnosis

- Wood constitutional imbalance
- Heat in the Blood (causing the heavy bleeding)
- Heat in the Liver

Treatment

Treatment 1: GB 38 *yangfu*, Liv 2 *xingjian* – sedation and Fire points of the Liver and Gallbladder to both clear Heat in the Blood and in the Liver, and treat the constitutional imbalance.

Treatment 2: GB 41 *zulinqi*, Liv 1 *dadun* – Wood points on the Liver and Gallbladder channels to stop bleeding and treat the constitutional imbalance.

Freya had a period after these first two treatments. She reported that there was no change in the bleeding, which was just as heavy as before. She (and I) did think that her acne was looking less red and angry, however.

Treatment 3: GB 15 *toulinqi*, GB 40 *qiuxu*, Liv 3 *taichong* – a spirit point and the source points of the Liver and Gallbladder channels to free constraint of Freya's emotions and treat the constitutional imbalance.

Treatment 4: GB 9 *tianchong*, GB 37 *guangming*, Liv 5 *ligou*, Sp 10 *xuehai* – a spirit point, plus the *luo* junction points on the Liver and Gallbladder channels, with Sp 10 to cool the Blood.

Freya's next period was still just as heavy, although for the first time this cycle was twenty-seven days, as opposed to her normal twenty-one days.

As treatment progressed, Freya began to relax and show me more of who she really was, rather than keep her polite 'performance'. She began talking about her frustrations at school and revealed one day in a flood of tears that she was fed up with spending all her spare time practising her various instruments and just wanted to have more time to hang out with her friends. Freya herself seemed almost as surprised as her mother that she had said this, as if she had not really known it was what she felt.

Freya's next period was noticeably less heavy. She came in for her next treatment beaming as she told me that she had decided to continue playing her three instruments for enjoyment, but to stop doing any more instrumental exams. She had also decided to leave an orchestra which she said she found 'really boring'.

> Her mother told me that Freya was more emotional than she had ever known her to be. She was crying more often and getting cross about things. However, she said that in a strange way this felt like a good thing and that Freya seemed more 'alive'.
>
> I continued treating Freya for several more months along the same lines as described above. After six months, her periods were consistently much less heavy and she managed to avoid going on the pill. Equally, or arguably even more importantly, Freya was a much happier and relaxed girl.

Bleeding between periods

Bleeding between periods is surprisingly common in teenage girls. As well as being a sign of an imbalance, it is also inconvenient and difficult for a girl to manage. Furthermore, it may contribute to Blood deficiency.

Bleeding between periods may be due to:

- Heat in the Blood

- Kidney *yin* deficiency with Empty Heat

- deficient Spleen *qi* not controlling Blood

- Blood stagnation.

(See 'Patterns involved in menstrual problems' below.)

 Bleeding between periods in teenage girls is commonly due to a combination of Heat in the Blood with a background of Kidney *yin* deficiency, or to Spleen *qi* not controlling Blood (which is also sometimes seen in conjunction with Heat in the Blood).

Heat in the Blood will cause the blood to be bright red. Kidney *yin* deficiency with Empty Heat is likely to cause bleeding around ovulation with red blood. The blood from Spleen *qi* deficiency bleeding will be pale red. Blood stagnation tends to cause bleeding outside period time with dark blood.

No periods or scanty periods

Some girls may come for treatment because they have never had a period and are beyond the age when menstruation would normally have begun (generally considered to be sixteen years old). Others may have started menstruating, but then stopped.

No periods may be due to:

- extreme Blood deficiency

- Kidney *yin* or *jing* deficiency

- Cold stagnation

- Blood stagnation.

(See 'Patterns involved in menstrual problems' below.)

The most commonly seen patterns in girls who have no periods or scanty periods are Blood deficiency and Kidney deficiency. They may co-exist. The most common aetiologies are poor diet (including dieting and anorexia) and over-scheduling.

Pre-menstrual syndrome

Pre-menstrual syndrome includes a wide range of both physical and emotional symptoms. The fact that a woman's emotions may be different at this time of her cycle is generally joked about, and laughed at. A woman is taught to dismiss what she feels at this time as just being due to the fact that she is pre-menstrual. It is just 'due to her hormones' and therefore somehow not real or significant. Christiane Northrup explains, 'The luteal phase is when women are most in tune with their inner knowing and with what isn't working in their lives.'[49] Therefore, rather than dismissing the feelings that may come to the surface during the pre-menstrual phase, we should help a teenage girl to see them as useful signals pointing towards what is not working in her life and what needs to be changed.

Pre-menstrual syndrome may be due to:

- Liver *qi* stagnation
- Liver *yang* rising from Liver Blood and/or Kidney *yin* deficiency
- Blood deficiency
- Heat in the Blood.

(See 'Patterns involved in menstrual problems' below.)

Liver *qi* stagnation is the pattern most commonly seen in teenage girls who suffer from pre-menstrual syndrome. It often occurs in girls who have a tendency to suppress their anger.

Qi stagnation, Liver *yang* rising and Heat in the Blood tend to cause emotions in the 'anger family' pre-menstrually. They are likely to be depression, moodiness, flying off the handle, lack of tolerance and agitation. Blood deficiency is likely to cause emotions to do with upset and vulnerability, and a propensity to tearfulness. Of course, the two may co-exist and the girl may oscillate between these two families of emotions.

Sandy's mother rang me in desperation because of her daughter's extreme pre-menstrual symptoms. She said that, for a week before her period, Sandy became so angry that the rest of the family felt they were treading on eggshells. Last month she had trashed her bedroom in a fit of rage. At school, Sandy was a model student who had many friends and was thought of as easygoing and gentle. After several appointments and time chatting to Sandy, she said that she felt like 'a volcano inside' and was 'fed up with always being a good girl'. Treatment to take Heat out of her Liver and discussions about how she could express herself more authentically meant her symptoms gradually eased. She took up karate and found it really useful to express her more *yang* side in a constructive way.

Patterns involved in menstrual problems

Before looking at the Organ/Pathogen patterns involved, it is worth remembering that one of the best ways to support a girl during times of flux is to treat the Element of her constitutional imbalance. It is akin to placing a supportive hand gently on a toddler's back as she takes her first steps. It makes the process a little easier and can prevent things from going too far off course.

Treatment of the constitutional imbalance is sometimes enough on its own, even when there are one or more patterns present not directly related to that Element. At other times, it can be combined with treatment of the Organ/Pathogen patterns below.

The most commonly seen patterns in menstrual conditions in teenagers are:

- Liver *qi* stagnation
- Cold stagnation
- Blood stagnation

- Heat in the Blood

- Spleen *qi* deficient and not controlling Blood

- Blood deficiency

- Liver *yang* rising from Liver Blood and/or *yin* deficiency

- Kidney *yin* deficiency

- Kidney *yang* deficiency

Liver *qi* stagnation

Liver *qi* stagnation may cause:

- irregular periods

- painful periods

- pre-menstrual syndrome.

Liver *qi* stagnation is the most common cause of irregular periods and pre-menstrual syndrome in teenage girls. It may simply be a result of the monthly ebb and flow of *qi* and Blood not yet having established a rhythm. It may also, of course, be exacerbated by the inherent frustrations of being a teenager. A girl with a Wood constitutional imbalance may be particularly prone to *qi* stagnation.

Menstrual symptoms

- moodiness, depression, irritability

- irregular periods with a tendency towards a long cycle

- small clots in the menstrual blood and cramping pain during the period

- pain tends to come in waves and is eased by movement

- menstrual flow erratic

- all symptoms improve once bleeding begins

Other symptoms: abdominal bloating and distension, irregular bowel movements especially before period

Pulse: wiry

Tongue: normal, possibly slightly purple, possibly red sides, slightly distended sub-lingual veins

Treatment principles: smooth the Liver and move *qi*

SUGGESTED TREATMENT

Two distal points, such as Liv 3 *taichong* and GB 34 *yanglingquan*, together with one local point such as Ren 6 *qihai*, is often enough to regulate the cycle. The distal Spleen points may be added if there is also menstrual pain, as they directly affect the Uterus. Ki 13 *qixue* may be added if the girl feels anxious or panicky, especially in the pre-menstrual phase.

Points

Liv 3 *taichong*
Liv 6 *zhongdu*
Liv 12 *jimai*

> GB 34 *yanglingquan*
> Sp 8 *diji*
> Sp 6 *sanyinjiao*
> St 29 *guilai*
> St 28 *shuidao*
> Ren 6 *qihai*
> Ki 13 *qixue*

Method: sedation needle technique

Cold stagnation

Cold stagnation may cause:

- painful periods

- irregular cycle

- no periods.

Cold stagnation is the most common cause of severe period pain in teenage girls. The Uterus is energetically 'open' in the years leading up to menarche. If Cold invades (because of exposure to cold when playing sport or swimming), it congeals the Blood. Over time, it will also deplete Kidney *yang*. Infertility in an adult woman may be traced back to an invasion of Cold in the teenage years. Therefore, if left untreated, it may lead to years of physical and emotional pain.

Menstrual symptoms

- severe, tight, gripping or contracting pain

- pain relieved only by the application of warmth

- irregular periods with a tendency towards a long cycle

- small, dark clots in the menstrual blood

- no onset of periods at puberty

Other symptoms: there may be a general feeling of cold. If the Cold is confined just to the Uterus, symptoms in other parts of the body will be determined by whichever other patterns are present.

Pulse: may be tight (although the Cold will not usually show on the pulse if it is only in the Uterus)

Tongue: may be pale blue or bluish-purple (again, the Cold may not show on the upper surface of the tongue if it is confined to the Uterus)

Treatment principles: warm the Uterus; expel Cold; regulate Blood

> **SUGGESTED TREATMENT**
>
> It is often necessary to use two or three distal points, and one local point. Points should be combined with moxa. A moxa box on the abdomen is the most effective way of eliminating Cold from the Uterus. There are usually underlying deficiencies which need to be addressed too, most commonly of Spleen and/or Kidney *yang*. If there are signs of Kidney *yang* deficiency, then a moxa box on the back may be used too.
>
> **Points**
>
> Liv 3 *taichong*

GB 34 *yanglingquan*
Sp 6 *sanyinjiao*
Sp 8 *diji*
Sp 10 *xuehai*
St 28 *shuidao*
St 29 *guilai*

Method: sedation needle technique

Other techniques: moxa is essential

Blood stagnation

Blood stagnation may cause:

- painful periods

- heavy periods

- irregular cycle

- no periods.

Blood stagnation tends to be more straightforward to treat in a teenage girl than it does in an adult woman. As the girl's body is still in a state of flux, and because the stagnation has not had so many years to become established, Blood is more easily invigorated.

There are three main causes of Blood stagnation in a teenager. The first is trauma, such as an accident or sexual abuse. When this is the case, the practitioner should be aware that, during treatment, emotions that have been held in as a result of the trauma may come to the surface. Second, Blood stagnation may arise as a result of Blood deficiency, which is a commonly seen pathology in this age group. Third, Blood may be stagnant simply because the monthly ebb and flow of *qi* and Blood is not yet established. In a sense, this is not true Blood stagnation but more of a 'hesitancy'.

Menstrual symptoms

- severe, stabbing and fixed pain during the period

- pain is not eased by movement, nor significantly alleviated by pain-relief medication

- periods will be irregular with a tendency towards a long cycle

- large, dark clots in the menstrual blood

- a mix of fresh blood and dark blood

- heavy bleeding or no periods

Other symptoms

- If the Blood stagnation derives from **qi stagnation**: moodiness, depression, irritability, abdominal bloating and distension, irregular bowel movements.

- If the Blood stagnation derives from **Blood deficiency**: tearfulness, difficulty sleeping, light-headed when stands up, blurred vision, dry eyes, floaters, pins and needles, easily startled.

Pulse: wiry (if from *qi* stagnation) or choppy (if from Blood deficiency)

Tongue: distended sub-lingual veins

Treatment principles: invigorate Blood. If from *qi* stagnation: move Liver *qi*. If from Blood deficiency: nourish Blood.

> **SUGGESTED TREATMENT**
>
> In most teenage girls, moving *qi* will mean that Blood moves. However, there are occasional stubborn cases. These are often ones where there has been a history of trauma or the mother has had a history of painful periods. Then it may be necessary to open the *chong mai*. This is done by using the opening and coupled points (Sp 4 *gongsun* and Pc 6 *neiguan*) combined with points along the channel such as Ki 14 *siman*.
>
> **Points**
>
> To invigorate Blood and move *qi*:
>
> > Liv 3 *taichong*
> > GB 34 *yanglingquan*
> > Sp 6 *sanyinjiao*
> > Sp 8 *diji*
> > Sp 10 *xuehai*
> > St 29 *guilai*
> > St 28 *shuidao*
>
> **Method:** sedation needle technique
>
> To nourish Blood (when stagnation comes from Blood deficiency):
>
> > Ren 4 *guanyuan*
> > Liv 8 *ququan*
> > Bl 17 *geshu*
>
> Other points will depend on which Organ or Organs the Blood deficiency stems from.
>
> **Method:** tonification needle technique

Heat in the Blood

Heat in the Blood may cause:

* heavy periods.

In teenagers, Heat in the Blood may have built up in the years leading up to menarche. As *yang* increases, it has no means of discharging until the first period starts and the Heat begins to affect the Blood. Heat is often compounded by intense emotions and *qi* stagnation that are characteristic of adolescence.

It is important to ascertain whether the Heat in the Blood is affecting the Heart as well as the Liver. If it is affecting the Heart, there will be more symptoms of *shen* disturbance, such as poor sleep and agitation.

Menstrual symptoms

* heavy menstrual bleeding with 'flooding' of menstrual blood

* blood tends to be bright red, perhaps with small clots

* feels very hot during the period

Other symptoms: poor sleep which worsens in the pre-menstrual phase, mentally restless and agitated, fiery temper, thirst

Pulse: overflowing on the Wood pulses and possibly Fire pulses, may be rapid

Tongue: red, may have red spots on the side, yellow coat

Treatment principles: clear Heat from the Blood

SUGGESTED TREATMENT

The two key points to treat Heat in the Blood are Sp 10 *xuehai* and Liv 2 *xingjian*. These two points are often effective on their own. If the Heat affects the *shen*, then He 8 *shaofu* should be added. Any underlying deficiencies will need to be addressed with treatment too.

Points

Sp 10 *xuehai*
Liv 2 *xingjian*
GB 38 *yangfu*
He 8 *shaofu*
Bl 17 *geshu*
LI 11 *quchi*

Method: sedation needle technique

Spleen *qi* deficient and not controlling Blood

Spleen *qi* deficient and not controlling Blood may cause:

- heavy periods.

This is an extremely common cause of heavy, prolonged periods in teenage girls. Poor dietary habits, too much studying, lots of worry and sometimes over-exercising can mean that the Spleen is sorely taxed.

Menstrual symptoms

- heavy and/or prolonged periods

- pale and dilute blood

- feels tired and washed out during and after the period

Other symptoms: easily tired, may have a poor appetite or crave carbohydrates and sugar, tendency to worry, easily feels overwhelmed, loose stools

Pulse: deficient

Tongue: pale

Treatment principles: tonify Spleen *qi*

SUGGESTED TREATMENT

Two points per treatment, such as St 36 *zusanli* and Sp 3 *taibai*, needled with the tonification technique and treated with moxa cones, is often sufficient. The points used should be varied at each treatment. The aspects of the child's life that are causing the Spleen deficiency ideally should also be addressed. It is particularly useful to treat during the period in order to stem the bleeding.

Points

St 36 *zusanli*
Sp 1 *yinbai*

> Sp 3 *taibai*
> Sp 6 *sanyinjiao*
> Bl 20 *pishu*
> Du 20 *baihui*
> Ren 6 *qihai*

Method: tonification needle technique

Other techniques: moxibustion

Blood deficiency

Blood deficiency may cause:

- no periods

- scanty periods

- long cycle

- pre-menstrual syndrome.

Blood deficiency is another extremely common pathology seen in teenage girls. Although there are often lifestyle factors that are causing it, the simple fact of starting menstruation can itself cause Blood deficiency. When a girl begins menstruating, her daily required intake of iron increases from 8mg to 15mg.[50] Therefore, unless her diet includes lots of iron-rich foods, it is easy for her to become Blood deficient. It is particularly hard for vegetarian, vegan or dieting girls to get the iron they need from their diet.

 In some girls, Blood deficiency symptoms are worse at the end of and in the few days after menstruation. In others, Blood deficiency symptoms are worse pre-menstrually. This is because Blood is 'diverted' to the Uterus at this time and there is less available for all the other physiological functions in the body.

Menstrual symptoms

- periods do not start or start and then stop again

- if there are periods the bleeding is light and short

Other symptoms will depend on the Organ that the Blood deficiency stems from.

 Often, the Blood deficiency is related to and/or stems from the Organs related to the girl's constitutional imbalance. For example, if she has an Earth constitutional imbalance, the Blood deficiency will usually be most effectively treated via the Spleen. If she has a Wood constitutional imbalance, the Blood deficiency will probably be most effectively treated via the Liver.

LIVER

Light-headed when stands up, an imbalance in the expression of anger, blurred vision, floaters, dry or tired eyes after a lot of studying or looking at screens, numbness and tingling.

SUGGESTED TREATMENT
Points

> Liv 3 *taichong*
> Liv 8 *ququan*
> Ren 4 *guanyuan*

Bl 17 *geshu*
Bl 18 *ganshu*

Method: tonification needle technique

KIDNEY DEFICIENCY LEADING TO BLOOD DEFICIENCY

Prone to anxiety, may not sleep well (especially during the latter part of the night), physically unrobust, easily tires, dark circles under the eyes, late onset of periods.

SUGGESTED TREATMENT
Points

Ki 3 *taixi*
Ki 13 *qixue*
Bl 23 *shenshu*
Ren 4 *guanyuan*

Method: tonification needle technique

Other techniques: moxibustion

SPLEEN DEFICIENCY LEADING TO BLOOD DEFICIENCY

Small appetite, irregular eating, cravings for sugary foods or carbohydrates, prone to overthinking, easily feels overwhelmed, tearfulness, loose stools, may easily tire.

SUGGESTED TREATMENT
Points

St 36 *zusanli*
Sp 6 *sanyinjiao*
Bl 20 *pishu*
Sp 3 *taibai*

Method: tonification needle technique

Fifteen-year-old Kate had a very short, light menstrual bleed about once every six or eight weeks. She slept badly and was very anxious. She had been finding friendships at school difficult and easily felt upset by what she perceived as exclusion from her friendship group. Kate had a Fire constitutional imbalance. Treatment to tonify her Pericardium and Triple Burner, as well as general Blood-nourishing points such as Ren 4 *guanyuan* and Bl 17 *geshu*, helped her feel less anxious and sleep better. Her periods remained light but came regularly every month. She came for weekly treatments for two months, then fortnightly for another two months. After that, she just came for occasional top-ups if her anxiety showed signs of returning.

Liver *yang* rising from Liver Blood and/or *yin* deficiency

Liver *yang* rising from Liver Blood and/or *yin* deficiency can cause:

- pre-menstrual syndrome.

Liver *yang* rising is fairly commonly seen in teenage girls. There is a propensity for *yang* to rise as the girl adjusts to the abundance of *yang* that is characteristic of this phase. As already mentioned, Blood deficiency is also common, which further increases the propensity of *yang* to rise. Finally, studying, too much time spent on screens and activities that encourage girls to be 'in their heads' all draw *yang* upwards.

Emotional symptoms

- outbursts of anger or irritability
- otherwise tearful and weepy
- may be agitated and anxious if there is underlying *yin* deficiency

Physical symptoms

- headaches
- dizziness
- insomnia
- neck and shoulder tension

Other symptoms will depend on whether there is underlying Blood deficiency or *yin* deficiency.

Pulse: thin, choppy or wiry

Tongue: may be pale if underlying Blood deficient, or red if underlying *yin* deficiency

Treatment principles: subdue Liver *yang*; nourish Liver Blood or *yin*

SUGGESTED TREATMENT

If a girl has symptoms of Liver *yang* rising at the time of treatment, two or three points to subdue Liver *yang* may be used. An effective combination is the first three points suggested below. If she comes for treatment on a day when no Liver *yang* rising symptoms are present, it is usually best to focus on nourishing the underlying deficiency.

Although most books describe that Liver *yang* rising always stems from an underlying deficiency of Blood or *yin*, in practice (and in teenage girls especially) it sometimes seems to arise purely from Liver *qi* stagnation. The pulse is crucial in determining whether or not this is the case.

Points

To subdue Liver *yang*:

GB 20 *fengchi*
GB 43 *xaixi*
Liv 2 *xingjian*
TB 5 *waiguan*

Method: sedation needle technique

To nourish Liver Blood and/or *yin*:

Liv 3 *taichong*
Liv 8 *ququan*
Ren 4 *guanyuan*
Bl 18 *ganshu*
Ki 3 *taixi*

Method: tonification needle technique

Kidney *yin* deficiency

Kidney *yin* deficiency manifests somewhat differently in teenage girls than it does in adult women. There may be few or no signs of Heat. There is nearly always, however, anxiety, restlessness, poor sleep and a lack of internal calm and stability. Apart from when it is constitutional, it nearly always occurs in girls who have been pushed, have very full lives or who are naturally very driven.

Kidney *yin* deficiency tends to make bleeding light. If the *yin* deficiency has led to a significant amount of Empty Heat, however, the bleeding may be heavy. This is very rare in teenage girls, however.

Kidney *yin* deficiency may cause:

- no periods
- irregular cycle.

Menstrual symptoms

- irregular periods
- periods tend to be light and short
- menstrual cycle is likely to be long

Other symptoms: prone to anxiety, poor sleep (especially during the latter part of the night), appears to be physically unrobust, easily tires, may have dark circles under the eyes, onset of periods may have been late

Pulse: floating and empty

Tongue: red with a redder tip

Treatment principles: nourish Kidney *yin*, calm the *shen*

SUGGESTED TREATMENT

Severe *yin* deficiency may benefit from treatment of the *ren mai*. This may be done using the opening and coupled points (Lu 7 *lieque* and Ki 6 *zhaohai*) as well as points along the channel such as Ren 4 *guanyuan*.

Points

> Ki 3 *taixi*
> Bl 23 *shenshu*
> Ki 13 *qixue*
> Ren 4 *guanyuan*
> Liv 8 *ququan*

Method: tonification needle technique

To calm the *shen*:

> Du 24 *shenting*
> M-HN-3 *yintang*

Method: sedation needle technique

CASE HISTORY: FOURTEEN-YEAR-OLD GIRL WITH ALMOST CONSTANT BLEEDING

The following case history illustrates how treatment of the constitutional imbalance may help to establish a girl's menstrual cycle.

Nora's periods had started when she was thirteen. A year later, she was brought to the clinic because she bled almost constantly. She had a 'proper' bleed for ten days every month, which was neither particularly heavy nor painful. In between times, she had continual, heavy spotting. The blood was fresh, not dark.

Nora was a very anxious girl who found the social aspects of school challenging. She tended to wake early and found it hard to relax. Her mum reported that she 'flew off the handle' on a regular basis.

Observations: Nora was pale but had red cheeks and quite pronounced spots. She had blue beside her eyes. Her eyes flitted around the room and she seemed as if she was constantly on 'red alert'.

- Pulse: floating and thin
- Tongue: red

Diagnosis

- Water constitutional imbalance
- Kidney *yin* deficiency

Treatment principles: strengthen Water, nourish Kidney *yin*

Treatment
Treatment 1

Yuan source points Bl 64 *jinggu*, Ki 3 *taixi* (tonification needle technique)

Treatment 2

Ren 4 *guanyuan*, Bl 58 *feiyang*, Ki 4 *dazhong*

Treatment 3

Moxa cones (11 on each side) on Sp 1 to stop bleeding

Bl 28 *pangguangshu*, Bl 23 *shenshu*

Treatment 4

Moxa cones (11 on each side) on Sp 1 to stop bleeding

Ki 14 *simian*, Bl 62 *shenmai*, Ki 6 *zhaohai*

At this point Nora's spotting began to improve. She had several days in a row without any spotting at all. I continued using the same treatment principles as above, with a variety of points. After three months of treatment, Nora's cycle was normalised and she had no more spotting. She continued to come for treatments for a while longer as her mother had noticed other benefits. Nora had been less anxious and was sleeping better too.

Kidney *yang* deficiency

Kidney *yang* deficiency may cause:

- no periods
- short cycle.

Kidney *yang* deficiency, unless it is constitutional, may stem from long-term Spleen *yang* deficiency. When this is the case, it is important to treat the Spleen too. Another common cause of Kidney *yang* deficiency in teenage girls is that *yang* has been consumed in order to fuel the physiological changes associated with puberty. Unless the girl's lifestyle allows her time to build up her resources again, the *ming men* may remain deficient. It is like a fire that struggles to get going, rather than one which strongly flames.

Menstrual symptoms

- short cycle

- periods tend to be light and short

- fluid retention, especially in the pre-menstrual phase

Other symptoms: prone to lethargy and feeling low, lack of motivation, tends to feel cold, wants to sleep a lot, dark circles under the eyes, onset of periods may have been late

Pulse: deep, weak and possibly slow

Tongue: pale, wet, swollen

Treatment principles: warm and tonify Kidney *yang*

SUGGESTED TREATMENT

It is helpful to use points both on the abdomen and the lower back. Points on the abdomen directly affect the gynaecological system. Points on the lower back particularly affect the *ming men*. Combining one point on the abdomen, one point on the lower back and one or two distal points per treatment is usually effective.

Points

Ki 3 *taixi*
Bl 23 *shenshu*
Ki 13 *qixue*
Ren 6 *qihai*
St 36 *zusanli*
Du 4 *ming men*

Method: tonification needle technique

Other techniques: moxa may be applicable

SUMMARY

» There is a surge of Kidney *yang* during puberty, which fuels the developmental changes.

» In a deficient child, the surge may be too weak to fuel both the necessary changes and all the other physiological processes.

» In an excess child, the surge in *yang* may mean there is an excess of Heat 'trapped' in the body.

» Treating a girl in the lead-up to and beginning stages of menstruation can help to 'set' her cycle in order to prevent years of problems.

» The most commonly seen menstrual problems in teenage girls are: irregular periods; painful periods; heavy periods; bleeding between periods; no periods; and pre-menstrual syndrome.

» The most commonly seen patterns that cause these problems are: *qi* stagnation; Blood stagnation; stagnation of Cold; Heat in the Blood; Spleen *qi* deficient and not controlling Blood; Blood deficiency; Liver *yang* rising; Kidney *yin* deficiency; and Kidney *yang* deficiency.

Chapter 69

DIFFICULT OR EARLY
PUBERTY IN GIRLS

. . . .

> This chapter relates only to girls because this reflects my clinical experience. My strong suspicion is that there are just as many boys who struggle during puberty but they are less likely to come for treatment. It could be that the difficulties men experience in talking about and seeking help for their problems begins at this young age and that they therefore often suffer in silence. My hope is that in the future this will change or that there are practitioners who are already helping boys navigate puberty, and that they will share their experiences.

The topics discussed in this chapter are:

- Aetiology and Organs involved in puberty

- Patterns commonly seen at puberty

- Patterns involved in early puberty

- Lifestyle advice

Introduction
What is puberty?

Contrary to popular belief, the first period in a girl does not signify the start of puberty. Puberty begins silently many years before with hormonal secretions from the pituitary gland. It is a long process, rather than a one-off event, and it plays out differently in every girl. It often has a 'stop–start' quality to it, rather than being smooth.

The key milestones of puberty are:

- the production of oestrogen by the ovaries

- the onset of breast development in girls

- growth of pubic hair, followed by armpit hair, often accompanied by acne and body odour

- the onset of menstruation.

These physical milestones are often accompanied by:

- increased drive towards independence and autonomy

- changes in mood, which may involve heightened intensity of emotions.

When and why does puberty need treatment?

Puberty is a rite of passage, not an illness. When everything goes well, the child does not need treatment. Increasingly, however, children (who are in nearly all cases girls) come to the clinic for treatment with puberty-related problems. This is for two reasons. First, puberty is beginning at an age that is considered too young. Second, the transition is not smooth and the child is struggling through it either physically or emotionally, or both.

What is the normal age for puberty?

Until the 20th century, puberty usually coincided with the early teenage years. This has since changed significantly, and the greatest changes have been within the past two decades. However, whilst it is often thought that girls begin menstruating much earlier than they used to, the facts paint a somewhat different picture. The average age at which girls get their first period has fallen only slightly since the 1970s (by approximately six months). However, there has been a much more dramatic and noticeable change in the age at which the first signs of puberty, such as breast budding and the growth of pubic hair, begin. On average, girls in Europe and America develop breasts up to two years earlier than they did just forty years ago.[51]

Providing a medical imbalance has been excluded, the question of whether or not puberty is 'early' is not one which is straightforward to answer. What once would have been considered early is quickly becoming the new norm. It is relatively common for puberty to be knocking on the door for many eight- and nine-year-old girls. Rather than simply labelling this as 'early puberty', it is probably more realistic and helpful to accept that this is now a common age for puberty to begin and to turn our focus towards helping girls to navigate it.

 Western medicine differentiates between 'normal puberty', 'normal early puberty' and 'abnormal early puberty'. An abnormal early puberty is one where there is an underlying hormonal or medical issue that needs to be addressed by a Western medical physician. Normal early puberty is one that starts at an age that is considered young but where there is no underlying hormonal or other medical issue.

Another aspect of puberty that has changed is the length of time it often takes. It may be up to four years from the earliest signs, usually breast budding, until the first period. It may be a couple more years from then until a girl's menstrual cycle becomes regular. This means there is a long period of transition, during which a girl is especially susceptible to outside influences, be they emotional stress or environmental pollutants.

Why does puberty now begin at a younger age?

This question is one which numerous researchers around the world are devoting their lives to answering. Almost the only fact that everyone is in agreement about is that the answer is, as yet, unknown. However, some broad categories of triggers for early puberty have been identified. They are:

- being overweight or obese

- exposure to chemicals that disrupt the hormonal system

- social and psychological stressors (e.g. early childhood trauma, poor familial relationships).[52]

It is believed that genetics also plays a role, and that the factors mentioned above interact with a girl's genetic make-up.

In what ways may puberty be problematic?

Although puberty (when not caused by an underlying disease) is physically neither harmful nor painful for the child, it may bring emotional and psychological challenges. Puberty at any age can be a testing and tumultuous time. For a child to go through it at a relatively young age, when the disparity between physical and emotional maturity is even greater than usual, is harder. Added to this is the discomfort of being different from her peers. This can bring feelings of isolation and, in some children, shame. A child with very obvious signs of early puberty may be a target for bullies. The parent is often as unready emotionally to face her child going through puberty as the child herself.

Physical and emotional symptoms that may arise for the first time during puberty are:

- headaches
- insomnia
- anxiety and depression
- acne
- urinary tract infections.

What can we do as acupuncturists to help a girl navigate puberty?

Treat the physical and/or emotional symptoms
The patterns that cause the physical and emotional symptoms that may arise at puberty are discussed in the relevant chapters.

Treat the Organ/Pathogen imbalance
Many girls come for treatment during puberty without a specific symptom but because they are not thriving either physically or emotionally. In these cases, the practitioner must always determine whether there is an underlying Organ/Pathogen imbalance present. The patterns that may trigger early puberty are described later in the chapter. Addressing these imbalances can help to slow down the pubertal changes that are taking place if they are happening at a very early age. However, if puberty is happening at an appropriate age, but is causing difficulty for the child in some way, then any Organ/Pattern imbalance may be present.

Treat the constitutional imbalance
Puberty is a time both of enormous internal flux and change, and myriad external stressors (for example, changing schools, exposure to social media, increased academic pressure, divorce, family discord, etc.). It is also when the 'scaffolding' of childhood is gradually dismantled and a girl is expected to cope with more areas of life on her own. Treating a girl's constitutional imbalance helps to bring her back to herself and to find her own internal support structures as the external ones are diminishing. It can help to prevent imbalances becoming ingrained and maximise the chances of a girl riding this time and entering the next phase of her life in as healthy a state as possible.

Give lifestyle advice
It is hard for both parents and children who are struggling with this transitional phase to keep a sight of what is really important, what will help and what will hinder the process. The practitioner is in an ideal position, as an outsider, to give the family pointers and suggestions. It is often the case that the child will take on board lifestyle advice from a practitioner much more readily than she will a parent.

Lifestyle advice, of course, needs to be tailored to the individual and should be based on the unique situation of each girl. However, there are also some general suggestions which are universally relevant for any girl going through puberty. Please see the section 'Lifestyle advice' at the end of this chapter for a discussion of these.

Aetiology and Organs involved in puberty

The Kidneys

Kidney *jing* is said to govern birth, growth and development. One key aspect of development, in this context, is the highly significant changes that occur during the changeover phase between the seven- and eight-year cycles. According to the *Su Wen*, 'At two times seven years, fertility arrives, *ren mai* functions fully while the powerful *chong mai* rises in power.'[53]

A deficiency in the Kidneys, whether it be of *jing*, *yin* or *yang*, may mean that puberty arrives either too early or too late. It is interesting to note that it has become the norm for the first signs of puberty to begin around the time of the first changeover of cycles: that is, a full cycle before the time when the *Su Wen* described the onset of menstruation.

Kidney deficiency may also underpin teenage anxiety and depression, as well as physical symptoms such as headaches.

The aetiologies, functions and imbalances associated with the Kidneys during puberty are summarised in Figure 69.1.

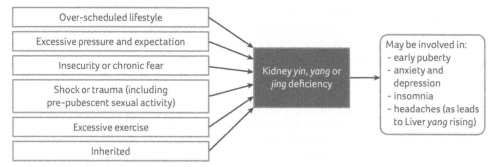

Figure 69.1 The Kidneys and puberty

The Liver

The Liver is involved in several ways in the onset of puberty. First, the Liver channel runs through the genitals. Second, the Liver receives Blood for menstruation from the *chong mai* which becomes replete with Blood ready for menstruation to begin in girls. Deficiency of Liver Blood may mean that menstruation is delayed. Heat in the Liver may be a factor in the early onset of puberty. Liver patterns may also be involved in teenage anxiety and depression as well as symptoms such as insomnia and headaches.

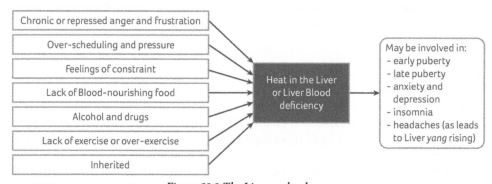

Figure 69.2 The Liver and puberty

The Spleen

The Spleen has the job of digesting the increased intake of food that usually accompanies puberty. An already weak Spleen may become weaker, and a Spleen that was just about coping beforehand may no longer cope. An imbalance in the Spleen may affect the nature of periods when they first start (see Chapter 68), as well as causing digestive problems and anxiety.

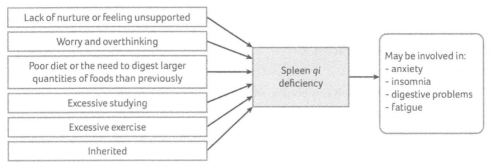

Figure 69.3 The Spleen and puberty

The Heart

Although many Chinese medicine books do not mention the Heart in relation to puberty, I mention it here for two reasons. First, the Heart of a girl is sorely tested because this is a time when friendships become crucial and she begins to become more conscious of and concerned with what people think of her and whether she is liked or not. Twenty-first-century girls have to withstand more social pressures than ever before, and it is often the Heart that bears the brunt of this.

Second, the Heart goes through changes during puberty because of its close connection with the gynaecological system. The Heart is connected to the Uterus via the *bao mai* and to the Kidneys via the *bao luo*.

A deficiency of Heart Blood or *yin* can cause insomnia and anxiety. An excess of Heat in the Heart may cause more severe mental–emotional problems. Any Heart imbalance may affect the regularity of menstruation.

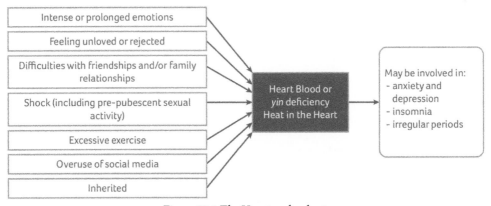

Figure 69.4 The Heart and puberty

Patterns commonly seen at puberty[*]

- Heart and Kidney *yin* deficiency
- Liver and Kidney deficiency
- Spleen *qi* and Heart Blood deficiency
- Rebellious *qi* in the *chong mai*

Heart and Kidney *yin* deficiency
Symptoms

- low-grade anxiety which may become more intense at times of stress
- easily feels insecure
- mental restlessness and agitation
- may take a long time to get to sleep
- may wake early in the morning and/or sleep may be interrupted

Pulse: floating and empty

Tongue: red prickles on the tip of the tongue

Treatment principles: nourish Heart *yin*; nourish Kidney *yin*; calm the *shen*

> **SUGGESTED TREATMENT**
> **Points**
> To nourish Heart *yin*:
>
> > He 6 *yinxi*
> > He 7 *shenmen*
> > Bl 15 *xinshu*
> > Ren 14 *juque*
>
> To nourish Kidney *yin*:
>
> > Ki 6 *zhaohai*
> > Ki 10 *yingu*
> > Bl 23 *shenshu*
> > Ren 4 *guanyuan*
>
> To calm the *shen*:
>
> > M-HN-3 *yintang*
> > Du 24 *shenting*
>
> **Method:** tonification needle technique

Liver and Kidney deficiency
Symptoms

- low mood
- slightly anxious or agitated

---

[*] These are by no means the only patterns but are the ones that, in my practice, most commonly occur in girls during this time.

- grumpy or moody
- lacking in motivation and drive
- lacking in a desire for independence
- delayed physical development
- tired or lacking in vigour

Pulse: thin, deficient

Tongue: may be pale or red

Treatment principles: tonify the Liver and Kidneys

> **SUGGESTED TREATMENT**
> **Points**
>
> > Bl 18 *ganshu*
> > Bl 23 *shenshu*
> > Du 4 *ming men*
> > Ren 4 *guanyuan*
> > Liv 3 *taichong*
> > Ki 3 *taixi*
>
> **Method:** tonification needle technique
>
> **Other techniques:** moxa may be applicable

Mary was sixteen years old. She had begun menstruating when she was fourteen and a half. She came for treatment because she was depressed. Her mother worried that Mary showed no signs of wanting more independence and seemed to lack any interest in doing things outside the family. She constantly complained of being tired and spent the weekends sleeping. Mary had dark circles under her eyes, her complexion was dull and her body frail. I diagnosed her as being Liver and Kidney deficient, with a Wood constitutional imbalance. She came for treatment every two or three weeks over a period of eighteen months. Progress was slow but, over this time, she gradually became more of a 'normal' teenager. She joined a drama club and saw her friends at weekends. Interestingly, between the ages of eight and twelve, she had been scouted for the junior team of a football club and had been training six days a week. I suspected this, together with a relatively poor physical constitution, was the cause of her deficiency.

Spleen *qi* and Heart Blood deficiency

Symptoms

- mild anxiety which is often worse at bedtime, when tired or when studying hard
- worry, overthinking and pensiveness
- tendency to feel misunderstood and uncared for
- dysfunctional relationship with food
- emotionally vulnerable and easily hurt
- takes a long time to get to sleep
- difficulty concentrating

- feels easily tired

- loose stools

Pulse: thin or choppy in the front position on the left-hand side, overall deficient

Tongue: pale

Treatment principles: tonify Spleen *qi*; nourish Heart Blood

SUGGESTED TREATMENT
Points
To strengthen the Spleen:

> St 36 *zusanli*
> Sp 3 *taibai*
> Bl 20 *pishu*

To nourish Heart Blood:

> He 7 *shenmen*
> Pc 7 *daling*
> Bl 14 *jueyinshu*
> Bl 15 *xinshu*

Method: tonification needle technique

Other techniques: moxibustion

Rebellious *qi* in the *chong mai*
Symptoms

- anxiety that waxes and wanes according to the phases of the menstrual cycle and is often worse just before the period

- a sense of anxiety rising up from the abdomen to the chest

- irregular periods or other menstrual difficulties

- discomfort in the abdomen

- tightness or discomfort in the chest

- a feeling of heat in the face with cold feet

Pulse: The pulse picture will depend upon the underlying patterns, which may be a deficiency of Blood or Kidney deficiency, or a full condition such as Blood stagnation. In some cases, Rebellious *qi* in the *chong mai* occurs on its own without any underlying pathologies.

Tongue: the tongue will depend on the underlying pathologies

Treatment principles: subdue Rebellious *qi* in the *chong mai*

SUGGESTED TREATMENT
Points

> Sp 4 *gongsun* and Pc 6 *neiguan* (the opening and coupled points of the *chong mai*) with the sedation technique

> Ki 21 *yeomen*, Liv 3 *taichong* (needled with the sedation technique in order to calm and subdue the Rebellious *qi*)
>
> St 30 *qichong*, Ki 13 *qixue*, Ki 14 *simian* (needled with the tonification technique in order to strengthen the Lower Burner to 'hold down' the Rebellious *qi*

Patterns involved in early puberty

As already mentioned, the fact that the first signs of puberty commonly occur at a much younger age than they used to may, at least in part, be a reflection of where we are in terms of our evolutionary process. Having said that, it is undeniable that *very* early puberty is usually unwelcome for a girl and makes her life more difficult. It is also true that the patterns most commonly seen in early puberty are due to lifestyle factors which, in the 21st century, are common.

Therefore, whilst on the one hand accepting that puberty is probably going to occur earlier in most girls today than it did a matter of only a few decades ago, we can on the other hand do what we can to prevent this trend becoming too marked.

- Kidney *yin* deficiency with Empty Heat
- Liver *qi* stagnation turning to Heat

> It is common for these two patterns to co-exist. Kidney *yin* deficiency often leads to Heat, and the long-term presence of Heat may deplete Kidney *yin*.

Kidney *yin* deficiency with Empty Heat

Symptoms

- bodily changes associated with puberty begin early
- agitation and restlessness
- anxiety
- poor sleep
- red cheeks

Pulse: floating, empty

Tongue: may be red, may be peeled or partially peeled, may be dry

Treatment principles: clear Empty Heat; nourish Kidney *yin*

> **SUGGESTED TREATMENT**
> **Points**
> To clear Empty Heat:
>
> Ki 2 *rangu*
> Liv 2 *xingjian*
> Ren 14 *juque* (to calm the *shen* if Empty Heat rises up and agitates the Heart)
>
> **Method:** sedation needle technique
>
> To nourish Kidney *yin*:
>
> Ki 3 *taixi*
> Ki 6 *zhaohai*
> Ki 9 *zhubin*

Bl 23 *shenshu*
Ren 4 *guanyuan*

Method: tonification needle technique

Liver *qi* stagnation turning to Heat

This pattern is commonly seen in girls around the time of puberty, even when it is not causing early puberty.

Symptoms

- bodily changes associated with puberty begin early
- coloured vaginal discharge with odour
- frequent urination
- irritable and moody
- quick to anger
- depressed

Pulse: wiry and possibly overflowing on the Wood pulses

Tongue: red spots on the sides

Treatment principles: smooth the Liver and move *qi*; clear Heat

SUGGESTED TREATMENT
Points

Liv 2 *xingjian*
Liv 3 *taichong*
Liv 14 *qimen*
GB 38 *yangfu*
GB 41 *zulinqi*

Method: sedation needle technique

Louise came for treatment at the age of eight. She had pronounced body odour and strong mood swings. She already had breast buds. I diagnosed Liver Heat and Kidney *yin* deficiency. The aetiology was very striking in Louise's case. Her parents had separated recently after what her mother described as 'years of living in a state of fear'. Her father was an alcoholic who became verbally and physically aggressive when drunk. Louise responded quickly to treatment to clear Heat from the Liver and nourish Kidney *yin*. After six treatments at weekly intervals, her body odour had gone and her moods were more stable. I continued to treat her every now and then for years. Her periods eventually started when she was twelve.

Lifestyle advice

The following pieces of lifestyle advice are useful for all girls approaching and going through puberty. They are particularly relevant for a girl who is starting puberty early, or who is struggling physically or emotionally through the process.

- **Promote emotional closeness:** A massive body of evidence supports the idea that a strong mother–child bond not only is the most important determining factor of how a girl navigates puberty, but also can even influence when a girl goes through puberty.[54] Nurturing this bond is no easy task for a mother or mother figure when a girl is riding the stormy waters of puberty. A discussion of how to do this is beyond the scope of this book, but acupuncture treatment can be a part of what helps a mother and child in this way. The better they feel in themselves, the stronger the position they are in to navigate their changing relationship.

- **Manage environmental risks:** Exposure to endocrine-disrupting chemicals (EDCs) can influence the age of onset of puberty. It is not known exactly which substances have the biggest impact, and it also depends on the dose of the exposure, the age at which a child is exposed and their route of entry into the body (e.g. whether they enter through the skin or via water). EDCs may be in foods, plastics, bath and beauty products,* household cleaning goods and household materials such as carpets. The goal is for a family to do the best they can in avoiding these substances based on what they can afford. It is not possible to avoid everything that may be an EDC, and it's important to keep things in perspective and not develop a mentality of being a 'victim' to our toxic world. That creates worry and stress which, arguably, have just as negative an impact on the body as the toxins themselves.

- **Reduce sugar, unhealthy fat and salt as far as possible in the diet:** Sugar, in particular, disturbs the body's metabolism, and can to lead to obesity which is likely to disturb the hormonal imbalance.

- **Get enough sleep:** The importance of sleep has been discussed in Chapter 8. It is particularly important during puberty as many of the hormones related to healthy development are released overnight.

- **Get regular, moderate exercise:** Being physically active helps to guard against obesity and also supports the maintenance of healthy hormone levels in the body.

CASE HISTORY: NINE-YEAR-OLD GIRL STRUGGLING WITH EARLY PUBERTAL CHANGES

This case history illustrates:

- how acupuncture can support a girl through a 'normal' puberty
- how treatment of the constitutional imbalance can help a girl to navigate pubertal change more easily.

Flo came to the clinic when she was nine years old. Her mother said that six months ago she had, seemingly overnight, transformed from being a happy, carefree girl who enjoyed home and school life, to being depressed, irritable, anxious and withdrawn. Flo was tearful during the initial appointment and said that she did not understand what was happening to her. She hated the fact that she now seemed to be always arguing with her mum and that school left her feeling frustrated, and also hated the changes that were taking place in her body.

Flo's mother had emailed me before the appointment to express her deep concern for the change in her daughter. She also worried that her daughter was a very 'early developer' as she already had pubic hair, body odour and breast buds.

Flo had also begun to struggle to get off to sleep for the first time in her life.

Observations: It was obvious from the start that both Flo and her mother were worried and anxious. Flo was very articulate about how she felt. She looked to be a normal weight and height for her age. She was a little pale, and had dark circles under her eyes.

Flo had thin pulses which were wiry in the Wood position. The Water pulses were particularly low.

---

* It is wrong to assume that 'natural' is always good. Tea tree oil and lavender are known to be EDCs, for example.

Although Flo was very open, I sensed an underlying fear in her. She expressed lots of catastrophic fantasies about the future (for example, that she would get her periods before any of her friends, that she and her mum were never going to get on again and that she was not going to be able to 'keep up' at school if she continued feeling like this).

Diagnosis: I diagnosed Flo as having a Water constitutional imbalance (dark around her eyes, groaning voice and 'leaks' of inappropriate fear) with Liver *qi* stagnation and Heart Blood deficiency.

Treatment: Before beginning treatment, I was able to explain to Flo and her mum that the changes that had happened over the past six months were very common for this age and that they did not mean that anything was 'wrong' with Flo or that she was an 'early developer'. I talked a little about the process of puberty and the fact that it may be years before Flo got her first period. I also explained that sometimes whilst the body is changing at a rapid pace, things become easily out of kilter and that acupuncture can help to smooth the process, make it a little easier and ensure that it does not go awry.

My treatments focused on the following:

- Treating Flo's constitutional imbalance in the Water Element (using a range of points on the Kidney and Bladder channels; see Chapter 30). I found that the Kidney chest points (Ki 24–Ki 27) were especially effective for Flo in that they helped her to feel brighter and less anxious.

- I found that, when I strengthened Flo's Water Element, her Wood pulses lost their wiry quality. Treating the mother Element in this way helped the child. I found I did not need to treat Flo's Liver *qi* stagnation directly.

- I also treated Flo's Heart Blood, using points such as Bl 15 *xinshu* and He 7 *shenmen*.

Lifestyle advice: I had a sense that Flo would be finding all of these changes easier if she had a bit of let-up in the rest of her life. She was naturally very driven and loved doing a lot of after-school activities. When I first began treating her, she was almost at the end of her academic year. We talked about her taking time over the summer holidays to reflect on what *really* gave her enjoyment and perhaps not spreading herself so thin when she started school again.

Flo's mum was very keen to know if there was anything she could do to help. Over the telephone, I reassured her further that what Flo was going through was entirely within the realms of normal. I suggested some books that she might want to read to help her understand the changes that Flo was likely to go through over the next few years.* I also explained that the best thing she could do for Flo was to be as relaxed as she could herself, and to give Flo the sense that there was nothing to worry about. Flo's mum shared that she had had a very difficult puberty herself and that she felt she had never really come to terms with some of the issues that had arisen for her. Shortly after I started treating Flo, her mum decided to see a psychotherapist to talk about these issues.

Outcome: I treated Flo on and off for several years. The first changes that became obvious were that she and her mother became less anxious and were able to navigate the changes that were going on within Flo more easily. Both Flo's mother and I felt that the treatment helped Flo to settle into the process of change she was going through and to take it in her stride. At times of stress, some of the original anxiety and irritability that Flo first came with would threaten to return, but a top-up treatment would stop it from taking hold. Flo got her first period when she was almost thirteen.

---

* For example, *Untangled: Guiding Teenage Girls Through the Seven Transitions into Adulthood* by Lisa Damour (2017; London: Atlantic Books).

SUMMARY

» Puberty tends to be a longer and more complicated process than it was a few decades ago.

» Acupuncture can help a child to navigate it more smoothly.

» The Organs that most commonly become imbalanced at puberty are: the Kidneys; the Liver; the Spleen; and the Heart.

» The patterns that most commonly arise in girls during puberty are: Heart and Kidney *yin* deficiency; Liver and Kidney deficiency; Spleen *qi* and Heart Blood deficiency; and Rebellious *qi* in the *chong mai*.

» The patterns that cause early puberty are: Kidney *yin* deficiency with Empty Heat; and Liver *qi* stagnation turning to Heat.

• Chapter 70 •

TREATMENT OF ACUTE CONDITIONS
· · · · · · · · · · · · · · · · · · · ·

The topics discussed in this chapter are:

- Cough

- Asthma attack

- Sore throat

- Acute diarrhoea

- Acute vomiting

- Fever

- Ear infection

- Acute febrile convulsions

Introduction

The following is meant as a quick reference guide to refer to when a child comes to the clinic in an acute episode of an illness. Although some kind of differentiation is needed, the focus should be on easing the acute symptoms. This is not the time to treat the underlying patterns. Once the child is through the acute episode, then the chapter relevant to that particular condition should be referred to so that ongoing treatment may be given.

Reasons to treat through an acute illness

Many people assume that acupuncture is not an appropriate treatment during an acute condition. Whilst it is true there may be times when leaving the house may exacerbate the child's condition, there are good reasons to treat in the acute stage of an illness:

- There is a Chinese saying that a treatment during an acute episode is worth two at any other time. The child's *qi* is 'mobilised' during an acute illness and therefore may more effectively be able to throw off a Lingering Pathogenic Factor than at any other time.

- It may mean the child avoids the need for strong medication.

- It can build confidence for the parent and child to have the experience of getting through an illness unaided by orthodox medicine.

There are some guidelines that apply in the treatment of acute illnesses:

- **Refer on when necessary:** There are times when a child is severely ill, and the first action should be to refer immediately to an orthodox medical professional. In most situations, it is still beneficial to treat the child with acupuncture whilst waiting for medical intervention.

For a list of red flag conditions, please see *The Acupuncturist's Guide to Conventional Medicine* by Clare Stephenson.[55]

- **Don't panic!** It can be alarming to see a small child in the midst of an asthma attack, having a convulsion or drowning in mucus. It is quite likely that the parent will, understandably, be anxious. An important role for the practitioner is to be a voice of calm. A child will pick up on panic and anxiety that she senses in the adults around her and will often then become fearful herself. Fear or panic will make any acute symptom worse. This can hardly be overstated.

- **Improvement should occur whilst the child is having the treatment:** Treating a child through an acute episode of an illness can have miraculous effects. If the treatment is going to work, the practitioner will usually see signs of improvement whilst still with the child. It is different to treating chronic conditions where the improvement may only be noticeable over time.

- **Know your limits:** Whilst there is enormous benefit in treating through an acute episode, if the practitioner does not feel able or confident enough to do it, then it is much better to say so and for the child to get help elsewhere.

Cough

Cough caused by an invasion of an External Pathogenic Factor

The EPF may be Wind-Cold, Wind-Heat or Wind-Dampness. The key sign that signifies the child has an External Pathogenic Factor is that the pulse is floating.

Key points

> Lu 7 *lieque*
> Bl 13 *feishu*
> LI 4 *hegu*
> Ren 17 *shanzhong*

Method: sedation needle technique

Additional techniques

> *Gua sha* on the upper back over the Lungs
> Cupping over Bl 12 *fengmen* or Bl 13 *feishu*
> Moxa on Bl 13 in the case of Wind-Cold

Additional points

If the cough is very Hot, or accompanied by fever:

> Lu 10 *yuji*
> Du 14 *dazhui*

If there is profuse Damp: Sp 9 *yinlingquan*

Cough characterised by huge amounts of mucus

This cough may actually be acute or chronic. The reason it is included in this chapter is because of the necessity to stop the cough as soon as possible. It probably means the child is becoming more and more depleted and nobody in the family is sleeping.

This treatment may need to be repeated several times. For what to do after the worst of the cough is over, please see Chapter 52.

Key points

> Ren 22 *tiantu*
> Ren 17 *shanzhong*
> Lu 7 *lieque*
> Bl 13 *feishu*

Method: sedation needle technique

Additional techniques: *gua sha* on the upper back over the Lungs

Phlegm-Heat cough

This cough will be barking and can be disturbing to listen to. It will *not* be accompanied by a floating pulse or other symptoms of an External Pathogenic Factor. As with the above cough, this may be acute or chronic. It can be severe and disruptive, and therefore it should be stopped as soon as possible.

This treatment may need to be repeated several times. For what to do after the worst of the cough is over, please see Chapter 52.

Key points

> Ren 17 *shanzhong*
> Lu 5 *chize*
> Bl 13 *feishu*

Method: sedation needle technique

Additional techniques: *gua sha* on the upper back over the Lungs

Asthma attack

The priority when treating a child with an asthma attack is to insert needles in the first three points immediately. Once they are in, then it is time to consider the differentiation of the asthma and add in additional points if necessary.

Key points

> *dingchuan* (M-BW-1)
> Bl 13 *feishu*
> Lu 6 *kongzui*

Method: sedation needle technique

Additional points

> Constrained Liver *qi* affecting the Lungs: Pc 6 *neiguan*, Liv 3 *taichong*
> Phlegm: Ren 22 *tiantu*, Ren 17 *shanzhong*
> Heat: Lu 10 *yuji*

Method: sedation needle technique

Sore throat

An acute sore throat is usually caused either by an invasion of Wind-Heat or Lung and Stomach Heat.

Key points

> Lu 10 *yuji*
> Lu 11 *shaoshang*
> LI 4 *hegu*

Method: sedation needle technique

Additional points

> Swollen tonsils: SI 17 *tianrong*
> Wind-Heat: GB 20 *fengchi*
> Internal Heat: LI 11 *quchi*
> Stomach Heat: St 44 *neiting*
> Fever: Du 14 *dazhui*

Method: sedation needle technique

Acute diarrhoea

Acute diarrhoea is usually caused by an invasion of either Cold-Damp or Damp-Heat. There are two key questions to ask to distinguish between these patterns:

- Are the stools smelly? If they are, it indicates Heat. If they aren't, there is no Heat.

- Does the child feel cold or is she slightly feverish? A cold child indicates Cold-Damp, and a feverish child indicates Damp-Heat.

The treatments below are *only* applicable in the first stages of acute diarrhoea. If the child had a sudden attack of diarrhoea and is now left with fatigue and diarrhoea which is less severe, then a different treatment is necessary. Please see Chapter 47 for a discussion of this.

Key points

> St 25 *tianshu*
> St 36 *zusanli*
> Sp 9 *yinlingquan*
> Bl 25 *dachangshu*

Method: sedation needle technique

Additional points

> Cold-Damp: Ren 6 *qihai*
> Damp-Heat: LI 11 *quchi*, St 44 *neiting*

Acute vomiting

A bout of acute vomiting in a child is most often caused by Cold or Heat invading the Stomach. The key distinguishing factor is whether or not the vomit is foul-smelling. If it is, it is a sure sign that Heat is present.

Key points

> St 21 *liangmen*
> St 34 *liangqiu*
> Sp 4 *gongsun*
> Ren 12 *zhongwan*
> Pc 6 *neiguan*

Method: sedation needle technique

Additional points

> Heat: St 44 *neiting*

Fever

Before looking at how to treat fevers, it is worth asking the question of whether a fever should indeed always be treated. A fever which is not particularly agitating the child, which has not been around for more than a day or two and which the child seems to be coping with may be best left. A mild fever may be a transformation and steaming (*bian zheng*) – a physiological leap in the child's development (see Chapter 3).

> **RED FLAGS: FEVER**
> If the parent or practitioner is in any doubt as to whether a child's fever is dangerous, she should immediately seek medical advice. Some of the key danger signs are:
>
> ✓ the fever persists for more than two days
>
> ✓ the fever is very high (more than 39° Celsius)
>
> ✓ the temperature rises very rapidly
>
> ✓ the child develops a purpuric rash
>
> ✓ the child is vomiting
>
> ✓ the child has convulsions

Key points

> Du 14 *dazhui*
> LI 11 *quchi*
> LI 4 *hegu*

Method: sedation needle technique

Additional techniques: cupping or *gua sha* on the upper back

Additional points

> When the fever is due to an External Pathogenic Factor: GB 20 *fengchi*
>
> The child is exhausted and no longer seems to be able to fight the fever: St 36 *zusanli* (tonification needle technique)
>
> When there is panic and nervousness: He 7 *shenmen*
>
> When there is a lot of mucus: Lu 7 *lieque*, Ren 17 *shanzhong*, St 40 *fenglong* (sedation needle technique)

Other ways of helping a fever

- The most effective remedy for any young child to get through a fever is for him to have the almost constant care of a main caregiver (providing that person remains calm).

- Rub vigorously and repeatedly down the *du* channel on the spine, from top to bottom.

- Boil the root of fresh ginger. Once cooled, put the child's feet in the water and then massage the soles of the feet. This will help to draw down the Heat from the head.

- If the child is very hot, putting a bag of frozen peas wrapped in a sock on the child's head will help to keep his brain cool.

- Ensure that the child keeps having a bowel movement, to avoid more Heat building up in the Intestines. This can be done by needling: TB 6 *zhigou*, GB 34 *yanglingquan* and Ren 6 *qihai*. It is also effective to do the abdominal massage described in Chapter 48.

- A young child going through a fever needs to avoid any degree of stimulation: no computers, no television, and so on.

Ear infection

Acute ear infections usually arise quickly and are excruciatingly painful for the child. A pre-verbal child will often hold or rub his ear during an attack, which helpfully tells the parent why he is in so much distress. Broadly speaking, ear infections arise either due to an invasion of an External Pathogenic Factor or from internal Heat.

Invasion of Wind

This can be recognised by the presence of other symptoms and signs of an external invasion, such as a floating pulse, fever and/or aversion to cold.

Key points

> TB 5 *waiguan*
> TB 17 *yifeng*
> GB 20 *fengchi*
> GB 2 *tinghui*
> LI 4 *hegu*

Method: sedation needle technique

Additional points

> If there are many Heat signs: Du 14 *dazhui*
>
> If there is blockage in the ear or pus coming out of the ear: GB 34 *yanglingquan*

Internal Heat in the Liver and Gallbladder

This pattern is more common in older children.

Key points

> TB 5 *waiguan*
> TB 17 *yifeng*
> GB 2 *tinghui*
> GB 41 *zulinqi*
> Liv 2 *xingjian*

Method: sedation needle technique

Acute febrile convulsions

The following protocols for treating acute, strong convulsions are taken from Scott and Barlow.[56] They suggest treating every two hours during acute attacks.

Protocol 1

> LI 4 *hegu*
> Liv 3 *taichong*

Method: sedation needle technique

Protocol 2

> Du 14 *dazhui*
> LI 11 *quchi*
> LI 4 *hegu*

Method: sedation needle technique

Protocol 3

> Pinch Ki 3 *taixi* and Bl 60 *kunlun*

SUMMARY

» If a child arrives at the clinic with a severe and acute illness, the practitioner should first assess whether or not he needs to be referred immediately to an orthodox medical practitioner.

» Keeping calm is essential when treating a child during an acute illness.

» Diagnosis need only focus on alleviating the acute symptoms of the illness. Underlying patterns can be diagnosed and treated after the acute episode.

» There is great value in treating a child through an acute illness. It may be an opportunity to expel an LPF which has caused the child intermittent health problems over a long period of time.

Appendix

Setting up a Paediatric Acupuncture Clinic

· ·

Whilst it is possible, of course, for a practitioner to treat the odd child here and there in between adult patients, some may wish to focus more strongly on creating a paediatric practice. The rhythm of treating children is different to that when treating adults. The practitioner is ideally in a different inner space. For these reasons, it may be desirable to have specific times of the week which are devoted solely to the treatment of children.

1. Decide that you want to treat children

Reading a book about paediatric acupuncture or going to lectures may be a good place to start but at some point it is necessary to actually commit to treating children. Everybody has to start somewhere. It is probably not possible for a practitioner to get to a point when she feels totally ready and prepared, so it is necessary to take a leap of faith and just start at some point.

2. Make space in your week

It is all very well for a practitioner to say that she wants to treat children, but not having any space in her week in which to do it means it will not happen. If someone's practice is full with adult patients, there will be no space to book in children. It may be helpful to leave a half-day of the week free in which children can be booked in when their parents call. School children will need to come after school during term times; pre-schoolers often prefer morning slots as they may sleep in the afternoons.

3. Sort out the logistics

It is important to think about how long appointments will be, and how much sessions will cost. On the one hand, the actual treatment of children will be shorter in time than with adults. On the other hand, everything else can take longer. Children hate to be rushed. The practitioner needs to factor in time for a child to take off and put on clothes, go to the loo, have a snack or a feed, and for the parents to deal with siblings. As a rough guide, at The Panda Clinic the initial slot is one hour. Follow-up sessions are thirty minutes, increasing to forty-five minutes for teenagers.

4. Find the right space

Before treating children, it is important to make sure that the clinic setting is suitable. The main prerequisites are the following:

- A space that is warm and welcoming to children, rather than one that is too clinical and smart that might make a child feel intimidated.

- Evidence of other children will also help a child to feel relaxed. Pictures on the wall that children have drawn are good.

- Toys and books for children to play with or read whilst waiting, or whilst the practitioner is talking to the parent, are essential.

- It is important that children feel they can express themselves rather than having to be hushed. Therefore, it might not be a good idea to work in a clinic where the practitioner in the room next door will be upset if there is a bit of noise.

- The treatment space needs to be big enough to fit in the practitioner, the parent and several children (as siblings may come too).

- It needs to be child-proof. The practitioner needs to make sure that sharps boxes cannot be grabbed, there are no plug holes for babies who are crawling around to put their fingers in and no other hazards.

5. Increase the number of tools in your tool box

As Maslow commented, 'if you only have a hammer, you tend to see every problem as a nail'.[57] As discussed in Chapter 33, it is advisable to be able to treat children with more than just needles. Techniques such as paediatric *tui na* and *shonishin* are relatively easy to learn. You may consider investing in a laser device, which can also be used with adult patients who are apprehensive about needles.

6. Spread the word

Many people assume that acupuncture is not a suitable form of medicine for children. Even those who receive it themselves may simply not have had the thought that it is something their children would either tolerate or benefit from. There are various simple ways a practitioner may spread the word that she can treat children with acupuncture:

- let current patients know

- let other local acupuncturists who may not want to treat children themselves know

- let therapists in other disciplines who work with children know

- create an online presence

- give talks to local groups attended by parents or in schools.

Once the ball has begun rolling, word will spread fast as communities of parents tend to share things they have found helpful.

7. Be prepared to be a beginner again

A practitioner may have decades of experience working with adults but feel that she is a novice when it comes to children. There are many aspects about working with children that are very different to working with adults. Each practitioner must find her own style with children, which may be somewhat different to the one she adopts with adults. She should be prepared to spend more time outside of the treatment room doing research, as children will come with conditions she has no experience of treating.

Some practitioners may find it helpful to find a colleague with some experience of treating children who offers supervision.

8. Anticipate what your challenges will be

The challenges involved in treating children are different to those that arise when treating adults. It can be useful for a practitioner to reflect on what her individual challenges might be and to prepare for them. For example:

- staying focused on the treatment when chaos is going on all around

- responding to the needs of the parents (which may be a desire for a lot of reassurance or for definite answers that cannot really be given) whilst remembering that the child is the patient

- remaining robust in the face of a young child who is severely ill.

9. Perseverance furthers

'Never work with children or animals' is an old show business adage, alluding to their unpredictability (and the fact that they may steal the show). There will be times when a toddler thinks it is fun to spend the entire session trying to run away from you, a baby screams and cries non-stop or a teenager is intensely sullen and monosyllabic. Some children will not respond to treatment. Parents will sometimes insist on their children continuing the behaviours in their lives that you perceive are contributing to their illness. However, these frustrations should not deter the practitioner from continuing to treat children. They should be viewed as part of the rich tapestry of practising and will, in time, be vastly outweighed by the wonder of seeing children who come to the clinic thrive.

10. Connect with your inner child

As George Bernard Shaw is said to have commented, 'We don't stop playing because we grow old; we grow old because we stop playing.'

A child will generally not respond well to an adult who has a heavy, intense air and with whom she cannot have some fun. It will lead her to feel that her weekly appointments are an onerous event. However, if there is a light, jovial and fun atmosphere during her appointments, she will enjoy them and is less likely to think of them as something that is related to the fact that she is ill. If a practitioner fundamentally enjoys working with children, then both the children and parents will respond to this in a positive way.

Conclusion

There are many children in all parts of the world who would benefit hugely from receiving acupuncture. The more practitioners who successfully treat children, the more understanding will grow of what a wonderful form of medicine it is for them. I encourage anyone reading this book to embrace the challenge of treating children and trust that the experience of doing so will be hugely rewarding.

Bibliography

Apley J (1975) *The Child with Abdominal Pains*. London: Blackwell Scientific Publications.

Attwell-Griffiths S, Bovey M (2014) The Purpose of Self-Injury and the Clinical Implications for Acupuncturists. *European Journal of Oriental Medicine*, Volume 7, No. 5.

Attwood T (2008) *The Complete Guide to Asperger's Syndrome*. London: Jessica Kingsley Publishers.

Becker E (1973) *The Denial of Death*. London: Souvenir Press.

Biddulph S (2017) *10 Things Girls Need Most*. London: Thorsons.

Birch S (2011) *Shonishin: Japanese Pediatric Acupuncture*. Stuttgart: Thieme.

Blyth D, Lampert G (2015) *Chinese Dietary Wisdom*. Reading: Nutshell Press.

Brostoff J, Gamlin L (1989) *Food Allergies and Food Intolerance*. Rochester, VT: Healing Arts Press.

Cao J, Su X, Cao J (1990) *Essentials of Traditional Chinese Pediatrics* (trans J Huide). Beijing: Foreign Languages Press.

Cohn A (2007) *Constipation, Withholding and Your Child*. London: Jessica Kingsley Publishers.

Corkille Brigg D (2001) *Your Child's Self-Esteem*. New York: Broadway Books.

Cowan S (2012) *Fire Child, Water Child*. Oakland, CA: New Harbinger.

Cunningham H (2006) *The Invention of Childhood*. London: BBC Books.

Damour L (2017) *Untangled*. London: Atlantic Books.

de Saint-Exupéry A (2009) *The Little Prince*. London: Egmont.

Deadman P (1981) The Causes of Disease (Part One). *Journal of Chinese Medicine*, No. 7.

Deadman P (1981) The Causes of Disease (Part Two). *Journal of Chinese Medicine*, No. 8.

Deadman P (2014) Taijiao (Foetal Education). *Journal of Chinese Medicine*, No. 106.

Deadman P (2016) *Live Well, Live Long*. Hove: JCM Publications.

Deadman P, Al-Khafaji M, Baker K (1998) *A Manual of Acupuncture*. Hove: JCM Publications.

Dechar L (2006) *Five Spirits*. New York: Lantern Books.

Diamant A (2001) *The Red Rent*. London: Macmillan.

Donaldson M (2006) *Children's Minds*. London: Harper Perennial.

Duerk J (2004) *Circle of Stones*. Novato, CA: New World Library.

Enders G (2015) *Gut*. London: Scribe.

Fallon Morell S, Cowan T (2013) *The Nourishing Traditions Book of Baby and Child Care*. Washington, DC: New Trends.

Ferguson S (2015) *Stool Withholding*. London: Macnaughtan Books.

Flaws B (1985) *Turtle Tail and Other Tender Mercies*. Boulder, CO: Blue Poppy Press.

Flaws B (1996) *Keeping Your Child Healthy with Chinese Medicine*. Boulder, CO: Blue Poppy Press.

Flaws B (trans) (2004) *Li Dong-Yuan's Treatise on the Spleen and Stomach*. Boulder, CO: Blue Poppy Press.

Flaws B (2006) *A Handbook of TCM Pediatrics*. Boulder, CO: Blue Poppy Press.

Fromm E (1995) *The Art of Loving*. London: Thorsons.

Gascoigne S (2001) *The Clinical Medicine Guide*. Clonakilty: Jigme Press.

Gerhardt S (2004) *Why Love Matters*. London: Routledge.

Gigante P (2005) Paediatric Developmental Disorders. *The Lantern*, Volume 2, No. 3.

Gill D, O'Brien N (2007) *Paediatric Clinical Examination Made Easy*. Edinburgh: Churchill Livingstone.

Grant L (2003) Treating Young Adults with Acupuncture. *Journal of Chinese Medicine*, No. 73.

Greenspan L, Deardorff J (2014) *The New Puberty*. New York: Rodale.

Haddon M (2004) *The Curious Incident of the Dog in the Night-Time*. London: Vintage.

Hammer L (1990) *Dragon Rises, Red Bird Flies*. New York: Station Press.

Hawthorne N (1986) *The Scarlet Letter*. London: Penguin Books.

Hicks A, Hicks J, Mole P (2011) *Five Element Constitutional Acupuncture*. Edinburgh: Churchill Livingstone.

Higashida N (2013) *The Reason I Jump*. London: Sceptre.

Jarrett L (1998) *Nourishing Destiny*. Stockbridge, MA: Spirit Path Press.

Jarrett L (2003) *The Clinical Practice of Chinese Medicine*. Stockbridge, MA: Spirit Path Press.

Jolly H (1984) *The First Five Years*. London: Pagoda Books.

Kalbantner-Wernicke K, Wray-Fears B (2014) *Children at Their Best*. London: Singing Dragon.

Koo L (1982) *Nourishment of Life*. Kowloon: Commercial Press.

Kreisel V, Weber M (2012) *Laser Acupuncture*. Starnberg: Fuchtenbusch.

Larre C (1994) *The Way of Heaven*. Cambridge: Monkey Press.

Larre C, Rochat de la Vallée E (1995) *Rooted in Spirit*. New York: Station Hill Press.

Larre C, Rochat de la Vallée E (1996) *The Seven Emotions*. Cambridge: Monkey Press.

Larre C, Rochat de la Vallée E (1997) *The Eight Extraordinary Meridians*. Cambridge: Monkey Press.

Larre C, Rochat de la Vallée E (2001) *The Kidneys*. Cambridge: Monkey Press.

Lee A, Lenti R (2006) Treatment of Children in an Acupuncture Setting: A Survey of Clinical Observations. *Journal of Chinese Medicine*, No. 82.

Lister L (2015) *Code Red*. UK: She Press.

Loo M (2002) *Pediatric Acupuncture*. Edinburgh: Churchill Livingstone.

Lyttleton J (2004) *Treatment of Infertility with Chinese Medicine*. Edinburgh: Churchill Livingstone.

Macfarlane A, McPherson A (1996) *The Diary of a Teenage Health Freak*. Oxford: Oxford University Press.

Maciocia G (1998) *Obstetrics and Gynecology in Chinese Medicine*. Edinburgh: Churchill Livingstone.

Maciocia G (2005) *The Foundations of Chinese Medicine*. Edinburgh: Churchill Livingstone.

Maciocia G (2008) *The Practice of Chinese Medicine*. Edinburgh: Churchill Livingstone.

Maciocia G (2009) *The Psyche in Chinese Medicine*. Edinburgh: Churchill Livingstone.

Majebe M (2001) Chinese Medicine and Autism. *Journal of Chinese Medicine*, No. 66.

Miller A (1987) *The Drama of Being a Child*. London: Virago.

Miller N (2015) *Vaccine Safety Manual*. Sante Fe, NM: New Atlantean Press.

Milner J, Bateman J (2011) *Working with Children and Teenagers Using Solution Focused Approaches*. London: Jessica Kingsley Publishers.

Mole P (2007) *Acupuncture for Body, Mind and Spirit*. Oxford: How To Books.

Neustaedter R (2002) *The Vaccine Guide*. Berkeley, CA: North Atlantic Books.

Neustaedter R (2005) *Child Health Guide*. Berkeley, CA: North Atlantic Books.

Nielsen A (1995) *Gua Sha*. Edinburgh: Churchill Livingstone.

Northrup C (1998) *Women's Bodies, Women's Wisdom*. London: Piatkus.

Nuland S (1998) *How We Live*. London: Vintage.

O'Sullivan S (2016) *It's All in Your Head*. London: Vintage.

Odent M (2002) *Primal Health*. Forest Row: Clairview Books.

Pledger J (2014) A Feasibility Study of Acupuncture for the Treatment of Children with Autism Spectrum Disorder. *European Journal of Oriental Medicine*, Volume 7, No. 5.

Po-Tuan C (1986) *The Inner Teachings of Taoism*. Boston, MA: Shambhala.

Requena Y (1989) *Character and Health*. Brookline, MA: Paradigm.

Richardson N (2012) The Nation in Utero: Translating the Science of Fetal Education in Republican China. *Frontiers of History in China*, Volume 7, No. 1.

Rochat de la Vallée E (2007) *The Essential Woman*. Cambridge: Monkey Press.

Rochat de la Vallée E (2009) *Wu Xing*. Cambridge: Monkey Press.

Rossi E (2011) *Pediatrics in Chinese Medicine*. Barnet: Donica.

Scott J (1993) Accumulation Disorder. *Journal of Chinese Medicine*, No. 42.

Scott J (2009) Teenage Depression and Acupuncture. *Journal of Chinese Medicine*, No. 90.

Scott J, Barlow T (1999) *Acupuncture in the Treatment of Children*. Seattle, WA: Eastland Press.

Skynner R, Cleese J (1997) *Families and How to Survive Them*. London: Vermilion.

Slingerland E (2014) *Trying Not to Try*. Edinburgh: Canongate.

Smith J (2012) *The Parent's Guide to Self-Harm*. Oxford: Lion.

Solomon A (2014) *Far from the Tree*. London: Vintage.

Stephenson C (2017) *The Acupuncturist's Guide to Conventional Medicine*. London: Singing Dragon.

Stock Kranowitz C (2005) *The Out-of-Sync Child*. New York: Perigree.

Storr A (1968) *Human Aggression*. London: The Penguin Press.

Tolstoy L (1978) *Anna Karenina*. London: Penguin Classics.

Tsabary S (2010) *The Conscious Parent*. Vancouver: Namaste Publishing.

Walker S (2012) *Responding to Self-Harm in Children and Adolescents*. London: Jessica Kingsley Publishers.

Weiger L (1965) *Chinese Characters.* New York: Dover Publications.

Wernicke T (2014) *Shonishin.* London: Singing Dragon.

Wilks J (ed) (2017) *An Integrative Approach to Treating Babies and Children.* London: Singing Dragon.

Wilms S (2005) The Transmission of Medical Knowledge on 'Nurturing the Fetus' in Early China. *Asian Medicine: Tradition and Modernity,* Volume 1, No. 2.

Wilms S (trans) (2013) *Venerating the Root: Part 1.* Sun Simiao's *Bei Ji Qian Jin Yao Fang,* Volume 5. Corbett, OR: Happy Goat Publications.

Wilms S (trans) (2015) *Venerating the Root: Part 2.* Sun Simiao's *Bei Ji Qian Jin Yao Fang,* Volume 5. Corbett, OR: Happy Goat Publications.

Wilson B (2015) *First Bite.* London: Fourth Estate.

Winnicott D (2006) *The Family and Individual Development.* Abingdon: Routledge.

Xin-ming S (1986) The Treatment of Epilepsy by Acupuncture. *Journal of Chinese Medicine,* No. 20.

Ya-li F (1994) *Chinese Pediatric Massage Therapy.* Boulder, CO: Blue Poppy Press.

Yousheng L (2014) *Let the Radiant Yang Shine Forth.* Corbett, OR: Happy Goat Publications.

Zand J, Rountree R, Walton R (1994) *Smart Medicine for a Healthier Child.* New York: Avery.

Endnotes

·············

Part 1

1. Jung C (2014) *Modern Man in Search of a Soul*. Abingdon: Routledge Classics, p.62.
2. Quoted in Flaws B (2006) *A Handbook of TCM Paediatrics*. Boulder, CO: Blue Poppy Press, p.7.
3. Ibid.
4. Skynner R and Cleese J (1997) *Families and How to Survive Them*. London: Vermilion, pp.75–76.
5. Chen Wen Zhong (1241 CE) *A Treatise on Pediatric Etiology* (*Xiao Er Bing Yuan Fang Lun*). Quoted in lecture notes: Gigante P (2016) Clinical Applications of the Art of Nurturing the Young (County Dublin, 14 May).
6. Strachan D (1989) Hay Fever, Hygiene and Household Size. *British Medical Journal* Vol 299, No. 6710, pp.1259–1260. Retrieved from: www.ncbi.nlm.nih.gov/pmc/articles/PMC1838109 (September 2017).
7. Flaws B (2006) *A Handbook of TCM Pediatrics*. Boulder, CO: Blue Poppy Press, p.7.
8. Wilms S (2013) *Venerating the Root, Part 1*. Sun Simiao's *Bei Ji Qian Jin Yao Fang*, Volume 5: Paediatrics. Corbett, OR: Happy Goat Productions, p.123.
9. Ibid.
10. Skynner R and Cleese J (1997) *Families and How to Survive Them*. London: Vermilion, p.76.
11. Quoted in Birch S (2011) *Shonishin: Japanese Pediatric Acupuncture*. Stuttgart: Thieme, p.10.
12. Ibid., p.11.
13. Wilms S (2013) *Venerating the Root, Part 1*. Sun Simiao's *Bei Ji Qian Jin Yao Fang*, Volume 5: Paediatrics. Corbett, OR: Happy Goat Productions, p.15.
14. Ibid.
15. Enders G (2015) *Gut: The Inside Story of Our Body's Most Under-Rated Organ*. London: Scribe, pp.26–27.
16. Skynner R and Cleese J (1997) *Families and How to Survive Them*. London: Vermilion, p.274.
17. Nuffield Trust and Health Foundation (2017) How Does the Overall UK Infant Mortality Rate Compare to Individual UK Countries? Retrieved from: www.qualitywatch.org.uk/indicator/infant-mortality (August 2017).
18. Lu H (1972) *A Complete Translation of the Yellow Emperor's Classic of Internal Medicine (Nei Jing and Nan Jing)*. Vancouver: Academy of Oriental Heritage.
19. Yousheng L (translated by Zuozhi L and Wilms S 2014) *Let the Radiant Yang Shine Forth: Lectures on Virtue*. Corbett, OR: Happy Goat Productions, p.143.
20. Yang Shou-zhong and Duan Wujin (1994) *Extra Treatises Based on Investigation and Inquiry: A Translation of Zhu Dan-xi's Ge Zhe Yu Lun*. Boulder, CO: Blue Poppy Press, p.24.
21. Ibid., p.98.
22. Ibid., p.99.
23. Quoted in Deadman P (2014) Taijiao (Foetal Education). *Journal of Chinese Medicine*, No. 106, p.49.
24. Unschuld P (2011) *Huang Di Nei Jing Su Wen*. Berkeley, CA: University of California Press, p.47.
25. Gigante P (2005) Paediatric Developmental Disorders. *The Lantern* Vol 2, No. 3, p.15.
26. Quoted in Deadman P (2014) Taijiao (Foetal Education). *Journal of Chinese Medicine*, No. 106, p.49.
27. O'Connor T et al. (2013) Practitioner Review: Maternal Mood in Pregnancy and Child Development – Implications for Child Psychology and Psychiatry. *Journal of Child Psychology and Psychiatry* Vol 55, No. 2, pp.99–111.
28. Deadman P (2014) Taijiao (Foetal Education). *Journal of Chinese Medicine*, No. 106, p.51, quoting Sun Simiao.
29. Yousheng L (translated by Zuozhi L and Wilms S 2014) *Let the Radiant Yang Shine Forth: Lectures on Virtue*. Corbett, OR: Happy Goat Productions, p.176.
30. Skynner R and Cleese J (1997) *Families and How to Survive Them*. London: Vermilion, p.95.
31. Wordsworth W (1802) *Intimations of Immortality from Recollections of Early Childhood*.
32. Scott J and Barlow T (1999) *Acupuncture in the Treatment of Children*. Seattle: Eastland Press, p.12.
33. Ibid., p.328.
34. Veith I (1972) *The Yellow Emperor's Classic of Internal Medicine*. Berkeley, CA: University of California Press, p.117.
35. Larre C and Rochat de la Vallée E (1986) *Survey of Traditional Chinese Medicine*. Paris: Institut Ricci.
36. Quoted in Hicks A, Hicks J and Mole P (2011) *Five Element Constitutional Acupuncture*. London: Churchill Livingstone.
37. Ibid., p.113.
38. Ibid., p.130.
39. Ibid., p.159.
40. Ibid., p.145.

41. Ibid., p.90.
42. Weiger Dr L (1965) *Chinese Characters: Their Origin, Etymology, History, Classification and Signification*. New York: Dover Publications.
43. Larre C and Rochat de la Vallée E (1996) *The Seven Emotions: Psychology and Health in Ancient China*. Cambridge: Monkey Press, p.66.
44. Larre C and Rochat de la Vallée E (1995) *Rooted in Spirit*. New York: Station Hill Press, p.127.
45. Ibid., p.170.
46. Fromm E (1995) *The Art of Loving*. London: Thorsons, p.39.
47. Hawthorne N (1986) *The Scarlet Letter*. London: Penguin Classics, p.96.
48. Wilms S (2013) *Venerating the Root, Part 1*. Sun Simiao's *Bei Ji Qian Jin Yao Fang*, Volume 5: Paediatrics. Corbett, OR: Happy Goat Productions, p.83.
49. Skynner R and Cleese J (1997) *Families and How to Survive Them*. London: Vermilion, p.31.
50. Hawthorne N (1986) *The Scarlet Letter*. London: Penguin Classics, p.243.
51. Brummelman E et al. (2013) *My Child Redeems My Broken Dreams: On Parents Transferring Their Unfulfilled Ambitions onto Their Child*. University of Utrecht. Retrieved from: http://journals.plos.org/plosone/article?id=10.1371/journal. pone.0065360 (September 2017).
52. Storr A (1968) *Human Aggression*. London: The Penguin Press, p.45.
53. Ibid., p.44.
54. Solomon A (2014) *Far from the Tree: Parents, Children and the Search for Identity*. London: Vintage, p.2.
55. Skynner R and Cleese J (1997) *Families and How to Survive Them*. London: Vermilion, p.105.
56. Wilms S (2013) *Venerating the Root, Part 1*. Sun Simiao's *Bei Ji Qian Jin Yao Fang*, Volume 5: Paediatrics. Corbett, OR: Happy Goat Productions, p.235.
57. Ibid., p.259.
58. Barr C (2016) Who are Generation Z? The Latest Data on Today's Teens. *The Guardian*, 10 December. Retrieved from: www.theguardian.com/lifeandstyle/2016/dec/10/generation-z-latest-data-teens (December 2017).
59. Quoted in Flaws B (2006) *A Handbook of TCM Pediatrics*. Boulder, CO: Blue Poppy Press, p.8.
60. Enders G (2015) *Gut: The Inside Story of Our Body's Most Under-Rated Organ*. London: Scribe Publications, p.127.
61. Wilms S (2013) *Venerating the Root, Part 1*. Sun Simiao's *Bei Ji Qian Jin Yao Fang*, Volume 5: Paediatrics. Corbett, OR: Happy Goat Productions, p.81.
62. Yousheng L (translated by Zuozhi L and Wilms S 2014) *Let the Radiant Yang Shine Forth: Lectures on Virtue*. Corbett, OR: Happy Goat Productions, p.184.
63. Ibid., p.180.
64. Veith I (1972) *The Yellow Emperor's Classic of Internal Medicine*. Berkeley, CA: University of California Press, p.206.
65. McGrath K (n.d.) *The Good-Night Guide for Children*. Skipton: The Sleep Council. Retrieved from: https://search3. openobjects.com/mediamanager/coventry/fsd/files/the_good_night_guide_for_children.pdf (August 2017).
66. Retrieved from: https://sleepfoundation.org/sleep-topics/teens-and-sleep (August 2017).
67. Quoted in Deadman P (2016) *Live Well Live Long: Teachings from the Chinese Nourishment of Life Tradition*. Hove: JCM Publications, p.191.
68. Hammer L (1990) *Dragon Rises, Red Bird Flies: Psychology and Chinese Medicine*. New York: Station Hill Press, p.337.
69. Maciocia G (1998) *Obstetrics and Gynecology in Chinese Medicine*. London: Churchill Livingstone, p.63.
70. Hammer L (1990) *Dragon Rises, Red Bird Flies: Psychology and Chinese Medicine*. New York: Station Hill Press, p.338.
71. Deadman P (2016) *Live Well Live Long: Teachings from the Chinese Nourishment of Life Tradition*. Hove: JCM Publications, p.240.
72. Quoted in Maciocia G (1998) *Obstetrics and Gynecology in Chinese Medicine*. London: Churchill Livingstone, p.64.
73. Quoted in Deadman P (2016) *Live Well Live Long: Teachings from the Chinese Nourishment of Life Tradition*. Hove: JCM Publications, p.243.
74. Stephenson C (2017) *The Acupuncturist's Guide to Conventional Medicine*. London: Singing Dragon, p.77.
75. Ibid., p.116.
76. Maciocia G (2015) *The Foundations of Chinese Medicine*. Edinburgh: Churchill Livingstone, p.623.
77. Stephenson C (2017) *The Acupuncturist's Guide to Conventional Medicine*. London: Singing Dragon, p.627.
78. Ibid., p.627.
79. Ibid., p.636.
80. Hiller-Sturmhöfel S and Swartzwelder HS (2004/2005) Alcohol's Effect on the Adolescent Brain. *Alcohol Research and Health* Vol 28, No. 4. Retrieved from: https://pubs.niaaa.nih.gov/publications/arh284/213-221.htm (September 2017).
81. California Society of Addiction Medicine (2009) Impact of Marijuana on Children and Adolescents. Retrieved from: http://csam-asam.org/sites/default/files/impact_of_marijuana_on_children_and_adolescents.pdf (December 2017).
82. Wilms S (2013) *Venerating the Root, Part 1*. Sun Simiao's *Bei Ji Qian Jin Yao Fang*, Volume 5: Paediatrics. Corbett, OR: Happy Goat Productions, p.61.
83. Wilms S (2015) *Venerating the Root, Part 2*. Sun Simiao's *Bei Ji Qian Jin Yao Fang*, Volume 5: Paediatrics. Corbett, OR: Happy Goat Productions, p.3.

84. Wilms S (2013) *Venerating the Root, Part 1*. Sun Simiao's *Bei Ji Qian Jin Yao Fang*, Volume 5: Paediatrics. Corbett, OR: Happy Goat Productions, p.241.

85. Gersanhik O (2007) Trauma and Parkinson's Disease. *Handbook of Clinical Neurology* Vol 84, pp.487–499.

Part 2

1. Gide A (1959 [1903]) *Pretexts: Reflections on Literature and Morality*. London: Secker and Warburg.

2. Quoted in Solomon A (2016) *The Noonday Demon*. London: Vintage, p.328.

3. Quoted in Slingerland E (2015) *Trying Not to Try: The Art of Effortlessness and the Power of Spontaneity*. London: Canongate Books, p.144.

4. De Saint-Exupéry A (2009) *The Little Prince*. London: Egmont.

5. Scott J and Barlow T (1999) *Acupuncture in the Treatment of Children*. Seattle, WA: Eastland Press, p.60.

6. Ibid., p.73; Rossi E (2011) *Paediatrics in Chinese Medicine*. Barnet: Donica, p.34.

7. Stephenson C (2017) *The Acupuncturist's Guide to Conventional Medicine*. London: Singing Dragon, p.571 (original work published 2011).

8. Maciocia G (2004) *Diagnosis in Chinese Medicine*. Amsterdam: Elsevier, p.544.

9. Quoted in Gigante P (2016) Clinical Application of the Art of Nurturing the Young (Course notes; County Dublin, 14 May).

10. Wilms S (2013) *Venerating the Root, Part 1*. Sun Simiao's *Bei Ji Qian Jin Yao Fang*, Volume 5: Paediatrics. Corbett, OR: Happy Goat Productions, p.21.

11. Quoted in Unschuld P (1990) *Forgotten Traditions of Ancient Chinese Medicine*. Brookline, MA: Paradigm Publications, p.17.

12. Veith I (1972) *The Yellow Emperor's Classic of Internal Medicine*. Berkeley, CA: University of California Press, p.117.

13. Larre C and Rochat de la Vallée E (1986) *Survey of Traditional Chinese Medicine*. Paris: Institut Ricci, p.64.

14. Soulie de Morant G (1994) *Chinese Acupuncture*. Brookline, MA: Paradigm Publications, p.6.

15. Birch S (2011) *Shonishin: Japanese Pediatric Acupuncture*. Stuttgart: Thieme, p.23.

16. Scott J and Barlow T (1999) *Acupuncture in the Treatment of Children*. Seattle, WA: Eastland Press, p.87.

17. Quoted in Unschuld P (1992) *Medicine in China: A History of Ideas*. Brookline, MA: Paradigm Publications, p.283.

18. Veith I (1972) *The Yellow Emperor's Classic of Internal Medicine*. Berkeley, CA: University of California Press, p.215.

19. Hicks A, Hicks J and Mole P (2011) *Five Element Constitutional Acupuncture*. London: Churchill Livingstone, pp.202–207.

20. Larre C and Rochat de la Vallée E (1996) *The Seven Emotions*. Cambridge: Monkey Press, p.170.

21. Dahl R (1977) *Danny the Champion of the World*. London: Puffin, p.9.

22. Larre C and Rochat de la Vallée E (2004) *Spleen and Stomach*. Cambridge: Monkey Press, p.20.

23. Fromm E (1995) *The Art of Loving*. London: Thorsons, p.40.

24. Winnicott D (2006) *The Family and Individual Development*. Abingdon: Routledge, p.42.

25. Quoted by Hirsch A (2014) Maya Angelou Appreciation. *The Observer*. Retrieved from: https://www.theguardian.com/books/2014/jun/01/maya-angelou-appreciation-afua-hirsch. (April 2018).

26. Larre C and Rochat de la Vallée, E (1996) *The Seven Emotions*. Cambridge: Monkey Press, p.159.

27. Maciocia G (2008) *The Practice of Chinese Medicine*. London: Churchill Livingstone, pp.272–273.

28. Becker E (2011) *The Denial of Death*. London: Souvenir Press, p.13.

29. Nesbit E (1993) *The Railway Children*. Ware: Wordsworth Editions.

30. Fromm E (1995) *The Art of Loving*. London: Thorsons, p.34.

31. Larre C and Rochat de la Vallée E (1992) *The Secret Treatise of the Spiritual Orchid*. Cambridge: Monkey Press, p.54.

32. Gerhardt S (2004) *Why Love Matters: How Affection Shapes a Baby's Brain*. Hove: Routledge, p.70.

33. Fromm E (1995) *The Art of Loving*. London: Thorsons, p.44.

34. Solomon A (2014) *Far From the Tree: Parents, Children and the Search for Identity*. London: Vintage, p.404.

35. Szasz T (1973) *The Second Sin*. London: Routledge & Kegan Paul.

36. Dahl R (2013) *Charlie and the Chocolate Factory*. Puffin: London.

37. Larre C and Rochat de la Vallée E (1996) *The Seven Emotions*. Cambridge: Monkey Press, p.170.

38. Dechar L (2006) *Five Spirits: Alchemical Acupuncture for Psychological and Spiritual Healing*. New York: Lantern Books, p.174.

39. Maciocia G (2005) *The Foundation of Chinese Medicine*. London: Churchill Livingstone, Chapter 32.

40. Veith I (trans) (1966) *Huang Ti Nei Ching Su Wen* (*The Yellow Emperor's Classic of Internal Medicine*). University of California Press: Los Angeles.

41. Quoted in Maciocia G (2005) *The Foundations of Chinese Medicine*. London: Churchill Livingstone, p.488.

42. Quoted in Maciocia G (2005) *The Foundations of Chinese Medicine*. London: Churchill Livingstone, p.165.

43. Maciocia G (2005) *The Foundations of Chinese Medicine*. London: Churchill Livingstone, p.147.

44. Maciocia G (2005) *The Foundation of Chinese Medicine*. London: Churchill Livingstone, Chapter 33.

45. Flaws B (2006) *A Handbook of TCM Paediatrics*. Boulder, CO: Blue Poppy Press, p.8.

46. Wilms S (2015) *Venerating the Root, Part Two: Sun Simiao's Bei Ji Qian Jin Yao Fang, Volume 5: Pediatrics*. Corbett, OR: Happy Goat Productions, p.3.

47. Maciocia G (2008) *The Practice of Chinese Medicine*. Edinburgh: Churchill Livingstone, p.265.

48. Maciocia G (2005) *The Foundation of Chinese Medicine*. London: Churchill Livingstone, Chapter 34.
49. Scott J and Barlow T (1991) *Acupuncture in the Treatment of Children*. Seattle: Eastland Press, p.42.
50. Quoted in Maciocia G (2005) *The Foundations of Chinese Medicine*. London: Churchill Livingstone, p.158.
51. Larre C and Rochat de la Vallée E (1989) *The Kidneys*. Cambridge: Monkey Press, p.40.
52. Larre C and Rochat de la Vallée E (1989) *The Kidneys*. Cambridge: Monkey Press, p.73.
53. Maciocia G (2005) *The Foundation of Chinese Medicine*. London: Churchill Livingstone, Chapter 34.
54. Flaws B (2006) *A Handbook of TCM Pediatrics*. Boulder, CO: Blue Poppy Press, p.9.
55. Maciocia G (2005) *The Foundation of Chinese Medicine*. London: Churchill Livingstone, Chapter 35.
56. Flaws B (1985) *Turtle Tail and Other Tender Mercies: Traditional Chinese Pediatrics*.
57. Larre C and Rochat de la Vallée E (1992) *The Secret Treatise of the Spiritual Orchid*. Cambridge: Monkey Press, p.129.
58. Matsumoto K and Birch S (1993) *Five Elements and Ten Stems*. Brookline, MA: Paradigm Publications.
59. Maciocia G (2005) *The Foundations of Chinese Medicine*. London: Churchill Livingstone, p.207.
60. Ibid., p.665.

Part 3

1. Quoted in Unschuld P (1990) *Forgotten Traditions of Ancient Chinese Medicine*. Brookline, MA: Paradigm Publications, p.17.
2. Veith I (1972) *The Yellow Emperor's Classic of Internal Medicine*. Berkeley, CA: University of California Press, p.215.
3. Quoted in Larre C and Rochat de la Vallée E (1995) *Rooted in Spirit*. New York: Station Hill Press, p.33.
4. Apley J (1975) *The Child with Abdominal Pains*. London: Blackwell Scientific Publications, p.13.
5. Ibid., p.67.
6. Quoted in Scheid V and Bensky D (2006) Medicine as Signification – Moving Towards Healing Power in the Chinese Medical Tradition. *European Journal of Oriental Medicine* Vol 2, No. 6, p.35.
7. Sunu K (1985) *The Canon of Acupuncture*. Los Angeles, CA: Yuin University Press.
8. Quoted in Unschuld P (1992) *Medicine in China: A History of Ideas*. Berkeley, CA: University of California Press, p.337.
9. Hicks A, Hicks J and Mole P (2011) *Five Element Constitutional Acupuncture*. Edinburgh: Churchill Livingstone, p.248.
10. I developed this idea from one suggested by David Allan in an online seminar called 'Spotlight on Children's Health' which is available on ProD Seminars (www.prodseminars.net).
11. Scott J and Barlow T (1999) *Acupuncture in the Treatment of Children*. Seattle, WA: Eastland Press, p.85.
12. Birch S (2011) *Shonishin: Japanese Pediatric Acupuncture*. Stuttgart: Thieme, p.74.
13. The location of this point is described differently in various texts. I use the description given in Birch S (2011) *Shonishin: Japanese Paediatric Acupuncture*. Stuttgart: Thieme.
14. Ibid., p.88.
15. Ibid., p.46.
16. Deadman P, Al-Khafaji M and Baker K (1998) *A Manual of Acupuncture*. Brighton: Journal of Chinese Medicine Publications, p.543.
17. Birch S (2011) *Shonishin: Japanese Pediatric Acupuncture*. Stuttgart: Thieme, p.81.
18. Scott J (2012) Diploma in Paediatric Acupuncture course notes, College of Integrated Chinese Medicine, Reading.
19. Kreisel V and Weber M (2012) *A Practical Handbook of Laser Acupuncture*. Starnberg: Füchtenbusch, p.65.
20. Nielsen's book *Gua Sha – A Traditional Technique for Modern Practice* (1995; Edinburgh: Churchill Livingstone) contains a page that may be given to parents explaining *gua sha*. This may also be shown to any medical practitioner the child comes into contact with who may otherwise be concerned about the appearance of the *sha*.
21. Flaws B (1985) *Turtle Tail and Other Tender Mercies*. Boulder, CO: Blue Poppy Press, p.20.
22. Ya-li F (1994) *Chinese Pediatric Massage Therapy*. Boulder, CO: Blue Poppy Press, p.7.
23. Birch S (2011) *Shonishin: Japanese Pediatric Acupuncture*. Stuttgart: Thieme, p.3.
24. Ibid., p.13.
25. Birch S (2014) Workshop on *Shonishin*. London, March.
26. Wernicke T (2014) *Shonishin: The Art of Non-Invasive Paediatric Acupuncture*. London: Singing Dragon.
27. Birch S (2011) *Shonishin: Japanese Pediatric Acupuncture*. Stuttgart: Thieme, p.4.
28. Wernicke T (2014) *Shonishin: The Art of Non-Invasive Paediatric Acupuncture*. London: Singing Dragon, p.68.
29. Ibid., p.69.
30. Birch S (2011) *Shonishin: Japanese Pediatric Acupuncture*. Stuttgart: Thieme, p.45.
31. Ibid., p.45.
32. Ibid., p.46.
33. Deadman P, Al-Khafaji M and Baker K (1998) *A Manual of Acupuncture*. Hove: Journal of Chinese Medicine Publications, p.543.
34. Birch S (2011) *Shonishin: Japanese Pediatric Acupuncture*. Stuttgart: Thieme, p.52.

Part 4

1. American Psychiatric Association (2000) *Diagnostic and Statistical Manual of Mental Disorders: DSM-IV-TR*. Washington, DC: American Psychiatric Association.

2. Hicks A, Hicks J and Mole P (2011) *Five Element Constitutional Acupuncture*. Edinburgh: Churchill Livingstone, p.117.
3. Solomon A (2014) *Far from the Tree: Parents, Children and the Search for Identity*. London: Vintage, p.280.
4. Pledger J (2014) A Feasibility Study of Acupuncture for the Treatment of Children with Autism Spectrum Disorder. *European Journal of Oriental Medicine* Vol 7, No. 5, p.29.
5. Flaws B (2006) *A Handbook of TCM Pediatrics*. Boulder, CO: Blue Poppy Press, p.11.
6. Barron J and Barron S (1992) *There's a Boy in Here*. New York: Simon and Schuster, p.96.
7. Dechar L (2006) *Five Spirits: Alchemical Acupuncture for Psychological and Spiritual Healing*. New York: Lantern Books, p.175.
8. Hicks A, Hicks J and Mole P (2011) *Five Element Constitutional Acupuncture*. Edinburgh: Churchill Livingstone, p.92.
9. Attwood T (2007) *The Complete Guide to Asperger's Syndrome*. London: Jessica Kingsley Publishers, p.99.
10. Baron-Cohen S (1997) *Mindblindness: An Essay on Autism and Theory of Mind*. Denver, CO: Bradford Books.
11. Dechar L (2006) *Five Spirits: Alchemical Acupuncture for Psychological and Spiritual Healing*. New York: Lantern Books, p.240.
12. Haddon M (2003) *The Curious Incident of the Dog in the Night-Time*. London: Vintage, p.2.
13. Quoted in Solomon A (2014) *Far from the Tree: Parents, Children and the Search for Identity*. London: Vintage, p.272.
14. Maciocia G (2008) *The Practice of Chinese Medicine*. Edinburgh: Churchill Livingstone, pp.387–388.
15. Kim-Cohen J, Caspi A, Moffitt TE et al. (2003) Prior Juvenile Diagnoses in Adults with Mental Disorder. *Archives of General Psychiatry* Vol 60, pp.709–717.
16. Lu H (1972) *A Complete Translation of the Yellow Emperor's Classic of Internal Medicine (Nei Jing and Nan Jing)*. Vancouver: Academy of Oriental Heritage, Chapter 42.
17. Veith I (1972) *The Yellow Emperor's Classic of Internal Medicine*. Berkeley, CA: University of California Press, p.117.
18. Larre C and Rochat de la Vallée E (1992) *The Secret Treatise of the Spiritual Orchid*. Cambridge: Monkey Press, p.33.
19. Nicholls DE, Lynn R and Viner RM (2017) Childhood Eating Disorders: British National Surveillance Study. *British Journal of Psychiatry* Vol 198, No. 4, pp.295–301. Retrieved from: http://bjp.rcpsych.org/content/198/4/295 (September 2017).
20. Freeman H (2016) Don't Blame the Wellness Fad for Anorexia. *Guardian Magazine*, 11 June. Retrieved from: www.theguardian.com/commentisfree/2016/jun/11/hadley-freeman-dont-blame-the-wellness-fad-for-anorexia (September 2017).
21. Ibid.
22. Dechar L (2006) *Five Spirits: Alchemical Acupuncture for Psychological and Spiritual Healing*. New York: Lantern Books, p.250.
23. Doyle L, Treacy MP and Sheridan A (2015) Self-Harm in Young People: Prevalence, Associated Factors, and Help-Seeking in School-Going Adolescents. *International Journal of Mental Health Nursing* Vol 24, No. 6, pp.485–495.
24. Mental Health Foundation (2017) The Truth about Self-Harm. Retrieved from: www.mentalhealth.org.uk/publications/truth-about-self-harm (September 2017).
25. Attwell-Griffiths S and Bovey M (2014) The Purpose of Self-Injury and Clinical Implications for Acupuncturists. *European Journal of Oriental Medicine* Vol. 7, No. 5, pp.42–47.
26. Information taken from the Children's Sleep Clinic at http://millpondsleepclinic.com (September 2017).
27. Birch S (2011) *Shonishin: Japanese Pediatric Acupuncture*. Stuttgart: Thieme, p.157.

Part 5

1. Scott J (2012) Diploma in Paediatric Acupuncture course notes, College of Integrated Chinese Medicine, Reading; Scott J and Barlow T (1999) *Acupuncture in the Treatment of Children*. Seattle, WA: Eastland Press; Flaws B (2006) *A Handbook of TCM Pediatrics*. Boulder, Co: Blue Poppy Press.
2. Ya-li F (1994) *Chinese Pediatric Massage Therapy*. Boulder, CO: Blue Poppy Press; Rossi E (2011) *Pediatrics in Chinese Medicine*. Barnet: Donica.
3. Birch S (2011) *Shonishin: Japanese Pediatric Acupuncture*. Stuttgart: Thieme.
4. Wilson B (2015) *First Bite: How We Learn to Eat*. London: Fourth Estate, p.17.
5. Quoted in Apley J (1975) *The Child with Abdominal Pains*. Oxford: Blackwell Scientific Publications, p.89.
6. Birch S (2011) *Shonishin: Japanese Pediatric Acupuncture*. Stuttgart: Thieme, p.207.
7. Public Health England (2013) *Breakfast and Cognition: Review of the Literature*. London: Public Health England. Retrieved from: www.gov.uk/government/uploads/system/uploads/attachment_data/file/256398/Breakfast_and_cognition_review_FINAL_publication_formatted.pdf (September 2017).
8. Birch S (2011) *Shonishin: Japanese Pediatric Acupuncture*. Stuttgart: Thieme, p.141.
9. Ibid., p.135.
10. Maciocia G (2004) *Diagnosis in Chinese Medicine*. Edinburgh: Churchill Livingstone, p.705.
11. Birch S (2011) *Shonishin: Japanese Pediatric Acupuncture*. Stuttgart: Thieme, p.88.
12. For example, Shetreat-Klein M (2016) *Healthy Food, Healthy Gut, Happy Child*. St Louis, MO: Bluebird.
13. Sunu K (1985) *The Canon of Acupuncture*. Los Angeles, CA: Yuin University Press.
14. O'Sullivan S (2016) *It's All in Your Head*. London: Vintage, p.237.
15. Maciocia G (1989) *The Foundations of Chinese Medicine*. Edinburgh: Churchill Livingstone, p.139.
16. Birch S (2011) *Shonishin: Japanese Paediatric Acupuncture*. Stuttgart: Thieme, p.89.

17. Birch S (2011) *Shonishin: Japanese Pediatric Acupuncture.* Stuttgart: Thieme, p.88.
18. Ibid.
19. BBC News (2005, 30 August) How Emotions Spark Asthma. Retrieved from: http://news.bbc.co.uk/1/hi/health/4196478.stm (September 2017).
20. O'Farrell M (2016) 'I Have Three Seconds Before She Draws Blood': Life with Extreme Eczema. *Guardian Magazine,* 21 May. Retrieved from: www.theguardian.com/society/2016/may/21/life-with-extreme-eczema-maggie-ofarrell (January 2018).
21. For example, Scott J and Barlow T (1999) *Acupuncture in the Treatment of Children.* Seattle, WA: Eastland Press, p.353; Rossi E (2011) *Pediatrics in Chinese Medicine.* Barnet: Donica, p.187.
22. O'Farrell M (2016) 'I Have Three Seconds Before She Draws Blood': Life with Extreme Eczema. *Guardian Magazine,* 21 May. Retrieved from: www.theguardian.com/society/2016/may/21/life-with-extreme-eczema-maggie-ofarrell (January 2018).
23. Maciocia G (2008) *The Practice of Chinese Medicine.* Edinburgh: Churchill Livingstone, pp.130–135.
24. Scott J and Barlow T (1999) *Acupuncture in the Treatment of Children.* Seattle, WA: Eastland Press, p.345.
25. Maciocia G (2017) The Pathology and Treatment of Atopic Eczema. Online webinar, Chinese Medicine Online, 22 April.
26. Unschuld P and Tessenow H (2011) *Huang Di Nei Jing Su Wen: An Annotated Translation of Huang Di's Inner Classic – Basic Questions,* Volume I. Berkeley, CA: University of California Press, p.627.
27. Ibid.
28. Ibid.
29. Birch S (2011) *Shonishin: Japanese Pediatric Acupuncture.* Stuttgart: Thieme, p.118.
30. Maciocia G (2008) *The Practice of Chinese Medicine.* Edinburgh: Churchill Livingstone, p.149.
31. Scott J and Barlow T (1999) *Acupuncture in the Treatment of Children.* Seattle, WA: Eastland Press, p.328.
32. National Institute for Health and Care Excellence (2017) Most Common Ear Infections Should Not Be Treated with Antibiotics, Says NICE. Retrieved from: www.nice.org.uk/news/article/most-common-ear-infections-should-not-be-treated-with-antibiotics-says-nice (January 2018).
33. Scott J and Barlow T (1999) *Acupuncture in the Treatment of Children.* Seattle, WA: Eastland Press, p.293.
34. Flaws B (2006) *A Handbook of TCM Pediatrics.* Boulder, CO: Blue Poppy Press, p.179.
35. Ibid., p.191.
36. Stephenson C (2017) *The Acupuncturist's Guide to Conventional Medicine.* London: Singing Dragon, p.122.
37. Maciocia G (2005) *The Foundations of Chinese Medicine.* Edinburgh: Elsevier, p.207.
38. Wilms S (2013) *Venerating the Root, Part 1.* Sun Simiao's *Bei Ji Qian Jin Yao Fang.* Corbett, OR: Happy Goat Productions, p.111.
39. Tidy, C (2015, 25 June) Febrile Seizure. Patient: Making Lives Better. Retrieved from: https://patient.info/health/febrile-seizure-febrile-convulsion (September 2017).
40. Epilepsy Foundation (2017) What Happens During a Seizure? Retrieved from: www.epilepsy.com/learn/about-epilepsy-basics/what-happens-during-seizure (September 2017).
41. Xin-ming Dr S (1986) The Treatment of Epilepsy by Acupuncture. *Journal of Chinese Medicine,* No. 20.
42. Wilms S (2013) *Venerating the Root, Part 1.* Sun Simiao's *Bei Ji Qian Jin Yao Fang.* Corbett, OR: Happy Goat Productions, p.119.
43. Ibid., p.145.
44. Hammer L (1990) *Dragon Rises, Red Bird Flies: Psychology and Chinese Medicine.* New York: Station Hill Press, p.77.
45. American College of Obstetricians and Gynecologists (2015) 'Menstruation in Girls and Adolescents: Using the Menstrual Cycle as a Vital Sign.' Committee Opinion No. 651. Retrieved from: www.acog.org/Resources-And-Publications/Committee-Opinions/Committee-on-Adolescent-Health-Care/Menstruation-in-Girls-and-Adolescents-Using-the-Menstrual-Cycle-as-a-Vital-Sign (January 2017).
46. Biddulph S (2017) *10 Things Girls Need Most.* London: Thorsons, p.121.
47. Rochat de la Vallée E (2007) *The Essential Woman: Female Health and Fertility in Chinese Classical Texts.* Cambridge: Monkey Press, p.65.
48. Duerk J (2004) *Circle of Stones: Woman's Journey to Herself.* Novato, CA: New World Library, p.38.
49. Northrup Dr C (1998) *Women's Bodies, Women's Wisdom.* London: Piatkus, p.101.
50. Wilson B (2015) *First Bite: How We Learn to Eat.* London: Fourth Estate, p.212.
51. Greenspan L and Deardorff J (2014) *The New Puberty: How to Navigate Early Development in Today's Girls.* New York: Rodale.
52. Ibid., p.13.
53. Larre C and Rochat de la Vallée E (1989) *The Kidneys.* Cambridge: Monkey Press, p.38.
54. Ibid., p.188.
55. Stephenson C (2017) *The Acupuncturist's Guide to Conventional Medicine.* London: Singing Dragon.
56. Scott J and Barlow T (1999) *Acupuncture in the Treatment of Children.* Seattle, WA: Eastland Press, p.451.
57. Maslow A (1966) *The Psychology of Science.* New York: Harper and Row, p.16.

Subject Index

· · · · · · · · · · · · · · · · · · · ·

Author Index

· · · · · · · · · · · · · · · · · · · ·